PRIMARY CARE SECRETS
SECRETS
Third Edition

JEANETTE MLADENOVIC, MD
Senior Associate Dean, College of Medicine
Professor, Department of Medicine
The State University of New York Health Science
Center at Brooklyn
SUNY Downstate Medical Center
Brooklyn, New York

HANLEY & BELFUS
An Affiliate of Elsevier

HANLEY & BELFUS
An Affiliate of Elsevier

The Curtis Center
Independence Square West
Philadelphia, Pennsylvania 19106

DISCLAIMER

Although the information in this book has been carefully reviewed for correctness of dosage and indications, neither the authors nor the editor nor the publisher can accept any legal responsibility for any errors or omissions that may be made. Neither the publisher nor the editor make any warranty, expressed or implied, with respect to the material contained herein. Before prescribing any drug, the reader must review the manufacturer's current product information (package inserts) for accepted indications, absolute dosage recommendations, and other information pertinent to the safe and effective use of the product described.

Library of Congress Control Number: 2003113801

PRIMARY CARE SECRETS, 3rd edition

Permissions may be sought directly from Elsevier's Health Sciences Rights Department in Philadelphia, PA, USA: phone: (+1) 215 239 3804, fax: (+1) 215 239 3805, e-mail: healthpermissions@elsevier.com. You may also complete your request on-line via the Elsevier homepage (http://www.elsevier.com), by selecting 'Customer Support' and then 'Obtaining Permissions'.

ISBN-13: 978-1-56053-505-8
ISBN-10: 1-56053-505-9

Printed in the United States of America

Last digit is the print number: 9 8 7 6 5 4

CONTENTS

VIII. COMMON DISORDERS OF THE RENAL AND URINARY SYSTEM

IX. COMMON PROBLEMS OF THE BLOOD AND LYMPH SYSTEM

X. DISORDERS OF THE MUSCULOSKELETAL SYSTEM

CONTRIBUTORS

Irene Aguilar, M.D.
Senior Instructor, Department of Medicine, University of Colorado Health Sciences Center, Denver, Colorado

Mohammad R. Al-Ajam, M.D.
Clinical Instructor, Department of Internal Medicine, The State University of New York Health Science Center at Brooklyn, SUNY Downstate Medical Center; Veterans Affairs New York Harbor Health Care System, Brooklyn, New York

Stephen F. Albert, D.P.M., C.Ped.
Director, Podiatric Medical Education, Podiatric Section, Surgical Service, Denver Veterans Affairs Medical Center, Denver, Colorado

Catherine Amlie-Lefond, M.D.
Sacred Heart Children's Hospital, Spokane, Washington

C. Alan Anderson, M.D.
Associate Professor, Department of Neurology, University of Colorado Health Sciences Center; University of Colorado Hospital; Denver Veterans Affairs Medical Center, Denver, Colorado

Joseph C. Anderson, M.D.
Assistant Professor, Division of Gastroenterology, Department of Medicine, Stony Brook University; Stony Brook University Hospital, Stony Brook, New York

Elizabeth L. Aronsen, M.D.
Assistant Professor, Department of Medicine, University of Colorado Health Sciences Center; Presbyterian–St. Luke's Hospital, Denver, Colorado

Michael Augenbraun, M.D.
Associate Professor, Department of Medicine, The State University of New York Health Science Center at Brooklyn, SUNY Downstate Medical Center; University Hospital of Brooklyn; Kings County Hospital Center, Brooklyn, New York

Roberta K. Beach, M.D., M.P.H.
Professor Emeritus, Department of Pediatrics and Adolescent Medicine, University of Colorado Health Sciences Center, Denver, Colorado

Daniel H. Bessesen, M.D.
Associate Professor, Department of Medicine, University of Colorado Health Sciences Center; Denver Health Medical Center, Denver, Colorado

Joshua D. Blum, M.D.
Assistant Professor, Division of General Internal Medicine, Department of Medicine, University of Colorado Health Sciences Center; Denver Health Medical Center, Denver, Colorado

Edmund Bourke, M.D.
Professor, Department of Medicine, The State University of New York Health Science Center at Brooklyn, SUNY Downstate Medical Center, Brooklyn, New York

Simona Bratu, M.D.
Clinical Assistant Instructor, Department of Medicine, The State University of New York Health Science Center at Brooklyn, SUNY Downstate Medical Center; University Hospital of Brooklyn, Kings County Hospital Center, Brooklyn, New York

Jon M. Braverman, M.D.
Associate Clinical Professor, Department of Ophthalmology, University of Colorado Health Sciences Center; Denver Health Medical Center, Denver, Colorado

John F. Bridges, M.D.
Assistant Professor, Department of Psychiatry, University of Colorado Health Sciences Center, Denver, Colorado

Edmund Casper, M.D.
Associate Professor, Department of Psychiatry, University of Colorado Health Sciences Center; Director, Behavioral Health, Denver Health Medical Center, Denver, Colorado

Jonathan P. Castro, M.D.
Clinical Assistant Instructor, Division of Endocrinology, Diabetes, and Hypertension, Department of Medicine, The State University of New York Health Science Center at Brooklyn, SUNY Downstate Medical Center, Brooklyn, New York

Henry G. Chun, M.D.
Division of Gastroenterology, Department of Medicine, Kaiser Permanente California Richmond Medical Center, Richmond, California

David H. Collier, M.D.
Associate Professor, Department of Medicine, University of Colorado Health Sciences Center; University of Colorado Hospital; Denver Health Medical Center, Denver, Colorado

Iván Colón, M.D.
Assistant Professor, Section of Laparoscopy and Minimally Invasive Surgery, Department of Urology, The State University of New York Health Science Center at Brooklyn, SUNY Downstate Medical Center; University Hospital of Brooklyn; Long Island College Hospital, Brooklyn, New York

Lisa W. Corbin, M.D.
Assistant Professor, Department of Rehabilitation Medicine; Division of General Internal Medicine, Department of Medicine; Medical Director, Center for Integrative Medicine, University of Colorado Health Sciences Center; University of Colorado Hospital, Denver, Colorado

Colleen M. Crandell, M.D.
Clinical Assistant Instructor, Department of Dermatology, The State University of New York Health Science Center at Brooklyn, SUNY Downstate Medical Center; Kings County Hospital Center, Brooklyn, New York

Mary Ann De Groote, M.D.
Assistant Professor, Division of Infectious Diseases, Department of Medicine, University of Colorado Health Sciences Center, Denver, Colorado

Sarah J. D'Heilly, M.D.
Fellow, Division of Infectious Disease, Department of Medicine, University of Minnesota Medical School, Minneapolis, Minnesota

Susan J. Diem, M.D., M.P.H.
Assistant Professor, Department of Medicine, University of Minnesota Medical School, Minneapolis, Minnesota

B. Jane Distad, M.D.
Assistant Professor, Department of Neurology, University of Washington Medical Center, Seattle, Washington

Olga Dvorkina, M.D.
Assistant Professor, Division of Rheumatology, Department of Medicine, The State University of New York Health Science Center at Brooklyn, SUNY Downstate Medical Center; Kings County Hospital Center, Brooklyn, New York

Robert H. Eckel, M.D.
Charles A. Boettcher Endowed Chair in Atherosclerosis; Professor of Physiology and Biophysics; Professor of Medicine, Division of Endocrinology, Metabolism, and Diabetes, Department of Medicine, University of Colorado Health Sciences Center; University of Colorado Hospital, Anschutz Outpatient Pavilion, Denver, Colorado

Abdel-Rahman El-Bash, M.D.
Clinical Assistant Instructor, Department of Ophthalmology, The State University of New York Health Science Center at Brooklyn, SUNY Downstate Medical Center, Brooklyn, New York

Michele A. Ferguson, M.D.
Clinical Assistant Professor, Department of Neurology, University of Colorado Health Sciences Center; Denver Health Medical Center, Denver, Colorado; Boulder Community Hospital, Boulder, Colorado

Richard C. Fisher, M.D.
Associate Professor, Department of Orthopaedics, University of Colorado Health Sciences Center, Denver, Colorado

Carlos E. Girod, M.D.
Associate Professor, Division of Pulmonary and Critical Care Medicine, Department of Medicine, University of Texas Southwestern Medical Center; Parkland Memorial Hospital; Zale-Lipshy University Hospital, Dallas, Texas

James Goff, M.D.
Division of Gastroenterology, Sacred Heart Medical Center, Spokane, Washington

Loren E. Golitz, M.D.
Clinical Professor, Department of Pathology, University of Colorado Health Sciences Center; University of Colorado Hospital; Denver Veterans Affairs Medical Center, Denver, Colorado

Priya Grewal, M.D.
Assistant Professor, Division of Gastroenterology, Department of Medicine, New York University School of Medicine, New York, New York; Attending Physician, North Shore University Hospital, Manhasset, New York; Long Island Jewish Medical Center, New Hyde Park, New York

Alison B. Gruen, M.D.
Clinical Assistant Instructor, Department of Dermatology, The State University of New York Health Science Center at Brooklyn, SUNY Downstate Medical Center, Brooklyn, New York

Michael E. Hanley, M.D., FCCP
Associate Professor, Division of Pulmonary Sciences and Critical Care Medicine, Department of Medicine, University of Colorado Health Sciences Center; Denver Health Medical Center, Denver, Colorado

Robert H. Harris, M.D.
Assistant Professor, Department of Medicine, University of Colorado Health Sciences Center; Denver Health Medical Center, Denver, Colorado

Richard L. Hughes, M.D.
Chief, Division of Neurology, Denver Health Medical Center, Denver, Colorado

Juan C. Iregui, M.D.
Clinical Assistant Professor, Department of Medicine, The State University of New York Health Science Center at Brooklyn, SUNY Downstate Medical Center, Brooklyn, New York

Linda Ann Joseph, M.D.
Division of Endocrinology, Department of Medicine, The State University of New York Health Science Center at Brooklyn, SUNY Downstate Medical Center, Brooklyn, New York

Anne Kastor, M.D.
Assistant Professor, Department of Medicine, The State University of New York Health Science Center at Brooklyn, SUNY Downstate Medical Center; University Hospital of Brooklyn, Brooklyn, New York

Tatiana Khrom, M.D.
Clinical Assistant Instructor, Department of Dermatology, The State University of New York Health Science Center at Brooklyn, SUNY Downstate Medical Center, Brooklyn, New York

Joyce Seiko Kobayashi, M.D.
Associate Professor, Department of Psychiatry, University of Colorado Health Sciences Center; Staff Psychiatrist, Denver Health Medical Center, Denver, Colorado

Jennifer A. LaRosa, M.D.
Assistant Professor, Division of Pulmonary and Critical Care Medicine, Department of Medicine, The State University of New York Health Science Center at Brooklyn, SUNY Downstate Medical Center; Veterans Affairs New York Harbor Health Care System, Brooklyn, New York

Laura M. Lasater, M.D.
Assistant Professor, Division of General Internal Medicine, Department of Medicine, University of Colorado Health Sciences Center; Denver Health Medical Center, Denver, Colorado

David W. Lehman, M.D., Ph.D.
Assistant Professor, Division of General Internal Medicine, Department of Medicine, University of Colorado Health Sciences Center; Denver Health Medical Center, Denver, Colorado

Meg A. Lemon, M.D.
Clinical Professor, Department of Dermatology, University of Colorado Health Sciences Center; Denver Health Medical Center; Chairman, Department of Dermatology, St. Joseph Hospital, Denver, Colorado

Michael L. Lepore, M.D., FACS
Professor, Department of Otolaryngology–Head and Neck Surgery, University of Colorado Health Sciences Center; University of Colorado Hospital; Denver Health Medical Center; Denver Veterans Affairs Medical Center, Denver, Colorado

Allan Liebgott, M.D.
Staff Internist and Director, Correctional Care and Telemedicine, Denver Health Medical Center, Denver, Colorado

Stuart L. Linas, M.D.
Division of Nephrology, Department of Medicine, Denver Health Medical Center, Denver, Colorado

Terry Linn, D.O.
Formerly, Fellow in Gastroenterology, Department of Medicine, University of Colorado Health Sciences Center, Denver, Colorado

Richard P. Lofgren, M.D., M.P.H.
Professor, Department of Medicine; Senior Associate Dean for Clinical Affairs; Chief Medical Officer, Medical College of Wisconsin, Milwaukee, Wisconsin

Larry I. Lutwick, M.D.
Professor, Department of Medicine, The State University of New York Health Science Center at Brooklyn, SUNY Downstate Medical Center; Veterans Affairs New York Harbor Health Care System, Brooklyn, New York

Thomas D. MacKenzie, M.D., MSPH
Associate Professor, Department of Medicine, University of Colorado Health Sciences Center; Associate Director, Internal Medicine, Denver Health Medical Center, Denver, Colorado

Samy I. McFarlane, M.D.
Associate Professor, Division of Endocrinology, Department of Medicine, The State University of New York Health Science Center at Brooklyn, SUNY Downstate Medical Center; Kings County Hospital Center, Brooklyn, New York

Eric T. McFarling, M.D.
Hospitalist, Division of Internal Medicine, CentraCare Health System, St. Cloud, Minnesota

Philip S. Mehler, M.D.
Glassman Professor of Medicine, Department of Medicine, University of Colorado Health Sciences Center; Chief of Internal Medicine, Denver Health Medical Center, Denver, Colorado

Dawn A. Mellish, M.D.
Assistant Professor, Department of Medicine, The State University of New York Health Science Center at Brooklyn, SUNY Downstate Medical Center; Director of Service, Department of Medicine, Kings County Hospital Center, Brooklyn, New York

Rosalia Misseri, M.D.
Fellow in Pediatric Urology, Indiana University Medical School; Riley Hospital for Children, Indianapolis, Indiana

Jeanette Mladenovic, M.D.
Senior Associate Dean, College of Medicine; Professor, Department of Medicine, The State University of New York Health Science Center at Brooklyn, SUNY Downstate Medical Center, Brooklyn, New York

Kavita Nanda, M.D., M.H.S.
Fellow in Women's Health, Division of Health Services Research, Department of Medicine, Duke University Medical Center, Durham, North Carolina

Kristin L. Nichol, M.D., M.P.H., M.B.A.
Professor, Department of Medicine, University of Minnesota Medical School; Chief of Medicine, Minneapolis Veterans Affairs Medical Center, Minneapolis, Minnesota

Jerry A. Nick, M.D.
Associate Professor, Division of Pulmonary Sciences and Critical Care Medicine, Department of Medicine, University of Colorado Health Sciences Center; National Jewish Hospital, Denver, Colorado

Jeffrey Pickard, M.D.
Associate Professor, Division of General Internal Medicine, Department of Medicine, University of Colorado Health Sciences Center; Presbyterian–St. Luke's Medical Center, Denver, Colorado

Eduard V. Porosnicu, M.D.
Assistant Professor, Department of Medicine, The State University of New York Health Science Center at Brooklyn, SUNY Downstate Medical Center, Brooklyn, New York

Randall R. Reves, M.D., M.Sc.
Associate Professor, Division of Infectious Diseases, Department of Medicine and Department of Preventive Medicine and Biometrics, University of Colorado Health Sciences Center; Director, Denver Metro Tuberculosis Clinic, Denver Public Health Department; Staff Physician, Denver Health Medical Center, Denver, Colorado

Moro O. Salifu, M.D.
Assistant Professor, Department of Medicine, The State University of New York Health Science Center at Brooklyn, SUNY Downstate Medical Center, Brooklyn, New York

Iqbal S. Sandhu, M.D.
Assistant Professor, Department of Medicine, University of Utah School of Medicine; Gastroenterology Endoscopy Laboratory, University Hospital and Clinics, Salt Lake City, Utah

Archana Shrestha, M.D.
Instructor, Department of Neurology, University of Colorado Health Sciences Center; University of Colorado Hospital, Denver, Colorado

Lawrence G. Smith, M.D.
Dean for Medical Education, Mount Sinai School of Medicine; Attending, Department of Medicine, Mount Sinai Hospital, New York, New York

Andy W. Steele, M.D., M.P.H.
Associate Professor, Division of General Internal Medicine, Department of Medicine, University of Colorado Health Sciences Center; Denver Health Medical Center, Denver, Colorado

Stephen E. Steinberg, M.D.
Professor, Department of Medicine, The State University of New York Health Science Center at Brooklyn, SUNY Downstate Medical Center, Brooklyn, New York

Benjamin T. Suratt, M.D.
Assistant Professor, Department of Medicine, University of Vermont College of Medicine, Burlington, Vermont

Gina A. Taylor, M.D.
Clinical Assistant Instructor, Department of Dermatology, The State University of New York Health Science Center at Brooklyn, SUNY Downstate Medical Center, Brooklyn, New York

Thomas E. Trouillot, M.D.
Gastroenterologist in Private Practice, Denver, Colorado

Valerie K. Ulstad, M.D., M.P.A., M.P.H.
Clinical Associate Professor, Department of Medicine, University of Minnesota Medical School; Director of Cardiovascular Education, Cardiovascular Division, Hennepin County Medical Center, Minneapolis, Minnesota

Kevin T. White, M.D.
Division of Gastroenterology, Hepatology, and Nutrition, Department of Medicine, North Shore University Hospital, Manhasset, New York

Danny C. Williams, M.D., FRCPC, FACP, FACR
Assistant Professor, Division of Rheumatology, Department of Medicine, University of Colorado Health Sciences Center, Denver, Colorado

Reba Williams, M.D.
Assistant Professor, Department of Medicine, and Director of Ambulatory Care Services, The State University of New York Health Science Center at Brooklyn, SUNY Downstate Medical Center; Kings County Hospital Center, Brooklyn, New York

Timothy J. Wilt, M.D., M.P.H.
Professor, Department of Medicine, University of Minnesota Medical School; Center for Chronic Diseases Outcomes Research, Minneapolis Veterans Affairs Medical Center, Minneapolis, Minnesota

Nathaniel Winer, M.D.
Professor, Division of Endocrinology, Diabetes, and Hypertension, Department of Medicine, The State University of New York Health Science Center at Brooklyn, SUNY Downstate Medical Center; Attending Physician, Kings County Hospital Center; University Hospital of Brooklyn, Brooklyn, New York

Alicia L. Wolfert, M.D.
Assistant Professor, Division of General Internal Medicine, Department of Medicine, University of Colorado Health Sciences Center; Denver Health Medical Center, Denver, Colorado

PREFACE

Primary Care Secrets, 3rd edition, is designed for physicians, residents, students, and other health care providers who must develop and maintain a practical and scholarly breadth of knowledge to deliver the necessary daily care to their patients. As the first professional contact for both preventive and therapeutic needs, primary care providers are often faced with problems much different from those intensive experiences that provide educational opportunities on the classic inpatient service. For this reason, the abbreviated topics selected from this overwhelmingly broad subject matter were organized (where possible) according to problems commonly facing the health care professional in the outpatient setting. Answers to the questions posed are not meant to be proscriptive in nature, but rather to address approaches, rationales, and cost-effectiveness. In this third edition, additional questions have focused on the evidence base that is ever expanding to direct our care of patients. Additionally, a brief introductory chapter poses rudimentary questions about the process and safety of patient care. The contributors include medical and surgical specialists and subspecialists, in addition to generalists. They have, in many instances, provided opinions about which patients should be referred for the next level of care or admitted to the hospital. Although the subject matter does not specifically address the primary care of newborns and children, issues unique to the pediatric patient are discussed in several, especially nonmedical, chapters.

Primary Care Secrets is another text in the popular and unique Secrets Series® originated by the late Dr. Charles Abernathy, who cleverly acknowledged the time-honored Socratic educational approach in written format. Dr. Abernathy was a practicing academic surgeon whose energy and passion for life and medicine were infectious and apparent to all who were fortunate enough to cross his path. His intense commitment to the art of medicine, the fun of learning, and the fundamentals of teaching are embodied in The Secrets Series® books. These should serve as his reminder to us that the practice of medicine is based on "secrets" divulged within a relationship between physician and patient and interpreted in the light of sound clinical evidence.

I would like to express my appreciation to all the contributors for their time and efforts, to Janet Benjamin-Spence for her help in coordinating and collecting manuscripts, and to my project manager, Cecelia Bayruns, for her incredible patience and wonderful follow-up skills.

Jeanette Mladenovic, MD

DEDICATION

To my total support system,
Steve
and
Ben, Jessica, Amy, Jeffrey

I. Health Maintenance

1. PRINCIPLES OF PREVENTIVE MAINTENANCE AND TEST SELECTION

Richard P. Lofgren, M.D., M.P.H.

1. Why should laboratory or diagnostic tests be used?
  1. **Screening or case finding.** The purpose is to detect a condition before symptoms occur in the hope of altering the natural history of the disease.
  2. **Diagnosis of disease.** The purpose is to refine the diagnostic hypothesis either to "rule in" a disease if the likelihood of disease is high or to "rule out" a disease if the likelihood is low.
  3. **Patient management.** Tests can aid patient management by (a) monitoring the status of diseases, (b) identifying complications, (c) providing prognostic information, and (d) ensuring therapeutic levels.

2. What is the most important characteristic of a test used to monitor the status of a patient?
  The reproducibility of the test.

3. How is an "abnormal" test result defined?
  Differentiating normal from abnormal is often more difficult than it seems. A test result may be abnormal based on three different definitions:
  1. **Normal distribution:** For most analytic tests, normal limits are determined by measurements done in a large number of subjects and are arbitrarily defined as the range encompassed by 2 standard deviations from the mean. With a normal curve distribution, 95% of observations are within 2 standard deviations from the mean.
  2. **Biologically normal:** The results of tests that are statistically normal may not be biologically normal. The classic example is cholesterol. There is a threefold increase in the risk of cardiovascular disease with a high-normal cholesterol versus a low-normal cholesterol level.
  3. **Abnormal as treatable:** Abnormal refers not only to a value that increases the risk of bad outcome but also to a result that, if treated, results in improved outcome. Initially, hypertension was defined as a diastolic blood pressure above 105 mmHg because studies had shown that treatment at that level was beneficial. With further studies, the definition of "normal" has steadily decreased and may vary for different populations such as diabetic versus nondiabetic patients.

4. What are the limitations inherent in using the normal distribution as a definition of normal?
  1. **Chance phenomenon:** By definition, 5% of subjects will have results that lie at the extremes and will be labeled abnormal. With any given test, a normal individual has a 1 in 20 chance of having an "abnormal" result. The likelihood of having an abnormal result increases in proportion to the number of independent tests performed. Sixty-four percent of normal individuals will have at least one abnormal result on a chemistry panel of 20 tests. Therefore, it is distinctly abnormal for a normal person to have a normal screening "chem 20" panel.
  2. **Physiologic variable:** Some physiologic variables, such as alkaline phosphatase level, have a skewed distribution.

3. **Reference group:** Often the normal range is determined in young healthy volunteers (e.g., medical students). For many tests, the distribution varies by age, gender, or other important parameters. For example, alanine aminotransferase (ALT) is a sensitive indicator of liver disease. Levels can by affected by gender, obesity, and hypertriglyceridemia. The normal range was determined more than 20 years ago before problems such as mild chronic hepatitis C could be detected. Recent studies that account for these factors suggest that the upper limit of normal ALT level should be reduced from 40 U/L to 30 U/L. This would increase the sensitivity of the test to detect liver disease but would also produce more false-positive test results.

5. What are the sensitivity and specificity of a test?

Although the terms are often defined mathematically, it is helpful to remember what they mean in simple language:

Sensitivity is the probability that a test result will be positive if the disease is present.

Specificity is the probability that a test result will be negative if the disease is absent. The terms can also be defined using a 2 × 2 table:

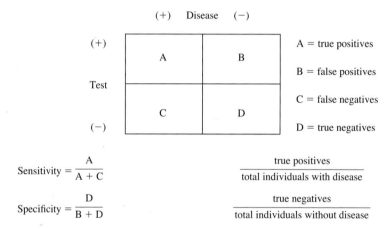

$$\text{Sensitivity} = \frac{A}{A + C} \qquad \frac{\text{true positives}}{\text{total individuals with disease}}$$

$$\text{Specificity} = \frac{D}{B + D} \qquad \frac{\text{true negatives}}{\text{total individuals without disease}}$$

6. If a test to detect a disease whose prevalence is 1/1000 has a 95% sensitivity and 95% specificity, what is the chance that a person found to have a positive result actually has the disease?

Less than 2%. There is a 95% chance that the test will detect the one individual out of 1000 with the disease. However, with a 95% specificity or a 5% false-positive rate, 50 normal individuals will have an abnormal result. Therefore, only 1 of the 51 individuals with a "positive" result will actually have the disease.

This question was asked of 20 students, 20 residents, and 20 attending physicians, and only 18% gave the correct answer. The most common answer given was "95%," a gross overestimation of the likelihood of disease! Appropriately interpreting test results is not intuitively obvious. In order to interpret test results properly, it is essential that the clinician make a "guesstimate" of the likelihood (or prevalence) of disease before obtaining a test. The most common mistake made in interpreting test results is failing to consider the probability of disease before the results are known. After the results are in hand, clinicians tend to be swayed by the findings and inflate the accuracy of the test.

7. What is predictive value?

Sensitivity and specificity are characteristics of a test. They tell you the likelihood a test result will be positive or negative if you already know the disease is present or absent. Knowledge of test characteristics does not, per se, permit the accurate interpretation of the test result. In practice, the clinician needs to know the likelihood that the disease is absent or present when the result is positive or negative. This is the **predictive value** of a test. It is determined by the sensitivity and specificity of the test and the prevalence of the disease in the population. **Positive predictive value** is the probability that the disease is present given a positive test result. **Negative predictive value** is the probability that the disease is absent given a negative test result.

In order to accurately interpret the test results (i.e., the positive and negative predictive value), one has to know (or make an *a priori* educated guess) about the prevalence of the disease before obtaining the test. The predictive value can be calculated using Bayes' theorem or a 2 × 2 table if the prevalence is known.

$$\text{Positive predictive value} = \frac{A}{A + B} \qquad \frac{\text{true positives}}{\text{total individuals with positive result}}$$

$$= \frac{(Se)(P)}{(Se)(P) + (1 - Sp)(1 - P)}$$

Se = sensitivity
Sp = specificity
P = prevalence of disease

$$\text{Negative predictive value} = \frac{D}{C + D} \qquad \frac{\text{true negatives}}{\text{total individuals with negative result}}$$

$$= \frac{(1 - P)(Sp)}{(1 - P)(Sp) + (P))(1 - Se)}$$

8. When ruling out a disease, what kind of test is needed?

When ruling out a disease, the clinician suspects that the probability of disease is low (i.e., "It is possible, but I doubt it"). In these situations, the clinician must select a test that almost always has a positive result when the disease is present (i.e., a sensitive test). If such a test result is negative, then the clinician can be confident that the likelihood of disease is remote. However, sensitive tests are not as specific and are subject to many false-positive results. If the pretest likelihood of disease is low and the test result is positive, then it is likely a false-positive result. When the probability of disease is low, a negative result using a sensitive test yields a very high negative predictive value.

Conversely, when ruling in a disease, the clinician strongly suspects the disease is present. In these situations, the clinician wants a test that rarely has a positive result in people without the disease (i.e., a specific test). A positive result confirms the diagnosis, whereas a negative result is likely a false negative. When the probability of disease is high, a positive result using a specific test yields a very high positive predictive value.

In summary, there are two important rules to remember when interpreting laboratory results. When ruling out a disease, you should select a very sensitive test, and you want the result to be negative. If it is positive, it is most likely a false-positive result and is not helpful (try to ignore the results). When ruling in a disease, you should select a very specific test. If the result is positive, the diagnosis is confirmed. However, if the result is negative, it is likely a false-negative result and is not useful. Armed with these two simple rules, the clinician can correctly interpret test results without necessarily calculating the exact predictive value. Clinicians must resist being unduly influenced if an "unexpected" result is obtained.

9. How can you increase the sensitivity and specificity of your diagnostic strategy?

Often, there is no single test that is sufficiently sensitive to rule out a disease (or sufficiently specific to rule in a disease). Clinicians can improve the sensitivity or specificity of the diagnostic approach by using multiple tests. Using several tests in combination or in parallel significantly increases the sensitivity (while decreasing the specificity) and, thus, the negative predictive value of the diagnostic strategy. If all of the tests used in combination have negative results, then it is unlikely the disease is present. Conversely, using multiple tests in sequence or series significantly increases the specificity (while decreasing the sensitivity). If you do test A and, if positive, do test

B and, if positive, do test C, then you can be fairly certain the disease is present if all three test results are positive (i.e., a strong positive predictive value).

10. When should you screen for a disease?
There are important factors to consider before screening for a disease.
1. **The disease should be common.** The disease must be relatively common for a screening program to be cost-effective. If the disease is rare, a significant number of normal individuals will have a false-positive result and the predictive value will be poor. Individuals with a false-positive result may be subjected to further expensive and perhaps invasive procedures.
2. **The disease should cause significant morbidity.** The disease must result in significant suffering. For example, tinea pedis may be common but does not cause sufficient problems to warrant a screening program.
3. **An effective screening test must exist.** A screening program needs to have a test with reasonable test characteristics (sensitivity and specificity) and be practical, convenient, and inexpensive with few side effects. Because the majority of individuals will not have the disease, the screening process has to be acceptable to patients. For example, although the complications of a cerebral aneurysm may be preventable, a screening program using complex imaging studies such as a magnetic resonance angiogram (MRA) is not practical or acceptable. However, screening for hypertension is simple and effective.
4. **Therapy must alter the natural history of disease.** Treatment early in the asymptomatic period should be superior to therapy started after symptoms develop. For example, data strongly suggest that removal of adenomatous colonic polyps decreases the incidence of colon cancer. Similarly, therapy of stage I breast cancer is superior to treatment of stage III disease. On the other hand, it is not clear that early treatment of asymptomatic localized prostate cancer improves patient outcomes. Because early therapy is not clearly beneficial, screening for this important disease has been questioned and is the source of great controversy.

11. What is the difference between primary, secondary, and tertiary preventive care?
Primary prevention is an intervention designed to prevent a pathologic condition or disease from occurring. Examples include immunizations to prevent specific infectious diseases or wearing a seat belt to prevent bodily injury during an accident.
Secondary prevention is an intervention designed to prevent future morbidity or mortality by treating a condition during the asymptomatic period. Early intervention is often relatively simple and more effective therapy. Screening and treating malignancies such as cervical, colon, and breast cancer are examples of secondary prevention.
Tertiary prevention is an intervention designed to prevent complications in patients with an established disease. For example, treating an elevated cholesterol level to prevent the progression of atherosclerosis in a patient with coronary artery disease is a tertiary preventive measure. Primary care physicians often spend considerable time delivering tertiary preventive services.
The distinction between the various types of preventive care can be blurred. For example, the treatment of hypertension could be primary intervention to prevent heart disease or tertiary intervention to prevent the progression of renal disease in a diabetic patient.

12. What is the purpose of the periodic health examination (PHE)?
1. **Preventing disease** (primary prevention), such as providing immunization
2. **Identifying risk factors** for common chronic disease, such as hyperlipidemia and obesity
3. **Case finding** (secondary prevention) to detect asymptomatic disease, such as screening for cervical or colorectal cancer, hypertension, and glaucoma
4. **Counseling and educating patients** to promote health behavior such as diet, exercise, and smoking cessation
5. **Updating the patient's clinical data,** including any new medical conditions, such as surgeries or allergies
6. **Enhancing patient–physician communication.** It is important that patients know and

trusts their physicians and become active partners in their own health. Periodic examinations can help nurture this relationship.

The PHE is a time-honored but often maligned practice. Few preventive medicine procedures have been demonstrated by randomized trials to reduce mortality and morbidity. However, patients who receive PHEs are more likely to receive the recommended preventive services. More than two thirds of adults think that PHEs are necessary. More than 90% expect to receive counseling and advice about diet, exercise, and alcohol and tobacco use. Similarly, the majority expect to receive tests to screen for common disorders such as breast cancer and hyperlipidemia. Discussions about the value of the PHE often fail to recognize the importance of points 5 and 6 and the psychological value of reassurance and the promotion of healthy habits.

13. What are the best methods to ensure that your patients receive the recommended immunizations and preventive services?

Many patients fail to receive the recommended immunizations, cancer screening, and other preventive services despite their and their physicians' best intentions. Several barriers can interfere with the delivery of preventive services, including knowledge, attitude, costs, convenience, health care beliefs, and competing agendas by both patients and physicians. Many strategies have been developed to overcome these barriers. These interventions include:

- **Reminders:** Send reminders (e.g., postcards, computer prompts, and flow sheets) to prompt patients or physicians about the need to update preventive services.
- **Provider feedback:** Supply providers with summaries about their performance in delivering preventive services.
- **Education:** Provide information about the preventative practices to patients, physicians, or both.
- **Financial incentives:** Provide financial incentives to patients or physicians.
- **Regulatory and legislative actions**
- **Organizational changes:** Change the work processes of the health care organization to promote teamwork and collaboration. Changes include separate screening clinics, planned visits for prevention, and using nonphysician staff members to deliver services.
- **Mass media campaigns**

Organizational changes are the most effective interventions for increasing the use of preventive services. Providing financial incentives such as eliminating copayments for preventive services is the next most effective. Patient reminder systems are less effective but still have a positive impact, especially if reminders are personalized rather than generic. Physician reminder systems and physician education are less consistent in their effectiveness.

14. What are the most common causes of death in teenagers and young adults?

The leading causes of death vary by age. The top causes of death in each age group are listed below. Because the causes of preventable death vary throughout life, the types of assessments and interventions performed during a PHEs should vary accordingly.

0–1 YEAR	1–4 YEARS	5–14 YEARS	15–24 YEARS
Conditions originating in perinatal period	Accidents	Accidents	Accidents
Congenital anomalies	Developmental and genetic	Cancer	Homicide
Sudden infant death syndrome (SIDS)	conditions that were	Homicide	Suicide
Unintentional injuries	present at birth		
Motor vehicle injuries	Cancer		

In teenagers and young adults, accidents and violence are the greatest risks to life, yet these problems are often not viewed as health problems per se. Specific changes in behavior can reduce the risk of injury and death. For example, between 50% and 85% of bicycle fatalities are the result of head trauma. Retrospective studies suggest that the risk of head injury can be reduced by as much as 75% by wearing a bicycle helmet. Death from a residential fire is two to three times more likely if the home does not have a properly functioning smoke detector. The proper use of lap and shoulder belts can reduce motor vehicle crash mortality by 40–50%. Alcohol-related vehicle crashes account for about half of all traffic fatalities each year. During a PHE with a teenager or young adult, it is recommended that the physician inquire about risky behaviors, including drug, alcohol, and tobacco use; use of seat belts and bicycle helmets; and the presence of firearms and smoke detectors in the home. Patients should be counseled about smoking cessation and avoiding smoking in bed, installing and maintaining a smoke detector, using seat belts and bicycle helmets on a regular basis, and keeping ipecac on hand. Additionally, any problems related to alcohol and drug use should be addressed.

15. Why and how do the recommended guidelines for preventive services vary?

Many professional organizations and societies, advisory panels, and federal organizations have issued guidelines. The content and frequency of the recommended preventive services are controversial and may vary significantly among published guidelines. In general, guidelines from specific professional societies, such as the American Cancer Society or the American Diabetes Association, are the most aggressive in recommending specific screening procedures.

On the other hand, the Canadian and U.S. Task Forces are more conservative in their recommendations. These task forces use explicit rules of evidence and criteria to generate recommendations. Recommendations to perform or not to perform a preventive service are based on the quality of the evidence that its performance would be beneficial. The strongest recommendations are reserved for interventions proved to be effective in well-designed studies. Measures are described as "clinically prudent" only if there is compelling *indirect* evidence. Many procedures receive no recommendations because the evidence of efficacy is lacking.

16. What is the difference between efficacy and effectiveness of preventive service?

Efficacy refers to the ability of an intervention to produce the desired outcome under optimal circumstances. **Effectiveness** is the performance of an intervention in a practice setting (i.e., if an intervention still works in the heterogeneous environment of clinical practice). Clinical studies usually involve highly motivated, selected patients with equally motivated health professionals. Often, preventive services are not nearly as effective when applied in "real-world" conditions. Unfortunately, the effectiveness of an intervention is rarely studied.

17. Why does domestic violence often go undetected in the medical setting?

Domestic violence is a serious and common health problem that affects more than 2 million women and 150,000 men each year. Violence or abuse between spouses and partners can occur in families from all demographic and economic strata. Women who are younger than 35 years, less educated, belong to a lower socioeconomic strata, or are unmarried appear to be at an increased risk. Histories of childhood family violence and alcohol problems are more common among the abusive partner. Women in various clinical settings report a prevalence of physical abuse of 6–15% in the previous 12 months with a lifetime prevalence of approximately 30%. Community surveys suggest that 3–4% of people older than 65 years are victims of physical or verbal abuse or neglect. However, data suggest that physicians correctly identify as few as 1 in 20 victims. Physicians recognize the need to screen for domestic violence, but < 10% do so on a regular basis. Physicians' lack of confidence in their abilities in recognizing and management of domestic violence correlates with lower screening rates.

To overcome the reluctance to address problems of abuse, it is recommended that medical settings display information about abuse. Physicians must become comfortable with asking and making inquiries about potential abuse as part of the clinical routine. Introducing screening questions about abuse makes the physician and patients more comfortable. It helps patients if they understand that the physician routinely asks such questions and they are not being singled out.

Sample of introductory questions included:

- "Unfortunately, violence often plays a role in our families and our community, so I am asking my patients the following questions."
- "We recognize that violence and abuse are common in our patients' lives, so I've begun asking about this routinely."

Sample of specific screening questions include:

- "Have you been physically abused by your spouse/partner/someone important to you?"
- "Have you been emotionally abused by your spouse/partner/someone important to you?"
- "Do you feel safe, or are your afraid in your personal relationships?"
- "Is your spouse/partner/someone important to you physically or emotionally hurtful to you?"
- "Have you or your spouse/partner/someone important to you ever used physical force when you were arguing?"

If a potential problem is identified, the physician should offer support, provide written materials about resources and options that are available that can remain private, and convey that the health care setting is a safe place to ask for help if violence or other abuse becomes a problem.

BIBLIOGRAPHY

1. Canadian Task Force on the Periodic Health Examination: The Canadian Guide to Clinical Preventive Health Care. Ottawa, Canada Communications Group, 1994.
2. Domestic violence. In ICSI Pocket Guidelines. Bloomington, MN, Institute for Clinical Systems Improvement, 2001, pp 208–212.
3. Elliott L, Nerney M, Jones T, Friedman PD: Barriers to screening for domestic violence. J Gen Intern Med 17:112–116, 2002.
4. Jaesschke R: Users guides to the medical literature. How to use an article about a diagnostic test. A. Are the results of the study valid? JAMA 271:389–391, 1994.
5. Jaesschke R: Users guides to the medical literature. How to use an article about a diagnostic test. B. What are the results and will they help me in caring for my patients? JAMA 271:703–707, 1994.
6. Kaplan MM: Alanine aminotransferase levels: What's normal? Ann Intern Med 137:49–50, 2002.
7. Laine C: The annual physical examination: Needless ritual or necessary routine? Ann Intern Med 136:701–702, 2002.
8. Sox HC Jr, Blatt MA, Higgins MC, Marton KI: Medical Decision Making. Newton, MA, Butterworth-Heinemann, 1988.
9. Stone EG, Morton SC, Hulscher ME, et al: Interventions that increase use of adult immunization and cancer screening services: A meta-analysis. Ann Intern Med 136:641–651, 2002.
10. US Preventive Service Task Force: Guide to Clinical Preventive Services: Report of the US Preventive Services Task Force, 3rd ed. Baltimore, Williams & Wilkins, 2000–2002.

2. EARLY CANCER DETECTION

Timothy J. Wilt, M.D., M.P.H.

1. Describe the four major biases that may result in invalid conclusions about the effectiveness of cancer screening methods.

1. Lead time is the length of time between detection of cancer with a screening test and the time at which the disease, by the presence of signs and symptoms, would have been detected in the absence of screening. **Lead-time bias** is a false increase in longevity associated with screening. The gain in longevity is apparent and not real. Lead-time bias occurs when survival appears to be lengthened because screening simply advances the time of diagnosis, lengthening the period between diagnosis and death without altering the natural history of the disease.

2. **Length bias** also may overestimate the benefits of cancer screening because less aggressive (slower-growing) tumors with relatively good prognoses are detected more frequently by screening programs. This occurs because of their longer detectable preclinical phase compared with more aggressive cancers. Therefore, less aggressive tumors are overrepresented in screening programs, resulting in apparent improved survival of screen-detected malignancies.

3. **Overdiagnosis bias** results when screening detects lesions that may not be clinically significant. Very early "cancers" detected during screening may never have caused symptomatic disease if they had been left undetected. Screening programs may overreport (overdiagnose) the number of malignancies. Some may not be clinically significant because they would not have caused problems if not found by early detection.

4. **Selection bias** refers to the fact that participants in screening programs are often different from the general population. They may participate because they are at higher risk for the disease, are more likely to comply with screening and treatment programs, and frequently have other health care practices that result in improved health outcomes independent of the screening program.

The only way to avoid these biases is to conduct randomized, controlled trials (RCTs) and then assess mortality rates for individuals screened versus those not screened. Ideally, RCTs should be of adequate size to detect reduction in all-cause mortality. In practice, this rarely occurs because the condition of interest effects relatively few individuals and interventions are postulated to relatively modest effects. In order to demonstrate that a screening intervention reduced all-cause mortality, trials would have to be extremely large. Therefore, screening trials traditionally are designed to evaluate reductions in disease specific mortality. Care should be taken to ensure the validity of cause-of-death ascertainment and ensure that the cancer screening, evaluation, and treatment process did not produce a corresponding increase in noncancer mortality.

2. The cancer detection and prevention guidelines of the United States Preventive Services Task Force (USPSTF) are based on a hierarchy of evidence in which greater importance is given to study designs that are less subjective to bias and misinterpretations. What study design provides the best evidence for effectiveness?

RCTs. Participants are assigned in a randomized fashion to a group receiving the intervention or a control group. Randomization depends on two related but separate processes: generation of an unpredictable randomized allocation sequence and concealment of that sequence until assignment occurs. Randomization provides at least three major advantages: (1) it eliminates bias in treatment assignment; (2) it facilitates blinding of the identity of treatments from investigators, participants, and assessors, including the possible use of placebo; and (3) it permits the use of probability theory to express the likelihood that any difference in outcome between treatment groups merely indicates chance. Generalizability and representativeness of results, however, may still be problematic.

3. Many cancers are rare. What type of study design is useful in investigating risk factors that may play a role in these diseases? Describe this type of study.

Case-control studies. Selection of study and control groups is based on whether participants have the disease rather than whether they have been exposed to a risk factor or intervention. By comparing people with and without the disease, investigators assess both groups for differences in risk factors preceding the onset of disease. Although useful for the study of rare diseases, this approach does not provide an estimate of incidence. In addition, representativeness of people with and without disease may be an issue. Five main concepts should guide assessment of case-control studies:

1. An explicit definition of the criteria for diagnosis of a case and any eligibility criteria for selection should be provided.

2. Control subjects should come from the same population as the cases, and their selection should be independent of the exposures of interest.

3. The data gatherers should be blinded to the case or control status of participants.

4. Exposure should be elicited in a similar manner from cases and controls.

5. Confounding should be addressed in the study design or analysis stage.

4. Current evidence supports the practice of screening chest radiographs or sputum cytology to reduce lung cancer mortality. True or false?

False. The USPSTF has concluded that screening does not reduce lung cancer mortality, even in high-risk smokers. Chest radiographs and sputum cytology have been proposed as tests for early detection of lung cancer. However, several RCTs, a nonrandomized controlled trial, and two case-control studies have failed to demonstrate a reduction in lung cancer mortality from frequent screening with chest radiographs and sputum cytology. The National Cancer Institute is conducting the Prostate, Lung, Colorectal, and Ovarian Cancers (PLCO) Screening Trial to again determine whether annual chest radiographic testing reduces lung cancer mortality compared with usual care. Another randomized trial is determining whether screening with chest radiographs versus spiral chest computed tomography (CT) reduces lung cancer mortality.

5. What is the best method for preventing lung cancer?

Counseling patients against tobacco use is the best method of preventing lung cancer. Lung cancer is the leading cause of cancer-related mortality in both men and women. There are an estimated 169,000 new cases of lung cancer and 155,000 lung cancer-related deaths annually in the U.S. The 5-year survival rate of patients with lung cancer is approximately 15%. Almost 90% of lung cancers are related to cigarette smoking; therefore, they should be preventable. Because smoking rates have increased in teenagers and women, efforts aimed at reducing smoking in these groups are particularly important. Interventions shown to be effective in helping patients to quit smoking include smoking cessation counseling by health care providers; nicotine replacement via patch, gum, or spray; and bupropion (Welbutrin, Zyban). Passive or second-hand smoke also has been demonstrated to be associated with an increased risk of chronic lung and cardiac disease. Therefore, efforts have focused on developing smoke-free environments in public areas such as workplaces, airports, and restaurants.

6. Does screening for colon cancer with fecal occult blood tests (FOBTs) reduce colon cancer mortality?

Yes. The results of three RCTs demonstrated that screening with FOBT reduces mortality from colorectal cancer by 15–33% compared with an unscreened control group. The reduction in colorectal cancer mortality was accompanied by a shift to detection at an earlier stage of cancer and improved survival in patients in whom cancer developed compared with the control group. Screening annually over a 13-year period with FOBTs and subsequent full colonoscopic evaluation for a positive FOBT result reduces colon cancer deaths by about 3 per 1000 persons. The number of people who need to be screened to prevent 1 colon cancer death over 10 years is about 1000. Colorectal cancer is one of the most common malignancies and the second leading cause of cancer-related death in the United States, with approximately 150,000 new cases and 60,000 deaths annually.

Although FOBT has been shown to prevent death from colon cancer, the reduction in all-cause mortality has not been clearly demonstrated. When the results from the 3 published RCTs of screening with FOBT ($n = 258,725$) were combined, they failed to show any trend toward overall mortality reduction. There were 186.41 deaths per 1000 people in the screened groups and 182.60 deaths per 1000 people in the unscreened groups. It is possible that the failure to demonstrate a reduction in all-cause mortality was attributable to an inadequate sample size of the combined results of these RCTs. However, it is equally plausible that there was an increase in non-colorectal cancer deaths in the screened group attributable to screening, diagnosis, and treatment. The best available information suggests that screening for colorectal cancer with FOBT changes the way people die, in that it modestly reduces the rate of deaths from colorectal cancer, but it fails to save lives.

7. What technical issues should be considered in conducting and interpreting FOBT results?

Screening with FOBTs involves many decisions, including (as noted above) whether screening actually saves lives, identifying persons who should not be screened, type of test chosen, frequency of screening, restriction of diet and medication during screening, number of specimens collected, whether to rehydrate samples, and management of persons with positive test results.

FOBT is recommended as a screening tool for adults at average risk for developing colon cancer. It should not be done in persons who are likely to have false-positive or -negative results (e.g., active hemorrhoidal bleeding or symptoms and signs suggestive of colorectal cancer) or are at increased risk of having colon cancer (e.g., first-degree family relative with colon cancer; personal history of adenomatous polyps). Screening should not be performed in people in whom additional evaluation and treatment are unlikely to be beneficial (e.g., life expectancy < 10 years because of advanced age or comorbid conditions).

In patients in whom colorectal cancer screening with FOBT is performed, two slides from each of three consecutive bowel movements should be obtained. Patients should abstain from substantial doses of nonsteroidal antiinflammatory drugs, red meat, poultry, fish, some raw vegetables, and vitamin C. The slides should not be rehydrated and should be developed within 7 days. The optimal frequency (annual vs. biennial) for FOBT is not clear, but annual FOBT is generally recommended. If a patient has a positive test result (i.e., one or more slide windows), the recommended approach is to proceed directly to complete colorectal evaluation, preferably by colonoscopy. Because the sensitivity of the FOBT is limited for neoplasms (30–50%), a negative FOBT result cannot rule out colorectal cancer. If signs or symptoms of colorectal cancer develop (e.g., overt blood in stool, iron deficiency anemia, change in bowel habits, unexplained weight loss), the patient should undergo colonoscopic evaluation rather than a "screening" FOBT.

8. Should flexible sigmoidoscopy or colonoscopy be used for colon cancer screening?

In addition to FOBT, evidence from case-control studies suggests that screening with a 65-cm flexible sigmoidoscopy every 3–5 years (and possibly as infrequently as every 10 years) detects additional lesions in the distal colon. It is associated with reduced colon cancer deaths. Currently, an RCT is evaluating the effectiveness of flexible sigmoidoscopy addition to FOBT to reduce colon cancer mortality. The USPSTF recommends that flexible sigmoidoscopy should be performed every 5 years for average-risk men and women between the ages of 50 and 75 years. There is no consensus about routinely screening with total colonic evaluation (e.g., colonoscopy or FOBT plus air-contrast barium enema). The U.S. Preventive Services Task Force recommends that total evaluation with colonoscopy can be used instead of FOBT and flexible sigmoidoscopy. If such a strategy is followed, colonoscopy should be repeated every 10 years in patients with normal examination findings. High-risk people (i.e., previous history of colon cancer, large adenomatous polyps, polyposis syndromes, ulcerative colitis, family history of colon cancer) should undergo a full colonic evaluation and are not considered to be part of the "screening population."

9. Has routine screening with digital rectal examination (DRE) or prostate-specific antigen (PSA) testing been demonstrated to reduce prostate cancer–specific mortality?

No. Despite widespread screening with DRE and PSA testing, neither early detection nor early treatment of prostate cancer has been demonstrated to reduce disease-specific morbidity or mortality. This has led to considerable controversy and confusion about the risks and benefits of early detection and treatment of prostate cancer.

The American Cancer Society and American Urological Association recommend that men at average risk for prostate cancer should be offered an annual DRE and PSA test beginning at age 50 years; men at high risk (i.e., African-American men and men with a family history of prostate cancer) should begin at age 40 years. Evidence-based guidelines from the USPSTF, National Cancer Institute, and American College of Physicians and American Academy of Family Practitioners either recommend against early detection of prostate cancer or state that interested men should be counseled about the unproven benefits and known harms of screening and treatment. All groups state that the efficacy of early detection and treatment in reducing morbidity and mortality has not been demonstrated.

Prostate cancer is the most frequently diagnosed cancer and second leading cause of cancer-related mortality in men. It was estimated that 180,000 men would be diagnosed and that 38,000 men would die from prostate cancer annually. From 1990 to 1997, the incidence of prostate cancer rose 200%, and the number of related deaths increased 39%. The marked increase in prostate cancer is most likely attributable to the greater frequency of PSA tests and subsequent prostate biopsy procedures that detect a large number of asymptomatic cancers. In recent years, prostate cancer deaths in the United States have declined. This has led to speculation that widespread early detection and treatment may be effective.

However, although potentially beneficial, the best available information indicates that early detection with DRE or PSA testing is not associated with improved survival. A large, RCT conducted in Ontario, Canada, failed to demonstrate a difference in survival between men randomly assigned to be invited to receive screening compared with men not invited. Similarly, a large, multicenter, case-control study demonstrated that screening was not associated with improved survival and that results did not support the effectiveness of PSA or DRE in screening for prostate cancer.

Furthermore, areas of the United States that have the highest rates of screening and early treatment do not have lowest prostate cancer mortality rates. Additionally, mortality rates in the United Kingdom are virtually identical to those observed in the United States despite wide differences between countries in their utilization of early detection and treatment. Large RCTs are being conducted in the United States and Europe to determine whether prostate cancer screening with annual DRE and PSA testing reduces prostate cancer and all-cause mortality.

10. Is PSA sensitive and specific for prostate cancer?

No. Although the PSA blood test is specific for the prostate, it is not specific for prostate cancer. In addition to prostate cancer, other factors that commonly result in increased PSA levels include age, acute urinary retention, benign prostatic hyperplasia (BPH), infection, and biopsy or surgery of the prostate. DRE does not produce clinically important elevations in PSA levels. The positive predictive value for prostate cancer in men older than age 50 years with PSA levels between 4 and 10 ng/mL is about 20%. This value does not vary substantially with age, suggesting that increased disease prevalence is balanced by decreased test specificity in older men. Use of PSA alone results in a cancer detection rate of about 3%. Elevations in PSA level of 4 and 10 ng/ml increase the odds of clinically significant intracapsular prostate cancer about 1.5–3.0-fold. Although PSA levels > 10 ng/mL may still reflect BPH, the odds of extracapsular cancer are increased by greater than twentyfold. Prostate cancer is no more likely to be present in men with lower urinary tract symptoms (LUTS) compatible with BPH. Because BPH leads to increased PSA values, the test actually has a worse predictive value in men with LUTS compared with asymptomatic men. Therefore, if the traditional cutoff value of 4.0 ng/mL is used to refer men for evaluation with prostate biopsy, approximately 400 of 1000 men will require a biopsy in order to detect 30 prostate cancers. Approximately 80% of men with prostate cancer would not have died of their prostate cancer even if not treated. PSA levels can be falsely negative and miss prostate cancer. Approximately 10–20% of men found to have prostate cancer have PSA values < 4 ng/mL. To rule out an occult prostate cancer even if the total PSA is < 4.0 ng/mL, some have advocated that patients be referred for a prostate biopsy if serial PSA values increase > 0.1 ng/mL/year.

11. What are acceptable treatment options for men with clinically localized prostate cancer?

There are at least three standard treatment options for early-stage or clinically localized prostate cancer: surgery to remove the entire prostate and surrounding tissue (i.e., radical prostatectomy), radiation to destroy the tumor (i.e., external beam or interstitial implants), and careful monitoring with palliative therapies (e.g., hormone treatment) if and when their is evidence of disease progression (i.e., watchful waiting). Results from a small clinical trial; case series of treatment with surgery, radiation, or watchful waiting; several structured literature reviews; and decision analysis modeling indicate that all three treatment approaches appear to provide similar survival rates. The American Urological Association concluded that all three treatments are considered options because the available evidence does not support the superiority of any one treatment in reducing disease-specific morbidity and mortality. Several RCTs are currently being conducted in the United States, Canada, the United Kingdom, and Scandinavia to determine which of these treatment options will provide the greatest length and quality of life in men with clini-

cally localized prostate cancer. Primary care physicians have the opportunity to serve as their patients' independent health care coordinators and consultants. They can help patients weigh the potential risks and benefits of treatment options, acknowledge treatment uncertainty rather than ad-
vocating a particular treatment option, facilitate the subsequent shared decision-making process,
and incorporate patient preferences into treatment plans.

12. How can men be effectively counseled about the potential risks and benefits of prostate cancer testing and treatment?

Rather then routinely testing men for prostate cancer with a DRE and PSA blood test, physicians should involve patients in medical decisions by providing balanced information about the
known risks and unproven benefits of early detection and treatment to men who express interest.
Men with LUTS compatible with BPH are at no greater risk of having prostate cancer than asymptomatic men. Therefore, testing should be considered a screening procedure (rather than a case
finding) regardless of the presence or absence of LUTS. Several methods can be used to efficiently
and effectively involve men in medical shared decision making regarding prostate cancer testing
and treatment. These include instructional videotapes, mailed printed pamphlets, and brochures
provided to patients at clinic appointments. The literature should include the following facts: (1)
prostate cancer is an important health problem; (2) the benefits of screening and aggressive treatment of prostate cancer have not yet been proven; (3) DRE and PSA measurement can both have
false-positive and false-negative results; (4) the probability is relatively high that further invasive
evaluation will be required as a result of testing; (5) aggressive therapy is necessary to realize any
benefit from the discovery of a tumor; (6) a small but finite risk for early death and a significant
risk for chronic illness, particularly with regard to sexual and urinary function, are associated with
treatments; (7) early detection may save lives; and (8) early detection and treatment may avert future cancer-related illness.

13. Does screening for breast cancer reduce mortality?

Considerable controversy exists regarding the effectiveness and risk associated with population-
based screening of women for breast cancer. The USPSTF recommends screening mammography
with or without clinical breast examination every 1–2 years for women aged 40 years and older. The
task force found fair evidence from RCTs that mammography screening significantly reduces mortality from breast cancer. The evidence is strongest for women aged 50–69 years. For women aged
40–49 years, the evidence that screening mammography reduces mortality from breast cancer is
weaker and the absolute benefit of mammography is smaller than in older women. No study has compared clinical breast examination with no screening. The USPSTF concluded that the reductions in
breast cancer mortality in studies using mammography alone were comparable to those using mammography plus clinical breast examination (CBE). Therefore, CBE does not appear to add any improvement in breast cancer–specific survival compared with mammography. Another systematic review and meta-analysis of randomized trials concluded that the currently available reliable evidence
does not show an overall survival benefit of mass screening for breast cancer (and the evidence is in-
conclusive for breast cancer mortality). However, mass screening lead to increased use of diagnostic
procedures and aggressive treatment. Additionally, annual mammography of 100,000 women for 10
consecutive years beginning at age 40 years would result in up to eight radiation-induced breast cancer deaths. Women, clinicians, and policymakers should consider these findings carefully when they
decide whether or not to attend or support screening programs.

14. Does breast self-examination (BSE) reduce mortality in women?

The best available information is that BSE does not reduce breast cancer mortality and is associated with an increased risk of false-positive results and biopsies. The role of BSE has been
evaluated in two RCTs and one nonrandomized, controlled trial. None have demonstrated a reduction in breast cancer mortality or significant improvements in the number or stage of cancers
detected. A nested case-control study from a Canadian screening study also failed to demonstrate
an association between BSE and reduction in mortality.

15. What is the accuracy of the Papanicolaou test in screening for and follow-up of cervical cytologic abnormalities?

The Papanicolaou smear (Pap smear), developed by George Papanicolaou in the 1930s, is the recommended screening test for cervical cancer. However, the best estimates suggest that it is only moderately accurate and does not achieve concurrently high sensitivity and specificity. In 2000, an estimated 12,800 women developed cervical cancer. Fortunately, the mortality rate of cervical cancer is relatively low compared with lung, breast, and colon cancer. Since the widespread practice of performing Pap smears, mortality has decreased from about 15 in 100,000 in the 1960s to approximately 8 in 100,000 women.

16. How often should Pap smears be performed?

Pap smears should be performed at least every 3 years in sexually active women who have a cervix. Screening should begin at the age of sexual intercourse. Screening can probably be discontinued at age 65 years if multiple smears have shown normal results. The frequency of examinations depends on the presence of risk factors, including early onset of sexual intercourse, multiple sexual partners, and low socioeconomic status.

17. What should be done if the results are "atypical"?

The principal goal of cervical smears is not to diagnose overt clinical cancer but to detect occult carcinomas and precancerous abnormalities that may lead to invasive cancer. Therefore, clinicians should conduct further evaluation rather than repeat a Pap smear in women who have "atypical" or "precancerous" lesions on Pap smear. In particular, the role of human papillomavirus (HPV) as a risk factor for cervical cancer has been considered. More than 99% of all cervical cancers contain high-risk HPV. Only a persistent infection with high-risk HPV of the cervical epithelium results in cervical cancer. Some organizations recommend that HPV testing be conducted in women with borderline and mild smears (e.g., atypical squamous cells of undetermined significance [ASCUS]). ASCUS may simply indicate inflammation or may be the first indicator of serious pathology. Therefore, following up abnormal Pap test results with HPV testing may reduce the use of unnecessary colposcopic examinations without missing potentially lethal cervical cancer. A randomized trial is evaluating the efficiency to detect CIN3 and cervical cancer by high-risk HPV testing in conjunction with cytomorphologic smear compared with screening by Pap smear.

18. Should CA-125 be used to screen women for ovarian cancer?

No. Although ovarian cancer is the fifth leading cause of cancer-related deaths in women (27,000 new cases and 14,000 deaths in 1995), routine screening with pelvic examination, Pap smears, transvaginal ultrasound (TVUS), or CA-125 blood testing is not recommended. The incidence of ovarian cancer increases with age, ranging from 14 per 100,000 women at age 50 years to 35 per 100,000 women at age 70 years. Additional risk factors include low parity and family history of ovarian cancer. Although hereditary cancer syndromes account for < 0.1% of women with ovarian cancer, the lifetime risk of developing ovarian cancer in women with a positive family history is ≤ 40%. Because the ovaries have a deep anatomic location, pelvic examination and Pap smear have poor sensitivity and specificity for detecting early-stage disease. The sensitivity and specificity of TVUS in the evaluation of a palpable ovarian mass are approximately 90% and 98%, respectively, but because of the low prevalence of the disease, TVUS is not practical for routine screening (positive predictive value = 3%).

The sensitivity of CA-125 for ovarian cancer increases with clinical stage but is only 50% for clinically localized stage I and II neoplasms. In addition, CA-125 is elevated in 1% of healthy women, ≤ 40% of women with benign cysts, and 30% of women with nongynecologic tumors. It may be possible to improve the accuracy by combining ultrasound measurements with CA-125; however, if this is done, the low prevalence of the disease will result in a large proportion of false-positive test results that require diagnostic laparotomy or laparoscopy. Recommendations for women at increased risk (e.g., those with presumed hereditary cancer syndromes) have included annual pelvic examinations or prophylactic oophorectomy. The effectiveness of any of these strategies has not been determined. An ongoing randomized trial is examining the effectiveness of multimodality screening (i.e., TVUS, CA-125, and pelvic examination) in reducing ovarian cancer mortality in 75,000 women aged 60–74 years.

19. What factors should physicians consider in screening patients for skin cancer?

The benefits from screening are unproven, even in high-risk patients. Clinicians should be aware that fair-skinned individuals aged > 65 years, patients with atypical moles, and those with > 50 moles constitute groups at substantially increased risk for melanomas. One third of newly diagnosed melanomas occur on non–sun-exposed areas that may not be routinely seen. Therefore, if screening is conducted, a complete skin examination is important at least once in an adult's lifetime. Clinicians should note skin lesions with malignant features such as asymmetry, border irregularity, color variability, diameter > 6 mm, or rapidly changing lesions. Suspicious lesions should be biopsied. In 1999, approximately 1 million new cases of basal cell and squamous cell carcinoma and about 44,000 new cases of malignant melanoma were diagnosed in the United States. Melanoma mortality is the sixth leading cause of cancer mortality, and incidence of melanoma and other skin cancers is increasing. Basal cell and squamous cell carcinomas cause limited morbidity or mortality even in the absence of screening.

20. Can a positive result FOBT result be interpreted if the patient is on a daily aspirin?

Evidence suggests that a daily aspirin (and even warfarin) does not produce false-positive results in clinical practice. Patients should restrict higher doses of aspirin, nonsteroidal antiinflammatory agents, iron, vitamin C, and high peroxidase-containing foods (beets) for 3 days before ordering FOBT. A high-residue, meat-free diet during testing also may be beneficial to reduce the number of false-positive test results.

21. Is routine screening for testicular cancer likely to improve overall mortality?

The United States Preventive Services Task Force does not recommend routine screening for testicular cancer. It is unlikely that screening for testicular cancer would substantially improve the already favorable outcome of this uncommon disease. For example, the overall cure rate in the absence of systemic screening is 92%. Testicular cancer is a relatively uncommon disease (annual incidence of 8–14/100,000 men aged 20–35 years). Therefore, a primary care physician who has 1500 men in his or her practice can expect to detect one testicular cancer every 15–20 years. The vast majority of test results would be normal or falsely abnormal. Screening and evaluation would result in considerable costs and possible morbidity with minimal benefit at best. Although men with a history of undescended testes or testicular atrophy are at increased risk for testicular cancer, the value of early detection has not yet been demonstrated.

22. What should primary care physicians do to reduce morbidity from oral cancer?

Identification and counseling of high-risk people against the use of tobacco or abuse of alcohol is probably the best strategy for reducing oral cancer complications. Because many patients have limited contact with dentists, the role of primary care providers in identifying and counseling the high-risk individuals is critical. More than 90% of deaths caused by oropharyngeal cancer are associated with smoking and alcohol. The use of snuff and chewing tobacco is also associated with oral cancer. The available screening tests are limited to oral examination of the mouth. Primary treatment of oral leukoplakia to prevent the development of oral cancer has not been widely accepted.

23. What are the potential harms of cancer screening?

Unlike diagnostic tests, screening is defined as tests done among apparently well people to identify those at an increased risk of a particular condition. Harms that might be accepted to treat a symptomatic patient with a known disease are less acceptable when they are caused by screening rests, which benefit only a few individuals but expose all screened individuals to the harms.

Promotional efforts at cancer screening usually emphasize death from the target disease. The main argument for this is that this is the condition that the screening test is intending to reduce mortality. Although the goal of cancer screening is to prevent deaths from the target cancer, screening may affect mortality in other ways. On the positive side, earlier detection of cancer could lead to increased use of milder and effective treatments and prevent some deaths. Screening could also prevent deaths from other diseases that are detected earlier incidentally. On the negative side, screening could lead to deaths from the evaluation of screening test results or from the earlier treatment (of the target or other disease) that would not have occurred without screening. However, disease-specific mortality may miss important harms (or benefits) of cancer screening because of misclassification in the cause of death. This can lead to overestimates of the impact that screening will have on the probability of dying. Evaluation of results from screening trials for cancer reveal two striking facts: (1) disease-specific mortality constitutes only a small proportion of all-cause mortality and (2) the differences in all-cause mortality between screened and unscreened participants is quite small. Specific adverse effects caused by screening include:

- Complications attributable to the screening test
- Complications from additional diagnostic procedures caused by inaccurate screening test results
- Identification and treatment of clinically unimportant or misdiagnosed cancers (patients may be treated unnecessarily or pathologists may disagree about the subtle abnormalities identified with screening)
- In effective treatment of cancers (screening tends to miss the most aggressive cancers)
- Psychological distress from screening either because of a diagnosis of cancer in patients whose livers were not extrended by screening or to the fear of a false-positive test result
- Costs of screening tests, diagnostic procedures, and treatments
- Physicians may not attend to other issues that are more important or of proven benefit to patients

Rather than routinely recommending certain screening strategies, especially in elderly patients or those with health conditions likely to result in a life expectancy less than 10 years, physicians should discuss potential risks and benefits of cancer screening. One could argue that given the information on all-cause mortality, the decision to be screened for a particular cancer would appear to be a very close call, at least in terms of living or dying. Knowing this may reassure the individual that whatever he or she decides, a major adverse outcome is highly unlikely. Even for the few cancer screening tests shown to be of demonstrated benefit on a population level, patient preferences often play a critical role in determining individual cancer screening decisions.

BIBLIOGRAPHY

1. Altman DG, Schulz KF, Moher D, et al: The revised CONSORT statement for reporting randomized trials: Explanation and elaboration. Ann Intern Med 134:663–694, 2001.
2. American College of Physicians: Screening for prostate cancer. Ann Intern Med 126:480–484, 1997.
3. American College of Physicians: Suggested technique for fecal occult blood testing and interpretation in colorectal cancer screening. Ann Intern Med 126:808–811, 1997.
4. Black WC, Haggstrom, Welch HG: All-cause mortality in randomized trials of cancer screening. J Natl Cancer Inst 94:167–173, 2002.
5. Concato J, Wells CK, Penson D, et al: Effectiveness of screening for prostate cancer: A nested case-control study. J Clin Epidemiol 2002:630, 2002.
6. Ernster VK, Barclay J, Kerlikowske K, et al: Incidence of and treatment for ductal carcinoma in situ of the breast. JAMA 275:913–918, 1996.
7. Friedman GD: Primer of Epidemiology, 3rd ed. New York, McGraw-Hill, 1987.
8. Grimes DA, Schulz KF: Uses and abuses of screening tests. Lancet 359:881–884, 2002.
9. Jemal A, Thomas A, Murray T, et al: Cancer statistics, 2002. CA Cancer J Clin 52:23–47, 2002.
10. Kerlikowske K, Grady D, Rubin SM, et al: Efficacy of screening mammography: A meta-analysis. JAMA 273:149–154, 1995.
11. Lederle FA, Niewoehner DE: Lung cancer surgery: A critical review of the evidence. Arch Intern Med 154:2397–2400, 1994.

12. Marshall KG: Population-based fecal occult blood screening for colon cancer: Will the benefits outweigh the harm? Can Med Assoc J 163:545–246, 2000.
13. Nanda K, McCrory DC, Myers ER, et al: Accuracy of the Papanicolaou test in screening for and follow-up of cervical cytologic abnormalities: A systematic review. Ann Intern Med 132:810–819, 2000.
14. Oboler SK, LaForce FM: The periodic physical examination in asymptomatic adults. Ann Intern Med 110:214–226, 1989.
15. Olson O, Gotzche PC: Screening for breast cancer with mammography. Cochrane Rev he Cochrane Library, issue 4, 2001.
16. Richert-Boe KE, Humphrey LL: Screening for cancers of the cervix and breast. Arch Intern Med 152:2405–2411, 1992.
17. Richert-Boe KE, Humphrey LL: Screening for cancers of the lung and colon. Arch Intern Med 152:2398–2404, 1992.
18. Schapira MM, Matchar DB, Young MJ: The effectiveness of ovarian cancer screening: A decision analysis model. Ann Intern Med 118:838–843, 1993.
19. Schulz KF, Grimes DA: Case-control studies: research in reverse. Lancet 359:431–434, 2002.
20. Towler B, Irwig L, Glasziou P, et al: A systematic review of he effects of screening for colorectal cancer using the faecal occult blood test, Hemoccult. Br Med J 317:559–565, 1998.
21. U.S. Preventive Services Task Force: Screening for skin cancer: Recommendations and rationale. Am J Prev Med 20(Suppl 3):44–46, 2002.
22. U.S. Preventive Services Task Force. Screening for Breast Cancer: www.ahrq.gov/clinic/uspstfix.htm.
23. Walter LC, Covinsky KE: Cancer screening in elderly patients. A framework for individualized decision making. JAMA 285:2750–2756, 2001.
24. Welch GH: Informed choice in cancer screening. JAMA 285:2776–2778, 2001.
25. Wilt TJ: Uncertainty in prostate cancer care: The physician's role in clearing the confusion. JAMA 283:3258–3260, 2002.

3. CARDIOVASCULAR DISEASE PREVENTION

Eduard V. Porosnicu, M.D.

Cardiovascular disease is the leading cause of death for both women and men in the United States, claiming nearly 1 million lives a year. It is estimated that 70 million Americans have one or more manifestations of cardiovascular disease, including high blood pressure (BP), stroke, and coronary heart disease (CHD). CHD alone affects more than 13 million Americans, and every year half a million people suffer an acute stroke. This chapter focuses on the actions that primary care physicians can take to reduce the risk of cardiovascular disease (specifically, CHD, cerebrovascular disease [CVD], and peripheral vascular disease [PVD]) in their patients. Treatment of hypertension and certain other cardiovascular risk factors (e.g., obesity and dyslipidemia) is covered in detail in other chapters.

1. What are the risk factors for CHD according to the 2001 National Cholesterol Education Program–Adult Treatment Panel (NCEP-ATP III)?

Major risk factors (exclusive of low-density lipoprotein [LDL] cholesterol):
Cigarette smoking
BP > 140/90 mmHg or taking antihypertensive medication
High-density lipoprotein (HDL) cholesterol < 40 mg/dL
CHD in first-degree relative (men < 55 years; women < 65 years)
Age: men > 45 years; women > 55 years
Life-habit risk factors:
Obesity
Sedentarism
Atherogenic diet

Emerging risk factors:
Lipoprotein α
Homocysteine
Prothrombotic or proinflammatory factors
Impaired fasting glucose
Ankle brachial index (ABI) < 0.9

2. How do I determine risk status for CHD events in an asymptomatic patient?
Count the number of major risk factors (listed in question 1).
- **0–1 risk factors:** low risk of coronary events (generally < 10% at 10 years)
- **≥ 2 risk factors:** Calculate the Framingham score (10-year risk based on gender, age, total cholesterol [TC], HDL cholesterol complex [HDL-C], smoking status, BP) (see NCEP-ATP III report)

Coronary risk can also be estimated based on the Sheffield tables or coronary artery disease (CAD) risk calculators (available at www.uptodate.com).

3. Name the three categories of coronary risk according to NCEP-ATP III and define the LDL cholesterol level goal and the cutoff level for therapeutic intervention for each named category.

RISK CATEGORY	LDL-C GOAL	LDL-C TO START LIFESTYLE CHANGES (mg/dL)	LDL-C TO CONSIDER MEDICATION (mg/dL)
CHD and CHD risk equivalents	< 100	> 100	> 130
Multiple (2+) risk factors	< 130	> 130	10-year risk 10–20%: > 130
			10-year risk < 10%: > 160
0–1 risk factors	< 160	> 160	> 190

4. What are CHD risk equivalents according to the NCEP-ATP III?
Clinical forms of atherosclerosis:
Peripheral artery disease
Abdominal aortic aneurysm
Symptomatic carotid artery disease
Diabetes mellitus
10-year risk for CHD > 20%

5. Should asymptomatic patients be screened for occult cardiovascular disease?
Screening for modifiable risk factors (e.g., hypertension, dyslipidemia, smoking) is strongly recommended, but screening asymptomatic people to detect occult atherosclerotic disease with modalities such as resting electrocardiography, exercise electrocardiography, or noninvasive carotid and peripheral vascular evaluation is not. Such tests have poor positive predictive value because of the low incidence of disease in asymptomatic populations; furthermore, the benefit of treating uncovered disease in asymptomatic patients is not established. In certain asymptomatic people, however, cardiac screening may be appropriate; this includes persons at very high risk for CHD (e.g., men older than age 40 years with several cardiac risk factors), persons in whom a catastrophic cardiac event would endanger public safety (e.g., airline pilots), and persons at moderate or high risk for CHD who wish to initiate a vigorous exercise program.

6. Who should be screened for dyslipidemia as a CHD risk factor according to NCEP-ATP III?
All adults age 20 years and older should be screened with a fasting lipoprotein profile (TC, LDL-C, total glucose [TG]); it should be repeated once every 5 years if found in optimal limits. If a nonfasting lipoprotein profile was initially done and TC is > 200 mg/dL or HDL-C is < 40

mg/dL, a follow-up fasting lipoprotein profile is needed for appropriate management based on LDL-C values.

7. What should be done about low levels of HDL-C and high triglycerides?

If HDL-C is < 40 mg/dL in men or < 50 mg/dL in women, initiate lifestyle changes (e.g., have the patient quit smoking, increase physical activity, and try to attain ideal body weight). For high-risk patients, consider drugs that raise HDL-C (e.g., niacin, if tolerated; fibrates, statins). If triglycerides are > 150–200 mg/dL, recommend decreased alcohol consumption, target ideal body weight, and obtain better diabetes control. Triglycerides > 200–500 is reflected in an increased non-HDL-C; it is an indication for statins in higher doses, niacin, or fibrates in addition to the lifestyle changes. If triglycerides are > 500 mg/dL, fibrate or niacin is indicated to reduce the risk of pancreatitis.

8. What advice should physicians give about alcohol and the risk of cardiovascular disease?

Moderate alcohol intake has limited cardioprotective effect. This might be partially explained by an increase in HDL cholesterol. Light alcohol intake (1–2 drinks/day) decreases stroke incidence, but the opposite is true for heavy drinking. Nonetheless, alcohol cannot be recommended as a cardioprotective substance because of the number of health hazards, including addictive potential, hypertension, liver damage, risk for breast cancer, physical abuse, and driving accidents. Based on epidemiologic data, the American Heart Association (AHA) recommends that alcoholic beverages be limited to the equivalent of 2 drinks per day (30 g of ethanol) for men and 1 drink per day for women. Physicians should not recommend that abstinent individuals begin drinking alcohol. Patients who drink light to moderate amounts with no associated medical or social problems may be reassured that that amount is acceptable and cardioprotective.

9. What are the dietary goals for the general population as stated in the AHA's 2000 guidelines?

The term *step 1 diet* (i.e., dietary goals for the general population) has been replaced in the AHA's 2000 guidelines by the term *major dietary guidelines*. The goals and advice on how to work toward them are summarized in the table below.

GOAL	STEPS TO ACHIEVING GOAL
Overall healthy eating pattern	Fruits and vegetables: > 5 servings/day
	Grain products: > 6 servings/day
	Low-fat dairy products
	Fish and lean meats
Appropriate body weight	Match energy needs with food intake
Desirable cholesterol profile	Saturated fat: < 10% of calories
	Cholesterol: < 300 mg/day
	Avoid transfatty acids (e.g., partially hydrogenated vegetable oils)
	Substitute unsaturated fatty acids (especially omega-3 fatty acids from fish, nuts, soybean and canola oil)
Desirable blood pressure	Salt: < 6 g/day
	Alcohol intake: < 2 drinks/day for men; < 1 drink/day for women
	Weight control
	DASH diet

DASH = Dietary approaches to stop hypertension.

10. What brief advice for a healthy diet should you give to your patients?

- Eat only when you are hungry (match energy intake with energy needs).
- Avoid foods that make you thirsty.
- Avoid processed meats and organ meats.
- Avoid fast food and prepackaged cookies, crackers, and baked goods.

- Use only low-fat dairy products.
- Use spray or liquid fats for cooking (e.g., canola oil).
- Increase intake of fruits, vegetables, legumes, grains, and nuts.
- Have fish twice or more a week.
- Have no more than two alcoholic drinks per day for men and no more than one for women.

11. What are the benefits of exercise?

Numerous observational studies indicate that physical activity is associated with a reduced risk of CHD and total mortality independently of its beneficial effect on other risk factors such as serum lipids, obesity, diabetes, and hypertension. Physical activity also protects against osteoporosis and promotes mental well-being. In the past, it was thought that only vigorous exercise would produce the desired health benefits; it is now believed that even a modest exercise program can have substantial positive effects.

12. When is it safe to start an exercise program?

The safety of starting an exercise program in an individual patient can be assessed with the Physical Activity Readiness questionnaire:

Physical Activity Readiness Questions

1. Have you ever been told that you have heart trouble?
2. Do you frequently get pain in your chest?
3. Do you often feel faint or have severe dizzy spells?
4. Have you ever been told that you have high blood pressure?
5. Have you ever been told that you have problems with bones or joints (such as arthritis) that may be made worse by exercise?
6. Do you have any other physical problem that may prevent you from exercising?
7. Are you older than 65 years and not used to regular, vigorous exercise?

Adapted from Harris SS, Caspersen CJ, DeFriese GH, Estes EH Jr: Physical activity counseling for healthy adults as a primary preventive intervention in the clinical setting. Report for the U.S. Preventive Services Task Force. JAMA 261:3588–3598, 1989.

A patient who answers no to all questions can safely undertake an exercise program without further testing or medical supervision. Patients who answer yes to any of the questions should be evaluated further. Exercise electrocardiography should be considered for older patients and patients with cardiac disease or risk factors who wish to undertake a vigorous exercise program. Screening exercise electrocardiography for young, asymptomatic patients with no cardiac risk factors is not necessary.

13. What should an exercise prescription include?

Prescriptions for exercise should specify intensity, duration, and frequency. Recommended intensity of exercise is in the range of 50–85% of maximal oxygen uptake (VO_2 max), which corresponds to 65–90% of the maximal heart rate. (The maximal heart rate is approximately equal to 220 minus the person's age.) Patients should be told their target heart rate and shown how to take their pulse; for example, for a sedentary 60-year-old person, it may be 104 ([220 − 60] × 0.65). The general recommendation for duration and frequency is 15–45 minutes three to five times per week. Patients should be told to gradually work toward their exercise goal. In many ways, brisk walking is the ideal exercise. It is easy, convenient, and free and has minimal risk of adverse effects (e.g., sudden death or musculoskeletal injury).

Patients should be told that increasing physical activity, even without embarking on a formal exercise program, has documented health benefits. A reasonable goal is to do 30 minutes a day of moderate-intensity activity, such as walking briskly, climbing stairs, mowing the lawn with a power mower, or general house cleaning. The 30 minutes can be accumulated through multiple shorter bouts of activity.

14. Is hormone replacement therapy (HRT) indicated for CHD prevention in post-menopausal women?

No. Two randomized, controlled trials published in July 2002 support this statement. The Heart and Estrogen-Progestin Replacement Study (HERS) evaluated HRT over 4.1 years in 2763 postmenopausal women with CHD (secondary prevention). There were no statistically significant benefits of HRT on any cardiovascular event rate.

The Women Health Initiative (WHI) estrogen plus progestin arm showed a relative risk increase in CHD events (29%) and strokes (41%) with HRT. This arm, which enrolled 16,000 healthy menopausal women, was stopped in May 2002 because of a significant 26% relative risk increase in invasive breast cancer and a doubling of venous thromboembolic events.

15. Which patients should take aspirin for primary prevention of cardiovascular disease?
- Individuals with a low risk of vascular events ($< 1\%$/year) derive no demonstrated cardiovascular benefit from aspirin.
- In those qualifying as CAD equivalents (ATP III), antiplatelet therapy reduces the risk for nonfatal myocardial infarction (MI), nonfatal stroke, and death from vascular or unknown causes. Consequently, the third Preventive Services Task Force "strongly recommends" the use of aspirin in adults at increased risk for coronary vascular disease ($> 3\%$/year), and the American Diabetes Association recommends aspirin for coronary vascular disease primary prevention in any diabetic with an additional vascular risk factor.
- The benefit-to-risk ratio is higher in younger patients, in those with lower systolic BP, and in those with lower cholesterol.
- Daily doses of 75–150 mg of aspirin were as effective as higher doses.
- The benefit of aspirin in coronary vascular disease primary prevention is far less than that derived from smoking cessation, dietary modification, or treatment of hypertension or hyperlipidemia.

16. Are vitamin supplements indicated for the prevention of CHD?

Randomized, controlled trials of antioxidants such as beta carotene and vitamin E in coronary vascular disease primary prevention failed to show any evidence of benefit. On the contrary, four randomized, controlled trials demonstrated a detrimental effect of beta carotene supplementation. From a practical standpoint, a healthy, diverse diet rich in grains, fruits, vegetables, and nuts supplies the needed vitamins.

17. What are the risk factors for stroke?

Factors such as age, race (increases in African Americans and Hispanic Americans), previous transient ischemic attack (TIA), and family history of stroke or TIA indicate a higher risk for stroke. These factors are not modifiable. Modifiable risk factors include hypertension, smoking, diabetes, hyperlipidemia, asymptomatic carotid stenosis, atrial fibrillation, and sickle cell disease. These should be targeted, especially in high-risk populations. Less well-documented risk factors are obesity, physical inactivity, alcohol abuse (> 5 drinks/day), drug abuse, hypercoagulable states, HRT, and oral contraceptive use.

18. What is the role of carotid endarterectomy for primary stroke prevention?

Endarterectomy should be considered in patients with high-grade ($> 60\%$ and $< 100\%$) extracranial carotid artery stenosis when performed by a surgeon with a $< 3\%$ morbidity or mortality rate. The benefit of endarterectomy for asymptomatic carotid artery stenosis is highly dependent on the surgical risk. A prior full evaluation for other treatable causes of stroke is needed. The patient selection should take into consideration comorbid conditions, life expectancy, and patient preference.

19. What are the indications for antithrombotic therapy for embolic stroke prevention in patients with atrial fibrillation?

The anticoagulation with warfarin (Coumadin) to an international normalized ratio (INR) range of 2–3 is the rule. As the exception, patients younger than 65 years with "lone" atrial fibrillation (i.e., none of the following risk factors: hypertension, diabetes mellitus, poor left ventricular function, rheumatic mitral valve disease, prior TIA or stroke, systemic embolism or stroke, prosthetic heart valve) can start aspirin therapy only. The cutoff age can be extended to 75 years if the patient prefers to avoid warfarin, but the provider and the patient should be aware that the risk of atrial fibrillation–associated stroke increases steeply with advancing age (annual risk from 1.5% in the 6th decade to 23.5% in the 9th decade of life).

20. Which preventive measures are indicated in people who have had an MI?
Many modifiable risk factors, including cigarette smoking, dyslipidemia, physical inactivity, obesity, hypertension, and diabetes mellitus, are important predictors of recurrent cardiac events among patients with a history of MI or other manifestations of CHD. Because the absolute risk reduction is directly proportional to the incidence of the events, secondary prevention is more cost-effective than primary prevention. Clinical trials demonstrating beneficial effects of secondary prevention have been reported for hypercholesterolemia, hypertension, exercise programs, and diabetes control. In addition, randomized, controlled trials have clearly demonstrated the benefit of early start and indefinite use of aspirin, clopidogrel, beta-blockers, and angiotensin-converting enzyme inhibitors after MI.

BIBLIOGRAPHY

1. Andersen RE, Blair SN, Cheskin LJ, Bartlett SJ: Encouraging patients to become more physically active: The physician's role. Ann Intern Med 127:395–400, 1997.
2. Biller J, Feinberg WM, Castaldo JE, et al: Guidelines for carotid endarterectomy: A statement for healthcare professionals from a Special Writing Group of the Stroke Council, American Heart Association. Circulation 97:501–509, 1998.
3. Booyse FM, Parks DA: Moderate wine and alcohol consumption: Beneficial effects on cardiovascular disease. Thromb Haemost 86:517–528, 2001.
4. Collaborative Group of the Primary Prevention Project (PPP): Low-dose aspirin and vitamin E in people at cardiovascular risk: A randomised trial in general practice. Lancet 357:39–95, 2001.
5. Fiore MC, Bailey WC, Cohen SJ, et al: Treating Tobacco Use and Dependence: Clinical Practice Guideline. Rockville, MD, U.S. Department of Health and Human Services, Public Health Service, 2000.
6. Fletcher GF: How to implement physical activity in primary and secondary prevention. A statement for healthcare-professionals from the Task Force on Risk-reduction, American Heart Association. Circulation 96:355–357, 1997.
7. Goldstein LB, Adams R, Becker K, et al: Primary prevention of ischemic stroke: A statement for healthcare professionals from the Stroke Council of the American Heart Association. Circulation 103:163–182, 2001.
8. Grady D, Herrington D, Bittner V, et al: Cardiovascular disease outcomes during 6–8 years of hormone therapy: Heart and Estrogen/Progestin Replacement Study follow-up (HERS II). JAMA 288:49–57, 2002.
9. Harris SS, Caspersen CJ, DeFriese GH, Estes EH Jr: Physical activity counseling for healthy adults as a primary preventive intervention in the clinical setting. Report for the U.S. Preventive Services Task Force. JAMA 261:3588–3598, 1989.
10. Heart Protection Study Collaborative Group: MRC/BHF Heart Protection Study of cholesterol lowering with simvastatin in 20,536 high-risk individuals: A randomised placebo-controlled trial. Lancet 360:7–22, 2002.
11. Karnath B: Smoking cessation. Am J Med 112:399–405, 2002.
12. Krauss RM, Eckel RH, Howard B, et al: AHA Dietary Guidelines: Revision 2000: A statement for healthcare professionals from the Nutrition Committee of the American Heart Association. Circulation 102:2284–2299, 2000.
13. Pearson TA, Blair SN, Daniels SR, et al: AHA Guidelines for Primary Prevention of Cardiovascular Disease and Stroke: 2002 Update: Consensus Panel Guide to Comprehensive Risk Reduction for Adult Patients without Coronary or Other Atherosclerotic Vascular Diseases. American Heart Association Science Advisory and Coordinating Committee. Circulation 106:388–391, 2002.
14. Smith SC Jr, Blair SN, Bonow RO, et al: AHA/ACC Scientific Statement: AHA/ACC guidelines for preventing heart attack and death in patients with atherosclerotic cardiovascular disease: 2001 update: A statement for healthcare professionals from the American Heart Association and the American College of Cardiology. Circulation 104:1577–1579, 2001.

15. Third Report of the National Cholesterol Education Program (NCEP) Expert Panel on Detection, Evaluation, and Treatment of High Blood Cholesterol in Adults (Adult Treatment Panel III). Bethesda, MD, National Institutes of Health, 2001, NIH publication 01–3670.
16. Writing Group for the Women's Health Initiative Investigators: Risks and benefits of estrogen plus progestin in healthy postmenopausal women: Principal results from the Women's Health Initiative randomized, controlled trial. JAMA 288:321–333, 2002.

4. IMMUNIZATIONS AND SCREENING FOR INFECTIOUS DISEASES

Sarah J. D'Heilly, M.D., and Kristin L. Nichol, M.D., M.P.H., M.B.A.

1. Which vaccines are recommended for children?

Current recommendations are for all children to receive the following vaccines:

VACCINE	REGIMEN
Diphtheria, tetanus, pertussis	5 doses
Polio	4 doses
Measles, mumps, and rubella (MMR)	2 doses
Haemophilus influenzae B (Hib; conjugate vaccine)	3–4 doses
Hepatitis B	3 doses
Streptococcus pneumoniae (pneumococcal conjugate vaccine)	4 doses
Varicella	1–2 doses

These vaccines are administered at various intervals from birth to age 12 years; 80% of injections are scheduled during the first 15–18 months of life. Several of these recommendations are new or have been modified within the past few years:

1. In 1996, routine varicella vaccination was recommended for all susceptible children.

2. In 1997, diphtheria-tetanus-acellular pertussis (DTaP) vaccine became the preferred vaccine for protection against diphtheria, tetanus, and pertussis in infants and young children because of the reduced frequency of adverse reactions and equal or increased efficacy.

3. In 1999, an all inactivated polio virus vaccine schedule was recommended because of the success of the global polio eradication project. Oral polio virus vaccine is still used in countries where polio is endemic.

4. In 1999, routine administration of hepatitis A vaccine was recommended for children who live in areas where rates of disease are at least 20 cases per 100,000 population.

5. In 2001, routine pneumococcal conjugate vaccine was recommended for all children younger than 23 months and for children 24–59 months at high risk for pneumococcal infection.

6. In 2002, influenza vaccination guidelines were changed to encourage routine administration of influenza vaccine to healthy children 6–23 months old.

7. In 2003, an intranasally administered live, attenuated influenza vaccine was approved for use in healthy people aged 5–49 years.

2. Which vaccinations are recommended for adults?

Vaccinations for adults, in contrast to those for children, are largely recommended only for persons in specific risk groups. The vaccines most often administered to adults include:

VACCINE	DOSE AND TARGET GROUP
Influenza vaccine	Yearly for people who are elderly, at high risk of influenza-associated complications, likely to be at high risk (i.e., ages 50–64 years), or likely to transmit disease to high-risk persons
Pneumococcal vaccine	Once for people 65 years or older and people at high risk; revaccinate certain groups at highest risk
Tetanus-diphtheria	Booster every 10 years after primary series has been completed
Hepatitis B	Three doses for people at high risk, including international travelers and health care providers
Hepatitis A	Two doses for people at high risk, including international travelers
Varicella	Two doses for people without a history of varicella disease or who are seronegative for varicella
Meningococcal	Routinely given to persons at high risk (terminal complement deficiency, asplenia) and in outbreaks; considered for college students
MMR	Two doses or other evidence of immunity (prior physician diagnosis of measles, laboratory evidence of immunity, or birth before 1957) for people at high risk, including health care providers

People aged 65 years and older and people with chronic medical conditions (especially chronic heart and lung disease) are at particularly increased risk for complications from influenza and pneumococcal disease and should be offered both vaccines. Tetanus-diphtheria boosters are recommended routinely for all adults who have previously completed the primary series of three doses. Hepatitis B vaccine is recommended for people with high-risk life-styles (e.g., intravenous drug users, bisexual or homosexual men, people with other sexually transmitted diseases), those with high-risk occupations (e.g., health care providers), and people who live or work in high-risk environments (e.g., prison inmates). Hepatitis B vaccination is also recommended for international travelers whose itineraries include much of eastern Europe, Asia, Africa, and Central and South America. Hepatitis A vaccination is recommended for people at increased risk for infection as well as for food handlers. People at increased risk for infection include international travelers whose itineraries include countries with moderate or high rates of hepatitis A, homosexual or bisexual men, users of street drugs, and people with chronic liver disease or clotting factor disorders. Mumps, measles, and rubella (MMR) vaccine is recommended for health care providers and students at colleges or other educational institutions after high school who have not previously received two doses of the vaccine and who lack evidence of adequate immunity (i.e., prior physician diagnosis of measles disease, laboratory evidence of immunity, birth since 1957).

Varicella vaccine is recommended for susceptible adults. Meningococcal vaccine is recommended routinely for those at high risk for disease, including people with terminal complement deficiencies, people with functional or anatomic asplenia, and travelers to hyperendemic or epidemic countries (particularly the "meningitis belt" of sub-Saharan Africa). Vaccination is also an important part of control of meningococcal outbreaks. In addition, college students, particularly those living in dormitories, are at increased risk for meningococcal disease. Currently, routine vaccination is not recommended for this group, but students and their parents should be educated about the disease so an individualized decision can be made.

In addition to routine immunizations, for travelers outside the United States, the need for any other vaccines should be assessed. Special immunization requirements are geographically defined and may include immunizations for yellow fever, cholera, typhoid fever, hepatitis B, hepatitis A, and other diseases. Local and state health departments and the Centers for Disease Control and Prevention may be consulted for up-to-date information on immunization recommendations for international travelers.

3. Do vaccine-preventable diseases continue to be a major cause of illness and mortality?

The past several decades have seen dramatic decreases in the numbers of reported cases of vaccine-preventable diseases in the United States. For example, with the introduction of the *Haemophilus influenza* type B (Hib) vaccine, cases of invasive disease have decreased by > 99% among young children. In 2000, the United States had a record low number of reported measles cases. Nevertheless, vaccine-preventable diseases continue to be major causes of illness and death each year in all age groups. Outbreaks of measles, congenital rubella syndrome, pertussis, and mumps continue to occur, underscoring the importance of these diseases among children. In addition, influenza and pneumonia continue to rank as the sixth leading cause of death in the United States, killing ≤ 50 times more people (≥ 85% of whom are elderly) than all other vaccine-preventable diseases in all age groups combined.

The major reason is that vaccination rates often fall far short of national goals. Among children aged 19–35 months, immunization rates have increased, with 90% coverage levels for diphtheria-pertussis-tetanus, polio, haemophilus B, hepatitis B, and measles-containing viruses. Nevertheless, even among such children, ≥ 22% are not up to date for all of the recommended vaccines, and the rates for pneumococcal vaccine are only 41%. The lowest vaccination rates may be seen especially in certain difficult-to-reach groups, including the urban poor and racial and ethnic minorities. Only 55% of elderly persons have received pneumococcal vaccine; only about 67% have received influenza vaccine; and ≤ 72% of adults aged 70 years and older may lack adequate immunity to tetanus.

Vaccine-preventable Diseases in the U.S.: Decrease in Morbidity Related to Vaccine-preventable Diseases in U.S., 1900–1998

DISEASE	AVERAGE NO. OF CASES PRIOR VACCINE USE	NO. OF CASES REPORTED, 1998	DECREASE IN MORBIDITY (%)
Congenital rubella	823	5	99.4
Diphtheria	175,885	1	100
Invasive *Haemophilus influenzae*	20,000	54	99.7
Measles	503,282	89	100
Mumps	152,209	606	99.6
Pertussis	147,271	6279	95.7
Polio (paralytic)	16,316	0	100
Rubella	47,745	345	99.3
Tetanus	1314	34	97.4

Adapted from Centers for Disease Control and Prevention: 10 Great public health achievements. MMWR 48(12):241–247, 1999.

Occurrences of Vaccine-preventable Diseases by Age Group, 1999

VACCINE-PREVENTABLE DISEASE	TOTAL REPORTED CASES, 1999	CASES BY AGE GROUP		
		< 25 YEARS	25–64 YEARS	> 65 YEARS
Pertussis	7288	5940	1253	80
Tetanus	40	5	26	9
Measles	100	74	25	0
Mumps	387	263	106	7
Rubella	267	146	117	1
Polio	0	0	0	0
H. influenzae	1309	370	415	504
Hepatitis B	7694	1447	5770	333
Hepatitis A	17,047	7287	8749	877

Adapted from Centers for Disease Control: Summary of notifiable diseases, United States, 1999. MMWR 48(53):12, 2001.

Deaths Due to Vaccine-preventable Diseases, United States, 1989–1998

DISEASE	CASES	DEATHS
Influenza	(millions)	350,000–500,000
Pneumococcal disease	(millions)	120,000*
Hepatitis A	282,650	1013
Hepatitis B	146,644	9694
Measles	60,189	132
Mumps	24,075	7
Rubella	4412	21
Pertussis	53,634	65
Tetanus	486	77

*85% of deaths are among the elderly.
Adapted from Centers for Disease Control and Prevention: Summary of notifiable diseases, U.S., 1999. MMWR 48(53):82–90, 2001.

4. How can vaccination rates be improved?

Many opportunities exist for improving levels of immunity by increasing vaccination rates among targeted persons in the United States. Strategies to improve vaccination rates should address barriers to and facilitators of successful vaccination efforts, including:

Patient issues
- Physician's recommendation
- Access and convenience, including use of nontraditional settings
- Cost
- Awareness of importance of vaccines, vaccine efficacy, and vaccine safety

Provider issues
- Up-to-date knowledge about vaccine recommendations, efficacy, and side effects
- Reimbursement
- Effective organizational structures in practice settings to ensure that vaccine is systematically offered and administered (including patient identification, tracking, standing orders, and recall systems)
- Feedback using objective measures of performance

Public policy issues
- Public and provider education
- Reimbursement
- Vaccine purchase and distribution
- Regulations requiring evidence of immunity in specific situations (e.g., school enrollment, college matriculation)

Studies have shown that a physician's recommendation for immunization is among the most potent predictors of patient behavior. For providers, strategies aimed at improving organizational structures within their practice seem to be most effective in improving vaccination rates. Age-based strategies for assessing vaccination needs also may be effective. Recently, recommendations have been made for assessment of immunization during routine health visits for adolescents aged 11–12 years. It also has been recommended that at age 50 years, all adults should be assessed for immunization as well as other preventive health services. By age 50 years, 12% of adults have chronic lung disease and more than one third have chronic heart disease, placing them in target groups for influenza and pneumococcal vaccinations.

5. What are special considerations with regard to vaccinations and immunocompromised hosts?

Immunocompromised people may be at increased risk for vaccine-preventable diseases. This risk is determined by the nature and severity of the underlying process. Such people may also be at increased risk for adverse reactions to live-virus vaccines because viral replication after administration of live-virus vaccines may be enhanced in severely immunocompromised persons. Killed or inactivated vaccines, however, do not represent a danger to immunocompromised people and generally should be administered as recommended for otherwise immunocompetent people.

Live versus Killed or Inactivated Vaccines

LIVE (ATTENUATED) VACCINES*	KILLED OR INACTIVATED VACCINES[†]
Measles[‡]	Diphtheria
Mumps[‡]	Pertussis
Rubella[‡]	Tetanus (toxoid)
Oral polio vaccine	Hepatitis B
Varicella	Hepatitis A
Live, attenuated influenza vaccine	Meningococcal
	Pneumococcal
	H. influenzae
	Inactivated influenza vaccine
	Enhanced inactivated polio vaccine

*May be contraindicated for certain immunocompromised persons.
[†]Generally considered safe for administration to immunocompromised people.
[‡]Including MMR.

6. Which three groups of immunocompromised patients should be specifically considered in choosing vaccine type?

1. People who are severely immunocompromised as a result of non-HIV diseases (e.g., congenital immunodeficiency, leukemia, lymphoma, generalized malignancy) or therapy with certain drugs (e.g., alkylating agents, antimetabolites, radiation, or large amounts of corticosteroids)

2. People with HIV infection

3. Persons with conditions that cause limited immune deficits (e.g., asplenia, renal failure) that may require the use of special vaccines or higher doses but do not contraindicate use of any particular vaccine, including live-virus vaccines

Live-virus vaccines are contraindicated for persons in group 1. In addition, oral polio vaccine should not be given to any household contact or nursing personnel in close contact with a severely immunocompromised person because of shedding of vaccine virus by the vaccine recipient. For persons in group 2, oral polio vaccine also should be avoided; if there is need for administration of polio vaccine, the enhanced inactivated form of the vaccine (eIPV) should be used. MMR vaccination of people in group 2 is recommended for all who do not have evidence of severe immunosuppression. Vaccination early in the course of HIV disease is desirable because the immunologic response may decrease as HIV disease progresses. Furthermore, routine MMR vaccination of people in group 2 who have severe immunosuppression may result in an increased risk for adverse events associated with replication of vaccine viruses. Children in group 2 who are asymptomatic or only mildly symptomatic should receive the varicella vaccine because they are at increased risk for complications from primary varicella and from zoster. For persons in group 3, live-virus vaccines may be administered according to the usual schedules.

People with certain medical conditions that impair immune responses, such as renal failure, asplenia, and diabetes, may be at increased risk for specific diseases. Bacterial polysaccharide (especially pneumococcal vaccine) and influenza vaccines are often recommended.

7. Can pregnant women be vaccinated?

All considerations about the use of vaccines during pregnancy should weigh the benefits to the mother and fetus against the possible risks; current immunization recommendations should be consulted before administering vaccines. There are, however, several general precautions for the use of vaccines during pregnancy. Because of potential risk to the developing fetus, live-virus vaccines (particularly MMR and varicella) usually should be avoided altogether for both pregnant women and women who are likely to become pregnant in the near future. However, no cases of congenital rubella or varicella syndrome have been reported among infants born to women who received these vaccines during pregnancy. For this reason, in 2001, the recommended period of time to avoid pregnancy after administration of rubella-containing vaccine was decreased from 3 months to 28 days. In addition, although no convincing evidence indicates an increased risk to the fetus from inactivated virus or bacteria vaccines or toxoids, it is a reasonable precaution to delay, if possible, administration of any necessary vaccine or toxoid until the second or third trimester to minimize any possible or theoretical risk of teratogenicity for the fetus. Tetanus-diphtheria toxoid, for example, may be administered to pregnant women in this fashion if indicated. Limited data from case reports and other studies suggest that pregnancy may increase the risk for hospitalization for serious complications of influenza as a result of increases in heart rate, stroke volume, and oxygen consumption as well as decreases in lung capacity and changes in immunologic function. Accordingly, routine vaccination with inactivated influenza vaccine is recommended for all women who will be in the second or third trimester of pregnancy during the influenza season.

8. Which vaccines are recommended for health care providers?

Health care providers, including medical students, residents, and practicing physicians, are at increased risk for contracting and transmitting vaccine-preventable diseases, including influenza, MMR, hepatitis B, and varicella. Accordingly, health care professionals should have adequate immunity against these diseases, not only for their own protection but also for the protection of their patients. Often, this means annual influenza immunization, two doses of MMR (unless they were born before 1957 or have other evidence of immunity as described above), and hepatitis B vaccine. Serologic screening before possible varicella immunization of health care workers with negative or uncertain histories may be cost-effective. In addition, it is prudent for health care professionals to receive tetanus-diphtheria boosters every 10 years.

9. What adverse events may occur after immunizations?

Modern vaccines are remarkably safe and effective. Although adverse events have been reported after the administration of all vaccines, the most frequent events are minor, local reactions. Hypersensitivity reactions are uncommon and are almost always caused by hypersensitivity to one or more vaccine components: (1) animal protein (e.g., residual egg protein from egg-grown virus vaccines such as measles, mumps, and influenza vaccines), (2) antibiotics (e.g., trace neomycin found in MMR), (3) preservatives (e.g., thimerosal in inactivated influenza vaccine), and (4) stabilizers. In 1999, the U.S. Food and Drug Administration (FDA) asked vaccine manufacturers to eliminate or greatly reduce the amount of thimerosal in vaccines; currently, pediatric vaccines contain no or only trace amounts of thimerosol. Although much has been made in the media of a link between MMR and autism, the data do not support this claim. Both MMR and DTaP can temporarily increase the risk for febrile seizures in some children, but there is no increased risk for subsequent seizures or neurodevelopmental delay. Other severe, systemic effects are rare; often a cause-and-effect relationship between symptom and vaccine is difficult or impossible to establish.

Although serious side effects are uncommon, health care providers may encounter patients who have temporally associated events serious enough to require medical attention. Since 1988, health care providers and vaccine manufacturers have been required by law to report adverse events associated with certain vaccines, including MMR or its component vaccines, DTP/DTaP or its component vaccines, and polio vaccines. Adverse events that require medical attention after administration of any vaccine should be reported to the Vaccine Adverse Event Reporting Service (VAERS) of the U.S. Department of Health and Human Services. In 1999, distribution of rotavirus vaccine was discontinued after a number of cases of intussusception were reported to VAERS among infants who had received the rotavirus vaccine.

10. Identify common contraindications to the administration of vaccines.

Contraindications to the administration of vaccines include certain disease states (e.g., live-virus vaccines are contraindicated for severely immunocompromised people), other medical conditions (e.g., live-virus vaccines are generally contraindicated during pregnancy), and known hypersensitivity to previous doses of vaccine or vaccine components (e.g., persons with a history of anaphylactic reactions to eggs or egg products should not receive egg-grown virus vaccines such as mumps, measles, and influenza vaccines). In addition, severe reactions to previous doses may preclude subsequent doses of certain immunizations (e.g., anaphylactic reaction or encephalopathy within 7 days of DTP/DTaP vaccination not attributable to another identifiable cause).

Certain conditions are commonly misunderstood to be contraindications to administration of vaccines. These are better characterized as precautions that may increase the risk for an adverse reaction or decrease the ability of the vaccine to produce immunity. Vaccination may be deferred under these circumstances if possible but should be given if the opportunity to vaccinate may be lost. Physicians and other health care providers should maintain up-to-date knowledge about vaccine components and the indications and contraindications for vaccine administration to ensure appropriate immunization activities. Sources for this information include current vaccine package inserts and vaccination recommendations from expert groups such as the Advisory Committee on Immunization Practices (ACIP) of the Public Health Service.

The following situations do *not* represent contraindications to vaccination:

- Reactions to a previous dose of DTP or other vaccine that involved only a mild to moderate local reaction or temperature < 40.5°C
- Mild acute upper respiratory or gastrointestinal illness with temperature < 38°C
- Current antimicrobial therapy or convalescent phase of illnesses
- Premature infant
- Pregnancy of household contact
- Recent exposure to infectious disease
- Breastfeeding
- Personal history of nonspecific allergies
- Family history of allergies or seizures

11. What are some of the reasons for the recent vaccine shortages?

Recently, several vaccines have been in short supply. The many complex reasons for these shortages include voluntary interruptions by the vaccine manufacturers (e.g., varicella and MMR), unexpected demand (e.g., pneumococcal conjugate vaccine), and withdrawal of vaccine manufacturers from the market (e.g., tetanus and diphtheria toxoids). In general, when a vaccine is in short supply, physicians should first target those most at risk from a given disease and delay later routine childhood doses and booster doses. For example, because of a shortage of tetanus and diphtheria toxoids (2000–2002), routine boosters in adolescents and adults were delayed to ensure that adequate vaccine was available for wound management, travelers visiting diphtheria-endemic countries, and the first three routine childhood doses.

Much attention has been given to influenza vaccine over the past several influenza seasons. Production of influenza vaccine is a very complicated process. It starts with the selection of the three virus strains that represent the viruses likely to circulate in the United States during the upcoming flu season. Those three viruses will be included in that year's vaccine. These strains then have to be grown in culture before mass production of the vaccine can occur. All of this must be done in approximately 8 months' time. Problems such as difficulty growing one of the strains or the loss of vaccine manufacturers from the market (both of which have occurred over the past several years) can lead to a delay in arrival of the vaccine and possible vaccine shortages. In years with decreased or delayed influenza vaccine production, vaccination efforts should focus on high-risk groups in October with vaccination of other groups beginning in November. Although October and November are the optimal months to receive vaccine, vaccination should continue to be encouraged as long as vaccine is available.

12. Who should be screened for HIV?

Mortality from HIV has dropped substantially in recent years. In 1999, HIV dropped out of the top 15 leading causes of death. However, HIV disease ranks fifth among leading causes of death in 25–44-year-old adults and first among African-American men aged 25–44 years. People at increased risk for HIV for whom screening may be indicated include persons receiving treatment for sexually transmitted diseases (STDs), homosexual or bisexual men, injection drug users, people with a history of multiple sexual partners or prostitution, residence or birth in an area with high prevalence of HIV infection, people undergoing treatment for tuberculosis or drug abuse, and history of a blood transfusion between 1978 and 1985. Because treatment of HIV-infected pregnant women with antiretroviral agents reduces perinatal transmission, routine HIV counseling and voluntary HIV screening are now recommended for all pregnant women.

Screening is usually performed initially with an FDA-approved enzyme immunoassay (EIA) that detects antibodies to HIV. Even though this test reportedly has a sensitivity and specificity of about 99%, because of the implications of false-positive results, the EIA test should be repeated before being reported as positive. Positive EIA results should then be confirmed by an FDA-approved supplemental test (e.g., the Western blot test or immunofluorescence assay [IFA]) before a diagnosis of HIV infection is made. If the true prevalence of HIV positivity in a population is 0.5%, even with 99% sensitivity and specificity, the positive predictive value of a single ELA would be only 33%. In addition, because antibodies are not normally detected for 2–8 weeks after exposure, people with a history of a recent, significant exposure and an initial negative EIA test result should be considered for retesting. A positive EIA result and indeterminate Western blot result can represent either an infected person with incomplete antibody response or an uninfected person with a nonspecific reaction. In this situation, testing should be repeated in approximately 1 month.

In the past few years, the FDA has approved other potential diagnostic tests, including a rapid antibody detection test, a home sample collection test, an oral fluid test, and a urine-based test. All of these tests still require a second confirmatory test, and their appropriate use in clinical practice has yet to be determined. The rapid test may have some clinical utility such as in screening pregnant women presenting in labor and in management of occupational blood exposure. In these situations, a rapid test result can be available typically within 60 minutes and, if negative, can direct clinical decisions. Positive test results must still be confirmed with an appropriate confirmatory test. Other tests, such as viral load and HIV-1 p24 antigen, are not intended for diagnostic use and should not be routinely used. All screening should be accompanied by appropriate counseling and informed consent; people with positive test results should receive additional information, counseling, and follow-up as appropriate and should be informed of the need to notify sexual partners, people with whom intravenous needles have been shared, and others at risk of exposure. All seropositive cases also should be reported to local public health officials according to state guidelines.

13. Describe current recommendations for tuberculosis screening.

In contrast to the steady decline in incidence of tuberculosis (TB) from 1953 to 1984, over the 9 years from 1985 to 1992, there was a 20% increase. More than 28,000 more cases than expected were reported in 1985–1990 alone. Since 1992, there has been a substantial decline in reported TB cases among U.S.-born persons and a slight increase among foreign-born persons. Adverse social and economic factors, the HIV epidemic, and immigration of persons with TB infection are important risk factors. The goal of screening programs is to identify patients with recent TB infection and those with latent TB at risk for developing active disease. Routine testing of low-risk persons should be discouraged. Screening programs represent a critical component of TB control and should focus on high-risk populations, including:

1. Household members and close contacts of persons with known or suspected TB, including health care workers with significant exposures (contact investigation)

2. People with HIV infection

3. People with medical risk factors known to increase the risk of disease, including diabetes mellitus, conditions requiring prolonged high-dose corticosteroid therapy, gastrectomy, and chronic renal failure

4. Foreign-born people recently arrived (within 5 years) from countries with high TB prevalence, including migrant and seasonal farm workers

5. Medically underserved, low-income populations

6. High-risk racial or ethnic minority populations, as defined locally

7. Persons who inject illicit drugs or other locally defined high-risk substance users (e.g., crack cocaine users)

8. Residents and employees of congregate settings (e.g., long-term-care facilities, correctional institutions, mental institutions, nursing homes and facilities, and homeless shelters)

9. Health care workers who care for high-risk patients

10. Infants, children, and adolescents exposed to adults in high-risk categories

Flexibility is important in defining high-risk, high-priority groups for screening. The changing epidemiology of TB indicates that the risk for TB among groups currently identified as high risk may change over time, and groups currently not identified as high risk may become high-priority groups for screening in the future.

14. What are the screening methods used for TB?

The tuberculin skin test is the standard method for demonstrating TB infection. The most commonly used formulation of tuberculin is purified protein derivative (PPD); the usual dose is 5 tuberculin units (TU) (0.1 mm of PPD). The tuberculin should be administered intracutaneously (Mantoux test) and read at 48 and 72 hours after injection. The Mantoux test best detects infection and is the preferred test for screening. The tuberculin skin test is interpreted according to the amount of induration at the injection site. Persons are considered to have positive reactions with the Mantoux test in the following situations:

- **Induration ≥ 5 mm:** people with HIV infection, close contacts of infectious cases, people with fibrotic lesions on chest radiographs, and people on immunosuppressive therapy
- **Induration ≥ 10 mm:** all other persons with risk factors for TB (including recent immigrants and health care workers)
- **Induration ≥ 15 mm:** all other persons (i.e., low-risk persons for whom screening is not recommended)

The multiple puncture test and use of other PPD strengths are not accurate and should not be used for TB screening. People with positive skin reactions should be evaluated further to assess whether they have active disease. This evaluation usually includes clinical examination, chest radiograph, and sputum smear examination. Based on this evaluation, decisions are then made about the need for antimicrobial prophylaxis or treatment. In general, a positive screening test result indicates a person at high risk for developing active disease who should be offered treatment, regardless of age. All cases of active TB should be reported to the local public health officials according to state guidelines.

15. What about false-negative TB skin tests?

False-negative Mantoux TB skin tests may be caused by nonresponsiveness to delayed-type hypersensitivity-inducing antigens such as tuberculin; they are common in persons with impaired immunity (e.g., HIV-infected people). Delayed-type hypersensitivity responsiveness can be assessed with other antigens such as *Candida* species. However, the scientific basis for such testing is tenuous, and most skin-test antigens have no standardization. Anergy testing, therefore, is usually not part of screening for TB infection.

16. How should a TB skin test be interpreted in someone who has received bacille Calmette-Guérin (BCG) vaccination?

BCG is a live attenuated mycobacteria strain derived from mycobacterium bovis that is used in many parts of the world as vaccination against TB. Studies have shown that its efficacy in preventing serious TB disease in children is > 80%. The efficacy in adolescents and adults is unknown. Vaccination with BCG can cause a false-positive TB skin test. Tuberculin reactivity, however, wanes with time and in general an adult with a positive TB skin test result should be considered to have latent TB, regardless of BCG status.

17. Who should be screened for STDs?

DISEASE	POPULATIONS TO BE SCREENED
HIV	See question 12
Hepatitis B	Pregnant women at first prenatal visit; test may be repeated in the third trimester for high-risk women (injection drug use, exposure to hepatitis B)
	Currently no recommendation for or against routine screening of high-risk asymptomatic individuals
Syphilis	Prostitutes, people with multiple sexual partners in areas where syphilis is prevalent, people undergoing treatment for STDs, sexual contacts of persons with syphilis, pregnant women at first prenatal visit with additional testing at 28 weeks or later for women at increased risk for acquiring syphilis during pregnancy
	Depending on local prevalence rates, other high-risk populations also may benefit from screening, such as prison inmates
Gonorrhea	Prostitutes, people with multiple sexual partners, sexual contacts of people with gonorrhea, people with history of repeated episodes of gonorrhea, people undergoing treatment for other STDs, pregnant women at first prenatal visit with repeat testing later in pregnancy for women at increased risk
Chlamydia	People who attend clinics for STDs, people who attend other high-risk health care facilities (e.g., adolescent and family planning clinics) or have other risk factors (age < 25 years, multiple sexual partners, history of STDs, inconsistent use of condoms)
	Pregnant women with other risk factors should be screened at the first prenatal visit

To ensure adequate partner notification, all newly identified cases of STDs should be reported to local public health officials according to state guidelines.

18. Who should be screened for hepatitis C (HCV)?

Hepatitis C is the most common chronic bloodborne infection in the United States. An estimated 3.9 million Americans are infected with HCV and are at risk for complications from the infection and a potential source of transmission to others. The primary route of transmission is through percutaneous exposure to blood. Before July 1992, this was primarily from blood transfusion. Since July 1992, donated blood has been routinely tested, and now the primary route of exposure is through injection drug use. The highest prevalence of disease is in people aged 30–49 years. Routine testing is recommended for the following groups:

- Persons who ever injected illegal drugs
- Persons who received clotting factor concentrate before 1987
- Persons who were ever on chronic hemodialysis
- Persons with persistently abnormal alanine aminotransferase levels
- Persons who received blood from a donor later found to be HCV positive
- Persons who received blood or an organ transplant before July 1992
- Children born to HCV-positive mothers
- Health care workers with exposure to HCV-positive blood

It is likely that risk for HCV infection is increased among people with multiple sexual partners and people with a long-term partner who is HCV positive. However, data on the risk of sexual transmission of HCV are conflicting, and routine testing of these groups is neither recommended nor discouraged. Providers should be aware of this and discuss counseling and testing with people in these categories.

Only tests that detect anti-HCV are currently approved by the FDA for diagnosis of HCV infection.

19. Which tests should be used for screening for syphilis?

Tests used for screening for syphilis include both treponemal tests, which detect antibodies against *Treponema pallidum* or its components, and nontreponemal tests, which detect antibodies directed against lipoidal antigens. The main nontreponemal tests are the Venereal Disease Research Laboratory (VDRL) and rapid plasma reagin (RPR) tests. The main treponemal tests are the fluorescent treponemal antibody absorption test (FTA-ABS) and microhemagglutination test (e.g., MHA-TP). The VDRL and RPR tests usually become reactive during primary syphilis, remain at a peak in the first year of infection, and then fall slowly thereafter. After adequate treatment, the patient usually becomes seronegative after 12–24 months, depending on the duration of infection. A persistent high-titer RPR or VDRL can occur in HIV infection secondary to polyclonal antibody stimulation. The FTA-ABS and MHA-TP tests usually become reactive during primary syphilis and remain reactive for the patient's lifetime, regardless of treatment. For asymptomatic persons, screening is usually done with the VDRL or RPR tests with confirmation of positive test results by a treponemal test.

20. For which infectious diseases should pregnant women be screened?

Screening during pregnancy should take into account the particular risk profile of the patient. All pregnant women should be tested for syphilis and hepatitis B at the first prenatal visit. For those at high risk, these tests should be repeated in the third trimester. Screening for *Neisseria gonorrhoeae* should also be performed at the first prenatal visit for women at risk for infection and those in high-prevalence areas. Voluntary HIV testing after appropriate counseling is also recommended for all pregnant women. Screening for other STDs, such as chlamydial infection, should be undertaken if the woman has specific risk factors. Routine herpes simplex virus (HSV) cultures should not be routinely performed in the absence of lesions. In addition to STDs, pregnant women also should routinely be screened for rubella. If the woman is seronegative, the vaccine should be administered after delivery but before discharge from the hospital (such women should be counseled to avoid conception for 28 days after vaccination).

BIBLIOGRAPHY

General Information
1. Advisory Committee on Immunization Practices: General recommendations on immunization. MMWR 51(RR-2), 2002.
2. Advisory Committee on Immunization Practices: Recommendations childhood immunization schedule-United States, 2003. MMWR 54(4):1–4, 2003.
3. Advisory Committee on Immunization Practices: Update: Vaccine side effects, adverse reactions, contraindications, and precautions. MMWR 45(RR-12), 1996.
4. American College of Physicians Task Force on Adult Immunization and Infectious Diseases Society of America: Guide for Adult Immunizations, 3rd ed. Philadelphia, American College of Physicians, 1994.
5. Centers for Disease Control and Prevention: Assessing adult vaccination status at age 50 years. MMWR 44:561–563, 1995.
6. Centers for Disease Control and Prevention: Immunization of health care workers: Recommendations of the Advisory Committee of Immunization Practices and the Hospital Infection Control Practices Advisory Committee. MMWR 46(RR-18), 1997.
7. Chin J (ed): Control of Communicable Diseases Manual, 17th ed. Washington, DC, American Public Health Association, 2000.
8. Fedson DS, for the National Vaccine Advisory Committee: Adult immunization. Summary of the National Vaccine Advisory Committee Report. JAMA 272:1133–1137, 1994.
9. Gardner P, Eickhoff T, Poland GA, et al: Adult immunizations. Ann Intern Med 12(1 Pt 1):35–40, 1996.
10. Immunization Practices Advisory Committee: Update on adult immunization. MMWR 40(RR-12), 1991.
11. Pickering LK (ed): 2003 Red Book. Report of the Committee on Infectious Diseases, 26th ed. Elk Grove Village, IL, American Academy of Pediatrics, 2003.
12. U.S. Preventive Services Task Force: Guide to Clinical Preventive Services, 2nd ed. Baltimore, Williams & Wilkins, 1996.

Specific Topics
1. Advisory Council for the Elimination of Tuberculosis: Tuberculosis elimination revisited: Obstacles, opportunities, and a renewed commitment. MMWR 48(RR-9), 1999.
2. Advisory Committee on Immunization Practices: Poliomyelitis prevention in the United States. MMWR. 49(RR05);1–22, 2000.

3. Advisory Committee on Immunization Practices: Prevention and control of influenza. MMWR 50(RR-4), 2001.

4. Advisory Committee on Immunization Practices: Prevention of pneumococcal disease. MMWR 46(RR-8), 1997.

5. Advisory Committee of Immunization Practices: Prevention of hepatitis A through active or passive immunization. MMWR 48(RR-12), 1999.

6. Advisory Committee of Immunization Practices: Prevention of varicella: updated recommendations of the ACIP. MMWR 48(RR-6):1–5,1999.

7. Advisory Committee on Immunization Practices: Revised ACIP recommendation for avoiding pregnancy after receiving a rubella-containing vaccine. MMWR 50(49):1117, 2001.

8. Advisory Committee on Immunization Practices: Update: Recommendations to prevent hepatitis B virus transmission—United States. MMWR 48(02):33–34, 1999.

9. Barlow WE, Davis RL, Glasser JW, et al: The risk of seizures after receipt of whole-cell pertussis or measles, mumps and rubella vaccine. N Engl J Med 345:656–661, 2001.

10. Centers for Disease Control and Prevention: Preventing pneumococcal disease among infants and young children. MMWR 49(RR-9):1–38, 2000.

11. Centers for Disease Control and Prevention: Measles, mumps and rubella: Vaccine use and strategies for elimination of measles, mumps, rubella, and congenital rubella syndrome and control of mumps: Recommendations of the Advisory Committee on Immunization Practices (ACIP). MMWR 47(RR-8), 1998.

12. Centers for Disease Control and Prevention: Sexually transmitted disease guidelines—2002. MMWR 51(RR-6), 2002.

13. Centers for Disease Control and Prevention: Prevention and control of meningococcal disease. MMWR 49(RR-7), 2000.

14. Centers for Disease Control and Prevention: Progress toward elimination of *Haemophilus influenzae* type b invasive disease among infants and children—United States, 1998–2000. MMWR 51(11):234–237, 2002.

15. Centers for Disease Control and Prevention: Recommendations for prevention and control of hepatitis C virus (HCV) infection and HCV related chronic disease. MMWR 47(RR-19), 1998.

16. Centers for Disease Control and Prevention: Revised guidelines for HIV counseling, testing and referral and revised recommendations for HIV screening of pregnant women. MMWR 50(RR-19), 2001.

17. Centers for Disease Control and Prevention: Targeted tuberculin testing and treatment of latent tuberculosis infection. MMWR 49(RR06);1–54,2000.

18. Centers for Disease Control and Prevention: Update: Supply of diphtheria and tetanus toxoids and acellular pertussis vaccine. MMWR 50(51):1159, 2002.

19. Centers for Disease Control and Prevention: Vaccine Adverse Event Reporting System—United States. MMWR 39(41):730–733, 1990.

20. Centers for Disease Control and Prevention: Withdrawal of rotavirus vaccine recommendation. MMWR 48(43):1007, 1999.

21. Colditz GA, Brewer TF, Berkey CS, et al: Efficacy of BCG vaccine in the prevention of tuberculosis: Meta-analysis of the published literature. JAMA 271:698–702, 1994.

22. Feikin DR, Schuchat A, Kolczak M, et al: Mortality from invasive pneumococcal pneumonia in the era of antibiotic resistance, 1995–1997. Am J Public Health 90:223–229, 2000.

23. Gergen PJ, McQuillan GM, Kiely M, et al: A population-based serologic survey of immunity to tetanus in the United States. N Engl J Med 332:761–766, 1995.

24. Thompson WW, Shay DK, Weintraub E, et al: Mortality associated with influenza and respiratory syncytial virus in the United States. JAMA 289:179–186, 2003.

25. United States General Accounting Office: Childhood Vaccines: Ensuring an Adequate Supply Poses Continuing Challenge. Washington, DC, GAO, 2002, GAO publ. GAO-02-987. Available at: www.gao.gov.

5. CULTURAL AND ETHNIC DIVERSITY IN PRIMARY CARE

Irene Aguilar, M.D., and Jeanette Mladenovic, M.D.

1. Why is culturally competent health care important?
Cultural competence in the delivery of health care has been linked to increased access to care and reduced disparities in health outcomes.

2. What three domains of cultural competence should physicians consider in all doctor–patient relationships?
1. Values and attitudes of both the patient and the physician
2. The importance of communication styles (including linguistic competence)
3. The necessity for population-based clinical practice

3. What areas of beliefs should specifically be considered in patients who come from cultures that may differ from our own?

Dietary practices

Religious beliefs

Rituals of death and dying

Expectations and traditions surrounding childbirth

Expression and meaning of pain

Importance and use of folk medicine

4. What changes in the diversity of the United States population are anticipated by the year 2030?
It is anticipated that the minority populations in total will approach majority level. The large populations will be those of Hispanic origin, followed by black and Asian Americans. Thus, it is imperative that the medical community address differences in disease natural history, therapeutics, and outcomes to provide high-quality health care in the future.

5. Which diseases have historically been associated with a higher mortality rate in blacks than in whites?
Cardiovascular disease, cancer, chemical dependency, diabetes, infant mortality, violent deaths from homicide, and HIV all occur with a higher rate of death in the black population.

6. Which chronic illness disproportionately affects Hispanics?
Diabetes. The age-adjusted death rate is twice as high in Hispanics as in non-Hispanic whites. The excessive prevalence is believed to be related to multiple factors, including the high incidences of obesity, hyperinsulinemia, and family history.

7. What is the major health problem of Native Americans?
Alcohol abuse is the major cause of morbidity and mortality in the Native American community. Alcohol abuse contributes to death and illnesses from accidents, suicide, homicide, diabetes, congenital anomalies in infants, pneumonia, heart disease, and cancer. Alcoholism has been implicated in 50% of adult crime on Indian reservations. There is a high rate of unintentional injuries as well as chronic liver disease and cirrhosis-related deaths in Native Americans. The incidence of fetal alcohol syndrome is 4 per 1000 live births in Native Americans and Alaska Natives compared with 0.8 per 1000 live births in African Americans.

8. Why is it difficult to study health patterns or to complete clinical research in ethnic groups?
Although technically different, ethnicity and social classes are closely interrelated in the United States, making it difficult to interpret clinical research about health patterns of ethnic groups and

even about their diseases. This is further complicated by attitudes toward the health care system and trust in the medical enterprise, given the past history of experimentation in some groups (e.g., Tuskegee) before the strict guidance and enforcement of regulations that protect human subjects.

9. How may common physical findings can be recognized in individuals whose skin is not white?

Few signs cannot be recognized in a dark-skinned person with proper technique. Lighting (nonglare daylight), positioning (examination of the part of the body at heart level), environmental temperature, and the patient's emotional state contribute to an accurate examination in any patient. Color changes are best observed at sites where pigmentation from melanin, melanoid, and carotene is least: sclera, conjunctiva, nailbeds, lips, buccal mucosa, tongue, palms, and soles (unless heavily calloused). African Americans commonly have brown, freckle-like pigmentation of the gums, buccal cavity, border of the tongue, and even the nailbeds.

Jaundice is best seen in sclera. However, many darkly pigmented patients have heavy deposits of subconjunctival fat, which may mimic jaundice. Therefore, if inspection of the portion revealed naturally by the eyelid slit demonstrates icterus, the edges of the cornea and the posterior portion of the hard palate should be inspected.

Pallor is best diagnosed by the absence of underlying red tones; brown skin appears more yellowish brown, and black skin appears ashen gray. The conjunctiva are also an excellent site to assess pallor.

Petechiae are more easily seen on the abdomen, buttocks, and volar surface of the forearm. In dark brown skin, they may be more difficult to see except in the mucous membranes.

Cyanosis is the most difficult to diagnose. The mucous membranes show bluish discoloration. Applying light pressure to create pallor, observing for return of color, and following the examination serially over time are helpful approaches.

10. A 62-year-old Native American with constipation has seen a medicine man and was prescribed medicinal herbs, but his wife insisted that he see you. Should you change his treatment?

Recognition of the health beliefs and practices of local ethnic groups permits physicians to gain patient trust and to avoid creating a feeling of alienation. Every effort should be made to combine folk treatment with standard Western treatment as long as the two are not antagonistic and as long as the patient will come to no harm with the prescribed folk therapy. If the regimen is harmful, you may suggest that because this treatment has not seemed to work, something else may be tried.

11. A 28-year-old Mexican-American woman comes to see you for the sixth time in 3 months, complaining of restlessness, insomnia, anorexia, anergia, and anhedonia. After a comprehensive evaluation, you treat her for depression with little apparent improvement in symptoms. To which specialist should you refer her?

She should be referred to a traditional Mexican-American healer, a *curandero*. Curanderos believe in both natural and supernatural illness and often refer patients to traditional physicians if they feel that they are unable to diagnose and treat a natural illness. Curanderos deal with problems of a social, psychological, and spiritual nature as well as physical ailments.

The most likely diagnosis here is *susto*, which involves "soul loss" and is a folk illness believed to arise from fright. The soul is believed to have left the body to wander freely as a result of a dream or a particularly traumatic event. The symptoms of the disease, listed above, also may include hallucinations and various painful sensations. The curandero coaxes the soul back into the body, using prayer, *barridas* (sweeping over the body), and herb teas. Other common Mexican-American folk illnesses are listed below.

Empacho: an illness caused by a ball of food sticking to the wall of the stomach. Symptoms include stomachache, cramps, anorexia, diarrhea, and vomiting. Massaging the stomach, pinching the spine, and drinking a purgative tea are commonly prescribed by the curandero.

Mal ojo (evil eye): an illness to which all children are susceptible. It results from an admiring or covetous look from a person with a "strong" eye. Symptoms are vomiting, fever, crying, and restlessness. The evil eye may be prevented by wearing protective amulets or if the person with the strong eye touches the child while admiring him or her. The illness is treated by a curandero with a barrida and prayer.

Envidia (envy): cause of illness and bad luck. If success provokes the envy of friends and neighbors, misfortune may befall the person and his or her family.

12. An elderly Cambodian woman presents with diarrhea. On physical examination, you notice cigarette burns on her abdomen. She is not a smoker. Should you report her family to adult protective services?

No. Cigarette burns are a traditional method of folk healing in Asian populations. Moxibustion and dermabrasive practices are among the Chinese folk remedies widely practiced among Vietnamese, Khmer, Hmong, and Mien peoples. The dermal methods are seen as ways to relieve headaches, muscle pains, sinusitis, colds, sore throat, coughs, difficulty with breathing, diarrhea, and fever. A cigarette or piece of burning cotton may be touched to the skin, usually the abdomen, to compensate for "heat" lost through diarrhea. Cupping involves placing a heated cup on the skin; as it cools, it contracts and draws the skin and excessive energy ("wind") or toxicity into the cup. This procedure leaves circular ecchymoses on the skin. Pinching produces bruises or welts at the site of treatment. Rubbing of skin with a spoon or coin is done to bring the toxic "wind" to the body surface and also produces bruises or welts. Other traditional practices used by Asians include acupuncture, massage, and herbal concoctions and poultices, which rarely present a threat to the person and often nurture a sense of being cared for and the ability to alleviate bothersome symptoms.

Such remedies relate to Chinese theories of health as a state of balance among the different components of the body and of the body with its environment. Therapeutic diets require considerations of the "hot" or "cold" natures of foods, cooking methods, and the person's ailment. The various parts of the human body correspond to the dualistic principles of "yin" and "yang" and must be kept in harmony.

13. A 24-year-old Laotian woman presents for a physical examination before getting pregnant. How does her ethnic background influence your search for possible disease or prevention considerations?

Knowledge of an ethnic group's genetic disorders and disease prevalence strongly influences evaluation. The following six potential diagnoses should be considered in light of her desire to become pregnant:

1. **Hemoglobinopathies.** Microcytosis in people of Southeast Asian origin is most commonly related to alpha- and beta-thalassemia and hemoglobin-E carrier states. A study of Southeast Asians in California found that 8% from Vietnam and 3% from Cambodia and Laos have the beta-thalassemia trait; 36% of refugees from Cambodia and 28% of refugees from Laos were carriers of the hemoglobin-E trait. Correct diagnosis is necessary to provide genetic counseling and to avoid inappropriate treatment of carriers with iron (risking iron overload) for microcytic anemia.

2. **G6PD deficiency**

3. **Lactose intolerance**

4. **Hepatitis B carrier state.** The carrier state for hepatitis B was as high as 8.6% in one study of Southeast Asians.

5. **Parasitic infection.** As many as 35% of Southeast Asian refugees have positive stool result for parasites.

6. **Tuberculosis.** The incidence of positive purified protein derivative ($> 50\%$) is very common, with age-specific incidence of tuberculosis several times higher. Additionally, drug resistance is common.

BIBLIOGRAPHY

1. Ayanian JZ: Heart disease in black and white. N Engl J Med 329:656–658, 1993.
2. Becker LB, Han BH, Meyer PM, et al: Racial differences in the incidence of cardiac arrest and subsequent survival. N Engl J Med 329:600–606, 1993.
3. Betancourt J, Carrillo JE, Green A: Hypertension in multicultural and minority populations: Linking communication to compliance. Curr Hypertens Rep 1:482–499, 1999.
4. Buchwald D, Carolis PV, Gany F, et al: Five vignettes of cross-cultural care. Pat Care 28:120–123, 1994.
5. Burkett G: Culture, illness, and the biopsychosocial model. Fam Med 23:287–291, 1991.
6. Chesney AP, Thompson BL, Guevara A, et al: Mexican American folk medicine: Implications for the family physician. J Fam Prac 11:567–574, 1980.
7. Ford E, Cooper RS: Racial/ethnic differences in health care utilization of cardiovascular procedures: A review of the evidence. Health Serv Res 30:237–250, 1995.
8. Galanti G: Caring for Patients from Different Cultures, 2nd ed. Philadelphia, University of Pennsylvania Press, 1997.
9. Gamble VN: Under the shadow of Tuskegee: African Americans and health care. Am J Public Health 87:1773–1778, 1997.
10. Harwood A (ed): Ethnicity and Medical Care. Cambridge, Harvard University Press, 1981.
11. Helman C: Culture, Health and Illness, 3rd ed. Oxford: Butterworth Heinemann, 1994.
12. Henderson G, Primeaux M (eds): Transcultural Health Care. Menlo Park, NJ, Addison-Wesley, 1981.
13. Lamarine R: The dilemma of Native American health. Health Educ 20:15–18, 1989.
14. Like R, Steiner P: Medical anthropology and the family physician. Fam Med 18:87–92, 1986.
15. Lin-Fu JS: Population characteristics and health care needs of Asian Pacific Americans. Publ Health Rep 103:18–27, 1988.
16. Muecke MA: Caring for Southeast Asian refugee patients in the USA. Am J Publ Health 73:431–438, 1983.
17. Nickens HW: The role of race/ethnicity and social class in minority health status. Health Serv Res 30:151–162, 1995.
18. Roach LB: Color changes in dark skin. In Henderson G, Primeaux M (eds): Transcultural Health Care. Menlo Park, NJ, Addison-Wesley, 1981.
19. Spector RE: Cultural Diversity in Health and Illness. Stamford, CT, Appleton & Lange, 1996.
20. Thomson GE: Discrimination in health care. Ann Intern Med 126:910–912, 1997.
21. Whittle J, Conigliaro J, Good CB, Joswiak M: Do patient preferences contribute to racial differences in cardiovascular procedure use? J Gen Intern Med 12:267–273, 1997.
22. Whittle J, Conigliaro J, Good CB, Lofgren RP: Racial differences in the use of invasive procedures in the Department of Veterans Affairs Medical System. N Engl J Med 329:656–658, 1993.

6. COMPLEMENTARY, ALTERNATIVE, AND INTEGRATIVE MEDICINE

Lisa W. Corbin, M.D.

1. What is alternative medicine? How does alternative medicine relate to complementary medicine and integrative medicine?

Alternative medicine is a broad term that includes any treatment used for healing that is not widely taught in U.S. medical schools or widely available in U.S. hospitals. Examples include acupuncture, chiropractic, and herbal medicine. The term *alternative* implies that people are using these therapies *in place of* conventional care, but studies have shown (see below) that most people who are using these treatments also use conventional care. Thus, the term *complementary medicine* arose, reflecting the true way that these additional practices are used by patients. The acronym CAM stands for *c*omplementary and *a*lternative *m*edicine and has been adopted by the National Institutes of Health (NIH) and industry as an easier catch-all term for any of these treatments, no matter how they are used.

The specialty of integrative medicine arose from the realization of the numbers of patients who use CAM therapies in addition to conventional medicine and from the realization that some CAM treatments may benefit patients and others may interfere with conventional medications or treatments. In integrative medicine, CAM and conventional therapies are explored, and care is *co-ordinated* by professionals to maximize benefits and minimize risks.

2. How many patients use alternative medicine?

A study in the *New England Journal of Medicine* found that 42% of adults in the United States use CAM (as defined above). In 1997, there were 629 million visits to CAM providers in the United States, which is more than the number of visits to primary care physicians over the same period. Fewer than 40% of people who used CAM told their conventional physicians.

3. What are the typical demographics of an CAM user?

The typical CAM user is white, aged 25–49 years, college educated, and from a higher socioeconomic status. Most CAM users also see conventional practitioners for the same problems. People with chronic health problems (e.g., cancer, arthritis, and AIDS) are also more likely to try CAM.

4. Why do people use CAM?

Patients perceive CAM to be a healthier alternative to conventional medicine, often because of reports in the lay press of toxicities of conventional treatments and the lack of such reporting on alternative treatments. Many people mistakenly believe that just because a therapy is natural, it is safe. In addition, patients often turn to CAM as a way to regain a sense of control over their own health care; they choose the treatment instead of their physician. When conventional options seem to have run out, patients with chronic health problems may turn to CAM as a last-ditch effort.

5. What are the most popular CAM treatments?

The *New England Journal of Medicine* study found relaxation techniques, chiropractic therapy, and massage therapy to be the most frequently used. Other studies have found the use of other treatments to be much higher. The differences are probably because of how the questions were phrased and how treatments were defined. For example, one study found that 95% of patients in a Kaiser system were using herbal medicine.

6. Why should primary care physicians ask all patients about their use of CAM?

Primary care providers need to know all of the treatments their patients are using because they may affect conventional treatments. A treatment may cause direct drug–drug or drug–treatment interactions, or the CAM treatment itself may be the cause of the condition. In addition, a patient who is using CAM may have misconceptions about the utility of conventional treatment; for example, the patient may be using CAM because she or he believes that no conventional treatment exists for a certain condition or that the conventional treatment is unsafe. By asking all patients about CAM use, misconceptions about conventional treatments may be discussed and open patient–physician relationships can be fostered.

7. In evaluating any treatment, alternative or conventional, what three questions should the physician try to answer before recommending for or against the treatment?

1. What is the safety of the treatment (what are the risks)?
2. What is the efficacy of the treatment (what are the benefits)?
3. Is the treatment cost effective?

8. What is meant by *primum non nocere*? How does it relate to CAM?

Primum non nocere means "first, do no harm" in Latin. Even if you do not have time or interest in learning more about CAM treatments, at the very least familiarize yourself with the types of therapies that have high potential for harm.

9. Which common CAM treatments, when practiced by trained practitioners, are generally accepted to be safe?

The treatments listed below have few risks. However, the use of any CAM treatment can be harmful to the patient's health when it is used in place of a known, effective conventional treatment. The most obvious examples are alternative treatments for a cancer that can be cured by resection or when a patient forgoes insulin therapy in favor of an alternative treatment for type I diabetes.

- **Chiropractic therapy:** Despite concern about damage to the spinal cord or nerve roots with chiropractic therapy, such damage is exceedingly rare, especially with manipulation of the lower back. There have been uncommon reports of stroke after chiropractic manipulation of the neck.
- **Acupuncture:** Risk of infection is basically negated by the use of disposable, sterile needles. Risk of pneumothorax is real but estimated at fewer than 1 in 250,000 patients. Patients are expected to feel relaxed after acupuncture treatment; for some patients, this feeling may be quite profound.
- **Therapeutic massage:** This is generally safe. Well-trained massage therapists will make modifications in technique for patients with certain chronic illnesses (e.g., congestive heart failure, cancer, osteoporosis) to avoid fluid shifts or fractures. Modification is also used for patients taking blood thinners or with bleeding disorders to avoid bruising. Massage therapy is relatively contraindicated in patients with soft tissue infection because of the theoretic risk of spreading infection.
- **Homeopathy**
- **Mind–body therapies** (e.g., biofeedback, yoga, relaxation techniques, tai chi): Mind–body therapies are safe but may precipitate a psychological crisis in a patient with an unstable or untreated mental illness.
- **Aromatherapy**
- **Reflexology**

10. Which CAM treatments have been shown to be beneficial?

Few CAM treatments have been extensively studied in scientific fashion because funding for such studies is difficult to obtain, the nature of the treatments makes blinded studies difficult, and CAM practitioners often do not have a background in the scientific method. In addition, there are currently *no requirements* for proof of the safety and efficacy of herbal medicines and other dietary supplements before marketing (in contrast to conventional medications, which must go through rigorous testing and ongoing quality control). Thus, manufacturers do not feel the need to do studies. Despite these limitations, some good CAM studies have shown benefit for the following conditions:

- Chiropractic therapy for acute low back pain
- Acupuncture for pain, addiction, and nausea
- Relaxation techniques for insomnia and behavioral problems
- Biofeedback for mild hypertension and irritable bowel disease
- Certain herbs for certain illnesses (e.g., St. John's wort for mild depression and *Echinacea pallida* extract to shorten the duration of a cold)

This is not an exhaustive list of the benefits of CAM treatments. See the Bibliography for resources to find out more about CAM.

11. Why are herbs and supplements not routinely recommended?

The use of herbs and supplements should not be routinely recommended for patients because of the lack of quality control and standardization within the industry. The Dietary Supplement and Health Education Act of 1994 requires no proof of safety, efficacy, or quality control for this category of medications; thus, consumers cannot be sure of the following:

1. The actual content of the product (adulterants, such as antibiotics, steroids, tranquilizers, heavy metals, and nonsteroidal anti-inflammatory drugs [NSAIDs] are not illegal)

2. Whether the right part of the plant has been picked (harvesters are often not well trained, and toxic parts of the plant or the wrong plant entirely may have been used)

3. The right dosage of the supplement (without industry standardization, the amount of active ingredient varies up to 10,000-fold in various preparations of the same product; what may be safe or effective in one dosage may be frankly toxic in another)

In the future, it may be possible for conventional physicians to encourage the use of certain supplements for patients with certain conditions, if requirements are made for standardization and quality control and if information about proper dosing can be more easily obtained. Some organizations, such as the United States Pharmacopeia (USP) and Consumerlab.com, are compiling standardization information for certain products; manufacturers that meet these standards will be allowed to publicize this information.

12. Which CAM therapies have a risk of harm high enough to dissuade patients from their use?

- **Colonic enemas.** The volume of infused hypotonic solution may cause massive fluid and electrolyte imbalances, bowel perforation, and gut flaccidity. There also have been outbreaks of gastrointestinal illness (e.g., giardiasis) from equipment that was not properly sterilized between uses.
- **Certain herbal medicines** (see question 11). In the future, we may be able to recommend certain agents with confidence because some supplements do appear safe and effective.
- **Chelation therapy**
- Intensive, **restrictive diet** therapy or megavitamin therapy (the patient may become malnourished or toxic)
- **Certain Chinese patent medicines** (herbs may be adulterated with steroids or heavy metals)

13. What is the placebo response?

When any treatment is studied against a placebo, a reproducible, measurable 20–30% placebo response rate is found. In other words, patients who receive a placebo instead of the active treatment show an improvement about 30% of the time. They also have side effects. Thus, in evaluating the efficacy (or side effect profile) of any given treatment, it is important to know how it compares with placebo. No one knows why the placebo effect exists, but it seems to support the idea of a mind–body connection. In other words, if a patient (or physician) perceives that a treatment will work, it is more likely to have an effect, perhaps related to release of endorphins and other chemicals. This also underscores the importance of a good doctor–patient relationship as the foundation of any medical treatment and may explain why some alternative treatments appear to work.

14. How much money is spent on CAM? How do CAM users pay for their treatments?

In 1997, $21.2 billion was spent in the United States on CAM. This amount is more than the costs of hospitalizations for a year in the United States. Most of the costs are paid directly out of pocket by consumers, but insurance plans are beginning to offer coverage for certain treatments. Also, coverage of certain CAM practices is mandated by law in some states.

15. How should a patient who inquires about the use of CAM be advised?

First, the patient should be cautioned about any treatments that are known to be unsafe. Next, the condition or symptom for which the patient is interested in trying CAM should be well defined by both the patient and clinician, and the risks and benefits of conventional options for diagnosis and treatment should be discussed. If the patient does not want to try these options or has already exhausted them, it may be advisable to encourage the use of CAM. Both the patient and the physician should research the particular method in which the patient is interested and try to find and interview reliable providers in the area (see below). The patient should define the symptom or problem for which he or she is seeking treatment and keep a symptom diary before, during, and after the treatment to allow a more objective assessment of response, including side effects. The primary physician should communicate with the provider of the treatment as with any referral to ensure the best continuity of care.

Many providers of alternative treatments are required to be licensed in certain states. Your state's local organizations or national organizations can be contacted for this information. The provider should be asked about his or her experience with the problem in question and what sort of outcomes can be expected. The patient also should ask the provider how many visits the treatment will take, how much it will cost, and how soon the patient should expect a response. Potential side effects should be explored. All conversations with the patient and any other providers should be documented in the chart as with any patient encounter.

16. Does the primary care physician need to worry about being sued for referring a patient to an alternative provider?

According to Eisenberg: "Although physicians have been prosecuted for malpractice when they have personally delivered alternative treatments, no cases have involved conventionally trained physicians who have advised patients about alternative medical therapies."

BIBLIOGRAPHY

1. Bratman S, Kroll D: The Natural Health Bible. Roseville, CA, Prima Publishing, 1999.
2. Eisenberg DM: Advising patients who seek alternative medical therapies. Ann Intern Med 127:61–69, 1997.
3. Eisenberg DM, Davis RB, Ettner SL, et al: Trends in alternative medicine use in the United States, 1990–1997: Results of a follow-up national survey. JAMA 280:1569–1575, 1998.
4. Ernst E, White A: Acupuncture: A Scientific Appraisal. Oxford, Butterworth-Heinemann, 1999.
5. Gevitz N: Three perspectives on unorthodox medicine. In Gevitz N (ed): Other Healers: Unorthodox Medicine in America. Baltimore, Johns Hopkins University Press, 1988.
6. Meeker WC, Haldeman S: Chiropractic: A profession at the crossroads of mainstream and alternative medicine. Ann Intern Med 136:216–227, 2002.
7. National Center for Complementary and Alternative Medicine: http://nccam.nih.gov.
8. NIH Consensus Conference: Acupuncture. JAMA 280:1518–1524, 1998.
9. Winslow LC, Kroll DJ: Herbs as medicines. Arch Intern Med 158:2192–2199, 1998.

7. PHYSICAL EXAMINATION CORRELATES

Mohammad R. Al-Ajam, M.D., and Abdel-Rahman El-Bash, M.D.

1. How is blood pressure (BP) correctly measured by the cuff inflation method?

Direct measurement of BP with an intra-arterial transducer is the gold standard, but it is not practical. The sphygmomanometer cuff inflation technique is an indirect measure that is more indicative of flow than of pressure and is generally less accurate and less reproducible. Nonetheless, it is more practical and correlates acceptably with intra-arterial measurement of BP when proper technique is followed.

The relaxed patient should be seated in a quite environment, with an appropriately sized cuff and inflatable bladder wrapped around the bare arm 2 cm above the antecubital fossa. The inflatable bladder within the cuff needs to have a width equal to 40% of the length of the arm and a length equal to 80% of the arm's circumference. If the cuff is too large, it underestimates BP. Conversely, if the cuff is too small, it overestimates BP. The midarm should be aligned with the heart. During inflation, palpation of the radial pulse helps to estimate the systolic pressure and to detect an auscultatory gap or an Osler's phenomenon (see question 3). The bell of the stethoscope is then placed in complete contact with the antecubital skin over the brachial pulse, and the cuff is deflated at 2 mmHg/sec.

The appearance of the first sound corresponds to the systolic BP. In nonpregnant adults, the disappearance of the sounds, not their muffling, correlates with diastolic BP. In children younger than 13 years, pregnant women, and patients with high cardiac output or peripheral vasodilation, intraarterial blood flow is turbulent and the Korotkoff sounds are heard well into low ranges of 0–10 mmHg. In these conditions diastolic pressure corresponds to the muffling of the Korotkoff sounds.

Initial screening should be performed in both arms and occasionally legs. The highest of these readings is recorded as the BP. For serial monitoring of hypertensive patients, measurements in the same arm should be taken. If repeat readings are necessary, they should be at least 30 seconds apart to allow for resolution of the arterial vasospasm that may result from the first reading.

2. What is the importance of an auscultatory gap?

The intermittent disappearance of Korotkoff sounds within < 10 mmHg around systolic and diastolic BP readings is a normal finding. A phasic decrease in systolic BP occurs because of decreased venous return to the left heart during inspiration. A similar change occurs around the diastolic BP with expiration.

A definite but as yet unexplained auscultatory gap occurs in the midst of BP cuff deflation (phase II) in up to 21% of hypertensive patients. This finding is more common in older individuals and women (male:female ratio is 44%:67%) but has no relation to duration of hypertension, prior antihypertensive therapy, or the presence of isolated systolic hypertension. The cuff needs to be inflated beyond this gap. If it is insufficiently inflated to a pressure within this gap, then upon deflation, the point at which the Korotkoff sounds resume will be falsely interpreted as the systolic BP, hence significantly underestimating it. Conversely, if the cuff is only deflated to the onset of this gap, the onset of the gap may be mistakenly interpreted as the diastolic BP, hence overestimating it. This auscultatory gap correlates with a twofold increase in incidence of carotid artery atherosclerosis, increased arterial wall stiffness, and increased pulse velocity. It bears no relation to cardiac ventricular mass or dimension, or to cardiac index. It correlates significantly, however, with increased total peripheral arterial resistance.

3. What is Osler's maneuver?

In the normal population, arteries distal to the sphygmomanometer cuff collapse and become nonpalpable as the pulse is no longer felt during cuff inflation. In 1892, Sir William Osler described an interesting phenomenon. While measuring BP by the cuff inflation method in a subgroup of his patients, he noted that the brachial, radial, and ulnar arteries distal to the sphygmomanometer cuff remain palpable and uncollapsed despite becoming pulseless. This phenomenon is attributed to calcification and hardening of the vessels (arteriosclerosis).

In 1985, Maserelli evaluated Osler's maneuver by comparing BP measurement obtained through intraarterial transducers with those concomitantly obtained by traditional cuff sphygmomanometer. Sphygmomanometer readings were 10–54 mmHg higher than intraarterial devices for both systolic and diastolic BP in patients with palpable yet pulseless arteries (positive Osler sign). The pulse pressure, however, stays the same. In brief, the formula is:

Pulseless + nonpalpable distal artery = "Osler negative" = correct BP reading

Pulseless + palpable distal artery = "Osler positive" = falsely elevated BP reading or pseudohypertension

The potential consequence of this phenomenon is overdiagnosing and overtreating high BP.

4. If you detect a difference in BP between the two arms in a patient with chest pain, what should you do?

If a hypertensive patient presents with acute onset of chest pain, acute thoracic aortic dissection needs to be considered. Compare the pulse in all major arteries, including the carotids, femorals, and radials, to check for asymmetry. In addition, assessing BP on the left versus right arm is required. Although a 20-mmHg systolic BP difference between the arms was found in 19% of patients without thoracic aortic dissection in one cross-sectional study, this physical finding was an independent predictor of aortic dissection in another prospective observational study. The pooled sensitivity of this sign is only 31%, but it has a specificity of around 94% and a positive likelihood ratio (LR+) of 5.7 (95% confidence interval [CI], 1.4–23). The presence of a neurologic deficit substantially increases the likelihood of aortic dissection (LR+ 6.6 and 33 in two studies). However, despite its high specificity, the sensitivity of a focal neurologic deficit was only 17%; hence, its absence does not rule out dissection.

The presence of a diastolic murmur was not reported to be helpful in detecting dissection with a pooled sensitivity of 28%, a specificity of 80%, and an LR+ of 1.4 (95% CI, 1.0–2.0). These numbers are subject to potential biases, including small sample size.

Surprisingly, acute elevation in BP during the pain episode was not helpful in detecting dissection, with a pooled sensitivity of 49%.

5. What are the clinical signs of temporal arteritis (TA) that most likely lead to a diagnosis by biopsy?

Temporal arteritis is predominantly a disease of older individuals. In fact, 99% of people with a positive biopsy for TA are aged 50 years or older. As of the year 2000, 12.4% of the U.S. population was aged 65 years or older. In this aging society, awareness of TA needs to be heightened. Incidence of TA has been reported in people older than 50 years as 24.2 per 100,000 for women and 8.2 for men in one study. This rises with increasing age to a prevalence of 2 per 1000 at 80 years of age.

Certain physical signs have been shown to be predictive of a positive biopsy. Beaded temporal artery had an LR+ of 4.6 (95% CI, 1.1–18.4), prominent or enlarged artery had an LR+ of 4.3 (95% CI, 2.1–8.9), and a tender temporal artery had an LR+ of 2.6 (95% CI, 1.9–3.7). The absence of a temporal artery pulse had an LR+ of 2.7, but it did not achieve statistical significance (95% CI, 0.55–13.4), possibly because of the small population studied.

Physicians may yet be unable to lay a hand on the head of the blind and cure them, but when they lay a hand on the temple of an elderly patient with a headache and fever, they may prevent blindness, the most dreaded complication of TA.

6. What physical findings help in diagnosing streptococcal throat infections?

Generous use of antibiotics for treating all sore throats has lead to resistant organisms. There is no single physical finding that can accurately establish the diagnosis of streptococcal throat infection. The constellation of tonsillar exudate, anterior cervical adenopathy, fever, and the absence of cough has an LR+ of 6.3. Alternatively, clinicians need to perform the rapid streptococcal antigen test (e.g., ACON Labs) or obtain cultures for accurate diagnosis.

7. Is transillumination of the sinuses helpful in diagnosing sinusitis?

Proper transillumination of the sinuses requires a dark room. The frontal sinuses are examined with a light source placed in contact with the skin over the medial ipsilateral supraorbital ridge and pointing it upward. The examiner looks for transmission of light over the frontal sinuses. The maxillary sinus is examined by placing a light source over the ipsilateral inferior orbital ridge and pointing it downward. The patient is asked to open the mouth, and the examiner looks for transmission of light over the hard palate. No transmission of light is caused by fluid-filled sinuses or thickened mucosa suggestive of sinusitis.

In one study, abnormal transillumination alone had a sensitivity of 73%, a specificity of 54%, and an LR+ of 1.6 in detecting sinusitis. Hence, it was not helpful. Nevertheless, a combination of abnormal transillumination, sinus tenderness, nasal speech, history of mucopurulent secretion, colored nasal discharge, and poor response to decongestants had an LR+ of 4.7 (95% CI, 2.8–7.9). One might conclude that transillumination alone yields little benefit but is a useful adjunct in diagnosing sinusitis.

8. Does jugular venous pressure (JVP) correlate well with central venous pressure (CVP)?

To measure JVP properly, the patient's torso should be placed 30–45° above the horizontal plane. The vertical distance from the sternal angle of Louis to the highest point of internal jugular venous pulsation during inspiration is measured. An estimate of the CVP is obtained by adding 5 cm to the JVP because the right atrium is roughly 5 cm below the sternal angle regardless of the patient's position.

When JVP is used as an estimate of CVP across the whole range of low, normal, or high CVP, physicians' estimates are correct approximately half the time, no better than flipping a coin. One meta-analysis study, however, found that in the setting of an elevated CVP, clinical estimates using JVP are correct in around 80% of the cases LR+ 4.1 (95% CI, 1.3–13.1).

9. How do you differentiate a left-sided from a right-sided systolic heart murmurs?

Systole begins with S_1, the first heart sound (the closure of the mitral and tricuspid valves, and ends with S_2, the second heart sound (the closure of the aortic and pulmonary valves). Palpating the carotid artery gently during cardiac auscultation helps to determine whether a murmur is systolic or diastolic. S_1 is synchronous with the carotid pulsation, whereas S_2 follows the pulse. The neck should be felt while listening to the heart.

In one study, an increase of murmur intensity during inspiration was 100% sensitive and 88% specific for detecting right-sided systolic heart murmurs. All the patients had known valvular abnormalities, and all the evaluators were cardiologists, which may limit the generalization of these findings.

10. Which characteristics affect the likelihood that a diastolic murmur is caused by aortic regurgitation (AR)?

The typical murmur of AR is an early diastolic, decrescendo, blowing murmur, best heard over the third or fourth intercostal space at the left sternal border. This murmur is classically thought to be accentuated when the patient sits in the upright position and leans forward. The second heart sound, S_2, may be obscured on occasions. A pulmonic regurgitation (PR) murmur is best heard over the second left intercostal space but is louder during inspiration. It is an early diastolic decrescendo murmur as well, but it tends to have a lower pitch. The pitch may be louder if pulmonary hypertension is associated. The astute observer may notice it occurring after the pulmonic component P_2 of S_2. An Austin Flint murmur, a late diastolic murmur, is sometimes associated with AR and is caused by the regurgitant blood jet colliding with the left ventricular endocardium

In multiple studies, the presence of an early diastolic murmur was the most useful finding for diagnosing a greater than mild AR. The LR+ ranged between 8.8 and 32.0. The absence of such a murmur was most useful in ruling out severe AR. The negative likelihood ratio (LR−) range was 0.2–0.3. Most hemodynamic signs and maneuvers such as the Corrigan water hammer pulse, Duroziez's femoral murmur, the Musset head bobbing, the brachial-popliteal pulse gradient, and the wide pulse pressure have not been subjected to the rigor of evidence-based investigation. Only arterial occlusion with multiple tourniquets applied to the limbs to increase the intensity of an AR murmur by increasing afterload was studied. Increased intensity of the murmur on this maneuver increased the likelihood of an AR by more than eight fold; LR+ 8.4 (95% CI, 1.3–81). The authors nonetheless feel that it is too cumbersome a technique for general use.

11. What characteristics make a systolic murmur likely caused by aortic stenosis (AS) versus hypertrophic cardiomyopathy (HCM)?

The murmur of AS is a crescendo–decrescendo murmur best heard over the second right intercostal space. A concomitant decreased or absent S_2 increases the likelihood of AS (LR+ 3.1 and 50; two studies). Similarly, a peak murmur intensity in midsystole (LR+ 8.0; 95% CI, 2.7–23) or late systole (LR+ 101; 95% CI, 25–410), as distinct from early in systole, increased the likelihood of AS. A slow rate of increase of carotid pulse (LR+ 2.8–130; three studies) and an apical carotid delay (LR+ > 2.4) also increase the likelihood of AS. Lack of radiation to the right carotid decreases the likelihood of AS (negative likelihood ratio LR− 0.05 and 0.1 in two studies).

Passive leg elevation to a 45° angle increases systemic afterload and decreases an HCM murmur because of increased resistance to left ventricular outflow. In one meta-analysis, a decrease in systolic murmur intensity 20–30 seconds after leg elevation had an LR+ 8.0 (95% CI, 3.0–21) in predicting HCM. Its absence had an LR− of 0.22 (95% CI, 0.06–0.77). Squatting while breathing normally to avoid a Valsalva maneuver has a similar hemodynamic effect. A decrease in murmur intensity after this maneuver had an LR+ of 4.5 (95% CI, 2.3–8.6) for HCM. Its absence had an LR− of 0.13 (95% CI, 0.02–0.81).

12. Which physical signs are useful in detecting obstructive airways disease?

Wheezing, on unforced expiration, is the most potent predictor of airflow obstruction with an LR+ of 36 and a specificity of 99.6%. By contrast, the absence of wheezing has limited utility in ruling out an airflow obstruction because the sensitivity of this sign is merely 15%. Severe airflow obstruction may present with diminished breath sounds and no wheezing whatsoever. Interobserver agreement (i.e., precision) is highest for wheezing among all signs of airflow obstruction (kappa 0.43–0.93).

Forced expiratory time is the time needed by a patient to exhale forcefully and fully through an open mouth. It is measured by listening with a stethoscope over the larynx of a patient. Measurements are best made using a stopwatch for better accuracy. Zero time is defined as the onset of expiration. When expiration exceeds 9 seconds, an LR+ of 4.8 for airway obstruction exists. The precision of this sign is good as well (kappa = 0.7).

The ability to extinguish a match placed 10 cm away from an open mouth in full forceful exhalation is another measure of airflow obstruction. If the patient cannot blow out the match, this sign is considered positive for airflow obstruction. It has a low but acceptable precision (kappa = 0.39) yet it had a sensitivity of 61%, specificity of 91%, and LR+ of 7.1.

Measurements of systolic BP usually differ between inspiration (the lower value) and expiration. If this difference exceeds 15 mmHg, the patient is said to have pulsus paradoxus. This sign has limited use in establishing airflow obstruction (LR+ 3.7; LR− 0.69). In addition, no data are available in the literature concerning interobserver agreement on pulsus paradoxus.

13. What is clubbing, how is it diagnosed, and does it have a role in detecting disease?

Hippocrates first described clubbing in a patient with empyema in the fifth century B.C. To this day, however, there is no universal agreement on what constitutes clubbing. Three signs (by diverse authors) taken alone or together to assess clubbing have been most studied so far:

- **Nail fold angle (NFA) of ≥ 180°:** Normally, the NFA, which is that angle at which the nail projects from the nail bed, is around 160° (see Figure, *A*).
- **Ratio of the distal phalangeal depth to the distal interphalangeal depth (PD/IPD) of > 1:** Normally this ratio is < 1 (see Figure, *B*).
- **Schamroth sign,** proposed in 1976, which refers to the obliteration of the diamond-shaped window normally observed when the dorsal surfaces of two nails are opposed.

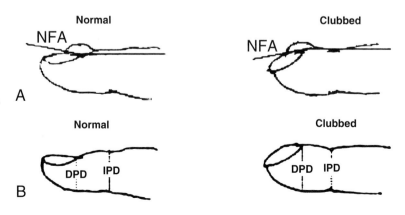

A, Nail fold angles. *B*, Phalangeal depth ratio.

The precision of clubbing, or interobserver agreement, varies depending on the experience of the physician. With fellows and residents, kappa values of 0.36 were obtained. When consultant pulmonologists were assessed, the kappa value was 0.9.

In one study by Baughman et al. involving patients with chronic obstructive pulmonary disease, the presence of clubbing (defined as DP/DIP ratio of > 1.0) indicated an increased likelihood of having bronchogenic carcinoma LR+ 3.9 (95% CI, 1.6–9.4).

14. What is the purpose of doing a clinical breast examination?

Clinical breast examinations must be done properly and thoroughly to have some value. The patient should be supine with the breast flat against the chest wall. Using the pads of the middle three fingers, the clinician should palpate a specific breast area with three small circular motions. The pressure and depth of palpation with each rotation should be gradually increased from superficial to intermediate to deep. After completion of three rotations, the hand is slid down, without lifting it up, to repeat the technique at an adjacent area. This continues until the entire breast is examined, including the axilla. Examining each breast should take a minimum of 3 minutes. Findings suggestive of breast cancer include, but are not limited to, a fixed, hard, or irregular mass. Any mass, however, requires further evaluation.

Clinical breast examination has a sensitivity of 54% and a specificity of 94% with an LR+ of 10.6 (95% CI, 5.8–19.2). Interestingly, clinical breast examination alone can detect from 3% to 45% of breast cancer missed by mammography. This does not apply, however, to self-breast examination, which differs in technique, sensitivity, and specificity. When clinical breast examination is performed with skilled hands and the proper technique, it can be highly specific for breast cancer. Alone, it is insufficient as a screening tool because of its low sensitivity.

15. What are Cullen's and Turner's signs?

A retroperitoneal or intraperitoneal hemorrhage may manifest itself by the appearance of a bluish-purple discoloration around the umbilicus (Cullen's sign) or in the flanks (Turner's sign). These bruise-like discolorations result from the catabolism of hemoglobin by the tissues. Cullen's sign was originally described in 1918 in a case of ruptured ectopic pregnancy. Turner's sign was described in 1920 in a case of acute pancreatitis. Although there are two names and the bluish-purple mark appears in two different places, they may be essentially considered as the same sign. Both signs have since been reported in many conditions that result in hemoperitoneum. Interestingly, the sensitivity of Cullen's for ruptured ectopic pregnancy, its original diagnostic utility, is 1%. Turner's sign has a 3% sensitivity for acute pancreatitis.

16. How useful is Murphy's sign in detecting acute cholecystitis?

The gallbladder fossa is located at the junction of the lateral border of the rectus muscle and the costal margin in the right upper abdominal quadrant just beneath the liver edge. While palpating that area, Murphy's sign may be elicited by asking the patient to inspire deeply, causing the gallbladder to descend toward the examining fingers. Patients with acute cholecystitis commonly experience increased discomfort and may halt their inspiratory effort, constituting a positive Murphy's sign. The utility of Murphy's sign was assessed in three studies. One population studied had a mean age of 38 years. Murphy's sign in that age group had a sensitivity of 62% and a specificity of 96%. The other two studies included populations with mean ages of 55 and 79 years. Sensitivity and specificity ranges were 44–48% and 62–79%, respectively. In the elderly, in whom cholecystitis is the most common cause of the surgical acute abdomen, a positive Murphy's sign may be useful, but a negative one must be treated with caution in this age group, given the low sensitivity.

17. Which physical findings help diagnose appendicitis?

Twenty-five percent of patients younger than age 60 years presenting to emergency departments for the evaluation of acute abdominal pain have appendicitis. The negative laparotomy rate in most series ranges from 15–35%. Computed tomography scanning had both a sensitivity and a specificity of 98% in one study. It will likely result in marked decrease in negative laparotomy rates in the future.

Helpful physical maneuvers include the psoas and obturator signs. The first is elicited by asking the patient to lie supine and flex the right hip against resistance applied by the examiner's hand just proximal to the knee. Alternatively, the patient may lie in the left lateral decubitus position and attempt to extend the right leg at the hip. If either of these maneuvers elicits pain in the right lower quadrant (RLQ), it is considered a positive psoas sign, which has a sensitivity of 16%, a specificity of 95%, and an LR+ of 2.38 (95% CI, 1.21–4.67). The obturator sign is elicited by internally rotating the right hip with the knee and hip flexed. The presence of RLQ pain with this maneuver constitutes a positive obturator sign, which has not been evaluated independently for evidence-based data. It is a common belief among clinicians, however, that it has a similar sensitivity and specificity to the psoas sign because both have the same mechanism of eliciting pain (i.e., irritation of the muscle by an inflamed appendix).

Another useful sign is RLQ rigidity (LR+ of 3.76; 95% CI, 2.96–4.78), but data on rebound tenderness (LR+ varied 1.1 to 6.3 in heterogeneous studies) and guarding (LR+ varied 1.6–1.8) were of limited utility. In meta-analyses, McBurney's point tenderness was not subjected to the rigor of evidence-based investigation.

18. What is the likelihood of detecting an abdominal aortic aneurysm (AAA) on physical examination?

In a study by Lederle et al., palpation of the abdomen was evaluated in high-risk patients. These were men aged 60–75 years with a history of hypertension or coronary artery disease. The finding of a definite or possible pulsatile mass had a sensitivity of 50%, specificity of 91%, and LR+ 4.4 in detecting an AAA > 5 cm in diameter. In thin patients whose abdominal girth was no more than 100 cm at the umbilicus, no AAAs were missed.

19. Does acanthosis nigricans correlate with insulin resistance and non-insulin-dependent diabetes mellitus (NIDDM)?

Acanthosis nigricans is a dark, rough patch of skin characterized histologically by hyperplasia of both the dermis and the epidermis, hyperkeratosis, and papillomatosis. It is found generally on skinfolds but most commonly on the back of the neck (99%), axilla (73%), antecubital fossa (47%), and inner thighs (35%). In nondiabetic patients, acanthosis nigricans correlates better with hyperinsulinemia than does obesity. This is consistent among all major U.S. ethnic groups: caucasians, Hispanics, African Americans, and native Americans. Adults with acanthosis nigricans report onset of skin changes at age 10–12 years. Beyond that, there is little progression. By age 40 years, prevalence of NIDDM among patients with acanthosis nigricans approaches 50%. African Americans with acanthosis nigricans have six times the prevalence of NIDDM compared with those without acanthosis nigricans. In caucasians, this ratio is tenfold.

20. Why should men endure digital rectal examinations (DREs)?

DRE is the least invasive and oldest method to screen for prostate cancer. Clinicians had routinely subjected men to this uncomfortable and sometimes embarrassing test. Is it worth the trouble?

A nonmalignant prostate is a smooth symmetrical structure with a uniform consistency, whether hypertrophied or not. A DRE that detects asymmetry, induration, irregularity, or nodularity points to cancer. In a meta-analysis of 22,000 patients, DRE was found to have a specificity of 97% (95% CI, 95–99%). Sensitivity for prostate cancer, however, was low at 4% (95% CI, 47–80%). Therefore, an abnormal finding on DRE is highly suggestive of cancer, but a normal finding has little clinical use.

Its high specificity, however, renders it a useful adjunct to prostate specific antigen (PSA) assay. Future refinements of the PSA assay may obviate the need to endure the uncomfortable finger.

21. What are Kernig's and Brudzinski's sign?

Vladimir Kernig first described the sign that bears his name in 1884. It is elicited by attempting to extend the knee when the hip is flexed at 90°. If the leg is halted by spasm of the hamstring muscles at a knee angle less than 135°, Kernig's sign is positive. In 1909, Joseph Brudzinski first described his "nape of the neck sign." A positive Brudzinski sign is present when the passive flexion of the neck in a supine patient results in reflexive flexion of the knees and hips.

One meta-analysis investigated signs of meningitis and found one small prospective study and nine retrospective ones. The presented data, however, are limited and do not permit definite conclusions. It is safe to conclude, however, that the presence of these signs in appropriate patients requires meningitis to be ruled out; the absence of these signs is not useful.

22. How do we test for anterior cruciate ligament (ACL) injury?

The lateral pivot shift test, the anterior drawer test, and the Lachman test (LT) are physical examination techniques used to assess injury to the ACL, one of the most common knee injuries.

Of these, only the LT has been proven by evidence-based methods to help in diagnosing ACL injuries. It is performed with the patient supine and the knee flexed at 20°. The examiner places his or her nondominant hand on the anterior distal femur just above the knee and the dominant hand on the posterior proximal tibia just below the popliteal fossa (see figure). The tibia is pulled anteriorly. The test is done on both knees. If the injured tibia is displaced more than the uninjured tibia, the test result is considered positive.

The LT has an LR+ of 25.0 (95% CI, 2.7–651.0) and is considered the most sensitive test for ACL injury. Severe pain sometimes precludes adequate completion of the test, necessitating appropriate analgesia.

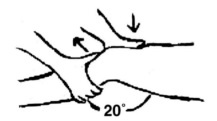

The Lachman test.

BIBLIOGRAPHY

1. Adedeji OA, McAdam WA: Murphy's sign, acute cholecystitis and elderly people. J R Coll Surg Edinb 41:88–89, 1996.
2. Barton MB, Harris R, Fletcher SW: Does this patient have breast cancer? JAMA 282:1270–1280, 1999.
3. Baughman RP, Gunther KL, Buchsbaum JA, Lower EE: Prevalence of digital clubbing in bronchogenic carcinoma by a new digital index. Clin Exp Rheumatol 16:21–26, 1998.
4. Cavallini MC, Roman MJ, Blank SG, et al: Association of the auscultatory gap with vascular disease in hypertensive patients. Ann Intern Med 124:877–883, 1996.
5. Choudhry NK, Itchells EE: Does this patient have aortic regurgitation? JAMA 281:2231–2238, 1999.
6. Ebell MH, Smith MA, Barry HC, Ives K: Does this patient have strep throat? JAMA 284:2912–2918, 2000.
7. Etchells E, Bell C, Robb K: Does this patient have an abnormal systolic murmur? JAMA 277:564–571, 1997.
8. Holleman DR, Simel DL: Does the clinical examination predict airflow limitation? JAMA 273:313–319, 1995.
9. Hoogendam A, Buntinx F, De Vet HCW: The diagnostic value of digital rectal examination in primary care screening for prostate cancer: A meta-analysis. Family Practice 16:621–626, 1999.
10. Klompas M: Does this patient have acute thoracic aortic dissection? JAMA 287:2262–2272, 2002.
11. Lederle FA, Walker JM, Reinke DB: Selective screening for abdominal aortic aneurysms with physical examination and ultrasound. Arch Intern Med 148:1753–1756, 1988.

12. Messerli FH, Ventura HO, Amodeo C: Osler's maneuver and pseudohypertension. N Engl J Med 312:1548–1551, 1985.
13. Myers KA, Farquhar DR: Does this patient have clubbing? JAMA 286:341–347, 2001
14. Smetana GW, Shmerling RH: Does this patient have temporal arteritis? JAMA 287:92–101, 2002.
15. Solomon DH, Simel DL, Bates DW, et al: Does this patient have a torn meniscus or ligament of the knee? JAMA 286:1610–1620, 2001.
16. Stuart CA, Gilkison CR, Smith MM, Bosma AM: Acanthosis nigricans as a risk factor for non-insulin dependent diabetes mellitus. Clin Pediatr 37:73–79, 1998.
17. Wagner JM, McKinney WP, Carpenter JL: Does this patient have appendicitis? JAMA 276:1589–1594, 1996.

II. Behavioral Medicine

8. DEPRESSION

Edmund Casper, M.D., and Allan Liebgott, M.D.

1. How frequently do primary care providers encounter patients with clinically relevant depression?

The prevalence of depressive disorders in primary care practice may be > 35% and even higher in patients with chronic medical illnesses. Among adolescents, the prevalence is approximately 20%. Thus, primary care providers must recognize the common symptoms of depression and feel confident in their ability to make the diagnoses. Most primary care physicians provide the treatment of depression and only refer to a psychiatrist in the event of suicidal behavior, which may require psychiatric consultation or hospitalization as part of the treatment plan.

2. Describe the spectrum of depression.

The diagnostic category of major depression varies from mild to severe with many cases of major depression being accompanied by onset of mania and frank psychoses. Major depression is usually an episodic illness, often beginning in adolescence, with remissions and exacerbations throughout life. A chronic form of less severe depression without acute major episodes is termed *dysthymia*. This is the patient who is mildly unhappy throughout his or her life.

3. What is the epidemiology of depression?

Depression has been diagnosed more in females than in males; however, this has been changing in recent years and as men age. People in relationships and commitments have a lower rate of depression. Major depressive episodes are frequently precipitated by stressful life events, such as a major loss from death or the failure of a relationship.

4. How can primary care providers recognize depression?

1. By recognition of classic symptoms: depressed mood accompanied by changes in sleep patterns, weight, or energy level and feelings of hopelessness, loss of self-worth, or disinterest in usual activities.

2. By the responses to screening questionnaires on routine physician visits. Routine questionnaires for new patients should include items related to depression or a standard depression screening test (such as the Center for Epidemiologics Studies Depression Scale).

3. By carefully pursuing concomitant depression in patients who abuse alcohol or drugs. Forty percent or more of substance abusers have concurrent mood disorders.

4. Patients who make frequent appointments with vague symptoms. More than 75% of patients who commit suicide have made a visit to a physician in the previous 4–6 months. Depressed individuals may present with physical symptoms that cannot be supported by a physical disorder. Common vague symptoms include dizziness, headache, palpitations, or other complaints that result in multiple physician visits.

5. What criteria lead to a diagnosis of a major depressive episode?

The diagnosis of depression have major symptoms and criteria that are fulfilled under the *Diagnostic and Statistical Manual of Mental Disorders,* 4th edition (DSM-IV), criteria. The criteria for classic depression require five or more of the following symptoms in a 2-week period:

- Thoughts of life being not worth living
- Extreme fatigue
- Poor concentration
- Depressed mood
- Significant alternation in weight, gained or lost
- Sleep disturbances
- Suicidal ideation or thoughts of death
- Feelings of guilt or worthlessness

The depression needs to be distinguished from grief reaction over the death of a loved one. Individuals with chronic mental illness also can develop a secondary disorder of severe depression.

6. Describe the manifestations of depression in the child or adolescent.

Children and adolescents have symptoms similar to adults' symptoms. Additional symptoms usually include irritability, agitation, difficulty in family relationships, truancy, and withdrawal from peer groups.

7. How does one distinguish between normal depressive reaction to loss of a loved one and a major depressive episode?

There is more support to accept grieving and grief reactions in the death of a loved one or a major change in life (e.g., divorce, loss of a relationship, death). The symptoms may appear to be the same initially: depressed mood, decreased interest, sleep disturbance, fatigue, and feelings of guilt and worthlessness. However, the person in a grief reaction will respond to interactions and outreach efforts by friends and family. A grief reaction could evolve into major depression, however, so this must be observed carefully by the treating physician.

8. Which medical diseases are associated with a high incidence of depression?

DISEASE	APPROXIMATE PREVALENCE (%)
Stroke	50
Chronic fatigue syndrome	50
Diabetes mellitus	30
Malignancies (especially of the pancreas or lung)	25
Myocardial infarction	25
Rheumatoid arthritis	20

Adapted from Katon W, Sullivan MD: Depression and chronic medical illness. J Clin Psychiatry 51(suppl 6):3–11, 1990.

9. Which drugs are particularly likely to induce depression?

Drugs that may frequently precipitate depression include alcohol, withdrawal from cocaine and amphetamines, steroids, isotretinoin, cimetidine, and narcotics, such as the opioid derivatives.

10. Which persons are at highest risk for suicide?

1. Any man older than age of 60 years who has a substance abuse problem, including alcoholism or other substance of abuse, with depressive symptoms

2. Divorced individuals

3. People with a combination of substance or prescription drug abuse and depression

4. People who are going through an acute loss or change in life are at risk for suicide

11. How does the patient's personal or family history aid in the diagnosis of depression?

Psychiatric illness, including depression, tends to run in families. If the person being evaluated has a relative who has suffered from depression, the examining physician should increase the suspicion for depression.

12. How should patients with major depression be treated?

The best treatment for patients with a major depressive episode is a combination of psychopharmacology and psychotherapy. Counseling or psychotherapy alone can be used to treat depression, and pharmacology antidepressants can be used alone to treat depression, but the combination of psychotherapy and antidepressants is superior to either one alone. Selective serotonin reuptake inhibitors (SSRIs) are the drugs of choice. However, if a person has responded to an antidepressant in the past, that antidepressant should be used first. Therapy should be continued for 9–12 months. If an individual has suffered two depressant episodes, consideration should be given for maintenance for an indefinite period of time or for life.

13. Does therapy for depression differ in patients with comorbid medical illness and other patients with major depression?

The therapy differs only in that the medical or underlining organic comorbid medical condition needs to be treated along with the depression. This is particularly an issue in individuals who suffer from alcoholism or other drug addiction. These patients may develop depression along with their addictive disorder and need to be treated for the depression concurrently with the substance abuse disorder.

14. What response is anticipated with treatment?

Two thirds of patients with depression respond to therapy with an antidepressant, psychotherapy, or the combination. Recurrences develop in one third of patients who have improved.

15. Describe the mortality and morbidity rates associated with major depression.

Fifteen to twenty percent of patients with recurrent major depressive disorders die of suicide, particularly those who have attempted suicide in the past. In medical patients, major depression causes greater disability than hypertension, diabetes, arthritis, and chronic lung disease. Patients with chronic depression function poorly and are increasingly disabled as they advance in age.

16. Which patients with major depression should be referred to a psychiatrist?

1. Patients who are acutely suicidal
2. Patients with accompanying psychosis
3. Patients who show no response to treatment after 4–6 weeks

17. What are the side effects of SSRIs?

The most common side effects of SSRIs are abdominal disturbance, agitation, insomnia, and sexual disorders. The side effects may be minimized by initiating therapy with lower doses. Although full therapeutic effectiveness may not reached for 2–4 weeks, many individuals with major depression respond within days of the initiation of therapy with SSRIs.

18. What is role of tricyclic antidepressant drugs (TCAs) in the treatment of depression today?

TCAs are reserved for treatment failures. TCAs have more side effects than SSRIs, and TCAs are more lethal than SSRIs if a patient tries to overdose with them. Some patients will not tolerate the side effects of tricyclics and will not take them. Amitriptyline (Elavil) is currently used more by neurologists. Other choices for individuals who do not respond to the SSRI include bupropion (Welbutrin), venlafaxine (Effexor), and other non-SSRIs, as well as mirtazapine (Remeron).

19. What is the advantage of newer second-generation agents such as the ones mentioned above, the SSRIs, and the combination adrenergic and serotonergic medications?
The greatest advantage is minimization of side effects and compliance with medication. The cost is higher, but the compliance is definitely improved with the newer generation of antidepressants.

BIBLIOGRAPHY

 1. Colorado Clinical Guidelines Collaborative: Major Depression Disorder in Adults: Diagnosis and Treatment Guidelines. Denver, Colorado Clinical Guidelines Collaborative, 2003. Available at www.coloradoguidelines. org.
 2. Frank E, Prien RF, Jarrett RB, et al: Conceptualization and rationale for consensus definitions of terms in major depressive disorder. Arch Gen Psychiatry 48:851, 1991.
 3. Jacobs D: The Harvard Medical School Guide to Suicide Assessment and Intervention. San Francisco, Jossey Bass, 1998, pp 417–435.
 4. Katon W, Sullivan MD: Depression and chronic medical illness. J Clin Psychiatry 51(suppl 6):3–11, 1990.
 5. McGreery JF, Franco K: Depression in the elderly: The role of the primary care physician in management. J Gen Intern Med 3:498–507, 1988.
 6. Michels R, Marzuk PM: Progress in psychiatry, part 1. N Engl J Med 329:552–560, 1993.
 7. Michels R, Marzuk RM: Progress in psychiatry, part 2. N Engl J Med 329:628–638, 1993.
 8. Reus V: Mental disorders. In Braunwald E, et al (eds): Harrison's Principles of Internal Medicine, 15th ed. New York, McGraw-Hill, 2001, pp 2542–2556.
 9. Stewart AI: Functional status and well-being of patients with chronic conditions. Results from the medical outcomes study. JAMA 262:907, 1989.
10. Thase M, Rush AJ, Howland RH, et al: Double-blind switch study of imipramine or sertraline treatment of antidepressant-resistant chronic depression. Arch Gen Psychiatry 59:233–239, 2002.

9. SLEEP DISORDERS

Lisa W. Corbin, M.D., and Eric T. McFarling, M.D.

1. Describe the stages of normal sleep.
By monitoring sleep in a laboratory using electroencephalography (EEG), electro-oculography (EOG), electromyography (EMG), and other recording methods, normal sleep patterns have been described. Sleep is divided into rapid eye movement (REM) sleep and non-REM sleep. REM sleep is characterized by eye movement bursts, a high-frequency EEG with low voltage, and atonia of skeletal muscles. In addition, REM is the stage of sleep during which most dreams occur.

Non-REM sleep is divided into four stages based on EEG patterns and accounts for the majority of time spent sleeping. Stages 1 and 2 (light sleep) are identified by a low-amplitude, high-frequency EEG tracing, and stages 3 and 4 (deep sleep) by a high-amplitude, slow (delta wave) pattern. Initial sleep is non-REM sleep.

A period consisting of stages 1 through 4 and REM sleep is a sleep cycle, and a night's sleep commonly consists of 3–5 cycles. As waketime nears, deep sleep is less prevalent, and a greater proportion of sleep is spent in REM.

2. How common are problems with sleep patterns in an otherwise healthy population?
Surveys show that approximately 1 in 3 people had problematic insomnia at some time during the past year. The prevalence is higher among women, elderly people, and people of high socioeconomic status. Approximately 1 in 20 adults complain of problems with excessive daytime sleepiness, which may include falling asleep at inappropriate times (e.g., during conversations, during work, or while driving).

3. Is insomnia a natural consequence of aging?
Older patients complain more about sleep difficulties than younger ones for a variety of reasons. The sleep–wake cycle changes with age and with less deep sleep, less REM sleep, and more nocturnal awakenings. The circadian rhythm advances so that older adults tend to get sleepier earlier in the evening and to wake up earlier in the morning. In addition, older people are more likely to have medical and psychiatric disorders that interfere with sleep. Patients tend to make up for less nocturnal sleep with daytime naps, preserving the overall amount of sleep time. Special attention to medical disorders and sleep hygiene (see question 7) and the use of sunlight or bright lights late in the afternoon may help elderly insomniacs.

4. What questions should be asked in taking a sleep history?
Primary care physicians often fail to ask patients about sleep problems, although these problems are common and often readily treatable. A sleep history results in diagnosis of the majority of sleep disorders. Useful adjuncts to the sleep history include talking to a sleep partner and having the patient keep a 1- or 2-week sleep log, including bedtime, arising time, naps, nighttime awakenings, and mood. The following specific questions supplement the medical and psychiatric history:
- Do you fall asleep during the day, or do others notice that you are excessively sleepy?
- Do you have problems getting enough sleep?
- When did the symptoms begin?
- What is your daily schedule, including work, meals, exercise, and naps?
- What is your bedtime routine?
- What medications are you taking?
- Do you know if you have any unusual movements, abnormalities in breathing, or snoring during sleep?
- What treatments have you tried in the past? Which were effective?

5. How does the time course of insomnia help with classification?
Insomnia is classified as **recent onset** (i.e., < 3 weeks ago) or **chronic.** Insomnia of recent onset is usually transient and may develop in patients with previously normal sleep that is altered because of a stressful life change. Examples are hospitalization, bereavement, academic examinations, and disturbance of circadian rhythms caused by air travel across time zones or shift changes at work. Chronic insomnia of months' or years' duration has a poorer prognosis and a high association with psychiatric or medical disorders.

6. Which medical disorders commonly interfere with normal sleep?
Many medical disorders cause symptoms that interfere with sleep (e.g., nocturia, pain, or dyspnea). Psychiatric disorders have a 40% cocominance of insomnia, and patients with insomnia have a high risk of developing depression within a year. Examples of medical conditions that specifically disrupt sleep include the following:

Respiratory disease, including asthma, emphysema, and cystic fibrosis
Congestive heart failure
Gastroesophageal reflux
End-stage renal or liver disease
Endocrine disease
- Hypo- or hyperthyroidism
- Addison's or Cushing's syndrome
- Diabetes mellitus (due to hyper- or hypoglycemia)
Severe anemia
Rheumatoid arthritis (pain)

Central nervous system neoplasms
Headaches, especially cluster headaches
Seizure disorders
Parkinson's disease
Fibromyalgia (associated with nonrestorative sleep)
Dermatologic disorders
Alzheimer's disease

Therapy directed specifically at the medical problem may relieve the insomnia. In addition, prescription and over-the-counter medications may interfere with sleep, either as a direct effect (e.g., certain antidepressants, theophylline, corticosteroids, decongestants, histamine$_2$ blockers, stimulants) or indirectly (e.g., diuretics may cause nocturia).

7. What is sleep hygiene?

Sleep hygiene is a set of behaviors used to promote sleep and improve sleep quality. The following measures are recommended:

- The bedroom should be dark, quiet, and comfortable in temperature.
- Reading, watching TV, or working in the bedroom should be avoided. Only sleep and sexual relations should occur there.
- Caffeine (present in tea, chocolate, some soft drinks, and some analgesic preparations) should be restricted for at least 8 hours before bedtime. Nicotine also should be minimized.
- Patients should attempt to keep a regular sleep–wake schedule with consistent bed and wake times, regardless of the amount of sleep achieved. Naps should be avoided.
- Regular exercise, finished at least 3–4 hours before bedtime, appears to promote sleep.
- Heavy meals at dinner should be avoided. A light snack before bedtime may aid sleep.
- Alcohol may hasten sleep onset, but its metabolites may cause sleep interruption later in the night, and its use should be avoided.
- If sleep is not achieved 10–20 minutes after bedtime, the patient should leave the bedroom and do a quiet activity such as reading. When sleepiness occurs, the patient should return to bed. If sleep is again not achieved, the cycle is repeated.
- Illuminated bedroom clocks (the insomniac's nemesis) should be removed.

The goal of sleep hygiene is to associate the bedroom with falling asleep quickly, minimizing frustration and anxiety.

8. What medications are used for the treatment of insomnia?

The most commonly used prescription hypnotics are benzodiazepines and sedating antidepressants. Barbiturates have a high incidence of tolerance, addiction, and death (if overdosed) and should not be used as hypnotics. Chloral hydrate (a "Mickey Finn," when mixed with alcohol) may be safer than barbiturates but can cause gastritis. Nonprescription medications sold as hypnotics include antihistamines, scopolamine (an anticholinergic), and salicylates. Tryptophan, in high doses, was used as a "natural" hypnotic before it was associated with the eosinophilia-myalgia syndrome. Melatonin is an endogenous hormone secreted by the pineal gland in concordance with the circadian sleep cycle in humans. It is sold as a supplement in health food stores and is derived from bovine brains or chemically synthesized. Small trials have presented subjective evidence that melatonin may have modest efficacy in sleep disorders that are caused by jet lag, shift work, and neurologic impairment, but no long-term studies have documented either efficacy or safety, including drug interactions. The Food and Drug Administration (FDA) does not review drugs classified as "supplements," nor is supplements' production regulated or standardized. For these reasons, melatonin cannot be routinely recommended.

9. When are medications appropriate in the treatment of insomnia?

All patients with short- or long-term insomnia should be instructed in good sleep hygiene as first-line therapy. Relaxation techniques and biofeedback also have been suggested, but clinically significant improvement in sleep has not been demonstrated. Sleep medication may be a useful adjuvant to good sleep hygiene in the management of short-term insomnia but should not be prescribed for chronic insomnia or used for more than 3–4 weeks; they should be prescribed only in the context of a secure doctor–patient relationship.

10. If medications to promote sleep are needed, which are most appropriate to prescribe?

Benzodiazepines are most commonly used and have a reasonable safety record. Benzodiazepines currently marketed as hypnotics are triazolam (Halcion), temazepam (Restoril), and flurazepam (Dalmane). They vary chiefly in rates of absorption and elimination, with triazolam having the shortest half-life and flurazepam the longest; temazepam has an intermediate duration.

Zolpidem is a nonbenzodiazepine hypnotic that reduces sleep latency with fewer side effects than benzodiazepines and is often used as a first-line agent for short-term treatment of insomnia.

Antihistamines are not as potent as benzodiazepines and may have anticholinergic side effects, such as urinary retention. Low-dose, sedating antidepressants (e.g., amitriptyline, trazodone) have advantages in that they are nonaddictive and safe in sleep apnea, but data about safety and efficacy for chronic insomnia are unavailable.

Agitation and insomnia in hospitalized elderly patients ("sundowning") may be paradoxically worsened by benzodiazepines; low-dose **haloperidol** is a more effective treatment in these patients.

Gabapentin has been shown helpful for sleep disorders associated with various neuropathies.

Melatonin is touted as a sleep-promoting supplement but has only shown to be helpful in a subset of elderly patients with low melatonin levels. Because of its classification as a supplement, it is not regulated by the FDA, and data on safety and efficacy are sparse.

11. What precautions must be observed when benzodiazepines are used for insomnia?

Most importantly, the insomnia should be fully investigated before prescribing sleep medications. Many medical and psychiatric disorders can present as insomnia and can be masked or worsened with benzodiazepines. These agents may depress respiratory drive and can worsen sleep apnea and emphysema. Rebound insomnia (worsening of sleeplessness after discontinuation of hypnotics) may occur after only one dose. It should also be kept in mind that any benzodiazepine can be addictive. Short-acting drugs (e.g., triazolam) may reduce sleep latency, but unwanted effects include early-morning awakening, anterograde amnesia, and increased daytime anxiety. Long-acting benzodiazepines (e.g., temazepam) may prevent early-morning awakening but can result in daytime sleepiness. Flurazepam has a long-acting metabolite that may cause daytime sedation after multiple doses, especially in elderly individuals. Drug interactions (e.g., alcohol, phenobarbital) may be dangerous. Tolerance to benzodiazepines is the rule, and no study shows a difference between hypnotics and placebo after 3–4 weeks of therapy.

12. My patient complains of falling asleep during the day. What diagnoses should be considered?

For patients with excessive daytime sleepiness, sleep apnea, narcolepsy, and idiopathic hypersomnolence (sleepiness of unknown cause but not meeting criteria for narcolepsy) should be considered. Medical disorders (e.g., thyroid disease, diabetes mellitus, hepatic or renal failure, anemia, hydrocephalus) and medications (e.g., clonidine, antihistamines, neuroleptics, tricyclic antidepressants) cause sleepiness. Schizophrenia and depression may present with somnolence. Patients with transient hypersomnia have excessive daytime sleepiness and loss of energy, usually caused by a stressful event, and recover in < 3 weeks. Also, some patients simply get insufficient amounts of sleep to participate in their daily schedules.

13. Describe classic narcolepsy.

Narcolepsy is characterized by the sudden onset of daytime sleep (lasting minutes to hours) with abnormally prompt entry into REM sleep. It may be caused by a low level of a recently discovered neuropeptide called *hypocretin*. Classic narcolepsy includes the following:

Cataplexy—the sudden, temporary loss of skeletal muscle tone, often following excitement or fear

Sleep paralysis—a transitory but frightening inability to move or speak occurring at transitions between wakefulness and sleep

Hypnagogic hallucinations—dreamlike visual or auditory hallucinations at the transitions of wakefulness and sleep

Abnormal nocturnal sleep—with frequent awakenings

The diagnosis is confirmed in the sleep laboratory by repetitively measuring the time from attempting sleep to sleep onset (multiple sleep latency testing [MSLT]). Sleep latency is usually < 5 minutes in narcolepsy and > 10 minutes in normal persons. The majority of narcoleptics also are found to have direct entry from wakefulness into REM sleep. Narcolepsy is uncommon in the United States, with an estimated prevalence of 1 in 2000 people, and usually presents in late adolescence to early 20s.

Current therapy includes stimulants to prevent daytime sleepiness (modafinil is the first-line agent), tricyclics such as imipramine or protriptyline to control cataplexy, and scheduled daytime naps.

14. What is sleep apnea?

Sleep apnea is the repetitive cessation of airflow through the nose or mouth during sleep. Apneic episodes and hypopnea (a marked reduction in tidal volume) are common in adults during sleep, but excessive apnea and hypopnea are pathologic. Sleep apnea may result from obstruction of the upper airway (obstructive sleep apnea), failure of respiratory drive (central sleep apnea), of a combination of the two. Obstructive sleep apnea is present in approximately 4% of the U.S. population.

15. When should obstructive sleep apnea be suspected?

Sleep apnea should be considered in any patients with excessive daytime sleepiness and a history of snoring. Suspicion is heightened in men, elderly and the obese individuals, and probably alcoholics. Other clues include long pauses without audible respirations (reported by the bed partner), frequent arousals, and early-morning headaches. Patients with obstructive sleep apnea may have large necks and a narrow upper airway on physical examination.

16. How is obstructive sleep apnea diagnosed?

Obstructive sleep apnea is diagnosed by high clinical suspicion along with sleep laboratory results. Polysomnographic monitoring measurement of airflow, respiratory effort, arterial oxygen saturation, heart rhythm, and monitoring to determine sleep stage. Simple ear oximetry is used by some centers for screening, but normal study findings do not rule out significant sleep apnea.

An **apnea–hypopnea index** (i.e., numbers of apneas and hypopneas per hour of sleep) of > 5, along with excessive daytime sleepiness, is diagnostic of obstructive sleep apnea.

17. What are the consequences of sleep apnea?

Complications of sleep apnea are believed to result from cessation of ventilation with acute oxygen desaturation and carbon dioxide retention. The immediate consequence is sleep disruption caused by intermittent nocturnal asphyxiation. Resulting daytime sleepiness may impair the ability to stay awake while working or driving; patients with obstructive sleep apnea have a risk for motor vehicle accidents that is three times the normal population. Short-term consequences include personality changes, intellectual deterioration, memory impairment, and impotence.

Systemic blood pressure (BP) increases during apneas, and sustained daytime hypertension, often refractory to medicines, is commonly found. Some studies have shown that treatment of sleep apnea can lower systemic BP. Effects on cardiac rhythm during sleep are commonly noted and probably contribute to the overall decrease in survival in patients with sleep apnea. Sleeping electrocardiogram may show bradycardia, sinus pauses, atrioventricular block, and ventricular premature beats. Chronic sleep apnea, usually in concert with primary pulmonary disease or severe obesity, may result in pulmonary hypertension and right-sided heart failure.

18. How is obstructive sleep apnea treated?

Conservative measures include weight loss (when modest weight loss may be effective), abstinence from alcohol and other sedatives, oxygen therapy to prevent severe desaturation, and training patients to sleep on their sides rather than supine. **Drugs** result in mild, if any, improvement in obstructive sleep apnea. The tricyclic antidepressant protriptyline appears to be the most effective. It appears to reduce REM sleep, during which the upper airway muscles are most relaxed. **Mechanical measures** are indicated for more severe cases. Nasal continuous positive airway pressure (CPAP) used during sleep appears to "splint" the upper airway and prevents soft-tissue collapse during inspiration. CPAP is delivered through a close-fitting nasal mask used at home. Although successful when used, patients often find the device uncomfortable, and long-term compliance is variable. Removals of parts of the soft palate (uvulopalatopharyngoplasty [UPPP]) results in improvement in < 50% of those treated, it is difficult to predict who will benefit, and postoperative complications are possible. Mandibular advancement may be a possible alternative but is not as good as CPAP. Experience with prostheses designed to hold the pharynx open during sleep has been limited but appears to be less effective than CPAP. Tracheostomy remains the definitive therapy for severe obstructive sleep apnea refractory to other therapies.

19. My patient complains that his legs jerk and keep him awake. How can I help?

Periodic leg movements of sleep are stereotypical leg jerks that occur after sleep onset and may cause frequent awakenings in the patient. They occur more commonly with age and are rare before age 40 years. They may be worsened by tricyclic antidepressants. Short-acting benzodiazepines do not reduce twitching but do suppress arousal from sleep.

Restless leg syndrome is a neurologic movement disorder that consists of unpleasant "crawling" muscular sensations in the legs that cause an almost irresistible urge to move the legs. The cause is usually idiopathic and may be familial, but secondary medical causes include iron deficiency, neurologic lesions, pregnancy, and uremia. This condition makes sleep onset difficult and may cause difficulty in sleep maintenance. Small doses of the antiparkinsonian drug Sinemet (carbidopa and L-dopa, 25/100 mg) may enable sleep onset. Other dopamine agonists have also been used, and benzodiazepines may be helpful as well. Opioid narcotics are effective but discouraged because of side effects and addiction potential.

Hypnic jerks are sudden movements that involve all the extremities and occur in the transition from wakefulness to sleep. They are commonly experienced by normal people and seldom impair sleep.

20. What are parasomnias?

Parasomnias are unpleasant or undesirable behavioral phenomena that occur predominantly during sleep. **Disorders of arousal,** which include sleepwalking and sleep terrors, are caused by rapid alternations between wakefulness and non-REM sleep. The patient is awake enough to carry out activities but not awake enough to be aware of the actions. **REM sleep behavior disorder** is more common in older people, in whom the paralysis that normally accompanies REM sleep is absent. It results in "acting out dreams" and can be dangerous. Small doses of clonazepam at night can be helpful.

21. Who should have a sleep study?

Most patients with excessive daytime sleepiness should be studied in a sleep laboratory (polysomnography). The evaluation may include an **MSLT** (usually on the day after polysomnography), during which the time from wakefulness to sleep during several daytime naps is measured. A mean sleep latency of < 5 minutes is evidence of pathologic sleepiness. Another sleep study technique, **actigraphy,** helps detect and quantify periodic leg movement disorders. Patients with clinical suspicion of a parasomnia should have the diagnosis confirmed by sleep study, often done with the aid of a video camera. Insomnia has not routinely been an indication for polysomnography. Other tests that may be considered are neuroimaging studies, pulmonary function tests, and other laboratory tests if clinical suspicion points to a comorbid cause of hypersomnia or insomnia.

BIBLIOGRAPHY

1. Aldrich MS: Narcolepsy. N Engl J Med 323:389–394, 1990.
2. American Academy of Sleep Medicine. www.aasmnet.org.
3. Ancoli-Israel S: Sleep problems in older adults: Putting myths to bed. Geriatrics 52:20–30, 1997.
4. Chase J, Gidal B: Melatonin: Therapeutic use in sleep disorders. Am Pharmacother 31:1218–1226, 1997.
5. Chokroverty S: Diagnosis and treatment of sleep disorders caused by comorbid disease. Neurology 54:S8–S15, 2000.
6. Flemons WW: Obstructive sleep apnea. N Engl J Med 347:498–504, 2002.
7. Gillin JC, Byerley WF: Drug therapy: The diagnosis and management of insomnia. N Engl J Med 322:239–348, 1990.

8. Hauri PJ, Esther MS: Insomnia. Mayo Clin Proc 65:869–882, 1990.
9. Hoffstein V, Szalai JP: Predictive value of clinical features in diagnosing obstructive sleep apnea. Sleep 16:118–122, 1993.
10. Krahn LE, Black JL, Silber MH: Narcolepsy: New understanding of irresistible sleep. Mayo Clinic Proc 76:185–194, 2001.
11. Krueger BR: Restless leg syndrome and periodic movements of sleep. Mayo Clin Proc 65:999–1006, 1990.
12. Kryger MH, Roth T, Dement WC: Principles and Practice of Sleep Medicine. Philadelphia, W.B. Saunders, 1989.
13. Lippmann S, Mazour I, Shahab H: Insomnia: Therapeutic approach. South Med J 94:866–873, 2001.
14. Mahowald M: Diagnostic testing for sleep disorders. Neurol Clin 14:183–200, 1996.
15. Nakra BRS, Grossberg GT, Peck B: Insomnia in the elderly. Am Fam Physician 43:477–483, 1991.
16. Reite MI, Nagel KE, Ruddy JR: The Evaluation and Management of Sleep Disorders. Washington, DC, American Psychiatric Press, 1990.
17. Restless legs syndrome: Detection and management in primary care. National Heart, Lung, and Blood Institute working group on restless legs syndrome. Am Fam Physician 62:108–114, 2000.
18. Schenck CH, Mahowald MW: Parasomnias: Managing bizarre sleep-related behavior disorders. Postgrad Med 107:145–156, 2000.

10. ALCOHOL AND SUBSTANCE ABUSE

Joshua D. Blum, M.D., and Philip S. Mehler, M.D.

1. What are the societal implications of alcoholism?

Alcohol abuse and its sequelae present some of the most serious social and medical problems in the United States. The toll on human life is staggering: approximately 100,000 Americans die each year as a result of alcohol abuse. One in 13 Americans either abuses alcohol or is an alcoholic. After heart disease and cancer, alcoholism is America's third largest health problem. Up to 25% of patients admitted to community teaching hospitals have alcohol dependence. Approximately 12 million Americans are hospitalized annually with manifestations of alcohol abuse. Moreover, the alcohol trauma syndrome is an enormous problem; 41% of patients experiencing trauma have measurable blood alcohol levels on initial evaluation in the emergency department. Alcohol is also involved in about 25% of suicides. The annual cost to society is estimated to be $185 billion.

2. Given the magnitude of alcohol abuse and the paramount importance of early detection, what types of screening instruments are available?

Two types of screening instruments are available: (1) self-report questionnaires and structured interviews and (2) clinical laboratory tests that detect pathophysiologic changes associated with excessive alcohol usage.

The CAGE questionnaire is a self-report screening instrument that appears to be suited to busy medical practices in which time for patient interviews is limited. Two "yes" answers correctly identify 75% of alcoholics. The specificity of the test is 95%. The sensitivity of the CAGE questionnaire is dramatically enhanced by an open-ended introduction as opposed to questions about the frequency and amount of drinking. Equivocal responses should be followed up with the question: "Have you ever been injured while drinking?" Another questionnaire, the Michigan Alcoholism Screening Test (MAST), is a formal 25-item test that requires 25 minutes to complete. A shortened 10-item MAST (B-MAST) has been constructed with items from the original test that are highly discriminating for alcoholism. A cut-off score of 6 is suggestive for the B-MAST.

CAGE Questionnaire

Have you ever felt you ought to *c*ut down on your drinking?
Have people *a*nnoyed you by criticizing your drinking?
Have you ever felt bad or *g*uilty about your drinking?
Have you ever had a drink first thing in the morning as an *e*ye-opener to steady your nerves or get rid of a hangover?

Brief MAST Questionnaire

POINTS	QUESTION
(2)	1. Do you think you are a normal drinker?*
(2)	2. Do friends or relatives think you are a normal drinker?*
(5)	3. Have you ever attended a meeting of Alcoholics Anonymous?
(2)	4. Have you ever lost friends or girlfriends/boyfriends because of drinking?
(2)	5. Have you ever gotten into trouble at work because of drinking?
(2)	6. Have you ever neglected your obligations, your family, or your work for 2 or more days in a row because you were drinking?
(2)	7. Have you ever had delirium tremens (DTs) of severe shaking, heard voices, or seen things that weren't there after heavy drinking?
(5)	8. Have you ever gone to anyone for help about your drinking?
(5)	9. Have you ever been in a hospital because of drinking?
(2)	10. Have you ever been arrested for drunk driving or driving after drinking?

*Negative responses are alcoholic responses.
Scoring: $\leq$ 3 points, nonalcoholic; 4 points, suggestive of alcoholism; 5 indicates alcoholism.

Clinical laboratory tests frequently are used to corroborate results of questionnaires. Several tests provide objective evidence of problem drinking, especially in patients who deny an alcohol problem. Increased levels of serum gamma-glutamyl transferase (GGT) are approximately 50% sensitive for alcohol use. Although serum GGT is the most widely used laboratory screening test for alcoholism, it lacks diagnostic specificity. Results are more specific in conjunction with elevated mean corpuscular volume (MCV), which increases with excessive alcohol intake. The ratio of the liver enzyme aspartate aminotransferase (AST) to alanine aminotransferase (ALT), if > 1, may be a useful marker of alcoholic liver disease.

3. **What major organ systems are affected by alcohol abuse?**
    Alcohol affects almost every organ system in the body.

    Cardiovascular system
    Hypertension
    Cardiomyopathy
    Atrial and ventricular dysrhythmias
    Endocrine system
    Testicular atrophy
    Feminization
    Amenorrhea and premature menopause
    Pseudo-Cushing's syndrome
    Gastrointestinal system
    Hepatitis and cirrhosis
    Esophagitis and gastritis
    Peptic ulcer disease
    Esophageal carcinoma
    Malabsorption with diarrhea
    Pancreatitis
    Immune system
    Increased susceptibility to bacterial infections
    Impaired macrophage function

    Hematologic system
    Anemia due to folate deficiency or sideroblastosis
    Thrombocytopenia
    Diminished neutrophil migration
    Nervous system
    Cognitive impairment
    Dementia
    Korsakoff's psychosis
    Wernicke's encephalopathy
    Peripheral neuropathy
    Musculoskeletal system
    Osteoporosis
    Avascular necrosis
    Skin
    Telangiectasias
    Palmar erythema
    Worsened rosacea, rhinophyma

4. Are gender differences observed in alcohol-related liver disease?

Yes. Although the cirrhosis-induced death rate is higher for men than women, women are more susceptible to alcohol-related liver damage and develop liver disease with shorter durations of alcohol abuse.

5. What are the consequences to the fetus of alcohol use during pregnancy?

Alcohol is a teratogen. Although a critical dosage or exposure level has not been determined, observations of human infants and experimental animals make it clear that a mother who drinks heavily during pregnancy, particularly during the first trimester, may severely damage her fetus. The distinct pattern of birth defects, known as the fetal alcohol syndrome, includes growth retardation, a characteristic constellation of craniofacial anomalies, central nervous system dysfunction, and malformations of major organ systems.

6. Describe the manifestations of alcohol withdrawal syndrome.

Alcohol withdrawal may have several different and occasionally overlapping manifestations. The clinical spectrum ranges from a "hangover" to life-threatening delirium tremens. Minor withdrawal may begin 6–12 hours after a significant decrease or cessation of drinking in heavy, chronic drinkers despite significant blood levels of alcohol. This stage may last 3–5 days and is characterized by tremors, sweating, anxiety, diarrhea, nausea, and insomnia. Patients may not require pharmacologic therapy. The degree of autonomic hyperactivity may progress to marked tremulousness, tachycardia, hyperactivity, and agitation after 12–24 hours. The patient may have visual and auditory hallucinations. The hallucinations are usually unpleasant and separated by a lucid interval.

Alcohol withdrawal seizures are not uncommon and usually occur within the first 48 hours. These are grand mal seizures without focality. Multiple seizures may occur in 2–5% of patients within a 6–10-hour period. Any focal findings on examination, seizures occurring during delirium tremens, and seizures occurring over several days or accompanied by fever should prompt a further neurologic evaluation. Alcoholic patients who remain asymptomatic for $\geq$ 36 hours after their last alcohol use are very unlikely to develop serious withdrawal symptoms.

7. Outline the principles of management in patients with alcohol withdrawal symptoms.

Although outpatient treatment of minor alcohol withdrawal has its place, pregnant women, older patients, and patients with hyperactivity of the sympathetic nervous system, marked tachycardia or hypertension, concurrent serious medical problems, lack of a social support system, and history of complications during previous withdrawal episodes require inpatient treatment. Delirium tremens requires management in the intensive care unit. Although patients experiencing mild withdrawal symptoms can be managed without adjunctive pharmacologic therapy, current guidelines recommend medicinal treatment for most patients experiencing alcohol withdrawal.

The proper management of alcohol withdrawal is aimed at alleviating patient suffering and preventing minor symptoms from progressing to major symptoms. Normalization of vital signs and moderate sedation are two desired endpoints of treatment. Sedation is accomplished by substituting for alcohol another sedative hypnotic agent, frequently a benzodiazepine, in a gradually tapering dose. The dosage of benzodiazepine for alcohol withdrawal is larger than usually given for anxiety or panic disorder. Patients should be assessed carefully to ensure adequate dosing to achieve sedation and amelioration of the hyperautonomic state. In patients with significant liver disease, lorazepam (Ativan) or oxazepam (Serax) should be used because neither is extensively oxidized by the liver. Intravenous use of benzodiazepines until mild sedation occurs prevents the physiologic storm that may be seen with delirium tremens. Whether symptom-triggered benzodiazepines are preferable to a fixed dosing schedule that is tapered over time is currently under debate, although evidence seems to favor the latter.

Adjunctive therapy also may be used. Haloperidol (Haldol) may be used to control agitation and belligerence but only after benzodiazepines have been given because haloperidol lowers the seizure threshold. Beta-blockers such as atenolol (Tenormin) also have been used successfully to reduce the adrenergic signs of withdrawal, especially in the outpatient setting. A daily dose of 50 mg during the withdrawal period shortens hospital stays and reduces the total dose of benzodiazepine required for treatment. In addition to beta-blockers, alpha$_2$-receptor agonists, such as clonidine (Catapres), also have been used to treat alcohol withdrawal because of their sedative as well as blood pressure–and pulse-lowering properties. The usual dosage is 0.2 mg twice daily. It is important not to use these adjunctive treatments without benzodiazepines because they do not prevent withdrawal seizures. In all stages of alcohol withdrawal, compulsive attention to fluid and electrolyte status is required, and most patients should receive thiamine and folate supplementation.

8. What pharmacotherapies are available to deter alcoholism?

Traditionally, **disulfiram** has been used to deter alcohol use. It blocks the enzyme aldehyde dehydrogenase, which results in an increased concentration of acetaldehyde. Therefore, patients who ingest alcohol while taking disulfiram get palpitations, dyspnea, headache, tachycardia, and flushing. The alcohol–disulfiram reactions are usually self-limiting; severe reactions are associated with dosages > 500 mg/day. Data about the efficacy of disulfiram in preventing relapse are poor, despite its widespread use. **Selective serotonin reuptake inhibitors** (SSRIs) have been investigated for their potential to decrease the desire for alcohol. Studies have shown some benefit in patients with coexisting depression. Buspirone has been noted to decrease alcohol craving in alcoholics with coexisting anxiety. Newer pharmacologic treatments center on narcotic antagonists that reduce alcohol craving and use. **Naltrexone** is the only one approved by the Food and Drug Administration (FDA), although its efficacy is uncertain. In one 12-week study, naltrexone compared favorably with placebo. There was a 23% relapse rate with naltrexone compared with a 54% relapse rate in the placebo group. Naltrexone should not be given to patients taking narcotics, because it may result in narcotic withdrawal symptoms. During routine use, the most common side effects are nausea, headache, constipation, fatigue, and somnolence. Elevations in liver enzyme level may occur, but levels return to baseline after the drug is stopped.

9. Which patients may benefit from disulfiram?

The ideal patient for disulfiram therapy is a daily rather than binge drinker who is committed to treatment but prone to relapse. The main contraindications to its use are heart disease, history of seizures, cirrhosis, diabetes, pregnancy, and significantly elevated levels of transaminase (greater than three times normal). Studies of disulfiram have never been definitively shown to increase rates of abstinence in patients not enrolled in a monitored treatment program.

10. Are there any newer medications for the treatment of alcoholism?

Acamprosate is a synthetic compound with a chemical structure that resembles homotaurine, a naturally occurring amino acid. Acamprosate acts centrally and appears to restore the normal activity of glutaminergic neurons, which become hyperexcited as a result of chronic alcohol exposure. Although acamprosate is currently under review by the FDA as an investigational drug, it has been available in France since 1989 and has been studied in several double-blind, placebo-controlled clinical trials in the outpatient setting. A recent review of these trials in the *Journal of Clinical Psychiatry* showed that patients treated with acamprosate exhibited significantly greater rates of treatment completion, time to first drink, abstinence rate, and cumulative abstinence duration compared with patients treated with placebo.

11. What's the difference between addiction and dependence?

Addiction is defined as the continued usage of a substance of abuse despite adverse consequences. **Dependence** is present when rapid reduction or withdrawal of a substance produces a recognized and predictable withdrawal syndrome.

12. What are brief interventions?

A brief intervention is a short counseling session focused on helping a person change a specific behavior. The interventions are often performed by a primary care provider at each outpatient visit, lasting up to several minutes. Methods may include brief assessment with feedback; behavioral modification; and setting goals, including contracting. The intervention is tailored to the patient's substance abuse problem and to the patient's readiness to change his or her behavior. Several clinical trials with alcoholics have shown that brief interventions reduce alcohol consumption and result in positive health behaviors such as reduced sick days at work. Perhaps even more than pharmacotherapies, brief interventions should be considered the cornerstone of addiction treatment in the primary care setting.

13. Which classes of drugs are characterized by potentially dangerous withdrawal syndromes?

Drugs of abuse are generally divided into the following categories: sedatives, stimulants, opiates, psychedelic agents, and phencyclidine (PCP). **Withdrawal** is defined as the predictable development of physical and psychological signs and symptoms in response to the abrupt discontinuation of a drug in dependent people. The only class of drugs connected with dangerous withdrawal syndromes is the central nervous system depressants, which include alcohol, benzodiazepines, barbiturates, chloral hydrate, and meprobamate.

14. Characterize the opiate withdrawal syndrome.

Mild withdrawal is characterized by yawning and dilated pupils. In more severe cases, vomiting, diarrhea, piloerection, rhinorrhea, and lacrimation are seen. Symptoms include anxiety, insomnia, abdominal cramping, irritability, and leg spasms. Withdrawal usually begins 6–12 hours after the last use of narcotics. Heroin withdrawal symptoms generally peak within 36–72 hours and may last 7–10 days. Although annoying, opiate withdrawal is generally not dangerous.

15. How is opiate withdrawal treated?

Opiate withdrawal can be treated by two different approaches. The first is to block the autonomic effects of the withdrawal using medications such as clonidine in dosages of 0.8–1.2 mg/day divided into four doses for a total of 10–14 days. Clonidine and other alpha-blockers block many of the physical symptoms but have no effect on craving.

The second approach is to use long-acting opiates to produce "cross-tolerance." Methadone, in dosages of 15–30 mg/day, is substituted for the opioid of abuse, whether it is heroin, meperidine, or codeine. This dose is maintained through the second or third day and then slowly tapered by 10–15% per day as guided by the patient's symptoms. Methadone can be used by any licensed physician on an inpatient basis but requires a special license to be administered as an outpatient.

16. What is opiate maintenance therapy?

Although pharmacologic withdrawal from opiates has never been shown to produce lasting abstinence, data support the use of long-term opiate therapy in the outpatient setting to reduce the use of illicit drugs. "Methadone clinics" have been shown to improve long-term abstinence and to reduce some of the other risks associated with intravenous drug use, such as transmission of HIV and criminal activity. Methadone, in dosages of 60–100 mg/day, is the most common only-opioid used in this capacity, but recent research has focused on the use of another long-acting medication, buprenorphine hydrochloride. Because the latter medication is a mixed agonist-antagonist, risk of abuse or serious respiratory depression is significantly reduced relative to methadone. In clinical trials, buprenorphine, 8–16 mg/day, compared with methadone, 20–30 mg/day, had similar effects on retention and illicit opioid use. Studies are currently underway to determine if use of this medication can be expanded outside of specialty clinics and into the primary care setting. Levo-alpha-acetylmethadol (LAAM) is another opiate approved for chronic maintenance therapy. Because of its longer half-life, it can be taken three times a week, avoiding the need for take-home medications on weekends.

17. What are the physiologic effects of cocaine?

Cocaine is obtained by adding hydrochloric acid to coca leaves. The water-soluble crystal that forms may be absorbed through the nasal mucosa or injected intravenously. "Crack" cocaine is a highly purified form of the cocaine free base that makes a popping sound when heated. When smoked, it produces immediate euphoria, but the effects last only for minutes, prompting repeated, frequent administration. The resulting craving makes it difficult for patients to abstain from cocaine use. The physiologic responses to and adverse effects of cocaine are primarily related to excessive catecholamine discharge: hypertension, tachycardia, hyperthermia, agitation, and seizures.

18. What medications are available to treat cocaine addiction?

No medication is currently approved for the treatment of cocaine addiction. Although retrospective data suggest that tricyclic antidepressants, SSRIs, and dopamine agonists (e.g., bromocriptine) may have some efficacy in reducing craving, addiction treatment is centered around psychotherapy, behavioral therapy, and twelve-step programs.

19. Which drug is contraindicated in cocaine-related chest pain?

If the chest pain is believed to indicate myocardial ischemia, beta-blockers are contraindicated because they result in unopposed coronary vasoconstriction mediated by alpha-adrenergic agents and may actually exacerbate cocaine-related cardiovascular toxicity. Nitroglycerin and calcium channel blockers are the mainstays of therapy along with the mixed alpha- and beta-adrenergic blocker labetalol. Heparin, aspirin, and thrombolytic agents also may have a role because of experimental evidence of cocaine-enhanced platelet aggregation and thrombosis.

20. Bidirectional nystagmus should suggest abuse of which recreational drug?

PCP is the only drug of abuse that produces bidirectional nystagmus; it has dopaminergic, anticholinergic, and adrenergic activities. Intoxicated patients present with hypertension, tachycardia, bidirectional nystagmus, hyperthermia, hallucinations, and marked agitation. The combination of a coma-like state with open eyes, diminished pain perception, intermittent periods of excitation, and severe muscle rigidity indicates a PCP reaction. Patients are at risk for hypertensive crisis, rhabdomyolysis, seizures, and bizarre, often violent, behavior. PCP is abused because of the sense of invincibility and power that it produces. It is most often smoked but also may be taken intravenously or orally. Management of acute PCP intoxication may be challenging. The patient should be placed in a quiet environment; in most instances, this suffices. Patients who are severely agitated, however, should be sedated adequately with benzodiazepines, cooled rapidly if indicated, and hydrated. Drugs such as haloperidol are effective for the treatment of terrifying hallucinations.

21. What drug of abuse imposes the largest health and economic burden on society?

The surprising answer is **nicotine,** one of the major preventable nemeses of public health. The 1989 Surgeon General's report estimated that 1 in 6 deaths in the United States was caused by cigarettes. In 1994, more than 430,000 deaths in the United States were directly attributable to smoking. Only recently have efforts been made to portray tobacco smoking as an addictive disease. Nicotine is a psychoactive drug associated with definite dependence, tolerance, and withdrawal syndrome. The withdrawal process is characterized by dysphoria, craving, irritability, and nervousness. Tobacco addiction is a complex process that involves nicotinic–cholinergic receptors in the brain. Because of the complexity of the addiction, many smokers are not able to quit by themselves. The pharmacotherapy of tobacco addiction involves maintaining a fairly consistent level of nicotine in the body through nicotine-substitution therapy. Thus, symptoms of abstinence are relieved. Nicotine chewing gum, inhalers, nasal sprays, and transdermal delivery systems are available to achieve this end. Sustained-release bupropion hydrochloride (marketed as Zyban) is a non-nicotine aid to smoking cessation approved for this use by the FDA. In placebo-controlled trials, use of this medication led to improved short-term and longer-term abstinence rates. However, without some form of concomitant behavioral support from a physician or other caregiver, pharmacologic therapies are frequently unsuccessful.

22. Characterize benzodiazepine withdrawal and its therapy.

Benzodiazepines are divided into **short-acting agents,** such as temazepam (Restoril) and triazolam (Halcion); **intermediate-acting agents,** such as alprazolam (Xanax), lorazepam (Ativan), and oxazepam (Serax); and **long-acting agents,** such as clorazepate (Tranxene), diazepam (Valium), and clonazepam (Klonopin). Dependence may develop rapidly, often within a few weeks. In general, the shorter the half-life, the more intense the withdrawal syndrome. Signs and symptoms of withdrawal occur within 24 hours of cessation with a short-acting benzodiazepine and by the fifth day with longer-acting drugs. Benzodiazepine withdrawal produces a highly excitable state that is contrary to the usual sedative effects and may include palpitations, diarrhea, polyuria, tremor, and seizures. Detoxification is predicated on the premise that benzodiazepines have mutual cross-tolerance. Conversions for equivalent doses are easily calculated. In general, a long-acting benzodiazepine is preferable for suppressing withdrawal symptoms. A schedule of 7–10 days of gradual tapering is set up if the abused benzodiazepine is short acting; a schedule of 10–14 days is used for longer-acting drugs, but clinical judgment may dictate a more prolonged tapering schedule.

Dose Conversions for Sedative Hypnotic Drugs

DRUG	DOSE (mg)	DRUG	DOSE (mg)
Barbiturates		**Benzodiazepines**	
Pentobarbital	100	Alprazolam	1
Secobarbital	100	Chlordiazepoxide	25
Butalbital	100	Clonazepam	4
Amobarbital	100	Clorazepate	15
Phenobarbital	30	Diazepam	10
Nonbarbiturates, nonbenzodiazepines		Flurazepam	15
Ethchlorvynol	300	Lorazepam	2
Glutethimide	250	Oxazepam	10
Methyprylon	200	Quazepam	15
Methaqualone	300	Temazepam	15
Meprobamate	400	Triazolam	0.25
Carisoprodol	700		
Chloral hydrate	500		

23. How accurate is urine drug testing?

Because of a determined effort to reduce drug abuse, drug testing has become more common. Most urine drug panels screen for marijuana, cocaine, opiates, PCP, and amphetamines. The cost of such tests is $50–100. Positive results are confirmed by gas chromatography–mass spectrometry (GC-MS). Almost one third of positive results on initial screening tests are found to be false. For example, sympathomimetic agents in over-the-counter decongestants test positive for amphetamines; confirmatory testing, however, is negative for the d-isomer of abused amphetamines.

In general, marijuana is detected for 1–3 days after occasional use and for up to 3–4 weeks in heavy smokers because of accumulation in fatty tissues. The major metabolite of cocaine, benzoylecgonine, may be detected for 2–3 days after use. A positive test result for PCP usually indicates drug use within the previous week.

24. What is a medical review officer (MRO)?

Another caveat with drug testing is that poppy seeds on baked goods contain sufficient amounts of morphine to produce a positive urine test result. The result is not a false-positive result because the drug is actually present. Errors in handling or analysis also may result in false-negative results. Therefore, decision making for formal drug testing requires the expertise of MROs with specific training in addiction medicine. MROs help to protect the rights of patients while contributing to the effort to reduce drug abuse.

CONTROVERSY

25. What is the role of anticonvulsants in preventing alcohol withdrawal seizures?

A seizure may herald the onset of a major withdrawal syndrome, and one third of patients with alcohol withdrawal seizures may later develop delirium tremens. Nonetheless, the routine use of phenytoin to prevent seizures in patients withdrawing from alcohol is controversial. Three studies have focused on this issue: two do not support the use of phenytoin, but one does. The efficacy of phenytoin in combination with a benzodiazepine thus remains uncertain. Current practice is to give phenytoin only to withdrawing patients with a documented history of non–alcohol-related seizures or a history of withdrawal seizures.

BIBLIOGRAPHY

1. Baldridge BE, Bessen HA: Phencyclidine. Emerg Clin North Am 8:541–549, 1990.
2. Barnes HN, Samet JH: Brief interventions with substance-abusing patients. Med Clin North Am 81:867–879, 1997.
3. Everett WD, Linden N: Drug testing in the workplace. Postgrad Med 91:164–170, 1992.
4. Ewing JA: Detecting alcoholism: The CAGE questionnaire. JAMA 252:1905–1907, 1984.
5. Hayner G, Galloway G, Wiehl WO: Haight-Ashbury clinic's drug detoxification protocols: Benzodiazepines and other sedatives. J Psychoact Drugs 25:331–335, 1993.
6. Henry JA, Jeffrey KJ, Dawling S: Toxicity and death from methamphetamine. Lancet 340:384–387, 1992.
7. Ling W, Wesson DR: Drugs of abuse—opiates. West J Med 152:565–572, 1991.
8. Mason BJ: Treatment of alcohol-dependent outpatients with acamprosate: A clinical review. J Clin Psychiatry 62(suppl 20):42–48, 2001.
9. Mayo-Smith MF: Pharmacological management of alcohol withdrawal. JAMA 278:144–151, 1997.
10. Mynor RL, Scott BD, Brown DP, Windford MD: Cocaine-induced myocardial infarction and patients with normal coronary arteries. Ann Intern Med 115:797–806, 1991.
11. O'Connor PG, Fiellin DA: Pharmacologic treatment of heroin-dependent patients. Ann Intern Med 133:40–54, 2000.
12. O'Connor PG, Schottenfeld RS: Patients with alcohol problems. N Engl J Med 338:592–602, 1998.
13. O'Connor RG, Selwyn PA, Stein MD: Management of the hospitalized intravenous drug users. Am J Med 96:551–558, 1994.
14. Saitz R, Mayo-Smith MF, Roberts MS: Individualized treatment of alcohol withdrawal: A randomized double-blind controlled trial. JAMA 272:519–523, 1994.
15. Saitz R, O'Malley SS: Pharmacotherapies for alcohol abuse. Med Clin North Am 81:881–907, 1997.
16. Swift RM: Effect of naltrexone on human alcohol consumption. J Clin Psychiatry 56(suppl 7):24–29, 1995.
17. Warner E: Cocaine abuse. Ann Intern Med 119:226–235, 1993.

11. ANXIETY

Joyce Seiko Kobayashi, M.D.

1. What portion of primary care office visits result in a diagnosis of anxiety disorders?

According to the 1997 and 1998 National Ambulatory Medical Care Surveys, a nationally representative, systematically sampled series of surveys of office-based physicians, the number of office visits with a recorded anxiety disorder diagnosis represented approximately 1.5% of all office visits in 1997–1998, or 12.3 million office visits per year in the United States. Conversely, almost half of all visits for anxiety disorders were to primary care physicians. These numbers are likely to be underestimates because anxiety is commonly underdiagnosed and undertreated in primary care settings. Although internal medicine residents approached general practitioners in rates of diagnosing depression, they were significantly less likely to diagnose anxiety.

2. Why do primary care physicians need to be knowledgeable about the evaluation and management of anxiety in the medical setting?

First, anxiety is accompanied by specific physical symptoms that may trigger a major diagnostic work-up. Astute clinicians can avoid this pitfall. Early diagnosis of anxiety spares expense and protects patients from unnecessary distress. Second, patients with a number of primary medical disorders may present with anxiety. In these cases, the physician should avoid premature diagnosis of an emotional disorder, which may delay proper medical treatment until the disease process worsens.

Finally, many patients react to a range of medical illnesses with significant anxiety, particularly in relationship to the acute diagnosis or later as symptoms become more severe or the illness becomes more life threatening. Management of anxiety as part of the adjustment to medical illness is best done by primary care physicians, who have long-term relationships with their patients and should be considered one of the most important tasks affirming the doctor–patient relationship in comprehensive primary care.

Patients who either express their anxiety through somatic symptoms or experience significant anxiety in reaction to medical illness frequently prefer to share their feelings with their primary care physicians and may feel abandoned if referred to a psychiatrist or other specialist. If a physician judges that a referral is necessary because of the severity of symptoms, suicidal ideation, acuity of presentation, or comorbid disorders, the patient should be assured that the physician will work closely with the psychiatrist and continue to follow the patient.

3. What are the three most common errors that a primary care practitioner can make with a patient who presents with significant anxiety?

1. The physician may be too quick to consider anxiety a psychiatric problem and either prematurely refer the patient to a mental health professional or rush to prescribe benzodiazepines. Routine treatment of anxiety with benzodiazepines is no more appropriate than routine treatment of a fever with antibiotics. Anxiety is often treated as the diagnosis rather than a signal to pursue the source of the anxiety or to attempt to understand its meaning. Physicians should not prematurely close diagnostic evaluations and should learn to feel comfortable with exploring patients' feelings with a few open-ended questions.

2. The physician may assume that he or she knows what the patient "must" be anxious about. A classic example is assuming that the patient about to undergo a course of chemotherapy is most concerned about the medically serious side effects rather than, for example, losing his or her hair or some other side effect that may feel more immediately threatening.

3. The physician may rush to reassure the patient that "there is really nothing to worry about." Instead, the physician should allow the patient to express his or her feelings, acknowledge that the patient must feel some reason to be anxious, and ensure the patient continued support as well as collaboration to identify and manage the source of anxiety.

4. What are the primary causes of anxiety in the medical setting?

- Anxiety as a normal alerting response to the perceived threat of medical illness and treatment interventions
- Anxiety as a symptomatic manifestation of medical illness
- Anxiety as a symptom of intoxication or withdrawal syndromes
- Anxiety disorders or other psychiatric disorders

5. What physical symptoms frequently associated with anxiety disorders may be confused with medical illness?

The variety of physical symptoms associated with anxiety may be classified into three general categories:

1. **Motor tension:** trembling, twitching, feeling shaky, muscle tension or aches, restlessness, easy fatigability

2. **Autonomic hyperactivity:** shortness of breath or smothering sensations, palpitations or tachycardia, sweating or clammy hands, dry mouth, dizziness or lightheadedness, nausea, diarrhea or other abdominal distress, hot flashes or chills, frequent urination, trouble with swallowing, "lump in throat"

3. **Vigilance of scanning:** feeling keyed-up or on edge, exaggerated startle response, difficulty in concentrating or "mind going blank," trouble with falling or staying asleep, irritability

Symptoms associated with panic attacks commonly precipitate major medical work-ups.

6. What aspects of medical illness and treatment are common sources of anxiety?

Many aspects of medical illness and treatment may cause anxiety, depending on the patient's history, capacity to cope, support network, and specific tasks of adjustment associated with a particular disease or its treatment. This may also vary according to the illness: the prevalence of significant anxiety in one AIDS clinic was 70%. It is essential to start by asking several open-ended questions about patients' reactions to diagnosis, experiences with proposed or related therapies, and major current concerns. Some patients may believe that their illness is a punishment; others may use it as an organizing focus for unmet dependency needs. Physicians should attempt to understand the meaning of illness for each person.

A number of predictable, deeper concerns are common, and physicians should listen for them in patients' discussions. Examples include fears of pain, abandonment, dependency, disfigurement, or social unacceptability; loss of control or function; and death. Asking about such deeper concerns too directly or prematurely, however, may increase the patient's anxiety; clinical judgment must be exercised. Reassuring the patient that he or she will not be abandoned, for example, does not require specific acknowledgment of this fear.

Some patients experience pathologic anxiety that is out of proportion to the situation. A common reason for this is an irrational expectation of a bad outcome based on the experience of a friend or relative whose medical situation might be completely unrelated. The physician should assess whether the level of anxiety is adaptive or signals the patient's need for further treatment. Reassurance focused solely on the medical aspects of the illness in these patients does not address their underlying concerns. Psychiatric consultation may be considered, with reassurance that the physician will continue to be involved.

Finally, patients also may feel anxious about the doctor–patient relationship or unable to trust the efficacy of medical treatment or the health care system in general because of prior experiences, sociocultural barriers, or personal histories of abuse or neglect. These patients often feel less anxious as the physician gains their trust through consistent caring and compassionate interaction.

7. List the medical disorders that may present with anxiety as a primary symptom.

- **Endocrine disorders:** hyperthyroidism, pheochromocytoma, hypoglycemia, hypo- or hypercalcemia
- **Cardiac disorders:** hypoxia, angina, arrhythmias, congestive heart failure, mitral valve prolapse
- **Pulmonary disorders:** hypoxia, chronic obstructive pulmonary disease, pneumonia, hyperventilation, pulmonary embolism
- **Neurologic disorders:** partial complex seizures, encephalitis, postconcussion syndrome, sleep disorders
- **Metabolic disorders:** vitamin B_{12} deficiency, porphyria
- **Stimulant toxicity:** caffeine, sympathomimetic medications or drugs
- **Withdrawal syndromes:** alcohol, benzodiazepines, barbiturates, opiates, or delirium of any etiology (see also Chapter 12, Psychoses)

8. Which psychiatric disorders present with anxiety as a major symptom?

Patients with several categories of psychiatric disorders may present with anxiety, including adjustment disorders, generalized anxiety, posttraumatic stress disorders, substance-induced anxiety disorder, and intoxication or withdrawal disorders (see Chapter 10, Alcohol and Substance Abuse). Less common underlying disorders include phobias, obsessive-compulsive disorder, and complicated bereavement. In addition, patients with somatoform, conversion, and certain personality disorders often seek help in the primary care setting with similar presentations. Finally, comorbid disorders are quite common. Generalized anxiety disorder, for example, does not commonly occur in isolation (current and lifetime prevalence: 1.2–6.6%) but has a lifetime comorbidity rate of 90%. One of the most common and treatable comorbid diagnoses that should always be kept in mind when anxiety is the presenting symptom is major depressive disorder. The reader is referred to the fourth edition of the American Psychiatric Association's *Diagnostic and Statistical Manual of Mental Disorders,* 4th edition, text revision (DSM-IV-TR) for a more specific listing of the diagnostic criteria of the above disorders.

9. What is a panic attack? What other disorders may be associated with panic attacks?

Patients with panic attacks often seek help first from their primary care physician. The essential element of a panic attack is a discrete period of intense fear or discomfort, in which four (or more) of the following symptoms develop abruptly and reach a peak within 10 minutes:

Palpitations	Feeling dizzy or faint
Sweating	Derealization (feelings of unreality) or
Trembling	depersonalization (being detached from
Sensation of shortness of breath or	oneself)
smothering	Fear of losing control or sanity
Feeling of choking	Fear of dying
Chest pain or discomfort	Paresthesias
Nausea or abdominal distress	Chills or hot flushes

Because patients experiencing a panic attack often feel as if they are having a heart attack or stroke and fear that they are dying, they are seen frequently in emergency departments and cardiac clinics. They may receive major medical work-ups (often at multiple sites) when an initial exclusionary work-up, thorough review of past records, and careful medical history may suffice. Accurate diagnosis may require psychiatric consultation and consideration of treatment with a selective serotonin reuptake inhibitor (SSRI) or a benzodiazepine. Continuity and collaborative care with a primary care physician and psychiatrist prevents further mismanagement of patients with panic disorder.

10. What clues help primary care physicians to recognize other common psychiatric disorders that present with anxiety?

1. **Major depressive disorder** is one of the most common and readily treatable disorders that may present with clinically significant anxiety, with or without panic attacks. Depressive disorders are commonly associated with *anhedonia* (loss of pleasure or enjoyment) and vegetative symptoms such as sleep, bowel, or appetite disturbances.

2. **Bipolar disorder (manic phase)** may present with agitation and irritability that may be differentiated from anxiety by rapid and pressured speech and easy provocation to anger.

3. **Adjustment disorder** with anxiety may be an acute or chronic condition and is characterized by the development of emotional or behavioral symptoms in response to an identifiable stressor or stressors occurring within 3 months of the onset of symptoms. The degree of distress exceeds what normally would be expected, or social or occupational functioning is significantly impaired.

4. A **substance-induced anxiety disorder** is diagnosed when the anxiety is judged to be caused by the direct physiologic effects of an illicit drug, medication, or toxin. Withdrawal syndromes from alcohol and sedating medications often make patients feel anxious.

5. **Post-traumatic or acute stress disorders** are diagnosed by characteristic symptoms in response to an extreme traumatic stressor.

6. **Phobias** are common in the general population but rarely reach the level of clinical significance. Lifetime prevalence of diagnosable specific phobias is around 10%. However, specific phobias (categorized as animal, natural environment, blood-injection injury, situational, and other types) may have significant effect on health care behavior (e.g., fears of blood, needles, and chok-

ing [medications]) and should be consciously assessed for clinical severity with an in-depth history. Patients with such disorders are aware that their fears are out of proportion to the situation but may not say so unless asked.

7. **Obsessive-compulsive disorders** are important to note (lifetime prevalence of 2–5%) because they are more common than is realized; effective pharmacologic treatments are available. These disorders are often disabling, and fears of contamination may bring a patient to the primary care physician.

The DSM-IV-TR provides a more specific listing of the diagnostic criteria of the above disorders.

11. What is the DSM-IV-TR?

The DSM-IV-TR, published in 2000, is a text revision of the fourth edition of the American Psychiatric Association's (APA) *Diagnostic and Statistical Manual of Mental Disorders* and is constantly in the process of updating and revision. This manual was the product of 13 work groups whose comprehensive literature reviews were critiqued by 50–100 advisers representing a diversity of clinical and research expertise; two methods conferences; 40 data reanalyses; and 12 field trials of the revised diagnostic criteria, involving 70 sites and more than 6000 subjects. The APA acknowledges the limitations of any categorical approach, given the heterogeneity of human behavior, but the DSM-IV has begun to incorporate different cultural perspectives and represents a major step in standardizing clinical diagnosis, communication, and research about mental disorders.

12. Which medications, substances, and toxic agents may cause anxiety as a symptom in either intoxication or withdrawal?

Although the term *intoxication and withdrawal syndromes* (see Chapter 10) appropriately brings to mind street drugs and alcohol, excessive caffeine ingestion and nicotine withdrawal are two of the most commonly overlooked causes or contributors to anxiety. Caffeine is frequently underestimated as a toxic agent, and a careful history of all sources of caffeine (e.g., coffee, sodas, over-the-counter stimulants) should be included in the evaluation of anxious patients. Symptoms may occur with 200 mg of caffeine daily (< 2 cups of coffee), and individuals vary in their susceptibility. Minor withdrawal from nicotine is usually self-medicated with more cigarettes, but patients who gradually increase tobacco consumption may not be conscious of withdrawal effects.

Withdrawal from benzodiazepines, barbiturates and other sedative/hypnotics, opiates, and alcohol commonly cause anxiety with or without tremulousness. Despite awareness of these pharmacologic effects, physicians may prescribe anxiolytics to patients who present in great distress without considering the possibility of a minor withdrawal syndrome.

Cocaine, phencyclidine, amphetamine, methamphetamine, and other stimulants, such as over-the-counter alpha-adrenergic medications (e.g., phenylpropanolamine, ephedrine, phenylephrine, and pseudoephedrine) may cause varying degrees of anxiety, irritability, agitation, and restlessness.

Among the major offending agents in causing anxiety, however, are commonly prescribed medications. The akathisia of neuroleptics is frequently accompanied by a subjective feeling of restlessness and anxiety that may be profoundly disturbing to sensitive patients. Antidepressants, such as fluoxetine or imipramine; xanthines, such as theophylline and other bronchodilators (e.g., epinephrine, isoproterenol, metaproterenol, albuterol, isoetharine); and calcium channel blockers (e.g., verapamil, nifedipine, diltiazem) may cause anxiety at therapeutic doses.

Other medications that have been reported to cause anxiety as a side effect include antihistamines, baclofen, cycloserine, indomethacin, oxymetazoline, and quinacrine.

13. What are some reasons primary care physicians may be hesitant to discuss an issue that causes anxiety in a particular patient?

1. Busy physicians may be concerned that such discussions will take too much valuable time. Simply acknowledging that a patient appears anxious may be sufficiently empathic to be calming. In general, this saves times because patients either may not return or may escalate their presenting symptoms (somatic, interpersonal, emotional) to ensure that they will be heard.

2. Conscientious physicians may feel "responsible" for solving the problem. Although few patients expect physicians to find solutions, most are grateful that someone is willing to listen. Often the more "helpless" the circumstances, the smaller the number of people who will listen; therefore, the patient is even more appreciative (and comforted) if the physician takes a few minutes to listen.

14. What clinical approaches to anxious patients may be useful?

The maxim **"Don't just do something; stand there,"** is important. Therefore, after ruling out medical etiologies, medication toxicity, and intoxication or withdrawal syndromes and reviewing the psychiatric history, the following guidelines may be considered for approaching anxious patients:

1. **Listen,** using a calm, responsive, but nondirect approach; do not rush to "solve" or "fix" the problem.

2. **Explore** the meaning of the illness, treatment, or situation for the patient.

3. **Target** the conscious reasons for the anxiety (e.g., fears of abandonment, dependency, and pain) by direct reassurance while continuing to listen for other concerns.

4. **Understand** that it may be difficult for the patient to identify the immediate cause of his or her anxiety but that the physician's willingness to listen may be directly calming.

5. **Assess** whether the anxiety is out of proportion to the situation and consider psychiatric consultation.

6. **Support** through continued discussions, marshalling the natural support network of friends and family or other support groups, trying to address concerns after they are identified, and considering pharmacologic approaches when indicated.

7. **Refer** to a psychiatrist if the patient is suicidal or symptoms continue to worsen despite initial interventions.

15. What conservative pharmacologic approaches may be safely used for anxiety?

When medical etiologies and intoxication or withdrawal syndromes have been ruled out, medication may be considered for a short time, along with supportive psychosocial and adjunctive approaches, such as meditation and relaxation exercises. SSRIs and benzodiazepines are highly effective agents, and patients should not be denied their benefits in bona fide circumstances. Benzodiazepines may be problematic because of their significant potential for tolerance and dependence; they should be used only after extensive patient education.

Paroxetine (Paxil), 10–30 mg, or sertraline (Zoloft), 25–50 mg, may be tried initially, with psychiatric consultation if further dosing adjustments are required.

Lorazepam (Ativan), 0.5–1.0 mg; clorazepate (Tranxene), 7.5–15 mg; or diazepam (Valium), 2–5 mg—all up to 3 times/day as needed for anxiety—may be considered when a trial with an SSRI has not worked or the severity of the anxiety or circumstances warrants. Lorazepam has the advantage of a relatively short half-life and metabolism through glucuronidation. Alprazolam (Xanax), 0.5 mg, also has a relatively short half-life, and patients occasionally experience minor withdrawal anxiety before the next scheduled dose. Patients should be warned about anxiety as a symptom of withdrawal and be educated about a time-limited course of medication in advance. Alprazolam may be difficult for patients to discontinue but may be considered specifically for severe panic attacks.

If the panic attacks are in the context of depressive symptoms, one of a variety of SSRIs such as paroxetine (Paxil), 20–60 mg, or sertraline (Zoloft), 50–150 mg, should be tried first. Clonazepam (Klonopin), 0.5 mg, is more useful for severe insomnia and agitation because of its relative potency and long half-life.

Buspirone (BuSpar), 5–20 mg three times/day, is a nonbenzodiazepine anxiolytic and may be tried before the benzodiazepines because of its lack of sedation and low abuse potential. However, the patient must generally follow a regular dosage pattern (three times/day) for several weeks before noticing a response. Buspirone is not useful on an as-needed basis and should not be used with monoamine oxidase inhibitors because of the possibility of hypertensive crisis. It may be effective in combination with an SSRI for combined anxiety and depression.

Low-dose atypical antipsychotics such as risperidone (0.5–1.0 mg), olanzapine (2.5 mg), or quetiapine (25 mg, administered at night) may be considered for patients with severe, disorganizing anxiety or incipient psychotic states, such as with borderline personality disorder or severe post-traumatic stress disorder.

Barbiturates are no longer indicated for anxiety or associated insomnia. Trazodone (Desyrel), 25–50 mg, may be useful for insomnia associated with anxiety if this is the primary symptom. A small dose of benzodiazepines for sleep or anxiety in patients suffering acute grief, on as as-needed basis for a few days, is often helpful.

After medications have been used, exploration of issues to identify sources of anxiety should continue, and nonpharmacologic approaches (e.g., meditation, self-relaxation exercises, support groups, counseling) should be encouraged.

BIBLIOGRAPHY

1. American Psychiatric Association: Diagnostic and Statistical Manual of Mental Disorders, 4th ed, text revision. Washington, DC, American Psychiatric Press, 2000.
2. Ballenger JC, Davidson JR, Lecrubier Y, et al: Consensus statement on transcultural issues in depression and anxiety from the International Consensus Group on Depression and Anxiety. J Clin Psychiatry 62 (suppl 13):47–55, 2001.
3. Barkin RL, Leikin JB, Barkin SJ: Noncardiac chest pain: A focus on psychogenic causes. Am J Ther 1:321–326, 1994.
4. Didden DG, Philbrick JT, Schorling JB: Anxiety and depression in an internal medicine resident continuity clinic: Difficult diagnoses. Int J Psychiatry Med 31:155–167, 2001.
5. Frank JB, Weihs K, Minerva E, Lieberman DZ: Women's mental health in primary care. Depression, anxiety, somatization, eating disorders, and substance abuse. Med Clin North Am 82:359–389, 1998.
6. Gater R, Tansella M, Korten A, et al: Sex differences in the prevalence and detection of depressive and anxiety disorders in general health care settings: Report from the World Health Organization Collaborative Study of Psychological Problems in General Health Care. Arch Gen Psychiatry 55:405–413, 1998.
7. Goldstein MZ: Depression and anxiety in older women. Prim Care 29:69–80, 2002.
8. Gross R, Olfson M, Gameroff M, et al: Borderline personality disorder in primary care. Arch Intern Med 162:53–60, 2002.
9. Harman JS, Rollman BL, Hanusa BH, et al: Physician office visits of adults for anxiety disorders in the United States, 1985–1998. J Gen Intern Med 17:165–172, 2002.
10. Jones GN, Ames SC, Jeffries SK, et al: Utilization of medical services and quality of life among low-income patients with generalized anxiety disorder attending primary care clinics. In J Psychiatry Med 31:182–198, 2001.
11. Kessler RC, McGonagle KA, Zhao S, et al: Lifetime and 12-month prevalence of DSM-III-R psychiatric disorders in the United States. Arch Gen Psychiatry 51:8–19, 1994.
12. Leon AC, Olfson M, Portera L: Service utilization and expenditures for the treatment of panic disorder. Gen Hosp Psychiatry 19:82–88, 1997.
13. Nisenson LG, Pepper CM, Schwenk TL, Coyne JC: The nature and prevalence of anxiety disorders in primary care. Gen Hosp Psychiatry 20:21–28, 1998.
14. Rickels K, Schweizer E: The clinical presentation of generalized anxiety in primary-care settings: Practical concepts of classification and management. J Clin Psychiatry 58:4–10, 1997.
15. Roy-Burne PP, Katon W: Generalized anxiety disorder in primary care: The precursor/modifier pathway to increased health care utilization. J Clin Psychiatry 58:34–38, 1997.
16. Wells K, Klap R, Koike A, et al: Ethnic disparities in unmet need for alcoholism, drug abuse, and mental health care. Am J Psychiatry 158:2027–2032, 2001.
17. Yudofsky SC, Hales RE (eds): The American Psychiatric Publishing Textbook of Neuropsychiatry and Clinical Neurosciences, 4th ed. Washington, DC, American Psychiatric Press, 2002.
18. Ziedonis D, Brady K: Dual diagnosis in primary care. Detecting and treating both the addiction and mental illness. Med Clin North Am 81:1017–1036, 1997.

12. PSYCHOSES

Joyce Seiko Kobayashi, M.D.

1. What are the common symptoms of a psychosis?

Psychotic symptoms generally reflect thinking that is out of touch with reality. Psychotic symptoms are often divided into **deficit symptoms,** which are discussed in relationship to schizophrenia (see question 11), and **positive symptoms,** which include the following:

- Auditory or visual hallucinations
- Delusions (paranoid, grandiose, romantic, jealous, mistaken identities, bizarre)
- Ideas of reference (e.g., a radio or television carrying a special message for an individual)
- Thought insertion
- Thought broadcasting
- Thought control
- Loosening of associations and disorganized thought process

2. How should primary care providers identify and assess positive psychotic symptoms?

Patients are often guarded about their unusual thoughts or may refer to their symptoms in colloquial or idiosyncratic terms. Frank psychotic symptoms may easily go unrecognized if not elicited by specifically asking about patients and observing unusual behaviors. Questions should be simple and nonthreatening, although the words used are less important than the customary ease in presentation, which the practitioner develops through routine and frequent use:

- Have you (ever) heard your name called, turned around, and no one was there? Do you ever hear voices or see things that others don't?
- Do you feel that strangers are staring at you, talking about you on the street, or know what you are thinking?
- Have you felt that you have special powers, such as being able to read other peoples' minds, or that your life has a special purpose or mission?
- Do you feel that the television or radio is talking directly to you or that people on television have special messages intended just for you?
- Do you (sometimes) feel that your thoughts are racing so fast that they feel out of control? Have you recently felt confused or had difficulty organizing your thoughts?

Observable behaviors include talking to oneself; sudden, intense staring in a different direction; hypervigilance; stereotypies; and compulsive or repetitive actions.

3. What are the most common psychoses or diagnoses that can present with psychotic symptoms in the primary care setting?

Delirium or dementia

Intoxication or withdrawal syndromes (substances or medications)

Schizophrenia or schizoaffective disorder

Mood disorder (depression, bipolar, or organic affective) with psychotic symptoms

4. Why should delirium be the first diagnosis considered in a patient with psychotic symptoms in the primary care setting?

1. It is often **iatrogenic,** particularly with medications in elderly individuals.

2. It may be the **initial presentation** of many serious and treatable medical disorders, but it must be recognized before treatment can start.

3. It is very **common,** particularly in high-risk populations (see question 11). A demented patient or a patient with an extensive history of alcohol abuse may become acutely delirious after taking a narcotic or anticholinergic medication. An elderly patient may present with delirium sec-

ondary to a simple urinary tract infection. In one study, up to 85% of terminally ill patients with cancer manifested delirium.

5. Define and characterize delirium.

Delirium is an acute change of mental status of organic cause with a primary disturbance of attention and cognition that may be associated with fluctuating levels of consciousness. It is characterized by abrupt onset (hours or days), distractibility or inability to sustain and focus attention, fluctuating course, confusion, and disorientation. Other common symptoms include visual hallucinations or perceptual disturbances, psychomotor agitation or retardation, disruption of sleep–wake cycles, and diurnal variation that is often referred to as *sundowning*. Although other common psychotic symptoms such as auditory hallucinations and delusions may be present, the diagnosis of *delirium should always be considered when a patient's speech is slurred, muttering, dysarthric, or incoherent* (see question 6).

6. What are some quick clues that can help differentiate a delirium from an axis I (DSM-IV-TR) psychiatric disorder? (See question 11 for more details about schizophrenia.)

DELIRIUM	PSYCHIATRIC DISORDER
The unfamiliar is misperceived as the familiar (e.g., mistaking a nurse for a relative).	The familiar is deemed unfamiliar (e.g., a relative replaced by an imposter).
Speech is dysarthric and muttering.	Speech is clearly articulated but bizarre.
Patients experience **illusions,** which are misperceptions of real stimuli.	Patients experience **hallucinations,** such as thinking a loud noise is gunfire or a light is a candle.
Disorientation and **emotional lability** fluctuate over the day and are often worse at night.	Disorientation and a changing level of consciousness are rare.
Distractibility is spurred by **external or physical** stimuli.	Distractibility is spurred by **internal or mental** stimuli.
Thought processes are **confused.**	Thought processes are connected by a **thread of associations.**
Thought content is **incoherent.**	Thought content is **nonsensical.**
Difficulties with word finding or memory fluctuate but are not the profound deficits observed with aphasia after a stroke or in dementia with profound memory loss.	
Specific motor symptoms such as **tremor, asterixis,** and **myoclonus** have sudden onset.	

7. Which conditions may predispose a patient to delirium?
- Age older than 65 years
- Underlying central nervous system disorders, including developmental disabilities, dementia, closed head injury
- Significant substance abuse history
- Advanced medical illness or organ failure
- Recent trauma or surgery

8. What are the common categories and some examples of the most common causes of delirium?
- Metabolic (hepatic or renal failure; fluid and electrolyte imbalance)
- Physiologic (hypoxia, hypertensive crisis)
- Infectious (meningitis)
- Trauma, structural, postsurgical
- Central nervous system or cerebrovascular disorders (tumor, stroke, hemorrhage)
- Toxins (medications, overdose, heavy metals)
- Intoxicants (illicit substances)

- Nutritional
- Hormonal (hyperthyroid)

9. List the most common categories of medications that may cause delirium in medically ill patients.

Although any psychoactive medication may cause a delirium at toxic levels, many medications are associated with delirium, even at therapeutic doses. It is also important to inquire about usage of herbal supplements.

Anticholinergics	Opiates
Antihistamines	Barbiturates
Antiparkinsonians	Benzodiazepines
Antiarrhythmics	Steroids
Antihypertensives	Sympathomimetics
Anticonvulsants	Beta-blockers

10. Are the terms *toxic psychosis, intensive care unit psychosis, organic psychosis,* and *metabolic encephalopathy* useful?

No. These earlier terms reflected the presumed etiology, but *delirium* should replace them. The term *organic mental syndrome* is still sometimes used when the condition is not defined clearly as delirium or dementia (or frequently a mixed picture). In general, however, terms such as *acute confusional state, reversible dementia,* and *cerebral insufficiency* should be discarded.

11. How is a delirium differentiated from schizophrenia?

	DELIRIUM	SCHIZOPHRENIA
Age at onset	> 5th decade of life	< 5th decade of life
Speech	May be dysarthric	Usually clear articulation
Hallucinations	Visual > auditory	Auditory > visual
Disorientation	Frequent	Uncommon
Memory	Often abnormal	May be normal
Confusion	Often complains about this	Rarely feels confused
Diurnal variation	May be worse at night (sundowning)	No change
Misinterpretation	Unfamiliar as familiar	Familiar as unfamiliar

The positive psychotic symptoms observed in schizophrenia usually occur in the context of a deteriorating level of function and are frequently associated with a more extensive course of deficit or *negative* symptoms, such as marked social isolation or withdrawal, peculiar or bizarre behavior, marked impairment in personal hygiene, blunted or inappropriate affect, poverty of speech or speech content, or marked lack of initiative. Formal diagnosis generally requires at least 1 week of positive psychotic symptoms within a 6-month period of deficit symptoms. If psychotic symptoms are not a result of delirium but are part of a schizophrenic or other formal psychiatric disorder, optimal management includes close collaboration with a psychiatrist, antipsychotic medications, and assignment of a case manager.

12. When are psychotic symptoms seen in a patient with dementia?

The diagnosis of dementia requires a primary disturbance in memory and new learning as well as secondary disturbances in higher cortical functions such as abstract reasoning, judgment, language, or personality. Patients are generally diagnosed with dementia before they experience frank psychotic symptoms. However, a surprisingly high percentage of patients with moderate to severe dementia of all causes may experience psychotic symptoms at some point in their illness, most commonly auditory or visual hallucinations or paranoid delusions.

Patients who are very forgetful or feel vulnerable because of becoming more disorganized may begin to believe that someone is taking their (misplaced) possessions or intends to harm them. Others who have difficulty hearing or who have little social contact may begin to talk to themselves or imagine visits from dead relatives. Diminished cognitive capacity may result in diminished ability to distinguish the real from the imaginary.

The possibility of superimposed delirium must always be considered in a demented patient with psychotic symptoms, particularly if the symptoms have an acute onset. In addition, many disorders that were historically described as secondary dementias because the cognitive symptoms are caused by a treatable or identifiable disease may present with mild cognitive dysfunction and prominent psychotic symptoms. Examples include porphyria, Huntington's chorea, endocrinopathies, nutritional deficiencies, temporal lobe epilepsy, and heavy metal toxicity.

Treatment of the delirium or secondary dementias obviously requires treatment of the underlying disorders, but psychotic symptoms of any cause are often ameliorated by very low doses of neuroleptics.

13. In which medical conditions may a mood disturbance be a prominent manifestation of delirium?

Steroid toxicity, hypo- and hypercalcemia, thyroid disease, and tertiary syphilis may result in prominent mood disturbances, although any delirious patient may intermittently manifest emotional lability.

14. In addition to schizophrenia and delirium, what disorders may present with psychotic symptoms?

1. **Mood disorders,** such as major depressive disorder and bipolar mood disorder (manic-depression), may or may not be associated with psychotic symptoms. Psychotic symptoms are usually congruent with the mood, such as delusions of guilt in depression or grandiose delusions in mania. Episodes frequently recur at variable intervals, but functioning generally returns to baseline with pharmacotherapy between episodes. There are seasonal affective disorders that are often triggered by the change of season, such as from winter to spring; mixed mood states (depressed mood with racing thoughts, manic irritability, or both); and rapid cycling disorders, which can vary from mania to depression within hours.

2. If psychotic symptoms persist in the presence and absence of a mood disorder (mood-incongruent psychotic symptoms), the diagnosis is usually **schizoaffective disorder,** which can present with a variety of mood subtypes.

3. The symptoms of a **brief reactive psychosis** are indistinguishable from psychotic symptoms that may occur in schizophrenia, but they appear in relationship to one or more markedly stressful events and resolve within a short period (usually within hours to a few weeks). Reactive psychosis is usually accompanied by significant emotional turmoil and is not associated with the gradual deterioration of function that often precedes a schizophrenic psychosis. A brief reactive psychosis may be observed in a patient who has been sexually assaulted, for example.

Formal diagnostic criteria for these and less common psychotic disorders may be found in the text revision of the fourth edition of the *Diagnostic and Statistical Manual of Mental Disorders* by the American Psychiatric Association (DSM-IV-TR). (See Chapter 11 for a description of DSM-IV-TR.) A discussion of psychotropic medication for each of these disorders is beyond the scope of this chapter.

15. What behavioral, environmental, and pharmacologic approaches are useful in treating the delirious patient with psychotic symptoms?

The initial treatment for a delirious patient must always be to treat all of the underlying medical conditions that could potentially cause the delirium. Other adjunctive approaches can be very helpful to patients while they stabilize because they are often frightened and confused. Some episodes of delirium have been so terrifying to patients who are afraid they may be "losing their minds" that they can develop a posttraumatic stress syndrome.

Interventions that help to orient the patient, structure activities, and make the environment feel more familiar are helpful. Strategies include introducing anyone who enters the patient's room and reminding the patient of the date and purpose of the visit; maintaining a regular daily schedule without abrupt changes in location; keeping a diary, appointment book, or calendar visible in the patient's room; having a night light, clock, and familiar objects nearby; asking friends or relatives to accompany or visit the patient frequently; keeping information and discussions simple, with frequent repetition; and writing down specific instructions about medications or activities.

Pharmacologic treatment for delirious patients, besides treating the underlying disorder, is usually a low-dose, antipsychotic medication such as risperidone (0.5–3.0 mg/day) in divided doses, which may be titrated slowly to the higher dose while monitoring for side effects (see question 16). For a highly agitated patient, limited use of a high-potency antipsychotic medication such as haloperidol (0.5–4.0 mg/day in divided doses) or trifluoperazine (1–4 mg/day in divided doses) may be considered. Olanzapine dissolvable wafers may be useful in patients who cannot swallow (2.5–5.0 mg/day). Quetiapine (25–50 mg) at night may be useful for nighttime sedation in addition to control of psychotic symptoms. Benzodiazepines may be useful (intramuscular injections of 1–2 mg) in the management of significant physical agitation, but the risk of further confusion requires restricting its use to these acute episodes.

16. What are common side effects of antipsychotic medications?

The most common side effects of antipsychotic medications derive from dopaminergic blockade of the extrapyramidal and tuberoinfundibular tracts causing movement disorders and hyperprolactinemia, respectively. Alpha-adrenergic blockade can result in orthostatic hypotension and anticholinergic (muscarinic) side effects, including dry mouth or sialorrhea and confusion. Movement disorders include acute dystonic reactions (stiffness) of the jaw, tongue, extraocular muscles, neck, back or extremities; Parkinsonian symptoms such as shuffling gait and flattened affect; akathisia (physical or subjective restlessness) and the long-term risk of tardive dyskinesia or choreoathetoid movements of the fingers, mouth, tongue, and feet. Hyperprolactinemia can be associated with galactorrhea and sexual dysfunction. Atypical or second-generation antipsychotic medications (risperidone, olanzapine, ziprasidone, quetiapine), which also affect serotonergic receptors, may be associated with significant weight gain, mood effects, and common extrapyramidal side effects, although usually to a lesser extent than high potency, first-generation antipsychotics such as haloperidol. The third-generation partial dopamine agonist antipsychotic aripiprazole is reported to have little weight gain and few extrapyramidal symptoms, but controlled trials are still limited.

17. What is the pathophysiology of delirium?

There are many differing hypotheses, based primarily on animal research involving neurotransmitter abnormalities; inflammatory response with increased cytokines; intraneuronal signal transduction or chemical messenger systems; increased activity of the hypothalamic-pituitary-adrenal axis; or changes in blood–brain barrier permeability.

Electroencephalographic studies correlate in severity of dysfunction with clinical symptoms and show general slowing in somnolent patients, but often low-voltage fast activity in agitated patients, such as in delirium tremens.

BIBLIOGRAPHY

1. American Psychiatric Association: Diagnostic and Statistical Manual of Mental Disorders, 4th ed., text revision. Washington, DC, American Psychiatric Press, 2000.
2. Bowles TM, Levin GM: Aripiprazole: A new atypical antipsychotic drug. Ann Pharmacother 37:687–694, 2003.
3. Desai MM, Rosenheck RA, Kasprow WJ: Determinants of receipt of ambulatory medical care in a national sample of mentally ill homeless veterans. Med Care 41:275–287, 2003.
4. Dolder CR, Lacro JP, Jeste DV: Adherence to antipsychotic and nonpsychiatric medications in middle-aged and older patients with psychotic disorders. Psychosom Med 65:156–162, 2003.
5. Duggan L, Fenton M, Dardennes RM, et al: Olanzapine for schizophrenia. Cochrane Database Syst Rev (1):CD001359, 2003.
6. Goetzel RZ, Hawkins K, Ozminkowski RJ, Wang S: The health and productivity cost burden of the "top

10" physical and mental health conditions affecting six large U.S. employers in 1999. J Occup Environ Med 45:5–14, 2003.

7. Jacobson SA: Delirium in the elderly. Psychiatry Clin North Am 20:91–110, 1997.
8. Krystal JH, D'Souza DC, Sanacora G, et al: Current perspectives on the pathophysiology of schizophrenia, depression, and anxiety disorders. Med Clin North Am 85:559–577, 2001.
9. Kumar C, McIvor RJ, Davies T, et al: Estrogen administration does not reduce the rate of recurrence of affective psychosis after childbirth. J Clin Psychiatry 64:112–118, 2003.
10. McCracken JT, McGough J, Shah B, et al: Risperidone in children with autism and serious behavioral problems. N Engl J Med 347:314–321, 2002.
11. Nasrallah HA, Tandon R: Efficacy, safety, and tolerability of quetiapine in patients with schizophrenia. J Clin Psychiatry 63(supp 13):12–20, 2002.
12. Rothschild AJ: Challenges in the treatment of depression with psychotic features. Biol Psychiatry 53:680–690, 2003.
13. Sajatovic M, Mullen JA, Sweitzer DE: Efficacy of quetiapine and risperidone against depressive symptoms in outpatients with psychosis. J Clin Psychiatry 63:1156–1163, 2002.
14. Trzepaca PT: Delirium: Advances in diagnosis, pathophysiology, and treatment. Psychiatry Clin North Am 19:429–448, 1996.

13. THE DIFFICULT PERSONALITY

John F. Bridges, M.D.

1. What is personality?

Although it is a common and intuitive concept, *personality* is a difficult term to define with specificity and completeness. Personality encompasses both internal perceptions of the self and the world and the activity of the self in the world (as objectively experienced and described by others). In addition, personality describes perceptions and actions that are consistent through time and characterize an individual with both biologic inborn traits and capacities (temperament) and acquired learned responses (character).

Most current understandings of personality suggest that inborn capacities and limitations interact with the accidents of environmental advantages and deficiencies to unfold the internal psychological structures and externally revealed patterns of behavior that we call personality.

2. When do personality traits become a personality disorder?

Constellations of personality traits that assume enduring, rigid patterns of maladaptive response to the stressors of life form the bases of a personality disorder.

3. Describe the salient features of the three major groups of personality disorders.

Ten personality disorders are grouped into three clusters (A–C). Disorders within clusters appear to share common features that suggest relationships among them. The clustering also acknowledges a high degree of overlap in symptomatology.

Cluster A: Persons who are unusual, odd, or eccentric in their thinking and appearance
- *Paranoid personality disorder*—characterized by a perception of others as motivated by a desire to harm or demean, a questioning of the trustworthiness of others, the bearing of grudges, and a tendency to be easily slighted and to find hidden meanings in the actions or words of others, confirming suspicions and mistrust.
- *Schizoid personality disorder*—characterized by a restriction in the capacity for social connection and an inability to feel or express emotions, the choice of solitary lifestyle, denial of the subjective experience of strong emotions, little affect expression, and apparent indifference to social, sexual, and emotional intimacy.

- *Schizotypal personality disorder*—characterized by the deficits in interpersonal connection of schizoid personality disorder with the additional features of oddities in thinking and behavior that share common themes with schizophrenia (though not as severe) and paranoid personality disorder, such as suspiciousness, ideas of reference, magical thinking, and additionally displaying quirky modes of speech, dress, and manner.

Cluster B: Persons who are dramatic and highly emotional and engage in erratic behaviors

- *Antisocial personality disorder*—characterized by irresponsible behaviors, beginning in adolescence and carrying through to an adulthood of inconsistent work and social relationships, failure to conform to social norms, disregard for truth, impulsiveness, aggression, reckless behaviors, and lack of remorse for injuries to others.
- *Borderline personality disorder*—characterized by unstable moods, relationships, and identity; impulsiveness, with intense emotional reactions leading to reckless self-damaging behaviors, suicide threats and attempts, an impaired ability to regulate moods and mood-dictated expressions of anger and other strongly felt feeling states, and transient paranoid ideation.
- *Histrionic personality disorder*—characterized by extreme and inappropriate emotionality, with seductive sexualized interactions with others, fluctuating extremes of feeling states often dramatically demonstrated, low frustration tolerance and preoccupation with immediate gratification, and vague, shallow, impressionistic speech.
- *Narcissistic personality disorder*—characterized by imagined or enacted grandiosity in the absence of empathic connection with others, an easily injured and highly overvalued sense of self-importance, an unrealistic sense of uniqueness in a context of interpersonal callousness, entitlement, and demand for attention.

Cluster C: Persons with excessive fearfulness and anxiety

- *Avoidant personality disorder*—characterized by social discomfort based on a pervasive fear of being negatively judged, an inability to tolerate disapproval, a need for guarantees of acceptance, and an unwillingness to engage in social and interpersonal engagements that risk exposure to these fearsome situations.
- *Dependent personality disorder*—characterized by pervasive dependent behavior and fear of interpersonal loss leading to an unwillingness to take chances, express opinions, make decisions, or undertake projects for fear of severing overvalued connections with others, with attendant feelings of abandonment and loss when even small rifts occur in relationships.
- *Obsessive-compulsive personality disorder*—characterized by inflexible demands for perfectionism that interfere with functioning; demands for submission by others to unreasonable standards; preoccupation with rules, details, right and wrong; and a marked lack of generosity in dealing with others.

Personality disorders under investigation for inclusion

- *Passive-aggressive personality disorder* (negativistic personality disorder)—characterized by a passive opposition to the demands of life, leading to an impaired capacity to work and accomplish goals, with irritable and oppositional responses to authority, deliberate procrastination, protestations of unreasonable expectations and personal misfortune, overevaluation of actual performance, and a concerted critical obstructionist stance to undertakings involving others coupled with feelings of being unappreciated.
- *Depressive personality disorder*—characterized by pervasive and nearly continuous feelings of gloom and hopelessness, low self-concept with a critical attacking attitude toward the self; persistent worry; blaming of others and self; and overall harboring a guilty, sad, unhappy view of life.

4. Are children and adolescents diagnosed with personality disorders?

Not usually. Because personality is presumed to be determined only partly by inborn traits or temperament, psychiatrists are wary of applying personality disorder diagnoses to youngsters. As defining criteria, such disorders have maladaptive long-term functioning and inflexible traits. It is the nature of human development over the entire life-span, and perhaps most prominently during the first 20 years of life, to try various methods of responding to and exploring the world. This process necessarily involves many responses that are less than ideally adaptive and fruitful.

5. Do excessive characteristics in childhood herald adult personality disorders?
Perhaps. Certain childhood disorders, diagnosed in persons under 18 years of age, appear to bear some relationship to the later development of personality disorders.

Disorder of childhood/adolescence	Personality disorder
Conduct disorder	Antisocial personality disorder
Avoidant disorder of childhood	Avoidant personality disorder
Identity disorder	Borderline personality disorder

6. What overall characteristics suggest the possibility of a personality disorder?
One of the hallmarks of a personality disorder is that the patient does not accept personal responsibility for the subjective distress that he or she experiences. A second hallmark is that the disorder is observable within the context of human relationships. The invisibility of the source of the problems to the patient is called *ego syntonicity*. To the patient, the problem lies not with the self but with others. Thus, the paranoid patient does not see suspicion and mistrust as excessive, out of context, or causing repeated failures in relationships. Such perceptions appear to be justified and reasonable responses to the measureless potential for injury in everyday life. Similarly, the narcissistic patient does not complain about the relentlessly alienating effects of grandiose and unempathic exploitation of others; rather, the patient complains about the infuriating and hurtful sense of living in a world of persons who do not afford him or her appropriate credit and admiration.

7. What reactions in the caregiver may suggest that the patient has a personality disorder?
Clinicians usually discover the presence of a personality disorder in the context of attempting to provide care for the patient. They find unexpectedly that delivery of care becomes increasingly difficult, apparently troublesome for both physician and patient. Such patients engender powerful responses from the caregivers, as they have from families, friends, and employers; they are irritating, frustrating, and maddening and evoke exaggerated responses from others. In addition, given the ego syntonicity of the symptoms, the caregiver may frequently be seen as the source of the patient's distress.

8. Before diagnosing a personality disorder, what common organic causes of abnormal behavior should be considered?
Personality disorders may be mimicked by various organic disorders as well as by other mental illnesses. Three common medical conditions may cause symptoms that appear similar to those described for personality disorders:
1. **Dementias of senile or presenile onset.** Such patients frequently present with behavioral problems, including irritability, paranoia, anger, and impulsiveness. They may demonstrate the exact symptoms of a disordered personality and elicit from family and friends the same avoidance and anger. The insidious onset masks such dementias, as does the tendency of patients, at least initially, to become exaggerated versions of their former selves. For example, the man who was occasionally irritable and picky gradually becomes an angry, hypercritical caricature of himself, or the sentimental, easily injured woman evolves into a weepy, irrationally inconsolable burlesque of her former self.
2. **Chronic use of certain prescribed medicines.** Chronic changes in mood and attitude may result from certain long-term drug therapies to which both patient and family have become inured. For example, even digitalis may induce chronic depression and paranoia. The differential diagnosis may require subtle questioning about the onset and progression of changes that are nearly invisible to patient or family.
3. **Substance abuse.** Substance abuse, especially alcohol abuse, in a patient or perhaps even in a patient's family may distort personality development and alter long-term patterns. Some re-

search suggests that commencement or cessation of substance use, over time, may radically alter personality style and functioning.

9. What classic patient–caregiver difficulties may occur with patients who have personality disorders or certain personality traits?

Patients with personality disorders can be extremely exasperating to treat. They approach the physician with admixtures of deep-seated fears and suspicions, unbounded wishes for dependency and caretaking, and profoundly distorted views of themselves and their doctors. Although the problems may not be appreciated by the clinician at the onset of the doctor–patient relationship, they soon manifest as characteristic and unwanted feelings and responses from the physician.

The hostile patient. Hostility from a patient is a surprise to clinicians accustomed to grateful and obedient responses. Patients who are paranoid or worried about their vulnerability easily perceive the doctor-patient relationship as unequal (as, in fact, it is) and compromising. They see the physician's ministrations as intrusive and threatening. Such anxiety is rationalized by attacking the physician, devaluing his or her motives, and questioning every decision. This response at first puzzles and later angers the doctor. It flies directly in the face of how physicians see themselves and prefer to be seen by others. Actual care for the patient quickly withers under the barrage of implied or expressed accusation. The doctor soon feels reluctant to pursue appropriate follow-up or to recommend difficult treatments, because he or she no longer wishes to be subjected to hostility and misunderstanding.

The dependent, demanding patient. Dependent patients with powerful wishes for unlimited nurturing initially may be welcomed by the physician, who is perceived as extremely competent and uniquely helpful. The physician responds by returning the patient's admiration and offering more explanations and thoroughness in treatment. Soon, however, such patients reveal an inexpressibly great need for attention. They increase their demands for time, advice, and contact. The physician begins to feel hounded and guilty for not responding wholeheartedly to the increasing demands. Eventually the physician withdraws, puts up barriers, and finds ways to avoid the patient. The patient responds with intensified demands for care and anger at the (accurate) perception of rejection. Thus rigorous medical care falters and fails.

The doctor defeater. Such patients may display paranoia, an exaggerated sense of self-worth, or wildly fluctuating attitudes toward themselves and the caretaker. Some patients seem to choose behaviors obviously in direct opposition to their own best interests. The common thread in their relations with physicians is the unremitting demand for care and the adamant refusal to acknowledge that any treatment is adequate or helpful. The physician becomes increasingly angry at such patients, often expressing the anger as jokes about the patient or benign neglect of the patient's complaints. The wish that the patient would "just go away" may be contrary to the physician's ideal self-image and may even result in stubborn attempts to "save" the patient.

In all of these cases—and their many permutations—the patient's mode of interaction is unexpected and misunderstood by the physician. The patient unknowingly frustrates and alienates the physician. The physician, also unknowingly, may take countermeasures in an attempt to proceed with "business as usual," not recognizing that medical reasoning and delivery of care are hampered by the deterioration in the relationship itself.

10. What guidelines should the physician use in caring for the patient with difficult personality traits or a frank personality disorder?

Dealing with patients whose illness manifests in the doctor–patient relationship is not easy. Nor is it easy for the patient, who has a lifetime of failed attempts to relate and to satisfy needs and whose pain over time is enormous. The following guidelines are useful:

1. Recognize the problem by using your own feelings as guides. Take note when you find yourself dreading a patient, imagining the patient on someone else's service, joking about the patient, or arguing with yourself about whether it is necessary to like a patient in order to provide adequate care.

2. Identify what behaviors are affecting the patient's medical care. Discuss the patient with a colleague. Step outside the dysfunctional relationship, and apply diagnostic thinking to the relationship itself. For example, the patient's relentless telephone contact may cause you to pull away, or the insistent demand for ever more and better tests to prove you "wrong" ("I'm sure you're hiding something from me, doctor") or the patient "right" ("I'm just another check in the mail for you, doctor, so I've got to watch out for myself") may force you into practicing defensively and therefore inefficiently.

3. Determine the best way to confront the patient's behavior and spell out its consequences. It is advisable to be consistent with your diagnosis of the problem. For example, the dependent worrier who fears abandonment may be told: "All of these phone calls are making it hard to determine when you really need my help, and they come at times when I cannot think as clearly as I'd like about your problems. I think it best if you save your unscheduled calls for clear medical emergencies, but why don't you give me a call each week when I can make sure that I will have time to talk with you? Wednesdays after my clinic hours make the most sense."

For the hostile patient whose angry accusations and demeaning attacks betray a fear of dependency and damage, a realistic and reassuring approach that shares control may help the relationship: "It can be very hard to feel that you are putting yourself in someone else's hands when you are ill. I want to make certain that you clearly understand what I'm recommending and that you have as much time as you need to ask questions about how the treatment will work. I want you to feel free to tell me what your worries are. We will need to work together closely on this."

For the self-defeating obstructor, awareness of his or her control and the physician's relative lack of power is essential. The approach to such patients must be both humble and frank with change in behavior couched as a choice rather than a demand: "Drinking as much and as often as you do puts you at great risk. I think that you understand by now how dangerous it is. I can offer some suggestions again for what measures you can take to stop drinking and offer my support, but finally you will have to decide whether or not to do what is best for your health."

11. Is it appropriate for a physician to refer to a colleague a patient who evokes irreconcilable conflict?

Yes. Patients are best treated by physicians who can care about them in a genuine way. This caring may find its highest expression in the ability to tolerate the patient's behavior without becoming personally upset. Each physician has certain strengths and weaknesses in this regard. Part of delivering the best possible care is recognizing limitations and the point at which the ability to offer thoughtful, objective care has become compromised. Just as physicians cannot expect to give good care when they are deprived of sleep or in the midst of a personal crisis, so they cannot expect to be capable of caring for every sort of problem patient.

If a patient presents impossible conflicts for the physician, it is the physician's right and responsibility to refer the patient to another practitioner from whom the patient may expect medical care uncompromised by negative feelings. This transfer should be undertaken openly, and the physician to whom the patient is referred should be told of the problems in advance. Alternatively, it may be helpful to share the care of such patients in an attempt to dilute the intensity of the conflicts.

12. Is referral to a psychiatrist appropriate in the care of patients with difficult personalities?

Yes. Although such patients frequently resent, and recoil from, referral to psychiatrists, it often is profitable to obtain a psychiatric consultation for the patient with a personality disorder or a difficult personality. A psychiatrist may be able to clarify the patterns of the patient's undermining of the relationship and offer suggestions about ways to deal with the conflicts.

13. Are personality disorders necessarily a predictor of medical outcome?

The *Diagnostic and Statistical Manual of Mental Disorders,* 4th edition, text revision (DSM-IV-TR), defines the interaction of psychological factors and medical conditions in a definite and prescribed manner. Without recognition of many specific ongoing disorders, treatment may be difficult, if not seemingly impossible. For a clinician this problem can be perplexing and seemingly insurmountable. The clinician must be aware of coexisting conditinos and understand their impact on attempts to care for the patient.

14. Do psychological disorders directly affect delivery of care?

Absolutely. Many varied psychological disorders other than depression can affect the delivery of care. An example is the patient with known disease who requires frequent follow-up but consistently misses appointments, even to the extent of endangering self and personal health. This pattern of behavior may be the result of true agoraphobia or other problems rather than denial of disease, "laziness," or noncompliance, as frequently stated by the provider.

15. What is somatoform disorder?

As opposed to factitious disorder or malingering, the symptoms are not intentionally produced, and secondary gain is often obscure if not nonexistent. The disorder begins before the age of 30 years and usually results in many visits to physicians in various areas and specialties with progressive deterioration in levels of function in interpersonal, social, employment, and other areas of life. The DSM-IV-TR describes specific criteria for the diagnosis:

1. **Four pain symptoms:** pain related to four different sites or functions.
2. **Two gastrointestinal symptoms** other than pain (e.g., bloating, vomiting, reaction to many different foods)
3. **One sexual symptom** other than pain (e.g., erectile dysfunction, menstrual problems)
4. **One pseudoneurologic symptom** (e.g., dizziness, local weakness, visual problems, taste problems)

For a definitive diagnosis, medical investigation of the above complaints must rule out substance abuse. If a medical condition does exist, the level of symptoms and their effect on the patient's life outweigh all physical findings.

16. Give examples of somatoform disorder.

Conversion disorder, pain disorder, hypochondriasis, and body dysmorphic disorder.

17. What are the ways in which a physician can treat patients with somatoform disorders?

Somatoform disorder is difficult to work with and frequently leads to feelings of frustration and helplessness on the physician's part. Despite frustration at numerous setbacks and seemingly unsuccessful outcomes, these disorders provide a great challenge in terms of treatment. Because little intentional behavior is associated with these disorders, helping patients recognize the psychological nature of their illness is of great importance. The most important point for the clinician to realize is that the often bizarre patterns of symptoms present a real problem for the patient. It is essential (as well as prudent both ethically and legally) to investigate all complaints in a reasonable and timely manner. However, one should not continually repeat previously negative tests if the same conditions recur with regular frequency. Likewise, repeating radiologic exams is wasteful and can feed into the fear and dependence with which these patients frequently exit their relationships with health care workers. Patients should be listened to and their complaints taken seriously, but it is essential to set limits. Frequent initial visits with gradual lengthening of intervals have proved highly effective. Directly addressing repetitive complaints with reassurance of negative testing may lead to anger on the part of the patient, but doing so in a nonthreatening, supportive manner can help decrease the level of the patient's complaints. It is also important to have strict rules in terms of visiting other clinicians for repetitive exams, receiving prescriptions from other sources, and frequency of calls and unscheduled visits.

18. What problems may the physician encounter when working with patients with somatoform disorder?

Perhaps the most common and difficult problems for the physician are related to personal attitudes and professional ego and self-image. Because these disorders often stem from early and deep psychological and physical abuse, the pattern of self-defeating behavior and unconscious sense of punishment leads to common and frequent treatment failures. Patients tend to experience many regressions, usually as their condition seems to be improving (the sense of "not deserving" to be well is a prime factor in this process), and may challenge the physician's expertise. Often the patient fires the physician, citing incompetence or other failings as the reason. Although such behavior can be frustrating (to say the least), the treating physician must not express feelings of anger against the patient, either directly or indirectly. Such control may seem difficult, but one must keep in mind the dictum "to do no harm" and treat the patient rather than oneself.

19. What is factitious disorder?

Factitious disorder and malingering are similar in that both involve the intentional expression of physical or psychological illnesses that in fact are not present. Generally, as defined in DSM-IV-TR, no external incentive (e.g., legal action, monetary gain, time from work) is related to factitious disorder. Rather, the incentive is to assume the sick role for attention or to gain sense of self-worth.

20. How does one approach a patient with chronic pain?

Chronic pain is another difficult situation for the clinician to manage. Many patients suffer from their condition for years and are shunted from practitioner to practitioner. Despite significant crossover with many of the situations discussed above, the patient with chronic pain is often mislabeled as having primarily a psychological problem. Yet the psychological problems generally result from the effect of the pain on the patient's life. The best approach is to believe what the patient tells you. Chronic pain differs from acute pain not only in duration of symptoms but also in the relatively normal results obtained from investigations. Many of these syndromes are related to injuries in the distant past that have healed yet predispose the patient to a constellation of progressive symptoms through pathways that at present are poorly understood. It is important to develop a frank relationship with such patients. From the beginning, reasonable expectations and plans should be developed. Any apprehensions or unreasonable hopes on the part of the patient should be addressed at the beginning of the relationship. Generally, an ongoing and open dialogue helps to facilitate interactions with such patients.

BIBLIOGRAPHY

1. American Psychiatric Association: Diagnostic and Statistical Manual of Mental Disorders, 4th ed, text revision. Washington, DC, American Psychiatric Association, 2000.
2. Cloninger CR, Svrakic DM, Przybeck TR: A psychobiological model of temperament and character. Arch Gen Psychiatry 50:975–990, 1993.
3. Morey L: Personality disorders in DSM-III and DSM-III-R: Convergence, coverage, and internal consistency. Am J Psychiatry 145:573–577, 1988.
4. Nestadt G, Romanoski AJ, Samuels JF, et al: The relationship between personality and DSM-III axis I isorders in the population: Results from an epidemiological survey. Am J Psychiatry 149:1228–1233, 1992.
5. Perry JC: Problems and considerations in the valid assessment of personality disorders. Am J Psychiatry 149:1645–1653, 1992.
6. Sadock BJ, Sadock VA (eds): Kaplan & Sadock's Comprehensive Textbook of Psychiatry, 7th ed. Philadelphia, Lippincott Williams & Wilkins, 2000.
7. Stone MH: Abnormalities of Personality. New York, W.W. Norton, 1993.
8. Svrakic DM, Whitehead C, Przybeck TR, Cloninger CR: Differential diagnosis of personality disorders by the seven factor model of temperament and character. Arch Gen Psychiatry 50:991–999, 1993.
9. Valliant GE: Adaptation to Life. Cambridge, Harvard University Press, 1998.
10. Widiger TA, Frances A, Spitzer RL, Williams JBW: The DSM-III-R personality disorders: An overview. Am J Psychiatry 145:786–795, 1988.

III. Primary Disorders of the Cardiovascular System

14. HYPERTENSION

Nathaniel Winer, M.D., and Stuart L. Linas, M.D.

1. When is a patient hypertensive?

Although a patient is considered to be hypertensive when the average of two or more measurements taken over 4 weeks detects systolic blood pressure of 140 mmHg and/or diastolic blood pressure of $\geq$ 90 mmHg, Framingham Heart Study data show that persons with high-normal blood pressure (135–139/85–89 mmHg) are at increased risk of major cardiovascular events, compared to those with optimal blood pressure (< 120/80 mmHg). Clinical trials will be required to determine whether pharmacologic or other treatment will benefit subjects with high-normal blood pressure. Patients with initial blood pressure of 140–159/90–99 mmHg (stage 1) should be reevaluated within 2 months; those with blood pressure > 180/110 (stage 3) should be referred for care within 1 week or referred for care immediately if risk factors or evidence of target organ damage are present.

2. Why should hypertension be treated?

Hypertension is a major risk factor for coronary, cerebral, and renal vascular disease. The Framingham Heart Study cohort demonstrated a statistically significant, progressive increase in coronary heart disease with increases in either systolic or diastolic blood pressure. Systolic blood pressure and pulse pressure correlate better with morbidity and mortality than diastolic blood pressure. Considerable evidence suggests that antihypertensive drug therapy reduces stroke and renal disease.

3. Does treatment of systolic hypertension alter outcome in elderly patients?

Yes. The Systolic Hypertension in the Elderly Program (SHEP), a large multicenter, randomized, placebo-controlled, blinded study, followed patients with a mean age of 72 years, an average systolic blood pressure of 170 mmHg, and diastolic blood pressure < 90 mmHg. Patients were randomized to treatment with a diuretic- and beta-blocker-based regimen aimed at reducing systolic blood pressure to less than 160 mmHg. Results showed a 36% reduction in the incidence of stroke and a 27% reduction in the incidence of nonfatal myocardial infarction and death in the treatment versus placebo groups. Treatment of a similar population with the calcium antagonist nitrendipine showed comparable reductions in strokes and heart attacks (Syst-Eur study). Recent clinical trials in older high-risk populations have shown that cardiovascular outcomes are significantly improved with either angiotensin-converting enzyme (ACE) inhibitor therapy (HOPE) or angiotensin II receptor antagonist treatment (LIFE).

4. What is the combined effect of elevated levels of serum cholesterol, smoking, and hypertension on the rate of death from coronary heart disease?

Of the 316,099 men screened in the Multiple Risk Factor Intervention Trial (MRFIT), the rate of death from coronary heart disease (CHD) was 230 times greater in smokers with a cholesterol level and systolic blood pressure in the highest quintile than in nonsmokers with a systolic pressure and cholesterol level in the lowest quintile. The study found a strong graded relationship between death due to CHD and an increase in systolic and diastolic blood pressure or cholesterol levels above 4.65 mmol/L (180 mg/dl).

5. Does therapy for hypertension influence left ventricular hypertrophy?

Yes. Major advances in understanding the relationship between hypertension and left ventricular hypertrophy (LVH) have been made. LVH, which is found in 50% of all hypertensive patients by echocardiography (5% by electrocardiogram), is a major risk factor for adverse cardiovascular outcomes, such as myocardial ischemia and infarction, congestive heart failure, and sudden death. Meta-analyses of clinical trial data show that ACE inhibitors are more effective in regressing LVH than calcium channel antagonists, beta-blockers, diuretics, or direct-acting vasodilators. The LIFE trial showed that angiotensin II receptor antagonist treatment also improved mortality and morbidity in high-risk older individuals with electrocardiographic evidence of LVH.

6. Describe the relationship between hypertension and abnormal carbohydrate metabolism.

Essential hypertension frequently clusters with insulin resistance, central obesity, glucose intolerance, hyperinsulinemia, overt diabetes, salt sensitivity, endothelial dysfunction, abnormal coagulation or fibrinolysis, LVH, and coronary artery disease (CAD). Although beta-blockers have been reported to increase the risk for developing diabetes, new-onset diabetes was decreased by approximately 30% with ACE inhibitor treatment in the HOPE trial and to a lesser extent with angiotensin II receptor antagonist therapy in the RENAAL trial.

7. When should secondary hypertension be suspected?

Traditionally, < 5% of patients with essential hypertension have been considered to have an identifiable, perhaps even curable, cause of hypertension; however, the increasing recognition of primary aldosteronism may expand this estimate. In patients with a diagnosis of essential hypertension, 8–10% may have underlying primary aldosteronism. Other causes of secondary hypertension include chronic renal insufficiency, renovascular stenosis, pheochromocytoma, Cushing's syndrome, oral contraceptive administration, illicit drug use, coarctation of the aorta, and rare monogeneic defects such as glucocorticoid-remediable hyperaldosteronism, Liddle's syndrome, and the syndrome of apparent mineralocorticoid excess. Secondary hypertension should be suspected in patients with (1) hypertension discovered at an early age (teenage or younger); (2) physical findings of Cushing's syndrome, (3) poorly controlled hypertension on three or more antihypertensive medications, one of which is a diuretic, and (4) spontaneous or diuretic-induced hypokalemia. Hypokalemia, formerly the hallmark of primary aldosteronism, is seen in less than one-half of patients with this disorder.

8. How may the history, physical examination, and initial laboratory data provide clues to the possible etiology of secondary hypertension?

A thorough history, physical examination, and laboratory studies should be performed to identify causes of secondary hypertension. Renovascular hypertension should be suspected in patients younger than 35 years, particularly women in whom fibromuscular dysplasia is more common, and in older patients with an abrupt worsening of blood pressure, especially in the presence of an abdominal bruit or evidence of other vascular disease (cerebral coronary or peripheral). Oral contraceptives are now an uncommon cause of secondary hypertension in women since the advent of low-dose estrogen pills. A history of the five P's (high blood *p*ressure, head *p*ain, *p*alpitations, *p*erspiration, and *p*allor) may suggest pheochromocytoma, but a Mayo Clinic retrospective study found that only about 25% of patients with pheochromocytoma at autopsy were diagnosed during life. The suspicion of Cushing's syndrome should be heightened in patients with centripetal obesity, moon facies, and striae who may have suffered a vertebral fracture or who present with an opportunistic infection. Coarctation of the aorta should be considered if blood pressures are lower in the legs than in the arms. Elevated serum creatinine or a decreased creatinine clearance suggests renal parenchymal disease.

9. When should the diagnosis of renovascular hypertension be pursued?

The prevalence of renovascular hypertension among a general population of hypertensive patients is 0.5%, a rate much lower than prior estimates of 5%, but the rate rises with increasing clinical suspicion. Renovascular hypertension should be considered in patients with:

- Severe hypertension (diastolic blood pressure > 120 mmHg)
- Hypertension refractory to treatment
- Abrupt onset of sustained moderate-to-severe hypertension at age < 20 years or > 50 years
- Hypertension with abdominal or femoral bruits
- > 25% increase of creatinine after initiation of ACE inhibitors
- Flash pulmonary edema with occlusive vascular disease

In these subsets of patients the incidence of renovascular hypertension is as high as 15%.

10. How should renovascular hypertension be evaluated?

Noninvasive tests have a high predictive value in diagnosing renovascular hypertension. Plasma renin activity (PRA) after administration of captopril and captopril renography have a sensitivity and specificity of > 90%. Random PRA, intravenous pyelography (IVP), and renography have not been shown to be useful. Magnetic resonance angiography (MRA) and duplex Doppler ultrasound of the renal arteries may be useful, but the latter procedure is highly operator-dependent.

11. Describe the most cost-effective evaluation of hypertension associated with hypokalemia.

Although diuretic therapy may give rise to hypokalemia, any patient who develops hypokalemia on diuretic therapy or has unprovoked hypokalemia should be investigated for primary aldosteronism. After potassium repletion and discontinuation of beta-blocker treatment, a random serum aldosterone and PRA should be obtained. If the aldosterone-to-renin (A/R) ratio is > 15 and serum aldosterone is ≥ 15 ng/ml, then further evaluation for primary aldosteronism is warranted. ACE inhibitor or diuretic therapy need not be discontinued prior to screening because suppression of renin activity in the face of these agents is even more persuasive evidence of primary aldosteronism. If the A/R ratio is elevated, a 24-hour urine collection for aldosterone, sodium, and creatinine should be obtained. Excretion of aldosterone > 14 µg/day and sodium ≥ 200 mg/day indicates lack of suppressability of aldosterone secretion and confirms the diagnosis of primary aldosteronism. If sodium is < 200 mEq/day, the 24-hour urine collection can be repeated after the patient has consumed a dietary sodium supplement of 10 gm/day for 3–5 days. An abdominal CT scan with thin slices through the adrenal glands can be performed; however, often an adrenal mass is not visualized or the findings are equivocal. The most reliable procedure for differentiating an adrenal adenoma from bilateral hyperplasia is adrenal vein sampling, provided an interventional radiologist experienced in this procedure is available. Laparoscopic adrenalectomy can be performed in patients with a unilateral adrenal adenoma; patients with bilateral adrenal hyperplasia can be treated with an aldosterone antagonist, such as spironolactone.

12. What is the significance of high-normal blood pressure?

As discussed above, patients with high-normal blood pressure (135–139/85–89 mmHg) are at increased risk for cardiovascular events. Because clinical trials evaluating pharmacologic intervention in this group have not yet been conducted, hygienic measures, such as the DASH diet (Dietary Approaches to Stop Hypertension; a menu consisting of salt restriction, fiber, fruits, and nuts), limitation of alcohol intake to two drinks per day, and weight reduction would be appropriate.

13. When and how should one initiate therapy for hypertension?

Patients with stage 1 hypertension (140–159/90–99 mmHg) may be treated with lifestyle modification for up to 12 months in the absence of risk factors, target organ disease (TOD), or clinical cardiovascular disease (CCD). Lifestyle modifications include the hygienic measures indicated above, regular, mild or moderate physical activity 3 times/week, and smoking cessation. If at least one risk factor is present but TOD and CCD are absent, lifestyle changes may be tried for up to 6 months. For patients with TOD, CCD, or diabetes with blood pressure > 140/90 mmHg, pharmacologic therapy should be initiated immediately. Because optimal blood pressure control will often require three or more antihypertensive drugs, initiation of therapy with combinations of antihypertensive agents may achieve target blood pressure goals more rapidly than a "stepped" care approach.

14. What is the single most important cause of inadequate blood pressure control?

Data from the National Health and Nutrition Examination Surveys (NHANES) indicate that about 27% of adults with hypertension in the United States have blood pressure controlled to < 140/90 mmHg. The major cause of poor control is patient nonadherence and physician reluctance to prescribe an adequate number of drugs in appropriate doses. Fewer than 50% of patients with high blood pressure keep follow-up appointments, and only 40% take their medications as prescribed. Barriers to adequate blood pressure control include poor doctor–patient communication, cost of medications, and side effects. Newer classes of antihypertensive agents, such as angiotensin II receptor antagonists, have favorable side effect profiles, which promote better patient adherence.

15. How do lifestyle modifications improve hypertension?

Lifestyle modifications may be used as primary treatment for stage 1 hypertension provided risk factors, TOD or CCD, and diabetes are absent. Such approaches have not definitively reduced morbidity or mortality but often lower blood pressure, reduce the number and dosage of medications, and improve the risk profile for cardiovascular disease.

16. Which hypertensive patient requires hospitalization?

Patients presenting with hypertensive emergencies may require hospitalization if there is evidence of actual or impending TOD. Conditions in which blood pressure must be rapidly reduced by the use of parenteral medications include hypertensive encephalopathy and dissecting aortic aneurysm. Situations that require less rapid blood pressure lowering, often with the use of oral antihypertensive medications, include severe hypertension with stroke, congestive heart failure, unstable angina, myocardial infarction, catecholamine excess (as in pheochromocytoma), eclampsia, substance abuse, and malignant or accelerated hypertension. Severe renal disease or extensive body burns with hypertension, hypertension with epistaxis, and over-the-counter sympathomimetic amine use also may require hospitalization.

17. What laboratory evaluation should all hypertensive patients undergo?

All newly diagnosed hypertensive patients should undergo basic laboratory studies, including:
- Urinalysis for protein, glucose, and blood
- Assessment of serum levels of creatinine, potassium, glucose, calcium, and uric acid
- A lipid profile
- A random serum aldosterone and PRA

Further studies may be added later either to evaluate the possibility of secondary hypertension or to analyze the effect of therapeutic interventions. Electrocardiograms should be performed on all hypertensive patients to exclude CAD, LVH, and other nascent heart diseases and to establish baseline values. Echocardiography may provide a more sensitive measure of LVH and LV function in selected patients.

18. How do age and race affect the choice of antihypertensive agents?

There are no persuasive data that support the notion that demographic variables such as age or gender affect the response to antihypertensive drugs. Both the Department of Veterans Affairs Cooperative Study Group on Antihypertensive Agents (Materson et al.) and the Treatment of Mild Hypertension Study (TOMHS) showed equivalent efficacy of antihypertensive drug classes across all demographic groups. However, the ALLHAT study showed that African Americans achieved greater blood pressure reduction with the diuretic chlorthalidone than non–African Americans.

19. How do concomitant medical conditions affect the choice of antihypertensive drugs?

Antihypertensive Drugs in Patients with Additional Medical Illnesses

CONDITION	PREFERRED AGENT	NOT RECOMMENDED
Asthma with COPD	ACE inhibitor AII receptor antagonist Calcium antagonist Thiazide diuretic	Beta blocker
Coronary artery disease	ACE inhibitor AII receptor antagonist Beta blocker Calcium antagonist	Vasodilators
Left ventricular dysfunction—systolic	ACE inhibitor AII receptor antagonist Calcium antagonist	Beta blocker
Left ventricular dysfunction—diastolic	Beta blocker	Calcium antagonist
Left ventricular hypertrophy	ACE inhibitor Calcium antagonist	Vasodilators Thiazides
Type 1 diabetes mellitus	ACE inhibitor	
Type 2 Diabetes mellitus	AII receptor antagonist	
Chronic renal failure (creatinine > 3 mg/dl)	ACE inhibitor Beta blocker Loop diuretic	Calcium antagonist (in African Americans)
Renovascular hypertension		ACE inhibitor

COPD = chronic obstructive pulmonary disease; ACE = angiotensin-converting enzyme; AII = angiotensin II

20. When should diuretics *not* be used in the treatment of high blood pressure?

Although diuretics are well tolerated, inexpensive, safe, and effective, they may be contraindicated in patients with gout, autonomic neuropathy with orthostasis, or urinary incontinence.

21. When is an ACE inhibitor contraindicated?

Contraindications to ACE inhibitor treatment include a history of angioedema or cough induced by ACE inhibitors, pregnancy, or potassium level > 5 mmol/L. ACE inhibitors also may be contraindicated in patients with a history of angioedema unrelated to ACE inhibitors, because there may be an increased risk of angioedema while taking an ACE inhibitor. ACE inhibitors may cause fetal or neonatal morbidity or mortality primarily in the second or third semester. Treatment with ACE inhibitors should be discontinued immediately after a patient learns that she is pregnant. The finding that an ACE inhibitor increases serum creatinine by 25–30% should not be a cause for concern, but rather should provide assurance that that the drug is having a salutary effect. By relaxing the efferent arteriole, ACE inhibitors reduce intraglomerular pressure and glomerular filtration rate. The decreased intraglomerular pressure may prevent the development of glomerular sclerosis and diabetic nephropathy.

22. List indications for ambulatory or continuous blood pressure monitoring.

- Discrepancy between home and office blood pressure readings
- Persistent elevation of blood pressure in the office without TOD
- Episodic elevation of blood pressure
- Hypertension resistant to treatment
- End-organ disease in the face of normal office blood pressure
- Evaluation of efficacy of treatment

23. Does smoking cessation influence hypertension?

Smoking cessation does not directly lower elevated blood pressure but does profoundly reduce cardiovascular mortality.

24. How do calcium antagonists differ in their hemodynamic effects?

Calcium antagonists lower blood pressure by preventing the entry of calcium into vascular smooth muscle cells, leading to vasodilatation and reduced systemic vascular resistance. Dihydropyridine calcium antagonists have greater vasoselectivity than verapamil and diltiazem, although the latter agents may slow atrioventricular conduction, which may be advantageous in treating patients with supraventricular arrhythmias.

25. When is hypertension considered to be drug resistant?

Resistance is usually defined as inadequate blood pressure control in patients receiving three antihypertensive drugs, one of which is a diuretic. As shown by the HOT study and other clinical trials, targeted blood pressure goals can be achieved in > 80% of patients if three or more antihypertensive agents are used.

26. When should hypertension be treated in diabetic patients?

Type 2 diabetes accounts for over 90% of all patients with diabetes and is increasing in prevalence as the incidence of obesity approaches 100 million individuals in the U.S. The natural history of type 2 diabetes is characterized by an early increase in glomerular filtration rate, due to efferent arteriolar constriction, and increased intraglomerular pressure, which leads ultimately to glomerular sclerosis and diabetic nephropathy. ACE inhibitors have been shown to delay the progression of this process. Although most experts agree that inhibition of the renin-angiotensin system should be instituted at the time of development of microalbuminuria, some advocate earlier intervention. Recent clinical trials of angiotensin II receptor antagonists (RENAAL, IDENT, and IRMA) show benefit in retarding the progression of diabetic nephropathy in type 2 diabetes. The only major clinical trial in type 1 diabetes (Lewis) indicated that the ACE inhibitor captopril delayed the progression of diabetic nephropathy.

BIBLIOGRAPHY

1. Antihypertensive and Lipid-Lowering Treatment to Prevent Heart Attack Trial (ALLHAT) Collaborative Research Group: Major outcomes in high-risk hypertensive patients randomized to angiotensin-converting enzyme inhibitor or calcium channel blocker vs. diuretic. JAMA 288:2981–2997, 2002.
2. Brenner BM, Cooper ME, de Zeeuw D, et al: Effect of losartan on renal and cardiovascular outcomes in patients with type 2 diabetes and nephropathy. N Engl J Med 345:861–869, 2001.
3. Dahlof B, Devereaux RB, Kjeldsen SE, et al: Cardiovascular morbidity and mortality in the losartan intervention trial for endpoint reduction in hypertension study (LIFE): A randomized trial against atenolol. Lancet 359:995–1003, 2002.
4. Grimm RH Jr, Flack JM, Grandits GA, et al: Long-term effects on plasma lipids of diet and drugs to treat hypertension. JAMA 275:1549–1556, 1996.
5. Hansson L, Zanchetti A, Carruthers SG, et al: Effects of intensive blood pressure lowering and low-dose aspirin in patients with hypertension: Principal results of the hypertension optimal treatment (HOT) randomized trial. Lancet 351:1755–1762, 1998.
6. Lewis EJ, Hunsicker LG, Clarke WR, et al: Renoprotective effect of the angiotensin II receptor antagonist, irbesartan, in patients with nephropathy due to type 2 diabetes (IDENT). N Engl J Med 345:851–860, 2001.
7. Lewis EJ, Hunsicker LG, Bain RP, Rohde RD: The effect of angiotensin converting enzyme inhibition on diabetic nephropathy. The Collaborative Study Group. N Engl J Med 329:1456–1462, 1993.
8. Neaton JD, Wentworth D, for the Multiple Risk Factor Intervention Trial Group: Serum cholesterol, blood pressure, cigarette smoking, and death from coronary heart disease. Arch Intern Med 152:56–64, 1992.
9. Parving, H-H, Lehnert H, Brochner-Mortensen J, for the Irbesartan in Patients with Type 2 Diabetes and Microalbuminuria Study Group (IRMA): The effect of irbesartan on the development of diabetic nephropathy in patients with type 2 diabetes. N Engl J Med 345:870–878, 2001.
10. SHEP Cooperative Research Group: Prevention of stroke by antihypertensive drug treatment in older persons with isolated systolic hypertension: Final results of the Systolic Hypertension in the Elderly Program (SHEP). JAMA 26:3255, 1991.
11. Sixth Report of the Joint National Committee on Prevention, Detection, Evaluation, and Treatment of High Blood Pressure (JNC VI). Arch Intern Med 157:2413–2446, 1997.

12. Staessen JA, Fagard R, Thijs L, et al: Randomized, double-blind comparison of placebo and active treatment for older people with isolated systolic hypertension. The Systolic Hypertension in Europe (Syst-Eur) Trial Investigators. Lancet 350:1632–1633, 1997.
13. Yusuf S, Sleight P, Pogue J, et al: Effect of an angiotensin-coverting-enzyme inhibitor, ramipril, on cardiovascular events in high risk patients. The Heart Outcomes Prevention Evaluation Study (HOPE). N Engl J Med 342:145–153, 2000.

15. CHEST PAIN

Valerie K. Ulstad, M.D., M.P.A., M.P.H.

1. What is the most important tool in distinguishing the cause of chest pain?

The history taken by the health care provider is without question the most valuable tool. It is important to have a systematic way in which to obtain the history.

2. What are the important components of the history in the evaluation of chest pain?

Remember the two C's when evaluating chest pain or discomfort—characterize and categorize.

1. **Characterize.** You are seeking a thorough description of the pain, including the *quality* of the sensation (crushing, burning, stabbing, tearing), the *location* and *radiation* of the pain, the *temporal intensity* of the discomfort, including how it begins (starts abruptly or builds up insidiously) and the *duration* (second, minutes, hours, days); the sources of *provocation* (exercise, emotional stress, eating, inhalation/exhalation, changing position); the *palliative features* (rest, nitroglycerin, food, change of position); and other *associated features* (pallor, diaphoresis, dyspnea, palpitations).

2. **Categorize.** What organ systems are you dealing with? Is there more than one type of pain? Is the discomfort cardiac, pulmonary, gastrointestinal, breast, musculoskeletal, neurologic, or psychological?

3. Name the most common cardiovascular causes of chest pain.

Common causes include atherosclerosis manifesting as ischemic heart disease (angina pectoris) and acute ischemic heart disease (myocardial infarction), pericarditis, dissecting aortic aneurysm, valvular heart disease, and hypertrophic cardiomyopathy. A careful history and physical exam are important in differentiating these individual and sometimes coexistent problems.

4. Describe typical angina pectoris.

Angina pectoris is a clinical syndrome characterized typically by a deep retrosternal pressure-like sensation that occurs during physical exercise (particularly in the cold), while eating, or during emotional excitement. In fact, patients may protest at the word *pain* and prefer *discomfort* as the most suitable descriptor. When the patient places a clenched fist over the sternum to describe the chest discomfort (Levine sign), angina is strongly suggested. The discomfort usually builds up gradually to its peak. Anginal discomfort usually does not radiate, but when it does, it may radiate to a variety of locations: the neck, jaw, teeth, left or right arm, or back. The ulnar aspect of the left arm is a particularly common site of radiation. There may be accompanying symptoms such as pallor, diaphoresis, nausea, dyspnea, and fatigue. The discomfort usually lasts 5–15 minutes and disappears with rest or sublingual nitroglycerin. The frequency of discomfort and level of exertion that precipitates the angina are important in determining the urgency for further diagnostic and therapeutic interventions.

5. List the risk factors for atherosclerotic cardiovascular disease.
Hypertension (systolic and diastolic)
Diabetes
Smoking
Male > 40 years of age
Postmenopausal woman
Family history of premature coronary artery disease (CAD)
Hyperlipidemia
Obesity
Physical inactivity

6. What physical findings support the presence of CAD?
The physical examination in a patient with severe angina may be completely normal. Relatively subtle findings such as an S_4, mitral regurgitation murmur, or sustained apical impulse may occur during an ischemic episode. Hypertension also may be present during pain.

7. Does a normal electrocardiogram (EKG) rule out CAD as the cause of chest pain?
Absolutely not. The EKG may be normal even during an acute myocardial infarction in up to 10% of patients. The history is more sensitive than the EKG. A normal EKG should never dissuade you from pursuing a worrisome history. Certainly, evidence of ST-T changes during an episode of pain can support the clinical diagnosis already made by the history, as would Q waves suggesting previous myocardial infarction.

8. How does the chest pain associated with acute myocardial infarction differ from that of angina pectoris?
The only real difference between these two syndromes is that angina pectoris is relieved relatively promptly with rest or nitroglycerin, whereas in acute myocardial infarction the pain may be prolonged (> 30 minutes), lasting potentially for hours. The pain of acute myocardial infarction also tends to radiate more widely.

9. What are anginal equivalents?
Anginal equivalents are symptoms that occur in place of typical anginal chest pain but represent the same pathophysiologic process. Examples include dyspnea; discomfort along the ulnar aspect of the left forearm; lower jaw, teeth, neck, or shoulder pain; nausea; indigestion; diaphoresis; or the development of gas or belching. The clinician should initially consider ischemic heart disease in the differential of these symptoms.

10. When is chest pain called "atypical"?
Atypical chest pain has two of the three following characteristics: (1) substernal location, (2) precipitation by exertion, or (3) relief by rest or nitroglycerin in 10 minutes or less.

11. What is Prinzmetal's angina?
Prinzmetal's angina occurs at rest or with ordinary activity and is precipitated by exercise. The discomfort tends to occur at night or in the early morning. The episodes may be severe and longer in duration than those of typical angina pectoris. This relatively rare situation is thought to be caused by coronary spasm. The clinician would be unable to distinguish between Prinzmetal's angina and an acute ischemic syndrome (e.g., unstable angina or acute myocardial infarction) while actually observing a patient having pain. A history that suggests recurrence, particularly at the same time of day, is suggestive of Prinzmetal's angina.

12. How does typical pericardial pain differ from angina?
Pericardial pain is sharper than angina. The patient may describe the pain as stabbing. The discomfort is often located on the left side of the chest and may radiate to the neck and left trapez-

ius ridge. Leaning forward may alleviate pericardial pain by causing the pericardium to fall away from the heart, and the pain may worsen when the patient lies flat on his or her back. Breathing, swallowing, and twisting the upper body may increase discomfort. The pain of pericarditis lasts for hours to days and is unaffected by exercise.

13. What physical findings support the diagnosis of pericarditis?

A low-grade fever may be present. High spiking fevers and a toxic-appearing patient should alert the clinician to possible purulent pericarditis that requires urgent draining. The classic cardiac examination in acute pericarditis is characterized by tachycardia and a friction rub. The rub may come and go. It is more likely to be heard with the patient lying on his or her back. Having the patient exhale and suspend respirations while one quickly listens maximizes the chances that the rub will be heard. Of course, one should look for evidence of systemic diseases that may be . associated with pericarditis.

14. What are the causes of pericarditis?

Pericarditis is usually idiopathic. Other etiologies include viral infection, myocardial infarction, aortic dissection rupturing into the pericardium, blunt chest trauma, malignancy, radiation, uremia, surgery, drugs (procainamide and hydralazine are the most common), and various connective tissue diseases.

15. Is an abnormal echocardiogram necessary to make the diagnosis of pericarditis?

No. Pericarditis is a clinical diagnosis. The absence of an effusion on the echocardiogram means just that. The echocardiogram is insensitive to inflammation. On the other hand, it is capable of detecting a very small amount of pericardial fluid.

16. What are the characteristic symptoms of aortic dissection?

The most striking feature of the classic presentation is abrupt onset with sudden severe pain. The pain is of maximal intensity immediately (as opposed to the crescendo nature of angina) and may be waxing and waning or unrelenting. The pain is frequently described as ripping or tearing. It commonly radiates from the anterior chest to the back, sometimes following the path of the dissection. The patient also may present with neurologic symptoms or limb ischemia, suggesting compromise of vessels leaving the aorta.

17. What are the risk factors for aortic dissection?

Hypertension is present in 70–90% of persons who develop dissection of the aorta. Other risk factors include Marfan syndrome, pregnancy, coarctation of the aorta, and trauma.

18. What types of valvular heart disease may present with chest pain?

An important valvular cause of chest discomfort is significant aortic stenosis. The pain is a typically anginal discomfort, probably due to inability to augment coronary blood flow to the hypertrophied myocardium. Angina is one of the classic symptoms of severe aortic stenosis.

Chest pain is no more frequent in patients with mitral valve prolapse than in healthy controls. When chest pain is present with documented mitral valve prolapse, it is most commonly stabbing and unrelated to exertion. The discomfort, however, may mimic angina pectoris.

19. How does hypertrophic cardiomyopathy cause chest pain?

This typical anginal pain is related to subendocardial ischemia with or without coexisting coronary artery disease. The demand of the hypertrophied myocardium outstrips the available myocardial oxygen supply, and ischemia results.

20. What features suggest a pulmonary or pleural etiology of chest pain?

An increase in chest discomfort with inspiration and sharp, well-localized pain with sudden onset of dyspnea should point to the lungs or pleura as the source of chest pain.

21. What features of the history suggest a musculoskeletal cause of chest pain?
Aggravation by moving or coughing suggests such a cause. Discrete superficial chest pain probably arises from a musculoskeletal injury. Pain lasting constantly for days or weeks suggests a musculoskeletal etiology, although space-occupying malignant processes in the mediastinum also should be considered.

22. What is Tietze syndrome?
Tietze syndrome consists of discomfort localized to swollen costochondral and costosternal joints that are painful on palpation.

23. Describe the chest pain associated with Da Costa syndrome (neurocirculatory asthenia).
This pain is functional or psychogenic. It is localized in the area of the cardiac apex, is dull and persistent, and lasts for hours with associated intervals of lancinating inframammary pain that lasts seconds. The pain may be associated with palpitations, hyperventilation, light-headedness, dyspnea, weakness, generalized numbness and tingling, and emotional instability.

24. How may gastrointestinal pathology masquerade as cardiac disease?
Esophageal spasm may closely mimic angina pectoris. The discomfort may be substernal, brought on by eating, and relieved by nitroglycerin; it also may radiate to the back. Relief of the discomfort with antacids, a water brash taste in the mouth, or dysphagia help point to the esophagus as the cause. Stooping or bending tends to provoke esophageal reflux. Indigestion due to peptic ulcer disease may imitate angina. Pain due to pancreatitis or cholecystitis may resemble acute myocardial infarction. Generally, there is no relationship between exercise and gastrointestinal causes of chest pain.

25. How often can the clinician determine a specific cause of chest discomfort?
Chest pain or discomfort is a common clinical problem. The priority is to rule out life-threatening causes promptly, realizing that after this is done no definite etiology for chest pain is found in as many as 50% of cases. Serial observation may provide other clues or simply resolution of the discomfort.

26. What is the immediate goal in the evaluation of the patient with acute chest pain?
Risk stratification into high, intermediate, or low risk for acute ischemic syndrome is the immediate goal. An ischemic cause of chest pain should always be considered first because the importance of early treatment of patients with acute myocardial infarction (MI) is well documented.

27. How does one assess the likelihood of significant CAD in patients with chest pain suggestive of unstable angina?
The majority of predictive information comes from the symptoms and the EKG. The likelihood of significant coronary disease is **high** with any of the following features:
- Known history of CAD
- Classic angina in men ≥ 60 or women ≥ 70
- EKG or hemodynamic changes with pain
- ST segment increase or decrease = 1 mm
- Marked symmetrical T-wave inversion in multiple precordial leads
- Variant angina

The likelihood of significant coronary disease is **intermediate** with absence of high-risk features and presence of any of the following features:
- Classic angina in men < 60 or women < 70
- Probable angina in men ≥ 60 or women ≥ 70
- Nonspecific chest pain in diabetic patients or nondiabetic patients with two or more other risk factors

- Evidence of other vascular disease
- ST depression of 0.05–1.0 mm
- T-wave inversion ≥ 1 mm in leads with dominant R waves

The likelihood of significant coronary disease is **low** with absence of any high- or intermediate-risk features:

- Chest pain probably not angina
- One risk factor but not diabetes
- Normal EKG
- T-wave flat or inverted < 1 mm in leads with dominant R waves

28. What characteristics suggest high, intermediate, and low short-term risk of death or nonfatal MI?

High risk of death or nonfatal MI (at least one of the following must be present):
- More than 20 minutes of ongoing rest pain
- Pulmonary edema
- Angina with new or worsening mitral regurgitation murmur
- Rest angina with dynamic ST changes ≥ 1 mm
- Angina with S_3 or rales
- Angina with hypotension

Intermediate risk of death or nonfatal MI (no high-risk features but any of the following):
- Rest angina now resolved but not a low likelihood of CAD
- Rest angina (> 20 minutes or relieved with rest or nitroglycerin)
- Angina with dynamic T-wave changes
- Nocturnal angina
- New-onset angina with walking < 2 blocks or at rest in past 2 weeks (but not a low or high likelihood of CAD)
- Q waves or ST depression ≥ 1 mm in multiple leads
- Age > 65 years

Low risk of death or nonfatal MI (no high or intermediate features):
- Increased angina in frequency, duration, or severity
- Angina provoked at a lower threshold
- New angina within 2 weeks to 2 months
- Normal or unchanged EKG

29. What is the cardiovascular response to cocaine use?

The cardiovascular responses to intravenous, intranasal, and inhaled cocaine are increased heart rate and increased blood pressure caused by inhibition of norepinephrine reuptake by sympathetic neurons.

30. What are the cardiovascular complications of cocaine use?

Myocardial ischemia with or without chest pain	Dilated cardiomyopathy
	Arrhythmias
Myocardial infarction	Conduction abnormalities
Myocarditis	Stroke

BIBLIOGRAPHY

1. American College of Emergency Physicians: Clinical policy for the initial approach to adults presenting with a chief complaint of chest pain, with no history of trauma. Ann Emerg Med 25:274–299, 1995.
2. Braunwald E, Zipes DP, Libby P (eds): Heart Disease: A Textbook of Cardiovascular Medicine, 6th ed. Philadelphia, W.B. Saunders, 2001.
3. Braunwald E, Jones RH, Mark DB, et al: Diagnosing and managing unstable angina. Agency for Health Care Policy and Research. Circulation 90:613–622, 1994.

4. Christie L, Conti CR: Systematic approach to the evaluation of angina-like chest pain. Am Heart J 102:897, 1981.
5. Constant J: The clinical diagnosis of nonanginal chest pain: The differentiation of angina from nonanginal chest pain by history. Clin Cardiol 6:11, 1983.
6. Duprez DA: Angina in the elderly. Eur Heart J 17(suppl G):8–13, 1996.
7. Gomez MA, Anderson JL, Karagounis LA, et al: An emergency department-based protocol for rapidly ruling out myocardial ischemia reduces hospital time and expense: Results of a randomized study (ROMIO). J Am Coll Cardiol 28:25–33, 1996.
8. Herlitz J, Karlson BW, Hjalmarson A: Ten-year mortality rate among patients in whom acute myocardial infarction was not confirmed in relation to clinical history and observations during hospital stay: Experiences from the Goteborg Metroprolol Trial. Int J Cardiol 44:217–224, 1994.
9. Hurst JW, Logue RB: Angina pectoris: Words patients used and overlooked precipitating events. Heart Dis Stroke 2:89–91, 1993.
10. Lange RA, Hillis LD: Cardiovascular complications of cocaine use. N Engl J Med 345:351–358, 2001.
11. Lee TH, Goldman L: Evaluation of the patient with acute chest pain. N Engl J Med 342:1187–1195, 2000.
12. Levine HJ: Difficult problems in the diagnosis of chest pain. Am Heart J 100:108, 1980.
13. Markiewicz W, Stoner J, London E, et al: Mitral valve prolapse in 100 presumably healthy young females. Circulation 53:464–473, 1976.
14. Martina B, Bucheli B, Stotz M, et al: First clinical judgment by primary care physicians distinguishes well between nonorganic and organic causes of chest pain. J Gen Intern Med 12:459–465, 1997.
15. Matthews MB, Julian DG (eds): Angina Pectoris. New York, Churchill Livingstone, 1985.
16. Miller A: Diagnosis of Chest Pain. New York, Raven Press, 1988.
17. Norell M, Lythall D, Coghlan G, et al: Limited value of the resting electrocardiogram in assessing patients with recent onset chest pain. Br Heart J 67:53–56, 1992.
18. Sampson JJ, Cheitlin MD: Pathophysiology and differential diagnosis of cardiac pain. Prog Cardiovasc Dis 13:507, 1971.
19. Shima MA: Evaluation of chest pain: Back to the basics of history and physical examination. Postgrad Med 91:155–158, 161–164, 1992.
20. Stubbs P, Collinson P, Moseley D, et al: Prospective study of the role of cardiac troponin T in patients admitted with unstable angina. BMJ 313:262–264, 1996.
21. Tarum JL, Jesse RL, Kontos MC, et al: Comprehensive strategy for the evaluation and triage of the chest pain patient. Ann Emerg Med 29:116–125, 1997.
22. Tibbing L: Issues in the treatment of noncardiac chest pain. Am J Med 92(5A):84S–87S, 1992.

16. AORTIC VALVE DISEASE

Valerie K. Ulstad, M.D., M.P.A., M.P.H.

1. How does aortic stenosis result in cardiac failure?

Aortic stenosis presents a fixed obstruction to the forward flow of blood. Thus, cardiac output cannot be augmented in times of need, potentially leading to inadequate blood supply to important vascular beds. The left ventricle hypertrophies to normalize the increased wall tension created by the stenosis. Left ventricular hypertrophy (LVH) results in abnormal ventricular filling, because the ventricle is less compliant. Filling pressure must then be elevated to maintain adequate ventricular filling. Finally the ventricle dilates when the muscle fails.

2. What are the common age-related etiologies of aortic stenosis?

In adults, aortic stenosis is nearly always the result of progressive leaflet calcification. When aortic stenosis becomes apparent in the 30–50 age group, an underlying congenital bicuspid or unicuspid aortic valve is usually present. After age 50, calcification is usually due to degeneration of the leaflets. The incidence of degenerative aortic stenosis increases with age. Rheumatic aortic stenosis is now relatively uncommon and is almost always accompanied by rheumatic mitral disease.

3. What is the pathophysiology of the symptoms in patients with severe aortic stenosis?

Patients with severe aortic stenosis are **SAD;** that is, they have **s**yncope, **a**ngina, and **d**yspnea. Syncope is due to reduced cerebral perfusion during exercise. Because cardiac output across the obstruction cannot be increased, the vasodilatation of exercise results in systemic hypotension.

Angina occurs because the myocardial oxygen demand of the hypertrophied ventricle exceeds the oxygen supply available via the coronary arteries, which themselves may be compressed by the hypertrophied myocardium. The subendocardium is the major site of ischemia in patients with thick hypertrophied ventricles.

Dyspnea or other evidence of congestive heart failure may be due to diastolic or systolic ventricular dysfunction. Systolic dysfunction may develop secondary to coexisting coronary artery disease or subendocardial fibrosis from recurrent subendocardial ischemia of the hypertrophied ventricle. Diastolic dysfunction may result from impaired relation to the hypertrophied ventricle.

4. Does chest pain in aortic stenosis always imply associated coronary artery disease?

No. In 50% of patients with critical aortic stenosis, angina occurs in the absence of coronary artery disease. The most likely mechanism for angina pectoris in aortic stenosis is tachycardia associated with shortened diastolic perfusion time in the face of LVH, impaired ventricular relaxation, and high diastolic wall stress. The result is a delay in the rise of diastolic perfusion to the endocardium.

5. List eight classic findings in aortic stenosis.

1. Narrow pulse pressure
2. Sustained apical impulse, which results from sustained outflow obstruction
3. Parvus et tardus pulse contour, which is small in volume and late in peaking. It results in a delayed carotid upstroke
4. Systolic ejection murmur, which is heard best at the right second intercostal space and often at the left sternal border, with radiation to the neck
5. Systolic ejection click, which may be heard at the moment of termination of the abnormal valve opening and is not heard when the aortic valve is no longer mobile
6. Paradoxically split S_2. Because emptying of the left ventricle is delayed, the aortic component now comes at the last part of the second heart sound. In inspiration, filling of the right side of the heart is augmented so that the two heart sounds are concordant.
7. Soft S_2, which occurs when the valve moves very little
8. S_4, which occurs with active diastolic filling into a hypertrophied ventricle

6. Does the intensity of murmur help in assessing aortic stenosis?

One should not be fooled by the intensity of the murmur, either soft or loud. However, the duration of the murmur and a later peak of intensity suggest more severe aortic obstruction.

7. How does the physician know when aortic stenosis has become critical?

The development of symptoms in a patient with aortic stenosis portends a poor prognosis. The average survival of patients with untreated aortic stenosis is 2–3 years after the development of angina or syncope and 1.5 years after congestive heart failure ensues. The natural history of aortic stenosis is characterized by a long asymptomatic period followed by a much shorter period. Although the rate of progression of aortic stenosis is unpredictable, once the valve is calcified, progression tends to become more rapid.

8. How should the physician follow patients with aortic stenosis?

Noninvasive assessment of the severity of obstruction with Doppler echocardiography should be carried out after a murmur radiating to the carotids is detected to establish the baseline degree of severity. The most important way to follow a patient is to closely monitor for the development of symptoms of angina, syncope, or congestive heart failure (CHF). Echocardiographic follow-up should be used in addition to clinical follow-up. Patients with **severe** aortic stenosis should have a yearly echocardiogram (echo), those with **moderate** aortic stenosis should have an echo every 2 years, and those with **mild** aortic stenosis should have echo follow-up every 5 years.

9. What should you tell the patient who has asymptomatic or mild aortic stenosis?

1. Become familiar with the possible symptoms.

2. Avoid vigorous physical activity.

3. Schedule regular yearly follow-up with the physician, and undergo echocardiography as directed.

4. Request subacute bacterial endocarditis prophylaxis for invasive and dental procedures.

10. What is the Gallavardin murmur?

It is a murmur of aortic stenosis heard best at the apex and left sternal border. Although it is ejection in quality, it has a high-pitched musical sound that may be confused with mitral regurgitation because of its location. It is associated with aortic stenosis in the elderly. It should not radiate to the axilla, as mitral regurgitation classically may do.

11. When is aortic valve replacement indicated in aortic stenosis?

When the patient starts to become symptomatic, aortic valve replacement is indicated. Aortic valve surgery is usually not indicated in asymptomatic patients even when the valve becomes critically stenosed, because the operative risk exceeds the nonoperative risk.

12. What are the indications for percutaneous balloon valvuloplasty of the aortic valve?

This technique is of limited value in adults. Restenosis occurs in 50% of patients within 6 months. The procedure may have a role in patients with severe aortic stenosis who are not operative candidates; in patients with cardiogenic shock due to critical aortic stenosis as a bridge to eventual surgery; for palliation of symptoms in selected nonoperable patients; or for pregnant patients with critical aortic stenosis.

13. How does chronic aortic insufficiency cause left ventricular failure?

In aortic insufficiency, the entire stroke volume is ejected into a high-pressure system (the aorta). The increase in diastolic volume due to regurgitation leads to ventricular dilatation. Ventricular hypertrophy occurs to normalize wall stress. The increased stroke volume causes enlargement of the left ventricle and the aortic root. Ventricular compliance is increased so that end-diastolic pressure does not become elevated until the ventricle can no longer keep up with the extra volume. End-diastolic volume then increases without an increase in the regurgitant fraction. End-systolic volume also increases, but both ejection fraction and forward stroke volume decrease. As the compliance of the ventricle falls, diastolic pressure rises and dyspnea occurs.

14. What are the most common causes of chronic aortic insufficiency?

Cusp abnormality	Aortic root distortion (aortitis)
Perforation from endocarditis	Ankylosing spondylitis
Scarring from rheumatic disease	Syphilis
Bicuspid aortic valve	Rheumatoid disease
Loss of valvular support	**Aortic root dilatation**
Aortic dissection	Marfan syndrome

15. Describe the potential physical findings in chronic aortic insufficiency.

1. Hyperdynamic apical impulse displaced laterally and inferiorly

2. Signs associated with the wide pulse pressure of aortic regurgitation (diastolic runoff into the left ventricle)

- Head bobbing—de Musset's sign
- Vigorous collapsing pulse—Corrigan's pulse

- Pulsations in capillary beds of nails—Quincke's pulse
- Systolic pulsations of the uvula—Müller's sign
- Femoral artery murmurs in systole when compressed proximally and diastolic murmur when compressed distally—Duroziez's sign

3. Murmurs
- High-pitched, blowing, decrescendo diastolic murmur immediately after S_2 heard best at the second right intercostal space, on expiration with the patient leaning forward
- Systolic ejection murmur due to increased flow across the aortic valve
- Mid-diastolic rumble—the Austin Flint murmur, caused by vibration of the anterior leaflet of the mitral valve in the regurgitant jet, may be heard at the apex

16. Once the diagnosis of aortic insufficiency is confirmed, what are the appropriate advice and follow-up?

Aortic insufficiency can be well tolerated for many years. Asymptomatic patients with severe aortic insufficiency and normal left ventricular function have been shown to remain symptom-free for long periods. In addition to subacute bacterial endocarditis prophylaxis, patients require serial clinical exams, periodic echocardiographic exams to detect early heart failure or deterioration in left ventricular function, and periodic exercise tests to confirm their asymptomatic status. Patients who are asymptomatic but who have moderate to severe aortic insufficiency and left ventricular enlargement benefit from vasodilator therapy to reduce the hemodynamic load on the chronically volume-overloaded ventricle. Nifedipine or angiotensin-converting enzyme (ACE) inhibitors are the best agents and have been shown to improve exercise capacity and delay the need for surgery.

17. When should you consider referral for aortic valve replacement in aortic insufficiency?

Asymptomatic patients with depressed left ventricular (LV) function need to be watched closely. If progressive deterioration in LV function is seen, aortic valve replacement should be considered. If LV dysfunction is truly present, most patients will have symptoms. Exercise testing may be useful to unmask the presence of symptoms in a sedentary individual.

Symptomatic patients should undergo valve replacement to improve ventricular function and survival. Patients with severe LV dysfunction are very high-risk surgical candidates, but the prognosis is dismal with medical therapy. It is impossible to predict which patients will have persistent LV dysfunction after surgery.

18. Can the rate of hemodynamic progression of aortic stenosis be predicted using echocardiographic data in asymptomatic patients?

Yes. Progression of clinical disease may be predicted by the aortic jet velocity, as assessed by Doppler echocardiography. Patients with an aortic jet velocity > 4.0 m/sec have a > 50% likelihood of death or onset of symptoms in the next 5 years compared with patients with a jet velocity < 3.0 m/sec, who are unlikely to develop symptoms due to aortic stenosis within the next 5 years. Patients with a jet velocity of 3–4 m/sec have an intermediate time to onset of symptoms.

19. What patient characteristics are associated with an increased rate of aortic stenosis progression?

Aortic stenosis progression appears to be accelerated by smoking, hypercholesterolemia, elevated serum creatinine, and elevated serum calcium.

20. How is the severity of aortic stenosis graded by echocardiography?

The aortic valve area determined by echocardiographic measurements is used to grade the severity of aortic stenosis.
- **Mild** aortic stenosis is an aortic valve area of > 1.5 cm^2 or > 0.9 cm^2/m^2.
- **Moderate** aortic stenosis is an aortic valve area of > 1.0–1.5 cm^2 or > 0.6–0.9 cm^2/m^2.
- **Severe** aortic stenosis is an aortic valve area of ≤ 1.0 cm^2 or ≤ 0.6 cm^2/m^2.

21. Does the aortic valve area or the aortic valve gradient determine the optimal time for aortic valve replacement surgery?

Neither. This decision should be made based on evaluation of the patient's symptoms. It may be challenging to detect the development of dyspnea on exertion in patients who have unconsciously decreased their physical activity. If the patient's exercise tolerance is difficult to assess, a carefully supervised exercise test may be helpful. The valve areas and gradients can be misleading if they are used alone. A low gradient, for example, may be present if heart failure has developed and the ventricle is incapable of generating high pressures.

BIBLIOGRAPHY

1. ACC/AHA guidelines for the management of patients with valvular heart disease. A report of the American College of Cardiology/American Heart Association. Task Force on Practice Guidelines (Committee on Management of Patients with Valvular Heart Disease). J Am Coll Cardiol 32:1486–1588, 1998.
2. Bonow RO, Lakatos E, Maron BJ, Epstein SE: Serial long-term assessment of the natural history of asymptomatic patients with chronic aortic regurgitation and normal left ventricular systolic function. Circulation 84:1625–1635, 1991.
3. Braunwald E, Zipes DP, Libby P (eds): Heart Disease: A Textbook of Cardiovascular Medicine, 6th ed. Philadelphia, W.B. Saunders, 2001.
4. Elayda MA, Hall RJ, Reul RM, et al: Aortic valve replacement in patients 80 years and older: Operative risks and long-term results. Circulation 88(pt 2):11–16, 1993.
5. Faggiano P, Aurigemma GP, Rusconi C, Gaasch WH: Progression of valvular aortic stenosis in adults: Literature review and clinical implications. Am Heart J 132(pt 1):408–417, 1996.
6. Gould KL: Why angina pectoris in aortic stenosis? Circulation 95:790–792, 1997.
7. Greenberg B, Massie B, Bristow JD, et al: Long-term vasodilator therapy of chronic aortic insufficiency: A randomized double-blinded controlled trial. Circulation 78:92–103, 1988.
8. Kennedy KD, Nishimura RA, Holmes DR Jr, Bailey KR: Natural history of moderate aortic stenosis. J Am Coll Cardiol 17:313–319, 1991.
9. Lombard JT, Selzer A: Valvular aortic stenosis: A clinical and hemodynamic profile of patients. Ann Intern Med 106:292–298, 1987.
10. Oakley CM: Management of valvular stenosis. Curr Opin Cardiol 10:117–123, 1995.
11. Otto CM, Burwash IG, Leggett ME, et al: Prospective study of asymptomatic valvular aortic stenosis: Clinical, echocardiographic, and exercise predictors of outcome. Circulation 95:2262–2270, 1997.
12. Palta S, Pai AM, Gill KS, Pai RG: New insights into the progression of aortic stenosis: Implications for secondary prevention. Circulation 101:2497–2502, 2000.
13. Rahimtoola SH: Perspective on valvular heart disease: An update. J Am Coll Cardiol 14:1–23, 1989.
14. Ross J: Afterload mismatch in aortic and mitral valve disease: Implications for surgical therapy. J Am Coll Cardiol 5:811–826, 1985.
15. Selzer A: Changing aspects of the natural history of valvular aortic stenosis. N Engl J Med 317:91–98, 1987.
16. Siemienczuk D, Greenberg B, Morris C, et al: Chronic aortic insufficiency: Factors associated with progression to aortic valve replacement. Ann Intern Med 110:587–592, 1989.
17. Sprigings DC, Forfar JC: How should we manage symptomatic aortic stenosis in the patient who is 80 or older? Br Heart J 74:481–484, 1995.
18. Stone PH: Management of the patient with asymptomatic aortic stenosis. J Card Surg 9(2 suppl):139–144, 1994.

17. MITRAL VALVE DISEASE

Valerie K. Ulstad, M.D., M.P.A., M.P.H.

1. What causes mitral valve prolapse (MVP)?

MVP occurs when part of a leaflet or both leaflets of the mitral valve extend above the plane of the atrioventricular junction during ventricular systole. The usual cause is an inherent abnormality of the leaflets and supporting chordae. Normal valves may demonstrate prolapse during conditions that make the left ventricle small, such as the Valsalva maneuver, dehydration, atrial septal defect (blood shunted to the right atrium away from the left atrium leads to underfilling of the left ventricle), and hypertrophic cardiomyopathy. Conditions in which the mitral valve is intrinsically abnormal are most likely to produce significant adverse consequences.

2. How common is mitral valve prolapse?

By strict echocardiographic criteria, approximately 2–5% of the population of the United States has MVP. Myxomatous degeneration of the mitral valve is hereditary as an autosomal dominant trait. Gene penetrance is stronger in women than in men, leading to the predominance of MVP in women.

3. What is MVP syndrome?

Most patients with MVP are asymptomatic. However, the MVP syndrome applies to patients with low body weight, low blood pressure, minor skeletal abnormalities (pectus excavatum, scoliosis, joint laxity), orthostatic hypotension, palpitations, and mild mitral regurgitation.

The pathogenesis of the symptoms is poorly understood but probably is related to autonomic dysfunction. Papillary muscle tension from billowing redundant leaflets may play a role in chest discomfort and development of certain arrhythmias. Patients tend to develop MVP syndrome in the second or third decade of life. Anxiety and panic attacks are no more common in patients with MVP than in the general population. Other names for MVP syndrome include *Da Costa's syndrome, soldier's heart, effort syndrome,* and *neurocirculatory asthenia.*

4. Does therapy always help patients with MVP syndrome?

Beta blockers slow the heart rate and increase diastolic filling, thereby increasing left ventricular size and reducing the degree of prolapse. The relief of symptoms with beta blockers is variable. Aerobic exercise has been shown to provide symptomatic improvement for some patients.

5. How is the diagnosis of MVP made?

The diagnosis is largely clinical; the hallmark is a midsystolic click with or without a late systolic murmur. The click occurs when the elongated chordae are snapped tight at the maximal excursion of the valve during closure in early systole. The regurgitant murmur most commonly is produced by abnormal coaptation of the leaflet edges. The Valsalva maneuver and the upright standing position make the ventricle smaller and thus may lead to a louder click earlier in systole and a longer, louder murmur. The auscultatory features may vary from day to day, according to changes in ventricular size.

Once the clinical diagnosis is made, an echocardiogram establishes baseline values and assesses the degree of prolapse, extent of leaflet thickening, and degree of mitral regurgitation. The echocardiographic diagnosis of MVP depends on the criteria used by the echocardiographer. Because the mitral annulus is shaped like a saddle, only in certain echocardiographic views can the prolapse be interpreted as genuine.

6. What risks are associated with MVP?

The major potential complications of MVP are (1) endocarditis, (2) development of severe mitral regurgitation (MR), (3) significant arrhythmias, (4) stroke due to thromboemboli, and (5) orthostatic syncope.

Endocarditis is more likely to occur in patients with thickened, deformed valves. The incidence of endocarditis in this subset of patients is 3.5–6%. Antibiotic prophylaxis for subacute bacterial endocarditis is recommended, especially if thick mitral leaflets and mitral regurgitation murmur are present on physical examination or echocardiogram.

Significant MR develops in 9–12% of patients with severely deformed valves. Progressive MR is related to various combinations of mitral annulus dilatation, chordal elongation, or chordal rupture. The risk of developing severe MR increases with age in men more than in women. Patients who develop significant MR should be followed echocardiographically. Once symptoms develop and the ventricular end-systolic dimension increases, surgery for mitral valve repair or replacement should be considered.

The incidence of **serious arrhythmia** is low enough that screening for arrhythmias is not indicated.

The abnormal surface of the myxomatous valve potentially predisposes to the development of **thromboemboli.** The presence of MVP increases the risk of stroke and transient ischemic attacks in patients under 45 years of age. Aspirin therapy is rational but unproved.

The risk of **sudden death** is slightly higher in patients with MVP than in the normal population. Ventricular fibrillation appears to be the mechanism of death.

The cumulative risk of all complications of MVP is 5–10% by age 75 in affected men and 2–5% by age 75 in affected women. Patients with MVP who have no auscultatory or Doppler evidence of MR should be reassured that their condition is benign.

7. List the causes of mitral regurgitation.
Primary mechanisms
Abnormalities of the leaflets
   Rheumatic valvulitis
   Endocarditis
   Myxomatous degeneration
Abnormalities of the chordae tendinae
   Spontaneous rupture from myxomatous degeneration
   Elongation from myxomatous degeneration
   Scarring and fusion from rheumatic inflammation
Abnormalities of the papillary muscles
   Ischemic dysfunction—disruption secondary to infarction
Secondary mechanisms
Left ventricular dysfunction and dilatation leading to malalignment of the mitral apparatus

8. Which cause of chronic MR most commonly requires surgery?
Myxomatous degeneration of the mitral valve.

9. What is the pathophysiology of chronic MR?
In MR, a portion of the left ventricular stroke volume is ejected backward into the relatively low-pressure left atrium. This part of the stroke volume is ineffective because it does not perfuse the body and deleterious because it adds works for the left ventricle. Increased diastolic stress produced by volume overload triggers myocyte hypertrophy and thus increases end-diastolic volume. Increased diastolic volume leads to an augmentation of stroke volume with a preservation of net forward flow. Eventually constant severe volume overload leads to left ventricular systolic dysfunction. Reduced emptying of the ventricle leads to pulmonary congestion and symptoms of dyspnea.

10. How does MR manifest itself?
MR presents with symptoms of left-sided heart failure, including dyspnea, orthopnea, and paroxysmal nocturnal dyspnea. In advanced disease, right heart failure also may be present.

11. What are the classic physical findings of chronic MR?

1. The apical impulse is diffuse and laterally displaced.

2. The intensity of the first heart sound is reduced, because the leaflets float relatively near the atrioventricular ring just before the onset of isovolumic contraction as a result of the large volume of blood entering the ventricle.

3. The second heart sound may be widely split, because the aortic valve closes early as a result of reduced stroke volume.

4. A holosystolic murmur, heard best over the apex, radiates to the axilla. A click and a late systolic murmur may be present with MVP. Loudness does not correlate with severity.

5. A third heart sound indicates a large left ventricular filling volume propelled into the left ventricle under higher than normal left atrial pressure. The absence of an S_3 suggests that the MR is not severe.

12. When is the optimal time for consideration of surgical intervention in patients with MR?

The correct timing for mitral valve surgery is immediately before the ejection fraction begins to fall, which is usually before the patient develops symptoms. It is hard for the clinician to anticipate the exact time. Close follow-up of patients with significant MR is important, because it is easy to wait too long, leaving the patient with heart failure even after surgery. The normal ejection fraction in MR is > 60–65%, with a hyperdynamic left ventricle emptying into the low-pressure left atrium. A "normal" ejection fraction in such patients is not normal. Regular echocardiographic evaluations are a reasonable way to follow ventricular function. When the echocardiographic evaluation shows that the ejection fraction is less than 55–60% or the end systolic dimension of the left ventricle is greater than 45 mm, the patient should be referred for consideration of mitral valve repair or replacement. The presence of atrial fibrillation or pulmonary hypertension on echocardiography despite an ejection fraction of > 60–65% and normal ventricular size should prompt the clinician to consider referral to a specialist.

Regular exercise testing also may be indicated to uncover early symptoms of exercise intolerance. The mildest symptoms of dyspnea on exertion are an indication to consider surgery. It is currently unclear whether vasodilators retard the progression of MR.

13. Why is mitral valve repair preferable to replacement?

- Better durability
- Lower risk of endocarditis
- Lower incidence of postoperative thromboembolism
- Better postoperative ventricular function
- Anticoagulation may be avoided
- Better operative and long-term survival

14. What is the most common cause of mitral stenosis?

Rheumatic heart disease is the cause of nearly all cases of mitral stenosis in the United States. In patients without a history of rheumatic fever, it is assumed that the acute episode was mild or misdiagnosed. The valvular stenosis results from the initial inflammation of the heart. Thickening of the leaflets and fusion and shortening of the chordae produce the stenosis several decades after the initial insult. The greater the original inflammation of the heart, the more likely the person is to develop significant valvular sequelae.

15. What is the pathophysiology of mitral stenosis?

The narrowed mitral orifice limits inflow into the left ventricle. The resulting elevation of left atrial pressure leads to pulmonary venous congestion and reactive pulmonary hypertension, which in turn may lead to right ventricular pressure overload and clinical right-heart failure.

16. What are the symptoms of mitral stenosis?

- Dyspnea
- Orthopnea

- Paroxysmal nocturnal dyspnea
- Hemoptysis, when high left atrial pressure causes rupture of the small bronchial veins
- Systemic embolism in patients with atrial fibrillation secondary to atrial dilation
- Hoarseness, when the enlarged left atrium impinges on the left recurrent laryngeal nerve

17. Describe the physical examination in patients with mitral stenosis.
- Normal left ventricular apical impulse
- Possible atrial fibrillation
- Loud first heart sound (S_1). The pressure gradient across the mitral valve holds the leaflets in a position deep into the ventricle throughout diastole. The leaflets close through a relatively wide excursion, with onset of isovolumic contraction giving a loud S_1. S_1 may become soft or absent when the valve becomes so diseased that it does not move at all in systole or diastole.
- Opening snap in diastole. The diseased valve reaches its maximal excursion in diastole and is stopped short by the valvular thickening.
- Diastolic rumbling murmur immediately after the opening snap. The murmur may become louder at the end of diastole in the patient still in sinus rhythm. The accentuation of the murmur is due to increased flow secondary to atrial coarctation. Such an increase in intensity is not heard in patients with atrial fibrillation.

18. What are the two common complications of mitral stenosis?
1. **Atrial fibrillation.** With an associated rapid ventricular response, atrial fibrillation is poorly tolerated, because shortened diastole limits the time for blood to cross the stenotic valve. Such patients may experience sudden onset of pulmonary edema, requiring prompt cardioversion. Medical therapy to achieve rate control is needed if the atrial fibrillation becomes chronic.

2. **Systemic embolization.** Chronic anticoagulation of patients with atrial fibrillation and mitral stenosis is clearly indicated to prevent systemic embolization of atrial mural thrombi. Many experts advocate anticoagulation for all patients with mitral stenosis, regardless of the rhythm, because 25% of nonanticoagulated patients with mitral stenosis suffer a systemic embolus.

19. What interventions are available for the patient with disabling symptoms due to mitral stenosis?
Patients who are asymptomatic can be managed medically with careful use of diuretics and control of heart rate. Once mild-to-moderate symptoms occur, three options are available:

1. **Percutaneous balloon valvuloplasty** is limited to patients with commissural fusion and noncalcified, pliable leaflets without evidence of left atrial thrombi (which may be dislodged during the procedure) or significant MR. Procedural morbidity is < 1%. This is a good option in pregnant women.

2. **Surgical commissurotomy** has the same indications as balloon valvuloplasty. Procedural mortality is < 1%. This option offers the opportunity for valve reconstruction.

3. **Mitral valve replacement** results in excellent long-term survival rates.

20. What preoperative clinical factors are associated with suboptimal outcomes (death, congestive heart failure) after mitral valve surgery?

Advanced age	Abnormal renal function
Poor functional class	Atrial fibrillation
Coronary artery disease	

21. Do marked pulmonary hypertension and right ventricular dysfunction preclude repair of the stenotic mitral valve?
No. Patients are at increased risk, but advances in perioperative management with the use of selective pulmonary vasodilators to improve right ventricular function have improved outcomes.

22. What is the significance of a flail mitral valve leaflet found on routine echocardiography in an asymptomatic patient with significant mitral regurgitation?

A flail leaflet means that there has been enough disruption of the chordal structures of the valve that a portion of the edge of the valve leaflet flips back into the left atrium in systole. An asymptomatic patient with a flail mitral valve leaflet discovered on echocardiography should be promptly referred to a cardiologist for consideration for mitral valve repair. The clinical threshold for referral is lower with a flail mitral leaflet because patients with mitral regurgitation due to flail leaflets, regardless of symptoms, have an excess mortality rate of 6.3% per year and high morbidity.

23. How should the asymptomatic patient with chronic severe MR be followed?

The patient should be seen for an evaluation of symptoms and an echocardiogram every 6 months.

BIBLIOGRAPHY

1. ACC/AHA guidelines for the management of patients with valvular heart disease. A report of the American College of Cardiology/American Heart Association. Task Force on Practice Guidelines (Committee on Management of Patients with Valvular Heart Disease). J Am Coll Cardiol 32:1486–1588, 1998.
2. Angell WW, Oury JH, Shah P: A comparison of replacement and reconstruction in patients with mitral regurgitation. J Thorac Cardiovasc Surg 93:665–674, 1987.
3. Antunes MJ, Franco CG: Advances in surgical treatment of acquired valve disease. Curr Opin Cardiol 11:139–154, 1996.
4. Ben Farat M, Maatouk F, Betbout F, et al: Percutaneous balloon mitral valvuloplasty in eight pregnant women with severe mitral stenosis. Eur Heart J 13:1658–1664, 1992.
5. Benjamin EJ, Plehn JF, D'Agostino RB, et al: Mitral annular calcification and the risk of stroke in an elderly cohort. N Engl J Med 327:374–379, 1992.
6. Boudoulas H, Kolibash AJ, Baker P, et al: Mitral valve prolapse and the mitral valve prolapse syndrome. Am Heart J 118:796–818, 1989.
7. Carabello BA: Mitral valve disease. Curr Probl Cardiol 18:421–480, 1993.
8. Cohen DJ, Kuntz RE, Gordon SPF, et al: Predictors of long-term outcome after percutaneous balloon mitral valvuloplasty. N Engl J Med 327:1329–1335, 1992.
9. Dajani AS, Bisno AL, Chung KJ, et al: Prevention of bacterial endocarditis: Recommendations by the American Heart Association. JAMA 264:2919–2922, 1990.
10. Devereux RB: Recent developments in the diagnosis and management of mitral valve prolapse. Curr Opin Cardiol 10:107–116, 1995.
11. Devereux RB, Kramer-Fox R, Kligfield P: Mitral valve prolapse: Causes, clinical manifestations, and management. Ann Intern Med 111:305–317, 1989.
12. Duran CM, Gometza B, Saad E: Valve repair in rheumatic mitral disease: An unsolved problem. J Card Surg 9(suppl 2):282–285, 1994.
13. Enriquez-Sarano M, Schaff HV, Orszulak TA, et al: Valve repair improves the outcome of surgery for mitral regurgitation: A multivariate analysis. Circulation 91:1022–1028, 1995.
14. Farb A, Tang AL, Atkinson JB, et al: Comparison of cardiac findings in patients with mitral valve prolapse who die suddenly to those who have congestive heart failure from mitral regurgitation and to those with fatal noncardiac conditions. Am J Cardiol 70:234–239, 1992.
15. Fenster MS, Feldman MD: Mitral regurgitation: An overview. Curr Probl Cardiol 20:1–280, 1995.
16. Galloway AC, Colvin SB, Bauman G, et al: Long-term results of mitral valve reconstruction with Carpentier techniques in 148 patients with mitral insufficiency. Circulation 78(suppl I):I-97–I-105, 1991.
17. Hochreiter C, Niles N, Devereaux R, et al: Mitral regurgitation: Relationship of noninvasive descriptor of right and left ventricular performance to clinical and hemodynamic findings and to prognosis in medically and surgically treated patients. Circulation 73:900–912, 1986.
18. Horstkotte D, Niehues R, Strauer BE: Pathomorphological aspects, aetiology and natural history of acquired mitral valve stenosis. Eur Heart J 12:55–60, 1991.
19. Jung B, Cormick B, Ducimetiere P, et al: Functional results 5 years after successful percutaneous mitral commissurotomy in a series of 528 patients and analysis of predictive factors. J Am Coll Cardiol 27:407–414, 1996.
20. Lehman KG, Francis CK, Dodge HT: Mitral regurgitation in early myocardial infarction: Incidence, clinical detection, and prognostic implications. TIMI Study Group. Ann Intern Med 117:10–17, 1992.
21. Llaneras MR, Nance ML, Streicher JT, et al: Pathogenesis of ischemic mitral regurgitation. J Thorac Cardiovasc Surg 105:439–442, 1993.

22. Reyes VP, Raju BS, Wynne J, et al: Percutaneous balloon valvuloplasty compared with open surgical commissurotomy for mitral stenosis. N Engl J Med 331:961–967, 1994.
23. Turu ZG, Reyes VP, Raju S, et al: Percutaneous balloon versus surgical closed commissurotomy for mitral stenosis: A prospective randomized trial. Circulation 83:1179–1185, 1991.
24. Wooley CF, Baker PB, Kolibash A, et al: The floppy myxomatous mitral valve, mitral valve prolapse, and mitral regurgitation. Prog Cardiovasc Dis 33:397–433, 1991.

18. SUPRAVENTRICULAR ARRHYTHMIAS

Valerie K. Ulstad, M.D., M.P.A., M.P.H.

1. When does a rhythm fall into the category of a supraventricular tachycardia (SVT)?
When the heart rate is greater than 100 beats per minute (bpm) and there is a narrow QRS complex.

2. What are the two most common mechanisms of SVT?
Abnormal automaticity and reentry.

3. Explain abnormal automaticity.
The sinoatrial (SA) node, elements of the atrioventricular (AV) node, and the His-Purkinje system spontaneously depolarize and thereby are said to demonstrate automaticity. These cells initiate the normal cardiac impulse and provide a hierarchy of subsidiary pacemakers ready to take over if the SA node fails. The SA node fires at the fastest rate and keeps the lower pacemakers suppressed. In certain pathologic situations, such as metabolic disturbances or certain drug toxicities, cells that do not usually exhibit spontaneous depolarization may become automatic and generate impulses that propagate through the heart.

4. What are the prerequisites for a reentry tachycardia?
Reentry is the most common mechanism producing SVT. A reentrant rhythm develops when a region of the myocardium is reexcited by one electrical impulse that returns to a given area by a circuitous route. There are three requirements for reentry to take place:

1. Two distinct parts of the heart must have different conduction velocities: two areas within the AV node, the conduction system and an accessory pathway, or two areas of the ventricular myocardium.

2. The two parts or paths for propagation of an electrical impulse must have the potential to form a circuit. Because they are different, one must conduct more slowly than the other; the path that conducts more rapidly takes longer to recover.

3. A premature beat enters the potential circuit and finds one path ready to conduct but the other blocked because it has not yet recovered. The impulse proceeds down one path and propagates through the tissue. At that point the second path may have recovered and is ready to conduct the propagated impulse. Thus the premature beat is the trigger. Under normal circumstances both pathways would have been ready to conduct the impulse. However, the premature beat exaggerated the difference between the two paths, finding one ready to conduct, the other still refractory. When the impulse comes around to the pathway that was initially refractory and finds it now ready to conduct, the reentrant circuit begins.

5. What are the five most common SVTs?
1. Atrial fibrillation
2. Atrial flutter
3. Multifocal atrial tachycardia (MAT)

4. Paroxysmal SVT
5. Sinus tachycardia

6. Which of the two major mechanisms accounts for each of the common SVTs?
1. **Reentry**
   Atrial fibrillation—multiple reentry circuits in the atrium
   Atrial flutter—reentry circuit within the atrium
   Paroxysmal SVT—reentry circuits within the AV node (AV node reentry) or via an accessory pathway (AV reentry as in Wolff-Parkinson-White syndrome [WPW])
2. **Accelerated automaticity**
   Sinus tachycardia
   MAT

7. What is paroxysmal SVT?
Paroxysmal SVT is a supraventricular rhythm that is regular at 120–220 bpm and has sudden onset and termination. The term is confusing, because it does not describe a specific arrhythmia mechanism but rather the clinical characteristics of the tachycardia. Paroxysmal SVT accounts for one-half of all patients with SVT. In the majority of patients, AV nodal reentry is the mechanism of the paroxysmal tachycardia. The second most common mechanism is AV reciprocating tachycardia via an extranodal bypass tract.

8. How may the P wave be helpful in diagnosing the type of SVT?

Use of P-Wave Morphology to Identify SVTs

P-WAVE MORPHOLOGY	SVT TYPE
No discreet P wave	Atrial fibrillation
Distinct sawtooth waves at 250–340 bpm (seen best in inferior leads)	Atrial flutter
P waves negative in inferior leads or buried within QRS	AV nodal reentry
Short PR and delta wave in sinus rhythm	WPW (potential for AV reentry)
Three different P-wave morphologies	MAT

9. Which rhythms usually have an irregular rate?
Atrial fibrillation, even at a rapid rate
Atrial flutter (which may be regular)
MAT

10. The QRS is usually narrow in SVTs. When may the QRS be wide in SVT?
1. Aberrant conduction, such as preexisting right or left bundle-branch block.
2. When an accessory connection (as in WPW) conducts antegrade, the AV node conducts retrograde, and the ventricular myocardium is depolarized cell to cell rather than along the conduction system.

11. In evaluating a patient with SVT, what historical and other medical information should be sought?
- History of palpitations or syncope
- Symptoms of possible hyperthyroidism or pheochromocytoma
- Habits and drug use: alcohol, caffeine, inhaled or oral beta agonists, over-the-counter cold medicines, illicit drugs
- Effect of a possible SVT on the patient's lifestyle (e.g., airplane pilot)

12. What are palpitations? What causes them?
Palpitations represent the patient's awareness of his or her own heart beat. The etiology of palpitations can be determined in a majority of patients. One-half of cases are due to cardiac dis-

ease, whereas one-third are due to psychiatric causes and a smaller number to other causes (habits, medicines, metabolic causes). Paroxysms of prolonged palpitations suggest a cardiac arrhythmia, either supraventricular or ventricular in origin.

13. How should patients with SVT be evaluated?

After a complete history and physical examination, the patient should have a chest radiograph and electrocardiogram (EKG). Thyroid function tests, hematocrit, and echocardiography to look for mitral valve prolapse or other evidence of valvular disease or occult myocardial disease should be considered.

14. How may carotid sinus massage or Valsalva maneuvers aid in the diagnosis and treatment of arrhythmias?

Carotid sinus massage and Valsalva maneuvers may have three major outcomes: abrupt cessation of the arrhythmia, slowing of heart rate during the maneuver, or no effect. Abrupt cessation of the arrhythmia with conversion to sinus rhythms is the most useful outcome. It may be seen when the arrhythmia is supraventricular and originates from an AV nodal reentrant or aberrant pathway mechanism. Sinus tachycardia slows during massage and subsequently regains speed. Other possible outcomes include accentuation of AV block or dissociation, atrial fibrillation in atrial flutter, and transient slowing of the ventricular rate.

15. When is carotid massage contraindicated?

In patients with possible digoxin toxicity, carotid massage may lead to fatal arrhythmias. Additional risks of carotid massage include stroke, syncope, seizures, asystole, or ventricular arrhythmias. Thus, carotid massage should be avoided in elderly patients.

16. When should a patient with supraventricular arrhythmias be hospitalized?

Patients who present with hypotension, chest pain, congestive heart failure, or sustained tachycardia should be hospitalized.

17. When should strategies to provide chronic prophylaxis against paroxysmal SVT be considered?

If the episodes are relatively slow, infrequent, and well tolerated, no therapy may be necessary. Patients should be counseled to limit use of caffeine, alcohol, and other drugs. When symptoms are frequent and bothersome, drug therapy and radiofrequency ablation of the arrhythmogenic focus are options. Drugs should slow AV node conduction; the most common drugs are beta blockers and calcium channel blockers.

18. When should drugs that block the AV node be avoided?

Beta blockers, calcium channel blockers, and digoxin are contraindicated in patients who may have tachycardias due to accessory pathways. In patients with MAT, digoxin may prove harmful.

19. When and why is it important to recognize WPW syndrome or accessory pathway arrhythmias?

WPW syndrome should be suspected in the presence of a delta wave on routine EKG or, more importantly, when the patient has atrial fibrillation that is conducted at a rapid rate (faster than the capability of the AV node), resulting in a rapid ventricular response of > 280. Of patients with WPW syndrome, 50% experience atrial fibrillation, which may deteriorate to ventricular fibrillation or present as sudden death. Thus, recognition of this rare entity is life-saving and requires referral to a cardiologist for appropriate management.

20. Which patients should be referred to a cardiologist for possible electrophysiologic testing?

1. Patients with uncontrolled symptomatic tachycardias of unknown diagnosis after preliminary work-up

2. Patients with symptomatic tachycardias with delta wave or other suspicion of aberrant conduction. The sole finding of delta waves is controversial.

3. Patients who respond poorly to initial medical management

21. What features in WPW suggest a low risk of rapid ventricular conduction, if atrial fibrillation should occur?

Two EKG features in WPW suggest that the accessory pathway conducts relatively slowly:

1. Intermittent preexcitation on the resting EKG (delta wave comes and goes)
2. Disappearance of delta wave with exercise

22. Is radiofrequency ablation (RFA) standard therapy for any SVTs?

Yes. RFA is more cost-effective than life-long drug therapy for some SVTs and can be performed safely with little discomfort to the patient. The most common applications are in patients with AV node reentry or WPW.

23. Is there an advantage to using an event recorder instead of a 48-hour Holter monitor to assess the patient with palpitations?

Yes. Event recorders are more cost-effective and provide better data. Holter monitoring is a poor diagnostic test for the evaluation of intermittent palpitations.

24. What is the role of adenosine in the diagnosis and therapy of narrow complex SVTs?

Adenosine is a rapidly metabolized, intravenously administered drug that causes inhibition of the AV node conduction by its effects on ion channels. Adenosine inhibits calcium channel opening and opens potassium channels. Adenosine is useful in the evaluation of narrow complex tachycardia because the transient AV block caused by the drug will allow the assessment of the atrial activity in SVTs perpetuated above the AV node (e.g., atrial fibrillation, atrial flutter, and MAT), and it will often terminate SVTs that rely on the AV node as part of the reentry circuit (AV node reentry and atrioventricular reentry or WPW). The effect of adenosine is similar to a very effective carotid sinus massage.

25. What are practical considerations in the administration of adenosine?

Adenosine must be given rapidly because it is metabolized very rapidly. The half-life of adenosine is 10–30 seconds. The initial dose is 6 mg followed by a saline flush to aid in the rapid delivery to the central circulation. If this does not work, the dose is doubled to 12 mg with the saline bolus afterward. A second 12-mg bolus can be given if necessary. The drug should be administered in the most proximal IV line available to facilitate its arrival at the heart. The effect should occur as soon as the drug reaches the AV node.

26. What are the side effects of adenosine?

The side effects are short lived due to it rapid metabolization; however, they include headache, chest pain, flushing, and shortness of breath.

27. What are the contraindications to the use of adenosine?

- Known asthma due to precipitation of bronchospasm in patients with reactive airways
- Conduction system disease with sick sinus syndrome or second- or third-degree AV block due to the potential to cause a serious bradyarrhythmia
- Cardiac transplant patients may be extraordinarily sensitive to the effects of adenosine with profound bradycardia.

BIBLIOGRAPHY

1. Benditt DG, Goldstein M, Reyes MJ, Milstein S: Supraventricular tachycardias: Mechanisms and therapies. Hosp Pract Aug:103–127, 1988.

2. Blackshear JL, Kopecky SL, Litin SC, et al: Management of atrial fibrillation in adults: Prevention of thromboembolism and symptomatic treatment. Mayo Clin Proc 71:150–160, 1996.
3. Camm AJ, Garratt CJ: Adenosine and supraventricular tachycardia. N Engl J Med 375:1621–1629, 1991.
4. Deering TF: The management of supraventricular tachycardias: Primary care considerations. J Med Assoc Ga 90:19–22, 2001.
5. Dreifus LS, Hessen S, Samuels F: Recognition and management of supraventricular tachycardias. Heart Dis Stroke 2:223–230, 1993.
6. Futterman LG, Lemberg L: Atrial fibrillation: An increasingly common and provocative arrhythmia. Am J Crit Care 5:379–387, 1996.
7. Ganz LI, Friedman PL: Supraventricular tachycardia. N Engl J Med 332:162–173, 1995.
8. Glatter KA, Cheng J, Dorostkar P, et al: Electrophysiologic effect of adenosine in patients with supraventricular tachycardia. Circulation 99:1034–1040, 1999.
9. Kalbfleisch SJ, El-Atassi R, Calkins H, et al: Differentiation of paroxysmal narrow QRS complex tachycardias using the 12-lead electrocardiogram. J Am Coll Cardiol 21:85–89, 1993.
10. Kinlay S, Leitch JW, Neil A, et al: Cardiac event recorders yield more diagnoses and are more cost effective than 48 hour Holter monitoring in patients with palpitations. A controlled clinical trial. Ann Intern Med 124(1 pt 1):16–20, 1996.
11. Manolis AS, Wang PJ, Estes NA III: Radiofrequency catheter ablation for cardiac tachyarrhythmias. Ann Intern Med 121:452–461, 1994.
12. Reiffel JA, Estes NA III, Waldo AL, et al: A consensus report on antiarrhythmic drugs. Clin Cardiol 17:103–116, 1994.
13. Waldo AL: An approach to therapy of supraventricular tachyarrhythmias: An algorithm versus individualized therapy. Clin Cardiol 17(suppl 2):II-21–II-26, 1994.
14. Wilbur SL, Marchlinski FE: Adenosine as an antiarrhythmic agent. Am J Cardiol 79:30–37, 1997.
15. Zimetbaum P, Josephson ME: Evaluation of patients with palpitations. N Engl J Med 338:1369–1373, 1998.

19. ATRIAL FIBRILLATION

Valerie K. Ulstad, M.D., M.P.A., M.P.H.

1. What are the common causes of chronic atrial fibrillation?
- Congestive heart failure
- Mitral stenosis
- Ischemic heart disease
- Hypertension
- Constrictive pericarditis

2. What evaluation should be performed in the patient with new-onset atrial fibrillation?
After a thorough physical examination, most patients should have the following tests:
- Assessment of electrolytes
- Assessment of thyroid-stimulating hormone (TSH)
- 12-lead electrocardiogram (EKG)
- Chest radiograph
- Echocardiogram

3. What are the clinical consequences of chronic atrial fibrillation?
- Increased risk of embolic stroke
- Increased mortality
- Bothersome symptoms
- Progressive impairment of ventricular function
- Progressive atrial myopathy

4. What four therapeutic goals should be considered in patients with atrial fibrillation?
1. Conversion to normal sinus
2. Maintenance of sinus rhythm if conversion is possible rhythm
3. Rate control for patients in chronic atrial fibrillation
4. Prevention of thromboembolism

5. What does rate control mean?
Cardiac output increases in most patients with atrial fibrillation to a mean rate of about 140 beats per minute (bpm). At faster rates, cardiac output begins to fall. A resting rate of 60–80 bpm is probably ideal, provided that it can be increased during exercise. The heart rate response to exercise also needs to be considered too before the rate is considered to be controlled. The rate should be 90–115 bpm during moderate exercise.

6. Which agents are available to control the rate in atrial fibrillation (AF)?
Rate control can be achieved with drugs that slow atrioventricular (AV) node conduction, such as beta blockers, calcium channel blockers, or digoxin. Sometimes combinations are necessary. These drugs rarely terminate atrial fibrillation. Digoxin provides good rate control at rest but poor rate control with exercise.

7. Which drugs are useful in pharmacologic cardioversion?
Patients with recent-onset (within 7 days) atrial fibrillation are more likely to be chemically converted. Agents that may be used for pharmacologic conversion of AF with a duration of ≤ 7 days include dofetilide, flecainide, ibutilide, propafenone, and amiodarone. The new oral agent dofetilide is probably the agent of choice for pharmacologic conversion of AF with a duration of longer than 7 days. Amiodarone and ibutilide can also be considered in this situation. Digoxin does not influence conversion to sinus rhythm.

8. Describe the practical guidelines for pharmacologic treatment of patients with AF.
1. Treat the symptomatic patient.
2. Treat underlying heart failure.
3. Correct metabolic disturbances.
4. The longer the patient has been in atrial fibrillation, the less likely spontaneous conversion to normal sinus rhythm (NSR) will be seen. Patients should not be pharmacologically converted to NSR until they have been adequately anticoagulated for 3 weeks with an international normalized ratio (INR) ≥ 2.0 or unless a transesophageal echo has shown no left atrial appendage thrombus.
5. The occurrence of proarrhythmia with antiarrhythmic agents during therapy is impossible to predict.
6. Consider hospitalizing and monitoring the patient when therapy is started, particularly if the patient has underlying structural heart disease (including left ventricular hypertrophy [LVH]) or a prolonged QT interval.

9. Which drugs are available for maintenance of normal sinus rhythm after conversion of AF?
Pharmacologic options include class IA antiarrhythmics, such as disopyramide, quinidine, or procainamide; class IC agents, such as flecainide and propafenone; and the class III drugs dofetilide, sotalol, and amiodarone. Any of these can be considered if there is no heart disease. LVH or other structural heart disease increases the susceptibility to proarrhythmia from class I drugs. For example, in the CAST study, class IC drugs were associated with increased mortality in patients with previous myocardial infarction (MI). In patients with LVH, previous MI, heart failure, or LV dysfunction, class III agents (i.e., dofetilide, sotalol, or amiodarone) should be considered.

10. What is the rate of ischemic stroke in elderly patients with atrial fibrillation compared with elderly patients without atrial fibrillation?
The stroke rate is 6 times higher.

11. List ten factors that increase the risk of stroke in patients with atrial fibrillation.

1. Mitral stenosis
2. Cardiomyopathy
3. Congestive heart failure
4. History of systemic emboli
5. Hypertension, including LVH
6. Mitral annular calcification
7. Left atrial size > 52 mm
8. Age > 60 years
9. Hyperthyroidism
10. Cardioversion and postcardioversion

12. List five independent predictors of embolic risk in patients with atrial fibrillation.

1. History of hypertension
2. Prior stroke or transient ischemic attack (TIA)
3. Diabetes
4. Age > 65 years
5. Recent heart failure

13. Is anticoagulation with warfarin effective in preventing stroke in patients with atrial fibrillation?
Yes. Five recent randomized clinical trials showed a 70% reduction in ischemic stroke when the INR ranged from 1.8 to 4.2. In general, INR from 2.0 to 3.0 is recommended. The elderly may be at increased risk for major bleeding. In the elderly the INR should be particularly closely monitored.

14. Which low-risk patients with atrial fibrillation may be considered for treatment with aspirin instead of warfarin?
Patients without diabetes, hypertension, heart failure, or previous stroke or TIA who are under age 65 may be given 325 mg of aspirin/day to prevent stroke. It should be noted, however, that clinical trials in low-risk patients are ongoing and that clinicians often tend to anticoagulate patients with atrial fibrillation.

15. How should anticoagulation be managed at the time of cardioversion?
Patients with atrial fibrillation of unknown duration or for more than 48 hours should be anticoagulated for 3 weeks before electrical cardioversion. Anticoagulation should be continued for at least 4 weeks after successful cardioversion to allow atrial contractile function to return to normal. Patients should then be assessed for the need for long-term anticoagulation.

16. When is it too late to consider cardioversion for atrial fibrillation?
It is probably never too late to try cardioversion. Increasing evidence indicates that atrial myopathy and LV dysfunction in progress patients with AF so that restoration of sinus rhythm is advantageous. Adequate anticoagulation before cardioversion is mandatory.

17. What is the goal of drug therapy to "maintain NSR"?
The goal is really to decrease recurrences of AF. It is unrealistic, however, to lead your patient to believe the AF will not recur.

18. What is meant by nonpharmacologic therapy of chronic atrial fibrillation?
Radiofrequency ablation of the AV node with permanent pacemaker implantation.

19. When should AV node ablation and permanent pacemaker implantation for chronic atrial fibrillation be considered?
This should be considered when the rate of AF cannot be controlled adequately with medications or when the patient cannot tolerate or has significant side effects from the medication. The patient also must be willing and able to take chronic anticoagulant therapy.

20. What are the negative aspects of AV node ablation and permanent pacemaker therapy?
- Need for chronic anticoagulation because the person is still in AF
- Loss of atrial kick to augment ventricular filling
- Lifelong reliance on a pacemaker due to the permanent alteration of the heart

21. What therapy should be considered in patients with paroxysmal AF?
- Suppressive antiarrhythmic therapy if symptoms are bothersome
- Medication that provides rate control when AF occurs
- Chronic anticoagulation to prevent stroke

22. What is the classification of AF and why is it important?
The management of AF depends on the pattern of presentation of the AF.
- **Paroxysmal AF**—lasts $\leq$ 7 days and is self-terminating. Most episodes last less than 24 hours.
- **Persistent AF**—is not self-terminating and continues until electrically or chemically converted.
- **Permanent AF**

23. Should all patients with AF be converted to NSR if it is possible?
This is an area of intense investigation. Studies so far suggest that symptom control is similar in patients with adequate rate control in chronic AF compared to patients treated aggressively to maintain NSR. Studies evaluating morbidity and mortality in large groups of patients are ongoing.

BIBLIOGRAPHY

1. Alber GW: Atrial fibrillation and stroke. Arch Intern Med 154:1443–1457, 1994.
2. Blackshear JL, Kopecky SL, Litin SC, et al: Management of atrial fibrillation in adults: Prevention of thromboembolism and symptomatic treatment. Mayo Clin Proc 71:150–160, 1996.
3. Boston Area Anticoagulation Trial for Atrial Fibrillation Investigators: The effect of low-dose warfarin on the risk of stroke in patients with nonrheumatic atrial fibrillation. N Engl J Med 323:1505–1522, 1990.
4. Cairns JA, Connolly SJ: Nonrheumatic atrial fibrillation: Risk of stroke and role of antithrombotic therapy. Circulation 84:469–492, 1991.
5. Connolly SJ, Laupacis A, Gent M: Canadian Atrial Fibrillation Anticoagulation (CAFA) study. J Am Coll Cardiol 18:349–355, 1991.
6. Ezekowitz MD, Bridgers SL, James KE, et al: Warfarin in the prevention of stroke associated with nonrheumatic atrial fibrillation. Veterans Affairs Stroke Prevention in Nonrheumatic Atrial Fibrillation Investigators. N Engl J Med 327:1406–1412, 1992.
7. Fiore LD: Anticoagulation: Risks and benefits in atrial fibrillation. Geriatrics 51:22–24, 27–28, 31, 1996.
8. Fuster V, Ryden LE, Asinger RW, et al: ACC/AHA/ESC guidelines for the management of patients with atrial fibrillation: Executive summary: A report of the American College of Cardiology/American Heart Association Task Force on Practice Guidelines and the European Society of Cardiology Committee for Practice Guidelines and Policy Conferences (Committee to Develop Guidelines for the Management of Patients with Atrial Fibrillation). Circulation 104:2118–2150, 2001.
9. Hohnloser SH, Kuck KH, Lilienthal J: Rhythm or rate control in atrial fibrillation: Pharmacological Intervention in Atrial Fibrillation (PIAF): A randomised trial. Lancet 359:1789, 2000.
10. Kahn ZU, Adolph RJ, Engel PJ: Persistent atrial mechanical dysfunction after spontaneous conversion of chronic atrial fibrillation to sinus rhythm. Am Heart J 131:606–608, 1996.
11. Klein AL, Grimm RA, Black IW, et al: Cardioversion guided by transesophageal echocardiography. The ACUTE Pilot Study. A randomized, controlled trial. Assessment of Cardioversion Using Transesophageal Echocardiography. Ann Intern Med 126:200–209, 1997.
12. Mackstaller LL, Alpert JS: Atrial fibrillation: A review of mechanism, etiology and therapy. Clin Cardiol 20:640–650, 1997.
13. Manning WJ, Silverman DI, Gordon SPF, et al: Cardioversion from atrial fibrillation without prolonged anticoagulation with use of transesophageal echocardiography to exclude the presence of atrial thrombi. N Engl J Med 328:750–755, 1993.

14. Man-Song-Hing M, Laupacis A, O'Connor A, et al: Warfarin for atrial fibrillation. The patient's perspective. Arch Intern Med 156:1841–1848, 1996.
15. Morley J, Marinchak R, Rials SJ, Kowey P: Atrial fibrillation, anticoagulation, and stroke. Am J Cardiol 77:38A-44A, 1996.
16. Petersen B, Boysen G, Godtfredsen J, et al: Placebo-controlled trial of warfarin and aspirin for the prevention of thromboembolic complications in chronic atrial fibrillation: The Copenhagen AFASAK Study. Lancet 1:175–179, 1989.
17. Reardon M, Camm AJ: Atrial fibrillation in the elderly. Clin Cardiol 19:765–775, 1996.
18. Singh S, Zoble RG, Yellen L, et al: Efficacy and safety of oral dofetilide in converting to and maintaining normal sinus rhythm in patients with chronic atrial fibrillation or flutter. The Symptomatic Atrial Fibrillation Investigative Research on Dofetilide (SAFIRE-D) Study. Circulation 102:2385, 2000.
19. Stein B, Halperin JL, Fuster V: Should patients with atrial fibrillation be anticoagulated prior to and chronically following cardioversion? Cardiovasc Clin 21:231–249, 1990.
20. Stroke Prevention in Atrial Fibrillation Investigators: Stroke Prevention in Atrial Fibrillation study: Final results. Circulation 84:527–539, 1991.

20. VENTRICULAR ARRHYTHMIAS

Valerie K. Ulstad, M.D., M.P.A., M.P.H.

1. Describe the electrocardiographic (EKG) characteristics of the premature ventricular contraction (PVC).

A PVC is an early (premature) QRS complex with a bizarre shape and a duration that exceeds the dominant QRS complex duration in the underlying rhythm. The T-wave deflection is large and in the opposite direction from the main QRS deflection. There is no preceding P wave.

The PVC is commonly conducted in a retrograde fashion toward the atria, but the sinoatrial (SA) node is rarely reset by the premature ventricular beat (in contrast to the premature atrial beat). A compensatory pause occurs after the premature beat until the next sinus beat arrives. The next sinus beat after the compensatory pause comes in time with the underlying sinus rhythm determined by the SA node. Another SA depolarization occurs simultaneously with the PVC, but its electrical activity is not seen on the EKG because it is hidden by the wide QRS complex.

2. How common are PVCs?

When a simple 12-lead EKG is used for screening, PVCs are documented in less than 1% of the population. If 24-hour Holter monitoring is used, PVCs are observed in 50–80% of normal people. The forms seen in normal people are usually single PVCs, but nonsustained ventricular tachycardia (NSVT) may be seen infrequently. The incidence of ventricular arrhythmias increases with age. They are also more common in men and in the presence of a low serum potassium.

3. Which everyday substances should patients with PVCs avoid?

Caffeine, tobacco, and alcohol increase the number of PVCs.

4. Define NSVT.

NSVT is defined as 3 or more ventricular beats in a row at a rate of at least 100 beats per minute (bpm), lasting 15–30 seconds. Longer runs are called *sustained ventricular tachycardia*.

5. List the two classes of ventricular arrhythmias.

1. Ventricular arrhythmias in the presence of a structurally **normal** heart
2. Ventricular arrhythmias in the presence of a structurally **abnormal** heart

6. What is the significance of ventricular arrhythmias in the presence of a structurally normal heart?

PVCs of low-to-moderate frequency in persons with normal ejection fraction and no organic heart disease are usually asymptomatic or present with mild dizziness or palpitations. The prognosis in such patients is excellent, even with nonsustained ventricular tachycardia (VT). Exercise-induced ectopy is not associated with an increased risk of sudden death in the normal population. The presence of symptoms with the arrhythmia does not alter the prognosis. The only indication for treatment is bothersome symptoms that ambulatory EKG monitoring clearly demonstrates are due to arrhythmia. For bothersome benign ventricular arrhythmias, beta blockers are the drugs of choice.

7. What does the presence of a PVC on a routine EKG mean?

PVCs may be the first evidence of underlying congenital, hypertensive, ischemic, or myopathic heart disease. Observation of PVCs should prompt an evaluation for cardiac pathology. A thorough history and physical examination are the first steps. Further testing should be done only if certain aspects of the history and physical exam need clarifying.

8. How does the presence of PVCs in patients with mitral valve prolapse influence prognosis?

Such patients have more simple and complex PVCs than the general population, but the prognosis is excellent in persons with structurally normal hearts. Reassurance is the best therapy. Bothersome symptoms may be treated with beta blockers if other lifestyle modifications fail. Class I agents are not advisable because of an unfavorable risk-benefit ratio.

The risk of sudden death is increased in the patient with a highly redundant mitral valve, severe mitral regurgitation, a history of syncope, a family history of sudden death, or a prolonged QT interval. In this small subgroup, runs of NSVT may be a marker of increased risk.

9. What is the risk associated with ventricular ectopy after myocardial infarction (MI)?

In the first weeks after an infarction, approximately 90% of patients have frequent PVCs. Complex forms have been documented in 20–40% of patients during this period. Simple PVCs are not associated with an increased mortality, but complex ectopy, particularly runs of NSVT, independently increases the risk of sudden cardiac death two- to fivefold. Left ventricular (LV) function is another independent prognostic factor in the postinfarction patient. LV dysfunction increases the risk of sudden death by two- to threefold. Patients with complex ventricular ectopy and LV dysfunction are at highest risk, with an incidence of sudden death in the first year after MI as high as 35%.

10. Is the suppression of PVCs with antiarrhythmic drugs beneficial for primary prevention of a first life-threatening arrhythmia in patients after an MI?

The Cardiac Arrhythmia Suppression Test (CAST) was a long-term, multicenter, placebo-controlled study designed to test the hypothesis that antiarrhythmic drugs for suppression of asymptomatic or mildly symptomatic PVCs reduce the risk of sudden cardiac death in postinfarction patients. After a 10-month follow-up, excessive mortality among patients randomized to encainide and flecainide therapy led to the removal of both agents from the trial. Even though the agents were shown to suppress asymptomatic or mildly symptomatic PVCs, suppression was associated with increased mortality. The benefit of antiarrhythmic drugs other than beta blockers after MI is unproved. Three placebo-controlled trials of amiodarone in postinfarction patients show no difference in mortality between treated patients and patients receiving placebo. Amiodarone does not increase mortality and may be advantageous in patients at high risk of sudden death. However, the routine use of amiodarone in postinfarction patients cannot be recommended.

11. Should patients with NSVT in the presence of dilated cardiomyopathy and congestive heart failure be treated with antiarrhythmic drugs?

We do not know. In patients with cardiomyopathy and clinical congestive heart failure (CHF), the 2-year mortality rate may be as high as 50%. Approximately 40% are sudden cardiac deaths, presumably due to a fatal arrhythmia. Ambulatory monitoring has shown that 70–95% of patients have frequent PVCs and 60–80% have NSVT. This group requires further study to determine whether antiarrhythmic agents offer a survival benefit. Unfortunately, no cohort of patients not receiving antiarrhythmic therapy for NSVT has been followed. The excessive mortality may be due to antiarrhythmic therapy rather than simply to the presence of the arrhythmia.

Current evidence does not support the use of antiarrhythmic agents to suppress the ectopy in such patients. Angiotensin-converting enzyme (ACE) inhibitors reduce mortality in patients with LV dysfunction and reduce the frequency of ventricular arrhythmias in patients with clinical heart failure. These drugs, therefore, are currently the best antiarrhythmic therapy for such high-risk patients. Amiodarone can be used to treat symptomatic arrhythmias. It does not improve survival in mild CHF but may improve survival in patients with class III and IV CHF and NSVT.

12. Is the implantable cardiac defibrillator (ICD) better than antiarrhythmic drugs in patients with life-threatening ventricular arrhythmias?

Yes. Several major studies have confirmed that ICDs are more effective than antiarrhythmic drugs in reducing mortality in high-risk patients. Antiarrhythmic drugs have not been shown to be effective in reducing sudden cardiac death in patients known to be at risk.

13. What is proarrhythmia?

Proarrhythmia is the appearance of a new arrhythmia or aggravation of an existing arrhythmia. In the broadest sense, the term refers to bradyarrhythmias, supraventricular tachycardias (SVTs), and VTs. Proarrhythmia is potentially seen with all antiarrhythmic agents; the incidence varies from 5% to 35%. The etiology is unclear, and occurrence is hard to predict. Proarrhythmia may be part of the mechanism of increased mortality in certain patients treated with antiarrhythmic drugs. The potential for proarrhythmia with antiarrhythmic agents must be considered whenever a patient is started on a new agent and each time the dose is adjusted. A fourfold increase in the number of PVCs and a tenfold increase in repetitive forms fit the criteria for identifying proarrhythmia with ambulatory monitoring.

14. What are the major side effects of antiarrhythmic therapy?

- Noncardiac side effects specific to each agent
- Organ toxicity specific to each agent
- Proarrhythmia
- Conduction defects
- Precipitation of congestive heart failure

There are so many antiarrhythmic drugs in part because they all pose potential problems. No antiarrhythmic drug is perfect. Beta blockers are probably the best. It is important to be completely familiar with the pharmacology of any prescribed antiarrhythmic drug.

15. When the physician is presented with a hemodynamically stable patient with a wide complex tachycardia, what is the likely diagnosis on the basis of statistics alone?

The differential diagnosis centers on VT or SVT conducted aberrantly through the heart. VT is more common by far and thus more likely.

16. What four clues does the EKG give to help differentiate VT from SVT with aberrancy?

1. Underlying heart disease favors VT.
2. Capture and fusion beats indicate VT.
3. AV dissociation indicates VT.
4. QRS width > 140 msec in the absence of preexisting bundle-branch block or accessory connection suggests VT.

17. What therapeutic considerations are important in patients with wide complex tachycardia?
1. Assume that the problem is VT, which is much more common.
2. Cardiovert the hemodynamically unstable patient.
3. Do not give verapamil, diltiazem, or adenosine; these may lead to profound hypotension and cardiovascular collapse in a patient with VT.
4. The drug of choice is amiodarone or procainamide, administered intravenously (loading dose followed by infusion).

18. How important is sudden cardiac death as a cause of cardiovascular death?
Very important. Approximately 50% of all cardiovascular deaths occur suddenly. The majority of these are caused by ventricular arrhythmias.

19. What is the major arrhythmia of sudden cardiac death?
The typical sequence of events is for ventricular tachycardia to degenerate to ventricular fibrillation, which degenerates further to asystole. The most common trigger of ventricular tachycardia is acute myocardial ischemia. Ventricular tachycardia can also develop related to scarring from previous ischemic injury to the heart. Coronary artery disease is responsible for 80% of fatal arrhythmias.

20. Is there any proof that ICDs are the best therapy to prevent sudden cardiac death in high-risk post-MI patients?
Yes. The MADIT and MUSTT trials evaluated post-MI patients with low ejection fraction; both trials documented nonsustained VT and inducible VT by electrophysiology study and showed that ICD therapy reduced mortality compared to drug therapy. It is now accepted therapy to implant ICDs in post-MI patients with low ejection fraction and nonsustained VT. It is less clear what the approach for primary prevention of arrhythmias should be in lower risk post-MI patients and in patients with dilated nonischemic cardiomyopathy.

21. What should be the approach to the patient who has survived a life-threatening arrhythmia in order to prevent recurrence of a potentially lethal arrhythmia or cardiac arrest?
The only evidence-based strategy in this situation is an ICD. This was shown in the AVID trial where ICD was better than drug therapy in patients with decreased ejection fraction who had a previous life-threatening arrhythmia. This has also been shown in at least two other trials.

BIBLIOGRAPHY

1. Antiarrhythmics Versus Implantable Defibrillators (AVID) Investigators: A comparison of antiarrhythmic-drug therapy with implantable defibrillators in patients resuscitated from near-fatal ventricular arrhythmias. N Engl J Med 337:1576–1583, 1997.
2. Brugada P, Brugada J, Mont L, et al: A new approach to the differential diagnosis of a regular tachycardia with a wide QRS complex. Circulation 83:1649–1659, 1991.
3. Buxton AE, Lee KL, Fisher JD, et al, for the Multicenter Unsustained Tachycardia Trial (MUSTT) Investigators: A randomized study of the prevention of sudden death in patients with coronary artery disease. N Engl J Med 341:1882–1890, 1999.
4. Echt DS, Liebson PR, Mitchell LB, et al: Mortality and morbidity in patients receiving encainide, flecainide, or placebo. The Cardiac Arrhythmia Suppression Trial. N Engl J Med 324:781–788, 1991.
5. Gregoratos G, Cheitlin MD, Conill A: ACC/AHA guidelines for implantation of cardiac pacemakers and antiarrhythmia devices: A report of the American College of Cardiology/American Heart Association Task Force on Practice Guidelines (Committee on Pacemaker Implantation). J Am Coll Cardiol 31:1175–1209, 1998.
6. Huikuri HV, Castellanos A, Myerburg RJ: Sudden cardiac death due to cardiac arrhythmias. N Engl J Med 345:1473–1482, 2001.
7. Julian DG, Camm AJ, Frangin G, et al: Randomised trial of effect of amiodarone on mortality in patients

with left-ventricular dysfunction after recent myocardial infarction: EMIAT. European Myocardial Infarct Amiodarone Trial Investigators. Lancet 349:667–674, 1997.
8. Moss AJ: Implantable cardioverter defibrillator therapy. The sickest patients benefit the most. Circulation 101:1638–1640, 2000.
9. Moss AJ, Hall WJ, Cannom DS, et al: Improved survival with an implanted defibrillator in patients with
coronary disease at high risk for ventricular arrhythmia. Multicenter Automatic Defibrillator Implantation Trial Investigators (MADIT). N Engl J Med 335:1933–1940, 1996.
10. Moss AJ, Zareba W, Hall WJ, et al, for the Multicenter Automatic Defibrillator Implantation Trial II Investigators: Prophylactic implantation of a defibrillator in patients with myocardial infarction and reduced ejection fraction. N Engl J Med 346:877–883, 2002.
11. Myerburg RJ, Castellanos A: Clinical trials of implantable defibrillators. N Engl J Med 337:1621–1623,
1997.
12. Myerburg RJ, Kessler KM, Bassett AL, Castellanos A: A biological approach to sudden cardiac death:
Structure, function and cause. Am J Cardiol 63:1512–1516, 1989.
13. Wellens JJ: The value of the electrocardiogram in the differential diagnosis of a tachycardia with a
widened QRS complex. Am J Med 64:27–33, 1978.

21. CORONARY ARTERY DISEASE

Valerie K. Ulstad, M.D., M.P.A., M.P.H.

1. What causes myocardial ischemia?

Myocardial ischemia is caused by an imbalance between myocardial oxygen supply and demand.

2. How may myocardial ischemia manifest?

Myocardial ischemia may manifest as angina pectoris, as ST-T changes on the electrocardiogram (EKG), and as left ventricular dysfunction due to inadequate supply of myocardial oxygen for normal contractile function.

3. What are the determinants of myocardial oxygen demand?

The need for oxygen delivery to the heart is increased when any of the following four conditions exist: (1) increased heart rate, (2) increased contractility of the heart, (3) increased afterload for the ejecting heart (crudely measured as the systolic blood pressure), and (4) increased preload (filling of the ventricles in diastole).

4. What are the most common clinical presentations of coronary artery disease (CAD)?

Typical angina pectoris
Unstable angina pectoris
Acute myocardial infarction
Sudden cardiac death

5. What is the pathophysiology of typical angina pectoris?

In typical exertional angina pectoris, ischemia results when myocardial oxygen demand is increased but supply is relatively reduced because of atherosclerotic obstruction of 50–70% of the coronary lumen. The affected individual has exertional chest discomfort relieved by rest. Because coronary reserve is reduced most in the subendocardium, ischemia occurs first in this region. An EKG during an episode of pain would likely show ST depression, which is indicative of subendocardial ischemia.

Some patients with chronic stable angina develop ischemia because of dynamic coronary vasoconstriction in the setting of fixed atherosclerotic disease. The eccentric lesions of atherosclerosis leave muscle in the neighboring vessel wall; thus, spasm in that area may suddenly worsen the stenosis. Such inappropriate coronary vasoconstriction has been shown to occur with cigarette smoking, exposure to cold, and exercise.

6. Describe the management of a patient with typical angina pectoris.

1. **Educate.** The patient needs to understand the disease process to be motivated to modify CAD risk factors and to seek medical attention promptly if symptoms worsen.

2. **Treat.** The patient should be started on therapy to relieve discomfort and to improve exercise tolerance. Sublingual nitroglycerin should be used as necessary.

3. **Evaluate.** An exercise stress test should be done to define objectively the level of exercise that precipitates myocardial ischemia and to provide the clinician with prognostic information. The patient who develops ischemia either clinically or on EKG during the first minutes of exercise has a poor prognosis. Such a patient should be referred for more invasive evaluation by coronary angiography.

7. What are the objectives in the medical treatment of angina?

- Reduction of myocardial oxygen demand during exercise or stress: nitrates, beta blockers, calcium channel blockers
- Promotion of maximal vasodilation of the coronary arteries: nitrates, calcium channel blockers

Severity of disease determines the amount of therapy. Usually nitrates are the first-line treatment, with other drugs added if more than episodic nitroglycerin is required.

Antianginal Therapy

AGENT	ACTION	IMPORTANT CONSIDERATIONS
Nitrates	Dilate coronaries Decrease preload	8–10 hr/day free of drug to avoid tolerance May cause headache
Beta blockers	Decrease heart rate Decrease contractility Decrease blood pressure	All agents potentially block beta$_1$ and beta$_2$ receptors; selective agents at low dose block beta$_1$ receptors more than beta$_2$ May precipitate CHF, bronchospasm, CNS side effects
Calcium channel blockers	Dilate coronaries Decrease contractility Decrease systolic pressure Decrease heart rate	Heterogeneous group Constipation

CHF = congestive heart failure; CNS = central nervous system.

8. What education should the patient receive about therapy with nitroglycerin?

Sublingual nitroglycerin prescriptions should be refilled every 6 months because the tablets become outdated. A patient who develops flushing or headache with sublingual therapy probably is using active nitroglycerin. Patients who use nitrates (either orally or by patch) to sustain blood levels must have a 10–12-hour nitrate-free period each day. This decreases the incidence of nitroglycerin tolerance and improves efficacy.

9. What is unstable angina?

The following situations suggest that the anginal pattern is unstable:

1. Rest angina or angina occurring with less effort than previously
2. More frequent angina with the same degree of exertion
3. More protracted discomfort that is less responsive to therapy or rest
4. Prolonged pain without evidence of myocardial infarction
5. Recent onset of angina

10. What is the pathophysiology of unstable angina?

Unstable angina is a clinical syndrome that falls between chronic stable angina pectoris and acute myocardial infarction. Studies suggest that myocardial oxygen supply is further reduced. The involved coronary artery in unstable angina tends to have an eccentric plaque with a fissure or crack and superimposed thrombus adherent to the site of the plaque crack or rupture. The precise factors that lead to plaque rupture are unknown. Platelets adhere to the disrupted thrombogenic intima and produce thromboxane A_2, which stimulates further platelet aggregation. The resultant thrombus is responsible for the sudden change in myocardial oxygen supply and subsequent change in symptoms. The thrombus may be intermittently occlusive, leading to waxing and waning discomfort at rest. If the thrombus completely occludes the vessel, a myocardial infarction follows, unless the vessel can be rapidly opened.

11. Describe the EKG in patients with unstable angina.

The majority of patients have transient ST-T changes (elevation or progression) or peaking or inverted T waves during pain. An EKG with ST-T segment deviation in two or more leads is highly predictive of adverse clinical events.

12. What therapy is indicated in patients with unstable angina?

Unstable angina is associated with a tendency to develop continually worsening pain, acute myocardial infarction, life-threatening ventricular arrhythmias, or sudden cardiac death. Patients should be hospitalized promptly for observation, monitoring, antianginal therapy (IV nitroglycerin if discomfort continues and beta blockers), and antithrombotic therapy (which may include enoxaparin or unfractionated heparin infusion, glycoprotein IIb or IIIa inhibitor, and aspirin or clopidogrel) to promote coronary artery patency. Thrombolytic therapy has no role in patients with unstable angina. Patients with EKG changes and chest pain or elevated troponin levels may be referred for early catheterization, whereas patients without EKG changes and normal troponin levels may be risk-stratified with exercise testing.

13. Describe the presentation of the patient with acute myocardial infarction (AMI).

The patient with AMI usually presents with discomfort similar in character to angina pectoris. The discomfort does not resolve promptly with rest and nitroglycerin. Continued discomfort at rest distinguishes AMI from a simple episode of angina. The EKG in patients with AMI typically shows ST segment elevation, suggesting transmural ischemia usually due to obstruction of an epicardial coronary artery. The presence of a new left bundle branch block on EKG should also be considered to represent evidence for acute MI in the clinical setting of ischemic chest discomfort.

14. What is the pathophysiology of AMI?

An intracoronary thrombus develops because of atherosclerotic plaque disruption and fissure. When the thrombus totally occludes the vessel, myocardial ischemia begins. If the vessel remains closed, myocardial infarction occurs. In more than 85% of patients with AMI, occluding thrombus can be demonstrated angiographically.

15. Why is prompt recognition of AMI so important?

The obstruction of a coronary artery quickly leads to abnormal ventricular wall motion in the distribution of the affected coronary artery. If the vessel remains closed for longer than 20–40 minutes, the ventricular muscle in the distribution of the coronary artery begins to become necrotic (infarction); the deepest layers of the myocardium are affected first.

The highest priority is to open the coronary artery. Emergent percutaneous coronary angioplasty with stent placement or thrombolytic therapy to lyse the occluding thrombus should be considered in every patient with AMI as soon as the diagnosis is made. When immediate percutaneous transluminal coronary angioplasty (PTCA) is available, immediate revascularization is preferable to thrombolytic therapy.

16. What is thrombolytic therapy?

Thrombolytic agents are capable of causing clot lysis directly or indirectly by accelerating the conversion of plasminogen to plasmin. Plasmin is a proteolytic enzyme that acts on fibrin to cause fibrinolysis, which results in thrombolysis and reperfusion. The three agents approved by the Food and Drug Administration for coronary thrombolysis include streptokinase, alteplase (a recombinant tissue-type plasminogen activator [TPA]), and anistreplase (an acylated plasminogen-streptokinase complex [APSAC]).

17. Does thrombolytic therapy work?

Yes. Intravenous thrombolytic therapy reduces early mortality from AMI by 25%, leads to an increase in postinfarction left ventricular ejection fraction, and reduces the likelihood of postinfarction congestive heart failure. Survival rates with various agents have so far been similar, although the role of adjunctive heparin with each has not been well studied. Using early patency of the coronary artery as an endpoint, randomized trials have shown that TPA is superior to streptokinase. In the GUSTO study, differences in early patency translated into a greater reduction in mortality in patients given TPA versus patients receiving streptokinase.

18. Who is the ideal candidate for thrombolytic therapy?

Ideal patients (who tend to be included in controlled trials) are younger than 75 years, with ST elevation in two or more contiguous leads, and present within 6 hours of the onset of chest discomfort. Many other patients may benefit from thrombolytic therapy, including patients with new left bundle-branch block, elderly patients with large infarctions, and patients presenting between 6 and 12 hours after the onset of pain.

19. What is the major side effect of thrombolytic therapy?

With all thrombolytic agents the major adverse effect is bleeding. Hemorrhage requiring transfusion occurs in 1–5% of patients and intracranial bleeding in 0.5–1.5%.

20. What is the role of aspirin in AMI?

Aspirin has been shown to reduce the incidence of reinfarction in patients treated with streptokinase and to double the reduction in mortality observed with streptokinase alone. Aspirin, 160–325 mg/day, should be started in the emergency department at presentation and continued indefinitely.

21. Should beta blockers be given after AMI?

Yes. Beta blockers have been shown to reduce mortality when started several days to several months after infarction. Both selective and nonselective forms of beta blockers reduce the incidence of sudden death after infarction.

22. Should beta blockers be started immediately upon presentation with AMI?

Yes. The immediate use of beta blockers, presumably to reduce myocardial oxygen demand by opposing the heightened adrenergic tone associated with AMI, has been shown to lead to a 13% reduction in 1-week mortality and a 19% reduction in nonfatal reinfarctions.

23. What is the role for angiotensin-converting enzyme (ACE) inhibitors in the postinfarction patient?

The Studies of Left Ventricular Dysfunction (SOLVD) and the Survival and Ventricular Enlargement (SAVE) trials suggest that postinfarction patients with an ejection fraction less than 40% have lower mortality, fewer hospitalizations for heart failure, and a lower incidence of recurrent infarction when treated with an ACE inhibitor.

24. What are the major complications of AMI?

- Arrhythmias (particularly ventricular)
- Systolic heart failure

- Mechanical complications (free wall, septal, or papillary muscle rupture)
- Left ventricular (LV) mural thrombus with embolization

25. What is the 1-year mortality rate after AMI?
The 1-year mortality rate after discharge is 4–7%. In patients younger than 70 years who are treated with thrombolytic therapy, the mortality rate may be as low as 3–5%.

26. List the factors associated with a poor prognosis after AMI.

1. Decreased LV ejection fraction— independent factor
2. Advanced age—independent factor
3. Female sex—independent factor
4. Complex or frequent PVCs— independent factor
5. Congestive heart failure
6. Postinfarction angina
7. Prior myocardial infarction
8. Large infarction
9. Atrial fibrillation
10. Extensive coronary artery disease
11. Diabetes
12. Hypertension
13. Continued smoking
14. Elevated serum cholesterol

27. What can be done to minimize the postinfarction risk?
1. Coronary angiography during acute hospitalization if the patient has continued ischemic symptoms in the hospital
2. Predischarge limited exercise testing to identify patients with residual ischemia for referral for coronary angiography and possible revascularization
3. Referral of patients with sustained ventricular tachycardia for coronary angiography and electrophysiologic evaluation
4. Smoking cessation (associated with a 40–60% decrease in mortality)
5. Lowering of cholesterol, usually with a statin drug
6. Use of beta blocker
7. Aspirin
8. ACE inhibitor if ejection fraction is ≤ 40%
9. Referral to cardiac rehabilitation (may reduce mortality by 20–50%)

28. Does lowering lipids in the patient with known CAD make a difference?
Yes. The Scandinavian Simvastatin Survival Study (4S) showed a 30% decrease in total mortality and a 42% reduction in cardiac mortality at 5 years in patients with known CAD and elevated total (= 261) and low density lipoprotein (LDL = 188) cholesterol. The Cholesterol and Recurrent Events (CARE) trial was an analysis of statin use in patients with known CAD and average cholesterol levels (mean total cholesterol = 209, LDL = 139). This study showed a 24% reduction in fatal CAD and nonfatal MI in the treated group after a follow-up of 5 years. The problem mechanism of the marked decrease in events is plaque stabilization.

29. What are the advantages of percutaneous coronary angioplasty with stent placement compared with thrombolytic therapy in patients with acute MI?
The former is:
- More likely to have an open infarct–related artery
- More likely to have normal blood flow in the infract related artery

30. What symptoms are women more likely to have than men when experiencing acute myocardial infarction?
Neck and shoulder pain
Nausea and vomiting

31. What four drugs should probably be part of every patient's discharge medications post-MI?
1. Aspirin
3. ACE inhibitor
2. Beta blocker
4. Statin

BIBLIOGRAPHY

1. American College of Cardiology/American Heart Association Task Force on Assessment of Diagnostic and Therapeutic Cardiovascular Procedures (Subcommittee to Develop Guidelines for the Early Management of Patients with Acute Myocardial Infarction): Guidelines for the early management of patients with acute myocardial infarction. J Am Coll Cardiol 16:249–292, 1990.
2. Braunwald E, Antman EM, Beasley JW, et al: ACC/AHA guidelines for management of patients with unstable angina and non-ST segment elevation myocardial infarction: A report of the American College of Cardiology/American Heart Association Task Force on Practice Guidelines (Committee on the Management of Patients with Unstable Angina). J Am Coll Cardiol 36:970–1062, 2000.
3. Braunwald E, Jones RH, Mark DB, et al: Diagnosing and managing unstable angina. Agency for Health Care Policy and Research. Circulation 90:613–622, 1994.
4. Clopidogrel in Unstable Angina to Prevent Recurrent Events Trial Investigators: Effects of clopidogrel in addition to aspirin in patients with acute coronary syndromes without ST-segment elevation. N Engl J Med 345:494–502, 2001.
5. Fuster V, Badimon L, Badimon JJ, Chesebro JH: The pathogenesis of coronary artery disease and the acute coronary syndromes: Part 1. N Engl J Med 326:242–250, 1992.
6. Fuster V, Badimon L, Badimon JJ, Chesebro JH: The pathogenesis of coronary artery disease and the acute coronary syndromes: Part 2. N Engl J Med 326:310–318, 1992.
7. Gibbons RJ, Chatterjee K, Daley J, et al: ACC/AHA guidelines for the management of patients with chronic stable angina: A report of the American College of Cardiology/American Heart Association Task Force on Practice Guidelines (Committee on Management of Acute Myocardial Infarction). Circulation 99:2828–2848, 1999.
8. Global Use of Strategies to Open Occluded Coronary Arteries in Acute Coronary Syndromes (GUSTO IIb) Angioplasty Substudy Investigators: A clinical trial comparing primary coronary angioplasty with tissue plasminogen activator for acute myocardial infarction. N Engl J Med 336:1621–1628, 1997.
9. Hamm CW, Braunwald E: A classification of unstable angina revisited. Circulation 102:118–122, 2000.
10. Heidenreich PA, Alloggiamento T, Melsop K, et al: The prognostic value of troponin in patients with non-ST elevation acute coronary syndromes. A meta-analysis. J Am Coll Cardiol 38:478–485, 2001.
11. Hochman JS, Tamis JE, Thompson TD, et al: Sex, clinical presentation and outcome in patients with acute coronary syndromes. N Engl J Med 341:226–232, 1999.
12. Pfeffer MA, Braunwald E, Moye LA, et al: Effects of captopril on mortality and morbidity in patients with left ventricular dysfunction after myocardial infarction: Results of the Survival and Ventricular Enlargement trial. The SAVE investigators. N Engl J Med 327:669–677, 1992.
13. Ryan TJ, Antman EM, Brooks NH, et al: 1999 Update: ACC/AHA guidelines for the management of patients with acute myocardial infarction: Executive summary and recommendations: A report of the American College of Cardiology/American Heart Association Task Force on Practice Guidelines (Committee on Management of Acute Myocardial Infarction). Circulation 100:1016–1030, 1999.
14. Sacks FM, Pfeffer MA, Braunwald E, et al, for the CARE investigators: Effect of pravastatin on coronary events after myocardial infarction in patients with average cholesterol levels. N Engl J Med 335:1001–1009, 1996.
15. Smith SC, Blair SN, Bonow RO, et al: AHA/ACC guidelines for preventing heart attack and death in patients with atherosclerotic disease: 2001 update. A statement for health care professionals from the American Heart Association and the American College of Cardiology. Circulation 104:1577–1579, 2001.
16. SOLVD Investigators: Effect of enalapril on mortality and the development of heart failure in asymptomatic patients with reduced left ventricular ejection fractions. N Engl J Med 327:658–691, 1992.
17. Weaver WD, Simes RJ, Betriu A, et al: Comparison of primary coronary angioplasty and intravenous thrombolytic therapy for acute myocardial infarction: A quantitative review. JAMA 278:2093–2098, 1997.
18. Wenger NK, Froelicher ES, Smith LK, et al: Cardiac Rehabilitation as Secondary Prevention: Clinical Practice Guideline: Quick Reference Guide for Clinicians No. 17. Rockville, MD, U.S. Department of Health and Human Services, Public Health Service, Agency for Health Care Policy and Research, and National Heart, Lung, and Blood Institute, 1995, AHCPR publication 96–0673.

22. CONGESTIVE HEART FAILURE

Valerie Ulstad, M.D., M.P.A., M.P.H.

1. What is congestive heart failure (CHF)?

CHF is a clinical syndrome related to cardiac dysfunction (systolic, diastolic, or both) and characterized by limited exercise tolerance, fluid retention, and reduced life expectancy.

2. What are the incidence and prevalence of CHF?

Three million people in the United States and 15 million people worldwide have CHF. There are approximately 400,000 new cases in the United States each year. The incidence is increasing despite the decline in mortality from cardiovascular disease, probably because an aging population has received benefit from improved therapies. CHF is the most common discharge diagnosis in patients age 65 years and older.

3. Describe the New York Heart Association (NYHA) classification of heart failure.

Class I: No limitation of physical activity; no dyspnea, fatigue, or palpitations with ordinary physical activity.

Class II: Slight limitation of physical activity; patients have dyspnea, fatigue, or palpitations with ordinary physical activity but are comfortable at rest.

Class III: Marked limitation of activity; less than ordinary physical activity results in symptoms, but patients are comfortable at rest.

Class IV: Symptoms are present at rest, and any physical exertion exacerbates the symptoms.

4. Characterize low-output cardiac failure.

Low-output failure, the most common form of heart failure, is characterized by reduced stroke volume, peripheral vasoconstriction, reduced pulse pressure, and increased arteriovenous (AV) oxygen difference.

5. What are the most important causes of low-output CHF in the United States?

Coronary artery disease: underlying
   cause in 50–75% of cases
Hypertension
Dilated cardiomyopathy
Valvular heart disease
Hypertrophic cardiomyopathy
Congenital heart disease
Cor pulmonale
Toxins: alcohol, doxorubicin (Adriamycin)
Infections

6. What is the most common cause of low-output CHF worldwide?

Chagas disease.

7. List seven prognostic indicators in CHF.

1. Ventricular function measured by ejection fraction
2. Peak exercise oxygen consumption
3. NYHA class
4. Plasma norepinephrine levels
5. Ventricular arrhythmias
6. Brain naturetic peptide levels
7. Serum sodium level

8. What is the mortality rate from CHF?

The 5-year mortality rate in men is 60%. Women do somewhat better, with a 5-year mortality rate of 45%. When the patient has symptoms of heart failure at rest (class IV), the 1-year mortality rate is about 50%. About 40% of deaths are sudden, presumably because of ventricular arrhythmias.

9. What is high-output cardiac failure?
High-output cardiac failure is characterized by widened pulse pressure, peripheral vasodilation, and an increased arteriovenous oxygen difference.

10. What conditions are associated with high-output heart failure?

Anemia	Paget disease
Hyperthyroidism	Hepatic disease
Systemic AV fistula	Dermatologic conditions causing high blood
Beriberi	flow in skin

11. Which symptoms of CHF are caused by isolated left ventricular dysfunction?

Dyspnea on exertion	Wheezing
Paroxysmal nocturnal dyspnea	Hemoptysis
Orthopnea	Fatigue
Cough	Weakness

12. What are the clinical signs of isolated left ventricular dysfunction?

Hypotension	Cardiomegaly (systolic dysfunction)
Weak pulses	S_3 gallop
Peripheral vasoconstriction	Rales
Cachexia	Pleural effusions
Cheyne-Stokes respirations	

13. Which symptoms of CHF are caused by isolated right ventricular dysfunction?
Right upper quadrant discomfort
Abdominal distention
Early satiety

14. What are the clinical signs of isolated right ventricular dysfunction?
Elevated jugular venous pressure
Hepatomegaly
Splenomegaly
Ascites
Peripheral edema

15. What is the most common cause of right-heart failure?
Left-heart failure.

16. Contrast systolic and diastolic dysfunction.
Systolic dysfunction occurs with a defect in the expulsion of blood from the ventricles or a decrease in ventricular contractility. Diastolic dysfunction occurs with abnormal resistance to ventricular filling in diastole.

17. How do Frank-Starling curves (stroke volume on the Y axis and end-diastolic volume on the X axis) differ for the normal heart and the heart with severe systolic dysfunction?
Note the effect of increasing preload. The normal heart augments its output with increases in preload. The heart with systolic failure is unable to augment its output further by increasing preload.

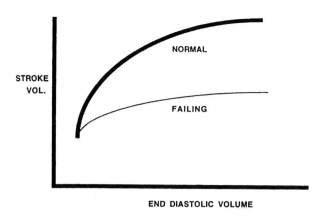

Frank-Starling curves for the normal heart and the heart with severe systolic dysfunction.

18. How do the function curves (stroke volume on the Y axis and afterload on the X axis) differ for the normal heart and the heart with severe systolic dysfunction?
    Note the effect of increasing impedance or afterload. The normal heart tolerates increased impedance well without a decrease in stroke volume. The heart with systolic failure fails further (i.e., stroke volume decreases further) with increased impedance.

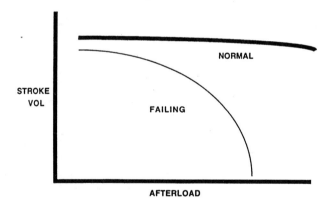

Function curves for the normal heart and the heart with severe systolic dysfunction.

19. Which is the more common cause of CHF syndrome, systolic or diastolic dysfunction?
    Systolic dysfunction is the more common cause. As a result, the terms *systolic dysfunction* and *CHF syndrome* tend to be used synonymously, but such usage is inaccurate.

20. Describe the vicious cycle of heart failure.
    A particular cardiac problem causes a decrease in cardiac output that leads to activation of the neurohormonal mechanisms, including the sympathetic nervous system, the renin-angiotensin-aldosterone system, and the arginine vasopressin system. The net effects are excessive vasoconstriction and increased sodium and water retention, which lead to increased vascular impedance to the already failing heart. Thus, the patient's condition worsens.

21. List the three major goals of therapy for CHF.
1. Improved quality of life
2. Prolonged survival
3. Improved natural history

22. What are the principles of treatment of CHF?
1. Remove or correct the precipitating cause. Always consider whether ischemia plays a role.
2. Correct exacerbating factors.
3. Using echocardiography, determine whether the dysfunction is predominantly systolic or diastolic.
4. Use pharmacologic therapy to effectively counteract neurohormonal activation.
5. Add diuretics if there is dyspnea and prescribe a low-sodium diet to control salt and water retention.
6. Encourage weight loss (if the patient is overweight) and regular exercise.
7. Prescribe digoxin in patients with atrial fibrillation or patients in normal sinus rhythm who are still symptomatic on angiotensin-converting enzyme (ACE) inhibitors, beta-blockers, and diuretics.

23. What common causes of cardiac decompensation should be considered in patients with previously stable CHF?
- Myocardial ischemia
- Mitral regurgitation
- Uncontrolled hypertension
- Increased dietary intake of sodium
- Superimposed medical illness, especially:
  Poorly controlled diabetes mellitus
  Pneumonia
  Pulmonary embolus

24. When should diuretic therapy be used in the treatment of CHF?
In chronic therapy of **CHF due to systolic dysfunction,** diuretics are used frequently, although they may not be necessary in some cases. Excessive diuresis may result in further activation of the neurohormonal system and intolerance of ACE inhibitors (hypotension).

In chronic therapy of **CHF due to diastolic dysfunction,** diuretics may be needed to decrease pulmonary congestion and to improve dyspnea. Diuretics must be given carefully to avoid an excessive decrease in preload because patients have stiff ventricles with intrinsic resistance to diastolic filling.

Loop diuretics are needed when renal function is abnormal (creatinine ≥ 2.0 mg/dL), because thiazide diuretics are ineffective in such patients. In patients with mild CHF, thiazide diuretics may have a role if renal function is normal. In refractory heart failure, a combination of thiazide and loop diuretics may be needed.

25. How should ACE inhibitors be used in CHF due to systolic dysfunction?
ACE inhibitors should be started in nearly all patients with symptomatic or asymptomatic left ventricular systolic dysfunction. Hypotension can be prevented by starting with low doses and by avoiding volume depletion before therapy institution. Marked subsequent increases in blood urea nitrogen (BUN) and creatinine (Cr) suggest renovascular disease, and the ACE inhibitor should be stopped. Angiotensin II receptor blockers should be tried in patients intolerant of ACE inhibitors or patients with side effects.

26. Should asymptomatic persons with left ventricular systolic dysfunction be treated with ACE inhibitor therapy?
Yes. This recommendation is based on the outcome of two major trials. The SOLVD trial showed that enalapril reduced the incidence of heart failure and the rate of related hospitalizations

in patients with asymptomatic decreased function (ejection fraction [EF] ≤ 35%). In the Survival and Ventricular Enlargement (SAVE) study, patients enrolled 3–17 days after infarction with EFs of < 40% and no clinical heart failure were randomized to captopril or placebo. Captopril prevented further reduction in EF and reduced the rates of recurrent infarction and mortality.

27. What is the difference in treatment of systolic as opposed to diastolic failure?
Although most of the trials looking at morbidity and mortality have been done in systolic dysfunction, pharmacologic treatment to blunt neurohormonal activation is indicated in both systolic and diastolic dysfunction. ACE inhibitors and beta-blockers are the cornerstones of therapy aimed at counteracting the neurohormonal activation associated with a decreased cardiac output.

28. How does one distinguish between systolic and diastolic dysfunction as the cause of the clinical syndrome of CHF?
The clinical syndrome is the same in both types of dysfunction. Echocardiography is a useful test in any patient with new heart failure. This test may demonstrate any important valvular or pericardial disease. Systolic dysfunction is evident with decreased contractility of the heart. If both left and right ventricular systolic functions are normal, restricted ventricular filling or diastolic dysfunction may be the culprit. Echo-Doppler studies may be used to look more carefully for diastolic dysfunction.

29. What endpoints should be evaluated in drug trials for treatment of CHF?
• Improved quality of life
• Improved exercise capacity
• Reversal of neurohormonal abnormalities
• Reduction of mortality

30. Describe the common types of cardiomyopathy.
Cardiomyopathy is a condition of varying and frequently unknown cause in which the dominant feature is cardiomegaly and low-output cardiac failure. Cardiomyopathies are categorized into three groups:
1. **Dilated**
   • Most common type; dilatation of all chambers
   • Decrease in systolic function of the ventricles
   • Causes include idiopathic factors, alcohol, Adriamycin, myocarditis, valve replacement, diabetes, thyroid disease, thiamine deficiency, pheochromocytoma, peripartum complications, and coronary artery disease
   • Chest radiograph shows enlarged heart; echocardiography shows enlarged chambers and reduced contractility; radionuclide ventriculography shows reduced EF
2. **Hypertrophic**
   • Less common; thickening of ventricular wall; small ventricular cavity
   • Abnormal diastolic function
   • Causes include genetic factors, hypertension, and acromegaly
   • Chest radiograph shows normal to mildly enlarged heart size, echocardiography shows small ventricular chamber, increased wall thickness, and increased contractility
3. **Restrictive (infiltrative)**
   • Rare
   • Systolic and diastolic function affected; both ventricles affected equally
   • Causes include amyloid and sarcoid disorders and hemochromatosis
   • Diagnosis often found only with biopsy after hemodynamic evaluation shows equal diastolic filling pattern (square-root sign) on right and left sides of heart

31. Which patients should undergo cardiac transplantation?
Transplantation should be considered in patients who remain severely compromised despite medical therapy. The 5-year survival rate for cardiac transplantation is 75–80%. Donor availability, however, limits widespread application.

32. What factors are associated with increased morbidity or mortality from cardiac transplant?

Obesity	Previous cardiac or thoracic surgery
Diabetes with organ damage	Chronic lung disease
Pulmonary hypertension	Intrinsic hepatic or renal disease

33. What is the role of ACE inhibitors after myocardial infarction (MI)?

In the presence of symptomatic or asymptomatic left ventricular dysfunction, ACE inhibitors provide additional benefit to aspirin, beta-blockers, and thrombolytic therapy. They should be given as soon as the physician believes that the patient is stable with an adequate blood pressure (BP). Reasonable times to start the ACE inhibitor are the morning after admission, if the patient is stable, and certainly before discharge. A meta-analysis of the use of ACE inhibitors after MI suggests a 24% reduction in mortality, a 27% reduction in hospitalization, and 20% reduction in recurrent MI.

34. What is the role of beta-blockers in the treatment of chronic heart failure?

Beta-blockers are a mainstay of therapy because they block the activation of the sympathetic nervous system. Sustained and chronic activation of the sympathetic nervous system leads to elevation of norepinephrine levels and downregulation of beta receptors, which have a negative impact on cardiac function and prognosis. Metoprolol, bisprolol, and carvedilol have been shown to provide significant reductions in morbidity and mortality in patients with chronic heart failure. A beta-blocker should be considered as part of the standard regimen for all patients with CHF ranging from mild to severe.

35. What is the best predictor of an individual's 1-year mortality from CHF?

Mortality in New York Heart Association Functional Classification

CLASS	1-YEAR MORTALITY
I	10%
II	10–15%
III	15–25%
IV	30–50%

36. What medications should be prescribed for patients with symptomatic CHF caused by reduced left ventricular systolic function?

- ACE inhibitor (or angiotensin II receptor blocker if intolerant of the ACE inhibitor)
- Beta-blocker (unless CHF is decompensated)
- Aldactone with more severe symptoms (if potassium handling is normal and renal function is normal)
- Furosemide if there is dyspnea or fluid retention
- Digoxin if there is persistent shortness of breath on the above medications

BIBLIOGRAPHY

1. Banerjee P, Banerjee T, Khand A, et al: Diastolic heart failure: Neglected or misdiagnosed? J Am Coll Cardiol 39:138–141, 2002.
2. Bristow MR, Gilbert EM, Abraham WT, et al: Carvedilol produces dose-related improvements in left ventricular function and survival in subjects with chronic heart failure. MOCHA investigators. Circulation 94:2807–2816, 1996.
3. Cohn J: The management of chronic heart failure. N Engl J Med 335:d490–498, 1996.
4. Cohn JN, Johnson GR, Shabeti R, et al: Ejection fraction, peak exercise oxygen consumption, cardiothoracic ratio, ventricular arrhythmias, and plasma norepinephrine as determinants of prognosis in heart failure. Circulation 87(suppl VI):VI-5–VI-16, 1993.

5. Cohn JN, Tognoni G: A randomized trial of the angiotensin-receptor blocker valsartan in chronic heart failure. N Engl J Med 345:1667–1675, 2001.
6. CONSENSUS Trial Study Group: Effects of enalapril on mortality in severe congestive heart failure: Results of the Cooperative North Scandinavian Enalapril Survival Study (CONSENSUS). N Engl J Med 316:1429–1435, 1987.
7. Eichhorn EJ, Bristow MR: Medical therapy can improve the biological properties of the chronically failing heart. A new era in the treatment of heart failure. Circulation 94:2285–2296, 1996.
8. Foody JM, Farrell MH, Krumholz HM: Beta blocker therapy in heart failure. JAMA 287:883–889, 2002.
9. Hunt SA, Baker DW, Chin MH, et al: ACC/AHA Guidelines for the evaluation and management of chronic heart failure in the adult: Executive summary. Report of the American College of Cardiology/American Heart Association Task Force on Practice Guidelines (Committee to Revise the 1995 Guidelines for Evaluation and Management of Heart Failure). J Am Coll Cardiol 38:2101–2113, 2001.
10. Latini R, Maggioni AP, Flather M, et al: ACE inhibitor use in patients with myocardial infarction. Summary of evidence from clinical trials. Circulation 92:3132–3137, 1995.
11. Levine TB, Francis GS, Goldsmith SR, et al: Activity of the sympathetic nervous system and the renin-angiotensin system assessed by plasma hormone levels and their relation to hemodynamic abnormalities in congestive heart failure. Am J Cardiol 49:1659–1666, 1982.
12. Lorell BH: Significance of diastolic dysfunction of the heart. Annu Rev Med 42:411–436, 1991.
13. McAlister FA, Teo KK: The management of congestive heart failure. Postgrad Med J 83:194–200, 1997.
14. McFate-Smith W: Epidemiology of congestive heart failure. Am J Cardiol 55:3A–8A, 1985.
15. Nohria A, Lewis E, Stevenson LW: Medical management of advanced heart failure. JAMA 287:628–640, 2002.
16. Packer M, Bristow M, Cohn JN, et al: The effect of carvedilol on morbidity and mortality in patients with chronic heart failure. N Engl J Med 334:1349–1355, 1996.
17. Pitt B, Zannad F, Remme WJ, et al: The effect of spironolactone on morbidity and mortality in patients with severe heart failure. Randomized Aldactone Evaluation Study Investigators. N Engl J Med 341:709–717, 1999.
18. Senni M, Redfield MM: Congestive heart failure in elderly patients. Mayo Clin Proc 72:453–460, 1997.
19. Senni M, Redfield MM: Heart failure with preserved systolic function: A different natural history? J Am Coll Cardiol 38:1277–1282, 2001.
20. SOLVD Investigators: Effect of enalapril on mortality and development of heart failure in asymptomatic patients with reduced left ventricular ejection fractions. N Engl J Med 327:685–691, 1992.
21. SOLVD Investigators: Effect of enalapril on survival in patients with reduced left ventricular ejection fractions and congestive heart failure. N Engl J Med 325:293–302, 1991.
22. Stevenson LW: Therapy tailored for symptomatic heart failure. Heart Fail 11:87–107, 1995.

23. CARDIAC TESTING

Valerie K. Ulstad, M.D., M.P.A., M.P.H.

1. How often is the initial electrocardiogram (EKG) diagnostic of myocardial infarction (MI)?

The initial EKG is diagnostic in 60% of patients. In 25% the EKG is abnormal but not diagnostic. In 15% the EKG is absolutely normal. Therefore, decisions about admission to the hospital should be based primarily on the history and current findings. The diagnostic accuracy of the EKG is enhanced by obtaining serial EKGs.

2. Does an EKG without Q waves rule out a previous MI?

No. A definitive diagnosis of a previous MI depends on the presence of pathologic Q waves. Within 6–12 months after an acute MI, about 30% of EKGs are still abnormal but no longer diagnostic for previous MI because the Q waves are absent. After 10 years, 6–10% of EKGs are completely normal.

3. List eight contraindications to exercise testing.

1. Uncontrolled hypertension
2. Critical aortic stenosis
3. Hypertrophic cardiomyopathy with significant obstruction
4. Untreated life-threatening cardiac arrhythmias
5. Decompensated heart failure
6. Advanced atrioventricular (AV) block
7. Acute pericarditis or myocarditis
8. Other acute illness

4. When should a stress test be stopped?

	REASON TO STOP EXERCISE TEST
Patient signs and symptoms	Severe fatigue
	Severe dyspnea
	Chest pain
	Marked elevation in systolic blood pressure (> 250 mmHg)
	Definite drop in systolic blood pressure (≥ 10 mmHg)
EKG changes	≥ 3 mm ST depression
	≥ 1 mm ST elevation in lead without abnormal Q wave
	Ventricular tachycardia
	Paroxysmal supraventricular tachycardia
	Decrease in heart rate
Noncardiac factors	Patient request
	Gait disturbance
	Technical problems interfering with test interpretation

5. In addition to exercise-induced chest pain, what signs and symptoms during an exercise test indicate an adverse prognosis and probable multivessel coronary artery disease (CAD)?

- Inability to exercise to 6 metabolic equivalents (METs) in an otherwise healthy patient
- Failure to increase systolic blood pressure ≥ 120 mmHg
- Definite drop in systolic blood pressure ≥ 10 mmHg
- ST depression > 2 mm
- Downsloping ST depression under 6 METs in 5 or more leads or persisting more than 5 minutes into recovery
- Exercise-induced ST elevation (excluding lead aVR)
- Sustained ventricular tachycardia

6. What is the value of a stress test in patients with an uncomplicated MI before hospital discharge?

A low-level exercise test to 5–6 METs or 70–80% of the age-predicted maximal heart rate is frequently performed before hospital discharge to assess the patient's functional capacity and to test for residual provocable myocardial ischemia at a relatively low level of myocardial oxygen demand. A negative submaximal stress test is associated with a 1-year mortality rate of 1–2%. An ischemic response indicates a poorer prognosis. Cardiac catheterization before discharge should be considered in such patients to assess revascularization options.

7. What are the major general principles to consider for stress testing?

1. Stress testing gives physiologic information, whereas angiography gives anatomic information.

2. Interpretation of the stress test requires integration of clinical data from the history and physical exam with data from the stress test.

3. Stress testing is done to identify patients who have a high risk of severe coronary disease. Stress testing is not done to rule out the presence of coronary disease.

8. What stress tests are available to aid in the assessment of patients with known or suspected CAD?
1. Standard treadmill testing with EKG monitoring
2. Bicycle ergometer with EKG monitoring
3. Myocardial perfusion imaging with thallium-201 or 99mTc sestamibi
4. Radionuclide angiography
5. Stress echocardiography
6. Cardiopulmonary exercise testing
7. Pharmacologic stress with dobutamine, dipyridamole, or adenosine and perfusion or echocardiographic imaging

9. List four advantages of stress imaging in comparison with standard exercise electrocardiography.
1. Greater accuracy when resting EKG is abnormal
2. Higher sensitivity
3. Ability to localize and characterize the extent of ischemia
4. Direct measurement of ventricular function

10. Should regular stress testing be done in patients with an abnormal baseline EKG?
The clinician may gain useful information about functional capacity by watching the patient exercise, although the interpretation of the EKG is difficult. In patients with baseline EKG abnormalities, perfusion imaging is preferred to regular treadmill testing because of its increased diagnostic accuracy. Baseline abnormalities include ST-T abnormalities, left bundle-branch block (LBBB), intraventricular conduction delay, paced ventricular rhythm, left ventricular hypertrophy, and Wolff-Parkinson-White syndrome.

11. Is a nondiagnostic treadmill study the same as a negative test?
No. It usually means (1) that the patient could not adequately exercise to address the clinical question or (2) that the baseline EKG was abnormal.

12. What is myocardial perfusion imaging?
Perfusion scanning provides physiologic information about coronary blood flow reserve, location of hypoperfusion, and extent and severity of the abnormality. Uptake of the agent by the myocardium is proportional to blood flow. Common perfusion agents include thallium-201 and the technetium agent sestamibi. Perfusion imaging can be used with treadmill, bicycle, or pharmacologic stress testing to assess the patient for myocardial ischemia.

13. Because the sensitivity for detecting CAD is similar for stress echocardiography and perfusion imaging, what are the important factors in selecting an imaging modality?
- Institutional expertise
- Body habitus of patient—can the heart be seen on echocardiography?
- Perfusion imaging is more expensive than echocardiographic imaging.
- Echocardiography provides other anatomic information.
- Myocardial perfusion imaging can detect ischemia in segments with abnormal wall motion at rest, whereas the significance of a worsening wall motion abnormality on exercise echocardiography is not well understood.
- Nuclear studies have been better validated for determining prognosis.

14. Which stress test should be used in patients with LBBB?
Exercise-induced ST depression cannot be used as a diagnostic or prognostic indicator in patients with LBBB. Most patients have ST depression with exercise, and the extent of ST depression is not meaningful. Pharmacologic stress testing with adenosine or dipyridamole is indicated in patients with resting or exercise-induced LBBB due to perfusion abnormalities that are sec-

ondary to the abnormal depolarization of the heart that mimic ischemia on exercise imaging studies.

15. How should patients on digoxin be evaluated for CAD?

Digitalis glycosides may produce exertional ST depression even with no evidence of digitalis effect on the resting EKG. Absence of ST depression during an exercise test in a patient on digitalis glycosides is considered a valid negative response. Digitalis should be withheld 1–2 weeks before exercise testing if one plans to rely only on EKG data. Having the patient remain on the drug is an option if one uses thallium perfusion imaging or stress echocardiography instead.

16. What are the options for stress testing in the patient who cannot exercise?

Pharmacologic stress testing with echocardiographic or myocardial perfusion imaging is an option for the patient who cannot exercise. Pharmacologic agents include dobutamine, dipyridamole, and adenosine. Dobutamine increases cardiac contractility and heart rate, thereby increasing myocardial oxygen demand and simulating physical stress. Dipyridamole and adenosine increase coronary blood flow and lead to redistribution of flow, producing a steal phenomenon in the distribution of significant coronary stenosis. Simultaneous echocardiographic imaging allows the detection, grading, and localization of wall-motion abnormalities due to ischemic provocation.

17. How does antianginal therapy affect the exercise treadmill test?

Nitrates, beta blockers, and calcium channel blockers prolong the time to the onset of ischemic ST segment depression and increase exercise tolerance. If the treadmill test is done for diagnostic purposes, cardiac drugs should be withheld for 3–5 half-lives. If the adequacy of drug therapy is being assessed, the test should be done with the patient taking the antianginal medication.

18. What diagnostic test should be ordered after a positive regular exercise treadmill test in a middle-aged woman with no risk factors and atypical chest pain to more accurately assess her for the presence of significant obstructive CAD?

In this setting, exercise-induced ST depression is more likely to be falsely positive for CAD. Myocardial perfusion imaging or stress echocardiography improves the diagnostic yield in patients with a suspected false-positive test.

19. What is the best way to assess the severity of aortic stenosis (AS)?

Two-dimensional echocardiography detects a thickened and calcified aortic valve with reduced opening. The LV size and wall thickness also can be assessed. Doppler echocardiography determines the transvalvular gradient and the valve area. AS is severe if the peak aortic flow velocity exceeds 4.5 m/sec, the aortic valve area is < 0.75 cm^2, and the LV outflow tract/aortic flow velocity is ≤ 0.25. A complete echocardiographic examination gives the clinician the necessary data to interpret the patient's complaints. Echocardiography can be done serially with minimal patient discomfort. Before the refinement of echocardiographic technology, it was necessary to cross the aortic valve in a retrograde fashion in the catheterization laboratory to confirm the presence of severe AS. Now the only reason to catheterize a patient with AS before surgery is to perform coronary angiography when coincident CAD is suspected. Such a patient may receive bypass grafts at the time of valve surgery.

20. Is there a reliable test to assess the presence of left atrial clot before cardioversion of atrial fibrillation?

Successful cardioversion is associated with a 5–7% incidence of embolism among patients who have not received anticoagulant therapy. Atrial thrombi are poorly detected by transthoracic echocardiography. A normal transthoracic echocardiogram does not rule out the presence of left atrial thrombi. The standard practice is several weeks of oral anticoagulation in patients with atrial fibrillation of unknown duration or duration > 2 days. Cardioversion of an anticoagulated patient carries an embolic rate of $< 1.6\%$.

Transesophageal echocardiography (TEE) is a highly accurate method of detecting atrial thrombi. If TEE excludes the presence of thrombi, early cardioversion can be performed safely without preprocedure anticoagulation. Anticoagulation during and after the procedure is still recommended until atrial contractility returns to normal.

21. Which imaging modalities can be used in patients in whom aortic dissection is suspected?

Potential imaging modalities include aortography, computed tomography (CT), magnetic resonance imaging (MRI), and TEE. The choice of test depends on the precise information that is sought by the surgeon and the expertise available in acquiring the images. Potentially available diagnostic information includes presence of dissection, involvement of the aortic root, sites of entry, extent of dissection, branch-vessel involvement, thrombus in the false lumen, aortic insufficiency, pericardial effusion, and coronary artery involvement.

All modalities are similar in specificity, but MRI and TEE tend to be more sensitive. Sensitivity is most important because aortic dissection is a rapidly lethal condition. MRI is probably better at defining the site of the intimal tear and recognizing intraluminal thrombus. Both modalities are noninvasive and easily identify the presence of pericardial effusion; neither requires the use of intravenous contrast material. TEE is superior at detecting and quantifying the degree of aortic insufficiency and in detecting involvement of the proximal coronary arteries. TEE tends to be more readily available and more rapid, because it can be performed at the patient's bedside.

22. What is the best test for rapid evaluation of potential cardiac etiologies in a hypotensive patient?

As fluid support is initiated, a simple transthoracic echocardiogram rapidly reveals the status of ventricular function. A hyperdynamic left ventricle suggests hypovolemia or sepsis as a cause of the hypotension. A poorly contractile left ventricle suggests low-output heart failure as the cause. A large pericardial effusion causing right and left ventricular diastolic collapse indicates a hemodynamically significant pericardial effusion that needs emergent drainage. A markedly dilated right ventricle leads to consideration of right ventricular infarction or large pulmonary embolus as the culprit. With such information the physician can begin to tailor therapy. A Swan-Ganz catheter eventually may be in order, but it should not be the starting point.

23. What does rest radionuclide ventriculography evaluate?

Rest radionuclide ventriculography provides a quantitative measurement of left ventricular ejection fraction. The red blood cells are tagged with a radioactive label, and counts in the left ventricle are obtained by a gamma counter in systole and diastole. The fraction of counts lost from diastole to systole is the ejection fraction. It can be obtained simply and requires no artificial assumptions about geometry of the left ventricle. It is reproducible on serial measurements and is the desired test for accurate measurement of the ejection fraction. The accuracy of the test may be affected by frequent premature atrial or ventricular beats or by atrial fibrillation.

24. What is the time course for troponin elevation in acute myocardial injury?

Onset of elevation: 4–6 hours
Peak: 8–24 hours
Duration of peak: up to 10 days

25. What is brain natriuretic peptide (BNP)? What is it used for?

BNP is made in the ventricles, and its concentration is raised in patients with symptomatic and asymptomatic left ventricular systolic dysfunction and is used to test for the presence and severity of congestive heart failure. Levels are increased in chronic heart failure in proportion to the severity of the congestive heart failure (CHF). The level of BNP may be an important prognostic indicator. Levels provide a guide to treatment of CHF.

26. How are pulmonary artery (PA) pressures measured with transthoracic echocardiography?

Most people (even those with normal hearts) have at least some tricuspid regurgitation when studied carefully by Doppler flow echocardiography. This can be used to estimate the pulmonary artery pressures noninvasively. The velocity of the tricuspid regurgitation jet is proportional to the pressure difference between the right ventricle (RV) and right atrium (RA) in systole by the relationship of $P = 4V^2$. Then the pressure difference is added to the RV diastolic pressure (which is estimated by the clinician by looking at the neck veins as a representation of RA pressure) to give the absolute number of the RV pressure in systole. In other words, the RV diastolic pressure is the floor from which the pressure difference in systole departs. Since RV diastolic pressure is equal to RA pressure, an echo report usually gives a number for PA pressure in the notation of some number plus RA pressure. RV systolic pressure should be the same as PA systolic pressure. In making this measurement you can usually assume that:

1. RV systolic pressure = PA systolic pressure (if there is no pulmonic valve stenosis)
2. RV diastolic pressure = RA pressure = pressure determined by assessment of the neck veins (if there is no tricuspid stenosis)

BIBLIOGRAPHY

1. Berman DS, Kiat H, Friedman JD, Diamond G: Clinical application of exercise nuclear cardiology studies in the era of health care reform. Am J Cardiol 75:3D–13D, 1995.
2. Bonow RO, Dilsizian V: Thallium-201 and technetium-99m-sestamibi for assessing viable myocardium. J Nucl Med 33:815–818, 1992.
3. Cerqueira MD: Diagnostic testing strategies for coronary artery disease: Special issues related to gender. Am J Cardiol 75:52D–60D, 1995.
4. Chang JA, Froelicher VF: Clinical and exercise test markers of prognosis in patients with stable coronary artery disease. Curr Probl Cardiol 19:533–587, 1994.
5. Cigarroa JE, Isselbacher EM, DeSanctis RW, Eagle KA: Diagnostic imaging in the evaluation of suspected aortic dissection: Old standards and new directions. N Engl J Med 328:35–43, 1993.
6. Douglas PS, Ginsburg GS: The evaluation of chest pain in women. N Engl J Med 334:1311–1315, 1996.
7. Eagle KA, Coley CM, Newell JB, et al: Combining clinical and thallium data optimizes preoperative assessment of cardiac risk before major vascular surgery. Ann Intern Med 110:859–866, 1989.
8. Gibbons RJ, Balady GJ, Beasley JW, et al: ACC/AHA guidelines for exercise testing: A report of the American College of Cardiology/American Heart Association Task Force on Practice Guidelines (Committee on Exercise Testing). J Am Coll Cardiol 30:260–315, 1997.
9. Jaffe AS, Ravkilde J, Roberts R, et al: It's time for a change to a troponin standard. Circulation 102:1216–1220, 2000.
10. Koglin J, Pehlivanli S, Schwaiblmair M, et al: Role of brain natriuretic peptide in risk stratification of patients with congestive heart failure. J Am Coll Cardiol 38:1934–1941, 2001.
11. Manning WJ, Silverman DI, Gordon SPF, et al: Cardioversion from atrial fibrillation without prolonged anticoagulation with use of transesophageal echocardiography to exclude the presence of atrial thrombi. N Engl J Med 328:750–755, 1993.
12. Mayo Clinic Cardiovascular Working Group on Stress Testing: Cardiovascular stress testing: Description of the various types of stress tests and indications for their use. Mayo Clin Proc 71:43–52, 1996.
13. McDonagh TA, Robb SD, Murdoch DR, et al: Biochemical detection of left ventricular systolic dysfunction. Lancet 351:9–13, 1998.
14. Nienabar CA, von Kodolistch Y, Nicolas V, et al: The diagnosis of thoracic aortic dissection by noninvasive imaging procedures. N Engl J Med 328:1–9, 1993.
15. Pellikka PA, Roger VL, Oh JK, et al: Stress echocardiography: Part II: Dobutamine stress echocardiography: Techniques, implementation, clinical applications, and correlations. Mayo Clin Proc 70:16–27, 1995.
16. Schiller NB: Pulmonary artery pressure estimation by Doppler and two-dimensional echocardiography. Cardiol Clin 8:277–287, 1990.
17. Schulman SP, Fleg JL: Stress testing for coronary artery disease in the elderly. Clin Geriatr Med 12:101–119, 1996.
18. Sox HC, Littenberg B, Garber AM: The role of exercise testing in screening for coronary artery disease. Ann Intern Med 110:456–469, 1989.
19. Tresch DD, Aronow WS: Clinical manifestations and diagnosis of coronary artery disease. Clin Geriatr Med 12:89–100, 1996.

IV. Disorders of the Eyes, Ears, Nose, and Throat

24. VISUAL IMPAIRMENT

Jon M. Braverman, M.D.

1. How is vision generally measured in the primary care office?

Most patients read an eye chart, which tests central visual acuity. Testing of standard acuity requires the equivalent of a 20-ft Snellen target. Several inexpensive devices are available that can be set up in an office hallway or examination room. Near cards (Rosenbaum variety) are also inexpensive and easy to stock. Keep in mind that near vision testing should be done with patients wearing their presbyopic correction (bifocal or reading glasses).

Peripheral vision can be tested grossly by confrontation. The examiner sits in front of the patient, and each closes the opposite eye to overlap respective fields. The examiner then asks the patient either to count the number of fingers presented within the field or to indicate when a finger is first seen entering the field. Most modern ophthalmologic practices use automated computerized perimeters to assess visual fields more accurately.

Several other components of vision can be measured, including color perception, dark adaptation, and contrast sensitivity. Changes in these parameters may occur secondary to eye disease; however, the tools and techniques required for evaluation are usually beyond the resources of primary care providers.

2. What three levels of visual processing should be considered in evaluating the possible causes of diminished visual acuity?

1. Loss of the ability to form a clear image on the retina
2. Loss of the ability of the retina to process the image
3. Loss of the ability to process the information from the retina to higher perceptual centers (optic nerve, chiasm, optic tracts, optic radiations, visual cortex, and visual association areas)

3. What are two of the most common causes of reversible blurring of vision?

1. **Dry eye syndromes** cause a deficiency of the tear film that covers the cornea. The resultant irregularity of the corneal surface interferes with normal, crisp focusing of light on the retina.

2. **Refractive error** (myopia, hyperopia, and astigmatism) affects more than half of the U.S. population. Pinhole testing of visual acuity often yields improved results, suggesting that the blurring is caused by refractive error.

4. List the four most common nontraumatic causes of progressive visual impairment in adults.

Cataracts, macular degeneration, chronic glaucoma, and diabetic retinopathy.

5. How can the ophthalmoscopic exam aid in defining the cause of decreased visual acuity?

The direct ophthalmoscopic exam is initially all that is necessary to identify the characteristics of the four most common causes of visual loss in adults. If necessary, a 1% tropicamide solution should be used to dilate the pupil in order to optimize visualization. These diagnoses may be suggested by the following abnormalities:

Cataract: A developing cataract is suggested by a cloudy view of the optic nerve and retinal vessels, along with loss of brightness or opacities within the red reflex. Often, cataractous changes appear as dark spots against the red reflex.

Chronic open-angle glaucoma: If the view of the optic nerve is clear but the ratio of the optic cup to the entire nerve head area (cup-to-disc ratio) is high, chronic open-angle glaucoma may be the cause.

Macular degeneration: In a patient with central visual impairment, the examiner has a clear view of the fundus details, and the optic nerve appears normal. Drusen of the retina (beige spots that may coalesce to cause pigment abnormalities in the macular region) are commonly seen in macular degeneration. Advanced cases demonstrate scarring and disorganization of the macular retina.

Diabetic retinopathy: Upon examination of the retina, one can observe areas of retinal hemorrhaging; cotton wool spots; exudate; and, occasionally, fronds of neovascular membranes emanating from the optic disc or retina near the vessels arching around the macula.

6. What causes vitreous opacification?

Vitreous opacification, as evidenced by poor visibility of the fundus on ophthalmoscopic exam (not caused by cataract), may result from hemorrhage; inflammatory or infectious infiltration; and, rarely, tumor (lymphoma). Common causes of hemorrhage include diabetic retinopathy and retinal tears. Infectious causes include bacterial endophthalmitis and parasitic infection (toxoplasmosis, toxocariasis).

7. What causes blurring of the optic disc?
- Papilledema due to increased intracranial pressure
- Optic neuritis (papillitis)
- Arteriolar ischemia to the optic disc, resulting in pale color and an edematous disc
- Acute hypertensive retinopathy, demonstrating a swollen optic nerve surrounded by hemorrhage and exudate

8. When should cataract removal be considered?

In the United States, 70% of people older than 75 years have an opacification of the lens, referred to as a *cataract*. The degree of visual acuity loss is proportional to the density of the cataract, provided that no other ocular disease is present. However, controversy surrounds the timing of cataract surgery, and the health care expenditure associated with removal is enormous. Detection of the cataract alone is not an indication for ophthalmologic surgery. Careful consultation with the patient is necessary to determine the degree to which the loss of visual clarity or glare induced by the cataract impairs normal function.

9. Can a cataract cause serious ocular problems other than visual limitations caused by poor light transmission?

Yes, but this is uncommon. Cataracts may contribute to various secondary disorders, including intraocular inflammation due to leaking of lens material inside the eye; chronic glaucoma resulting from the inflammatory response to liberated lens material; and acute glaucoma due to the physical apposition of the swollen lens with the iris and subsequent closure of the filtering angle. This last condition, acute secondary angle-closure glaucoma, is an emergency.

10. Which diseases can impair the ability of the retina to process visual images?

Age-related macular degeneration, retinal detachment, vaso-occlusive disease (retinal artery or vein occlusions), and certain acute infections of the retina (cytomegalovirus, herpes simplex or zoster, especially in an immunocompromised host) can interfere with the processing of retinal images.

11. What is the natural history of age-related macular degeneration?

Macular degeneration usually occurs in patients older than age 50 years and may progress with time. Patients may have no visual symptoms initially but may develop gradual blurring and distortion in the later stages of the disease. In 10–20% of cases, subretinal hemorrhage acutely compromises visual function and leads to scarring, causing permanent visual loss. Focal laser treatments have proven helpful in this subset of patients with the neovascular form of the disease. A growing body of literature suggests than vitamin and antioxidant supplementation may help to stabilize vision in some patients with the dry or atrophic form of the disease.

12. Why should patients be screened for glaucoma?

Chronic glaucoma causes damage to the optic nerve fibers as a result of an abnormal relationship between intraocular pressure and blood circulation. In its most common form (primary open-angle glaucoma), it is painless and visually asymptomatic until late in the course of the disease. Early visual loss occurs in the visual periphery and is typically not noticed by the patient. For these reasons, it is vital that patients be referred for glaucoma screening as part of a regimen of routine eye health care.

13. Who should be screened for glaucoma?

Risk factors for open-angle glaucoma include older age (> 40 years), high myopia, diabetes, and family history of glaucoma. The American Academy of Ophthalmology currently recommends routine yearly screening for patients at risk.

14. What is standard therapy for patients with chronic open-angle glaucoma?

Treatment of open-angle glaucoma begins with the use of topical agents to reduce intraocular pressure (IOP). Oral carbonic anhydrase inhibitors are second-line agents because of systemic side effects and are generally not used for long-term control of IOP. Laser therapy and intraocular surgery are reserved for patients whose condition is not controlled effectively by medical therapy, although studies to evaluate the efficacy of early surgical intervention are ongoing.

15. What causes floaters?

Opacities in the vitreous gel may throw shadows onto the retina, causing the patient to perceive dots or webs floating in space of front of the eye. Common causes of floaters include vitreous syneresis (mild degeneration of the vitreous collagen skeleton), hemorrhage, retinal tears, and vitreous detachment (a consequence of aging). Often the cause of floaters is not visible to the examiner. Acute onset of floaters, especially when associated with flashing lights (photopsia), should be referred to an ophthalmologist to rule out retinal tears or detachments.

16. What diagnoses should be considered in a patient who experiences sudden, painless unilateral loss of vision?

- Central retinal artery occlusion, often caused by an embolus
- Giant cell arteritis resulting in central retinal artery occlusion or ischemic optic neuropathy
- Central retinal vein occlusion
- Acute hemorrhage into the vitreous element
- Optic neuritis

17. What diagnoses should be considered in a patient who complains of sudden loss of vision in both eyes?

Sudden loss of vision in both eyes is an extremely uncommon event. If the fundi are normal, one must consider toxic optic neuritis, bilateral occipital lobe infarcts, or a possible conversion reaction (diagnosis of exclusion).

18. What is the classic cause of a bitemporal hemianopic visual defect?

Lesions, usually pituitary tumors, that compress the optic chiasm.

19. What is the most common cause of severe visual loss in adolescents and young adults?

Preventable ocular trauma remains a serious public health problem, especially in these age groups. Primary care physicians should counsel patients about the importance of proper eye protection during high-risk sports and other recreational or workplace activities.

20. What is a "lazy eye"?

The medical term for lazy eye is *amblyopia.* Amblyopia is the failure of the visual system to correctly "hardwire" during early childhood development. In some cases, amblyopia is an adaptive mechanism that prevents diplopia in the case of early-onset strabismus. Strabismic eyes do not develop normal vision because of suppression of the misaligned visual image, which prevents diplopia. When this suppression becomes permanent, the affected eye is amblyopic. Other mechanisms that produce amblyopia include monocular congenital cataract (or any congenital condition that blocks the formation of a clear retinal image) and highly asymmetric refractive error.

21. What are some common causes of acute-onset double vision?

Double vision, or *diplopia,* results from the misalignment of the visual axes and the loss of binocular fusion. Ocular motility problems are the most common cause of this symptom and include acute palsies of the cranial nerves (CNs) that control certain extraocular muscles (especially CN VI, III, and IV). Other less common causes of acute onset diplopia include myasthenia gravis, orbital inflammatory disease, cavernous sinus disease, and orbital tumors.

22. How debilitating is the loss of visual function in one eye?

The degree of disability often relates to the acuteness of the change in visual function. As two-eyed beings, we enjoy a highly developed visual system that allows for high-grade stereo perception, a rich appreciation of color and contrast, and the ability to see at low illumination. Our visual fields (the sum of central or macular vision and peripheral vision) overlap almost entirely, so the loss of input from one eye does not result in a 50% constriction of the field of visual perception. Likewise, the appreciation of color, contrast, and low-level illumination remains nearly intact even with input from only one eye. The most significant change relates to stereo perception, which can be quite disorienting for people newly introduced to monocular vision. The good news is that humans can adapt to judging depth by pseudo-stereo cues (e.g., size, shading) and live normal lives—just ask anyone you know who has a lazy eye. (Amblyopia causes functional monocular vision.)

BIBLIOGRAPHY

1. Bradford CA (ed): Basic Ophthalmology for Medical Students and Primary Care Residents, 7th ed. San Francisco, American Academy of Ophthalmology, 1999.
2. Ferris JD: Essential Medical Ophthalmology: A Problem-Oriented Approach. Philadelphia, Butterworth-Heinemann, 2001.
3. Kalina RE: Seeing into the future. Vision and aging. West J Med 167:253–257, 1997.
4. Kanski JJ: Clinical Ophthalmology: A Systematic Approach, 5th ed. Philadelphia, Butterworth-Heinemann, 2003.
5. Leese GP, Broadbent DM, Harding SP, Vora JP: Detection of sight-threatening diabetic eye disease. Diabet Med 13:850–853, 1996.
6. Newell FW, Patel S: Ophthalmology: Principles and Concepts, 8th ed. St. Louis, Mosby, 1996.
7. Shields SR: Managing eye disease in primary care. Part 3: When to refer for ophthalmologic care. Postgrad Med 108:99–106, 2000.
8. Sweet EH, Tark E 3rd: Eye care by primary care physicians: A survey of internists and family practitioners in the Sacramento, California, area. Ophthalmology 98:1454–1460, 1991.
9. Trobe J: The Physician's Guide to Eye Care, 2nd ed. San Francisco, American Academy of Ophthalmology, 2000.
10. Vaughan DG, Asbury T, Riordan P: General Ophthalmology, 15th ed. New York, McGraw-Hill, 1998.

25. EYE PAIN AND INFLAMMATORY DISEASES

Jon M. Braverman, M.D.

1. What are the usual sources of eye pain?

The eyelid, cornea, conjunctivae, and uveal tract (iris, ciliary body, and choroid) are inner-vated by sensory receptors; thus, lesions affecting these areas can produce pain. Pathology limited to the vitreous element, retina, or optic nerve is likely to be painless. Optic neuritis is an exception to this rule. Diseases of the sinuses and orbit also may cause referred pain to the eye.

2. Which diseases are associated with a red eye?

A red eye is the most common ocular complaint in the general population. The presence and severity of pain and visual changes are used to distinguish the many different entities that may account for this finding.

Possible Causes of Red Eye as Determined by Associated Findings

ETIOLOGY	PAIN	VISUAL CHANGES
Acute glaucoma	Yes, severe	Acute loss, often severe
Corneal inflammation (keratitis) or ulceration	Yes	Moderate blurring
Uveal tract or scleral inflammation	Yes, with photophobia	Variable blurring
Vascular or retinal disease	No	Acute or subacute loss; can be severe
Conjunctival inflammation (conjunctivitis)	Sometimes	Sometimes

3. Acute-angle closure glaucoma is an absolute ocular emergency. When should the primary care provider suspect this diagnosis?

Acute elevations in intraocular pressure (IOP) are far more damaging than slowly and chronically acquired elevations. The clinical presentation reflects this basic difference. Acute-angle closure glaucoma presents as an extremely painful eye (almost always unilateral) with loss of vision. The pupil is mid-dilated and nonreactive, and marked conjunctival injection is accompanied by clouding of the cornea attributable to edema. The fundus is poorly visualized. This constellation of symptoms and findings requires immediate referral to an ophthalmologist.

4. What is the significance of photophobia?

Photophobia, the avoidance of light caused by pain, may result from ocular or non-ocular processes. Ocular photophobia results from intraocular inflammation or congestion of the structures of the uveal tract, including the iris and ciliary body, and their associated contractile muscles. During exposure to light, pupillary constriction produces pain. Thus, inflammation in any of these structures (uveitis, iritis, cyclitis, choroiditis) is indicated by the complaint of photophobia. Non-ocular processes resulting in photophobia include migraine; meningeal irritation; and use of certain drugs, particularly those that cause pupillary dilation via anticholinergic properties.

5. What are the usual causes of uveitis? How is uveitis treated?

Inflammation of the uveal tract, presenting as photophobia and injection, is usually idiopathic. Abnormal pupils that react poorly to light may result from adhesions, called *posterior synechiae,* of the iris tissue to the lens surface. Several systemic diseases also are associated with uveitis or variable inflammation of the components of the uvea, including rheumatoid arthritis, sarcoidosis, lupus erythematosus, ankylosing spondylitis, Reiter's syndrome, inflammatory bowel disease, and juvenile rheumatoid arthritis. Infectious causes include syphilis, herpes simplex, varicella zoster, cytomegalovirus (CMV), and Lyme disease.

Treatment ranges from topical cycloplegics to systemic steroids or other immunosuppressive agents. Referral to an ophthalmologist is appropriate for workup and treatment.

6. What are the most common causes of conjunctivitis?

Bacterial, viral, allergic, and irritant causes are possible. Patients usually complain of red eyes and a sticky or watery discharge. Irritation is common, but severe pain and photophobia are not. Bacterial or viral conjunctivitis is usually self-limited, but it may be treated with a topical antibiotic without steroids, such as sulfacetamide (10% 3–4 times/day). Topical aminoglycoside should be reserved for more refractory disease. Patients with allergic conjunctivitis may be effectively treated with a new class of nonsteroidal topical anti-inflammatory agents. Irritant conjunctivitis, including dry eyes, may be treated with topical, nonpreserved lubricants.

7. When are topical steroids contraindicated in the treatment of eye disorders?

Topical steroids are absolutely contraindicated in patients who have a history of herpetic eye disease or who may have herpetic infection at presentation. Such patients require referral to an ophthalmologist.

8. What is ocular medicamentosus?

Ocular medicamentosus is iatrogenic or medication-induced conjunctivitis. Inflammation is a reaction to prescribed medication, any of its components or contaminants, or over-the-counter medicines or home remedies used by the patient to relieve the original conjunctivitis. This entity is improved by discontinuing all medications and using topical, nonpreserved lubricants if needed.

9. What conditions can produce the sensation of a foreign body in the eye?

- Corneal or conjunctival foreign body
- Corneal or conjunctival abrasion
- Punctate epitheliopathy commonly caused by dryness or chemical irritation
- Trichiasis (in-turned eyelashes)

10. What are the common infectious causes of keratitis (corneal inflammation)?

Numerous viral agents can cause infection of the corneal epithelium. Two of the more severe agents are herpes simplex and herpes zoster. Simplex disease is characterized by typical dendritiform epithelial ulcerations best seen with fluorescein staining, whereas zoster is associated with first division trigeminal dermatonal blistering eruptions. Many types of bacteria can also infect the cornea, but they usually require some kind of preexisting defects in normal host defense mechanisms (e.g., epithelial abrasion, indwelling foreign bodies, severe dryness, thermal or chemical burns) to take hold. *Neisseria gonorrhea* can cause a particularly aggressive infection that can rapidly proceed to corneal ulceration if not diagnosed and treated early.

11. What principles should guide therapy for a foreign body?

1. Attempt removal under topical anesthetic only with a cooperative patient and blunt-tip instruments (a cotton applicator moistened with anesthetic is best).

2. Ascertain the mechanism of injury. Any circumstance involving high-speed microprojectiles should be further evaluated by an ophthalmologist.

3. Patch the eye after treatment and refer the patient to an ophthalmologist. Topical 10% sulfacetamide ointment is an appropriate prophylactic antibiotic.

12. What is the difference between a sty and a chalazion?

A sty is acutely painful and suppurative due to a bacterial infection. A chalazion is a subacute process, typically a mildly to moderately painful swelling of the eyelid margin caused by granulomatous inflammation (sterile). Chalazions usually resolves spontaneously with warm soaks and time. Both are common inflammations of the sebaceous glands of the eyelid.

13. Name some potential eye diseases associated with acquired immunodeficiency syndrome (AIDS).

More than 50% of all patients with AIDS have ocular complications. Cotton wool spots, caused by retinal microvascular disease, are the most frequent physical finding. Ocular complications include the following:

- CMV retinitis, as evidenced by hemorrhage and infiltrate on funduscopic examination
- Retinal or choroidal infections due to toxoplasmosis and *Pneumocystis carinii*
- Retinal necrosis due to herpetic infections (simplex and zoster), with or without keratitis or iritis
- Orbital Kaposi's sarcoma and non-Hodgkin's lymphoma

14. What common ocular complaints should be interpreted with increased scrutiny in patients with HIV or AIDS?

Chronic dryness and foreign body sensation may be the only symptoms of corneal microsporidosis, which is often a systemwide infestation when ocular infection is diagnosed. Floaters are also a common benign complaint of healthy patients. In the HIV population, these symptoms may represent the early stages of retinitis, often caused by CMV.

15. What causes cotton wool spots in the fundus?

Cotton wool spots represent ischemic injury to the superficial nerve layer of the retina. Although frequently seen in diabetic retinopathy, they are not pathognomonic and also may occur with severe hypertension, anemia, leukemia, collagen vascular disease, endocarditis, and AIDS.

16. What is the significance of eye pain associated with paralysis of the third (oculomotor) cranial nerve?

Painful third nerve paralysis can be due to life-threatening intracranial aneurysms. Pain can also be caused by ischemic injury stemming from microvascular infarcts of the third nerve in diabetic and hypertensive patients. It is difficult to distinguish aneurysmal from nonaneurysmal causes without invasive testing; thus, these patients should be managed by neurologists in consultation with ophthalmologists.

17. What is the significance of a conspicuous absence of eye pain in the case of an injected and inflamed appearing eye?

The innervation that subtends pain sensation in the cornea also is a necessary component for normal corneal epithelial health and maintenance. A denervated (anesthetic) cornea can suffer a higher incidence of epithelial erosions and corneal infections than a normally innervated cornea. Patients do not typically appreciate a worsening corneal infection, so they do not seek medical attention early. People at risk for these complications include diabetics, people with prior herpetic infections of the cornea, and people with cranial neuropathies (especially those with concomitant cranial nerve V and VII palsies).

18. What can cause chronic eye discomfort in a patient with a normal appearing eye?

Burning, foreign body sensation, and blurring can occur in patients with keratitis sicca or dry eye syndrome. Various underlying causes of poor ocular wetting or lubrication should be identified in order to direct treatment. In mild to moderate forms, a dry eye may not express any obvious outward signs. The practitioner may elect to put the patient on a regimen of sterile lubricating drops or ointment to see if the symptoms improve. The most common reason for failure of a lubricating regimen is failure to use these agents frequently enough to restore optimal ocular surface health. Artificial tears have a duration of action of only a few minutes after application. Patients need to determine their own lubrication needs by using the drops more frequently than is probably necessary at first to eliminate the symptoms and then gradually tapering the frequency until the symptoms return.

19. A patient presents with a painful tender nodule along the lateral bridge of the nose about 1 cm from the medical canthus of the eye. There is mucopurulent discharge from the ipsilateral eye. What condition should be suspected with this presentation?

Dacryocystitis is an acute infection of the lacrimal sac, which is a structure the resides next to the nasion and above the maxillary bone on each side of the face. When normal tear flow through the lacrimal sac is impaired, secondary infection can occur, leading to the presentation described above. Treatment consists of antibiotic therapy. Incision and drainage of the suppurative lacrimal sac may appear to be indicated, but this is not recommended because a draining fistula will likely result from this intervention.

BIBLIOGRAPHY

1. Bradford CA (ed): Basic Ophthalmology for Medical Students and Primary Care Residents, 7th ed. San Francisco, American Academy of Ophthalmology, 1999.
2. Ferris JD: Essential Medical Ophthalmology: A Problem-Oriented Approach. Philadelphia, Butterworth-Heinemann, 2001.
3. Kanski JJ: Clinical Ophthalmology: A Systematic Approach, 5th ed. Philadelphia, Butterworth-Heinemann, 2003.
4. Karseras A: Ophthalmology and general medicine. Postgrad Med J 76:551–554, 2000.
5. Morrow GL, Abbott RL: Conjunctivitis. Am Fam Physician 57:735–745, 1998.
6. Newell FW, Patel S: Ophthalmology: Principles and Concepts, 8th ed. St. Louis, Mosby, 1996.
7. Shields SR: Managing eye disease in primary care. Part 3: When to refer for ophthalmologic care. Postgrad Med 108:99–106, 2000.
8. Sweet EH, Tark E 3d: Eye care by primary care physicians: A survey of internists and family practitioners in the Sacramento, California, area. Ophthalmology 98:1454–1460, 1991.
9. Vaughan DG, et al: General Ophthalmology, 15th ed. New York, McGraw-Hill, 1998.

26. HEARING LOSS AND TINNITUS

Michael L. Lepore, M.D.

1. What are the three types of hearing loss?

1. **Conductive hearing loss** is the most common type of hearing loss in children. It is manifested by a pathologic process that blocks the transmission of sound from the external auditory canal to the cochlear. Examples include cerumen impaction, otitis media in children, and otosclerosis.

2. **Sensorineural hearing loss** is the most common type of hearing loss in the elderly population. It results from an abnormality that affects the sensory cells of the cochlea or involve the neural distributions of the eighth cranial nerve. Patients with prior exposure to loud noises are more susceptible to sensorineural hearing loss and may experience the loss at an earlier age.

3. **Mixed hearing loss** is not as common as the other types of hearing loss. It is a combination of the above types. The patient has a neurosensory component and a conductive component on hearing tests. Mixed hearing loss is commonly seen in patients with a long history of chronic otitis media with intermittent otorrhea and evidence of cholesteatoma.

2. What is progressive sensorineural hearing loss?

This sensorineural hearing loss progresses over time if the patient is continuously exposed to conditions that affect the cochlea. This often occurs as part of the aging process. When patients' hearing loss becomes severe, amplification may be of benefit in order to enhance their communicative abilities.

3. Can autoimmune disorders cause progressive sensorineural hearing loss?

Progressive sensorineural hearing loss is associated with autoimmune disorders and is well documented in the literature in conditions such as Cogan syndrome, systemic lupus erythematosus, and other autoimmune rheumatologic disorders.

4. What percentage of adults older than age 65 years have a handicapping hearing loss?

Data from the National Health Interview Study in 1989 indicate that approximately 29% of people older than 65 years and 36% of people older than 75 years have a hearing loss severe enough to interfere with effective conversation. Presbycusis, the most common variety of hearing loss, may be defined as an unexplained, slowly progressive decline in aural sensitivity caused by the aging process. The hearing loss is usually symmetric, as is noise-induced hearing loss.

5. Why does hearing loss progress to a severe state before the patient seeks assistance?

The aging process may be accompanied by a number of chronic physical conditions of which the patient is acutely aware. Hearing loss, however, most commonly develops over many years and is, therefore, overshadowed by the acuity of concurrent conditions. Patients unknowingly develop coping mechanisms and do not notice an acute change in hearing until a severe loss is present.

6. What psychological effects of hearing loss may offer clues to its presence?

Patients often withdraw from their surroundings. They may demonstrate conversational manipulation, phobic behavior, paranoia, and mood disorders. The most frequent symptoms are mood disorders, as manifested by insomnia, loss of appetite, guilt, fatigue, anxiety, and uncontrolled emotional outbursts.

7. How does one evaluate a patient with presbycusis?

A careful history and a high index of suspicion in particularly susceptible patients are extremely important to identify warning signs. All elderly patients should undergo evaluation of hearing. Particularly important signs are difficulty with hearing in a room with other people and turning up the sound on the television set. Tinnitus is also an early symptom of hearing loss. A careful history of previous exposure to loud noise is important to ascertain. If hearing loss is suspected, an audiometric evaluation should be performed to determine the type and quality.

8. What level of noise exposure may contribute to hearing loss?

Long exposure to noise > 90 dB of sound pressure level (SPL) may cause progressive symmetrical hearing loss. Sources of chronic noise exposure with corresponding dB SPL are listed below:

SOURCE OF CHRONIC NOISE	dB SPL	SOURCE OF CHRONIC NOISE	dB SPL
Riveting steel tank	130	Boiler shop	100
Automobile horn	120	Hydraulic press	100
Sandblasting	112	Can manufacturing plant	100
Woodworking shop	100	Subway	90
Punch press	100	Average factory	80
Pneumatic drill	100		

9. How is sudden sensorineural hearing loss (sudden deafness) defined?

For research purposes, it is defined as sensorineural hearing loss of $\geq$ 30 dB over at least three contiguous audiometric frequencies within 3 days or less.

10. What is the most common cause of sudden deafness?

The incidence of sudden deafness is reported to be 5–20 per 100,000 persons per year. This figure, however, is probably higher because some patients recover so rapidly that they do not seek medical attention. The common cause of sudden deafness is idiopathic sudden sensorineural hearing loss. Characteristically, approximately one third of patients develop hearing loss upon waking in the morning, and about one half also notice disequilibrium or frank vertigo. The intensity of the vertigo usually corresponds to the severity of the hearing loss. Some of the predisposing factors associated with idiopathic sudden sensorineural loss include changes in the physical environment, such as altitude or atmospheric pressure; emotional disturbances; diabetes; atherosclerosis; pregnancy; use of contraceptive drugs; and stress of surgery, physical exertion, or general anesthesia.

11. What are the specific causes of acute hearing loss?

1. **Viral infections** may affect the cochlea by causing labyrinthitis or direct inflammation of the cochlear nerve. Measles, mumps, influenza, and adenoviruses have been associated with sudden deafness. Herpes zoster has been shown to produce a viral neuronitis or ganglionitis.

2. **Tumors** of the cerebellopontine angle may produce sudden deafness.

3. **Damage to the organ of Corti** may be induced by sneezing, coughing, bending, the Valsalva maneuver, or scuba diving.

4. **Rupture of the round or oval window** is usually accompanied by positional nystagmus. A positive fistula sign is demonstrated by applying positive pressure to the tympanic membrane, which causes ipsilateral nystagmus.

12. When should aggressive evaluation of a patient with sudden hearing loss be undertaken?

Initial evaluation of all patients should include a careful history, otologic and neurologic examination, audiologic testing, and routine laboratory studies. If hearing does not return in 1 month or if serial audiograms demonstrate progressive loss, computed tomography (CT) or magnetic resonance imaging (MRI) with gadolinium of the internal auditory meatus should be performed to rule out the presence of an acoustic tumor.

13. What is the anticipated natural history of idiopathic sensorineural hearing loss?

Age appears to play a significant role in recovery. Patients younger than age 40 years recover normal hearing approximately 50% of the time. The more severe the hearing loss, the less likely the recovery. The presence of vertigo is a bad prognostic sign. Spontaneous recovery may occur within days or weeks; if the loss persists beyond 1 month, there is little likelihood for recovery.

14. Why should patients with an idiopathic sensorineural hearing loss without resolution be tested for syphilis?

In its late phase, syphilis may cause sensorineural loss as the only manifestation of disease. Approximately 7% of patients with otherwise unexplained sensorineural hearing loss have a positive treponemal antibody test, as do 7% of patients with Ménière's disease. Thus, any patient with a positive treponemal antibody test and unexplained hearing loss should be treated for syphilitic otitis.

15. What other infectious disease may lead to hearing loss?

Tuberculosis may cause sensorineural and conductive hearing loss, although this is unlikely in the absence of pulmonary disease.

16. What commonly used medications may lead to hearing loss?

Aminoglycosides	Antineoplastic agents, such as cisplatin
Loop diuretics, such as furosemide	Interferon
Salicylates	Piroxicam

17. How do the Weber and Rinne tests help in delineating the origin of hearing loss?

Both tests are used to determine whether hearing loss is conductive or sensorineural. The **Weber test** is done by placing the stem of a tuning fork midline on the patient's skull and asking the patient whether the tone is heard in one ear better than in the other. The tone is louder on the side on which the balance of bone (sensorineural) to conductive hearing sensation is greatest. For example, if a patient has wax in the right ear, an ipsilateral conductive hearing loss causes a relative increase in bone (sensorineural) conduction. Thus, the Weber test lateralizes to the right. By contrast, an acoustic neuroma on the right side is accompanied by a relative decrease in bone conduction; thus, the Weber test lateralizes to the opposite side.

The **Rinne test** is done by placing a vibrating tuning fork on the mastoid process and asking the patient to acknowledge when the sound is no longer audible (bone conduction). At that point, the vibrating bells of the tuning fork are held at the external auditory canal. The patient normally should hear the tone better by air conduction than by bone conduction.

18. What precautions should be taken before removing impacted wax?

Before removing impacted ear wax by irrigation, the patient should be questioned about a history of perforated tympanic membrane or chronic otitis media. Care also must be exercised in diabetic patients to avoid trauma to the ear canal and secondary external otitis. In patients with perforations or previously draining ears, the cerumen must be removed by using a microscope. To avoid complications, such patients should be referred to an otolaryngologist.

19. What potentially life-threatening disorder is heralded by new-onset tinnitus?

Tinnitus, a common symptom in primary care practice, is characterized by the complaint of ringing or any other abnormal sound in the ear. Most disorders associated with tinnitus are not life threatening. However, tinnitus may be a prominent manifestation of one medical emergency: salicylate toxicity. Elderly patients who take aspirin chronically, as opposed to patients who take acute overdoses, experience the highest mortality rate from salicylism. One needs to ask specifically about aspirin intake because many patients do not consider it a prescribed medicine. When in doubt, an aspirin level is appropriate. Other manifestations of salicylism should be sought.

20. What is the incidence of tinnitus ?

It is estimated that tinnitus occurs in 10–15% of the general population. Approximately 30–40 million people suffer from this condition. Eighty-five percent of all ear complaints are related to tinnitus. Some forms of tinnitus may be transient (e.g., after exposure to a gunshot or a loud concert) and should resolve in a few hours.

21. What are the most common causes of tinnitus?

Tinnitus can be broadly divided into objective and subjective categories. **Objective tinnitus** is less common and often can be heard not only by the patient but also by the examiner. Causes of objective tinnitus include vascular abnormalities (e.g., arteriovenous shunts, arterial bruits, venous hums) mechanical abnormalities (e.g., disorders of the eustachian tube and stapedial muscle spasm). This type of tinnitus may be pulsatile in the case of vascular disorders or may change character based on the position of the head, pharynx, or jaw. **Subjective tinnitus** is far more common and most likely arises from damaged cochlear hair cells that discharge discontinuously. The vast majority of patients with subjective tinnitus have an otologic disorder.

22. What categories of medication have been implicated in causing tinnitus?

Diuretics (Diamox), beta-blockers (metoprolol), antibiotics (gentamicin), angiotensin-converting enzyme (ACE) inhibitors (enalapril), antimalarials (chloroquine), narcotics (pentazocine), nonsteroidal antiinflammatory drugs (NSAIDs; e.g., diclofenac), antihistamines (promethazine), and anesthetics (lidocaine). A miscellaneous group of medications can also cause tinnitus, including albuterol, carbamazepine (Tegretol), hydroxychloroquine (Plaquenil), lithium, priolec, and cyclobenaprile.

23. Which diseases are associated with unilateral tinnitus?

The majority of subjective tinnitus is bilateral. Unilateral tinnitus is usually due to an otologic disorder, such as chronic suppurative otitis, trauma, or Ménière's disease. In the absence of these diagnoses, workup should include an MRI scan in search of a central auditory lesion.

24. Who should be involved in the diagnosis and management of patients with severe tinnitus?

Primary care providers may need assistance from specialists in audiology, otolaryngology, neurology, and (occasionally) psychiatry. An audiologist localizes the pathology to the ear or to the central nervous system and, through special testing, detects the pitch and loudness of the tinnitus, the minimal masking level that eliminates the tinnitus, and the residual inhibition. An otolaryngologist or neurologist performs a thorough evaluation of the ears, nose, throat, head, and neck regions to determine the presence of any pathology that may explain the tinnitus. A neurologist may be required for diagnosis if a central lesion is suspected. In patients who are refractory to treatment or who have unexplained tinnitus, associated psychological disorders may require management.

25. How frequently can tinnitus be controlled?

About 30–40% of patients who report severe tinnitus may be treated, and 45–60% respond well to maskers or amplification instruments. In severe cases, tricyclic antidepressants may be of some benefit. Therefore, only 10–15% of patients are refractory to therapy. In addition to addressing local otologic problems as an etiology, any eustachian tube dysfunction should be corrected because it may significantly intensify tinnitus. Adequate ventilation of the eustachian tube and middle ear is achieved through the use of antihistamines and decongestants.

26. What advice should be given to patients with tinnitus?

1. Avoid loud noises, caffeine, drug use, alcohol excess, and tobacco.
2. Maintain an active lifestyle.
3. Join support groups such as the American Tinnitus Association (Portland, OR).

27. What is Ramsay Hunt syndrome?

Ramsay Hunt syndrome is a constellation of cranial nerve disorders resulting from recrudescence of latent varicella zoster virus infection of the facial nerve. The clinical presentation consists of severe otalgia associated with characteristic vesicular eruptions of the auditory canal and pinna. Complications of Ramsay Hunt syndrome arise from involvement of cranial nerves V, IX, and X and include facial paralysis, tinnitus, hearing loss, hyperacusis, vertigo, dysguesia, and decreased tearing. The syndrome is also called herpes zoster oticus. It is about one fifth as common as Bell's palsy.

BIBLIOGRAPHY

1. Adour KK: Otologic complications of herpes zoster. Ann Neurol 35:S62–S64, 1994.
2. Barker RL, Burton JR, Zieve PD, et al (eds): Principles of Ambulatory Medicine, 6th ed. Philadelphia, Lippincott Williams & Wilkins, 2002.
3. Bauer CA, Coker NJ: Update on facial nerve disorders. Otolaryngol Clin North Am 29:445–454, 1996.
4. Dobie RA: Noise-induced hearing loss. In Bailey BJ et al (eds): Head and Neck Surgery—Otolaryngology, 3rd ed. Philadelphia, Lippincott Williams & Wilkins, 2002.
5. Dobie RA: A review of randomized clinical trials in tinnitus. Laryngoscope 109:1202–1211, 1999.
6. Fetterman BL, Saunders JE, Luxford WM: Prognosis and treatment of sudden sensorineural hearing loss. Am J Otol 17:529–536, 1996.
7. Hughes GB, Freedman MA, Haberdamp TJ, Guay ME: Sudden sensorineural hearing loss. Otolaryngol Clin North Am 29:393–403, 1996.
8. Kohut RI, Hinojosak R: Sudden hearing loss. In Bailey BJ, et al (eds): Head and Neck Surgery—Otolaryngology, 3rd ed. Philadelphia, Lippincott Williams & Wilkins, 2002.
9. Koopmann CF Jr: Otolaryngologic (head and neck) problems in the elderly. Med Clin North Am 75:1373–1388, 1991.
10. Lavizzo-Mourey RJ, Siegler EL: Hearing impairment in the elderly. J Gen Intern Med 7:191–198, 1992.
11. Lichtenstein MJ: Hearing and visual impairments. Clin Geriatr Med 8:173–182, 1992.
12. Mattox DE, Wilkins SA: Tinnitus. In American Academy of Otolaryngology—Head and Neck Surgery Self-Instructional Package. Rochester, NY, Mosby, 1989.
13. Nadol JB: Hearing loss. N Engl J Med 329:1092–1102, 1993.

14. Patt BS, Meyerhoff WL: Aging and auditory vestibular system. In Bailey BJ, et al (eds): Head and Neck Surgery—Otolaryngology, 3rd ed. Philadelphia, Lippincott Williams & Wilkins, 2002.
15. Pensak ML, Adelman RA: Conductive hearing loss. In Cummings DW (ed): Otolaryngology—Head and Neck Surgery, vol 4, 2nd ed. St. Louis, Mosby, 1993.
16. Schleuning AJ: Management of the patient with tinnitus. Med Clin North Am 76:1225–1237, 1991.
17. Seidman MD, Jacobson GP: Update on tinnitus. Otolaryngol Clin North Am 29:455–465, 1996.
18. Shikowitz MJ: Sudden sensorineural hearing loss. Med Clin North Am 75:1239–1250, 1991.
19. Shulman A: Electrodiagnostics, Electrotherapeutics and Other Approaches to the Management of Tinnitus. American Academy of Otolaryngology—Head and Neck Surgery Instructional Courses, vol 2. St. Louis, Mosby, 1989, p 137.
20. Thurmond M, Amedee RG: Sudden sensorineural hearing loss: Etiologies and treatment. J Louisiana State Med Soc 150:200–203, 1998.
21. Vernon J, Schleuning AJ: Tinnitus: Its Care and Treatment. American Academy of Otolaryngology—Head and Neck Surgery Instructional Courses, vol 2. St. Louis, Mosby, 1989, p 131.
22. Vesterager V: Tinnitus: Investigation and management. Br Med J 314:728–731, 1997.

27. EAR PAIN AND INFECTIONS

Michael L. Lepore, M.D.

1. Which two cranial nerves are involved in the pathways for referral of ear pain?

Cranial nerves (CN) IX and X are the major nerves involved in causing referred ear pain (otalgia). The auricular nerve of Arnold and the internal branch of the superior laryngeal nerve provide sensory innervation from the ear and larynx, respectively; both are branches of the vagus nerve (CN X). The tympanic nerve (Jacobson's nerve), a branch of the glossopharyngeal nerve (CN IX) from the tympanic membrane and middle ear, and branches of the glossopharyngeal nerve from the oropharynx provide sensory innervation from their respective regions. Any pathologic condition involving the sensory innervations of these nerves may cause referred ear pain.

2. What entities cause ear pain?

Otalgia is a frequent complaint that has multiple possible causes. Patients may have a pathologic process confined to the ear (primary origin), or the pain may be referred to the ear from another source (secondary otalgia). Because most of the ear develops embryonically from the first (mandibular) and second (hyoid) branchial arches, any process in the distribution of the two arches from the larynx and pharynx to the skull base may refer pain to the ear. Some of the common causes of primary otalgia are:

Pinna and External Canal	Middle Ear and Mastoid
Furunculosis	Acute otitis media
External otitis	Acute mastoiditis
Foreign body in the external canal	Acute eustachian tube obstruction
Impacted cerumen	
Acute myringitis and myringitis bullosa	
Trauma to tympanic membrane	
Perichondritis	

Causes of secondary otalgia include dental pathology, cancer of the larynx and piriform sinus, tonsillitis, peritonsillar abscess, arthritis of the cricoarytenoid joint, nasopharyngeal pathology, temporomandibular joint disease, and lesions of the esophagus.

3. What is swimmer's ear?

Swimmer's ear is otitis externa, an extremely painful inflammatory process of the external ear canal and auricle. It is often associated with swimming and is a frequent diagnosis in primary care, especially in children. The disease is usually highly responsive to otic antibiotic therapy. However, prevention of recurrence may require the use of ear protection with swimming.

4. What are the types of otitis externa?

Acute localized otitis externa (forunculosis)
Mycotic external otitis (fungal): acute or chronic
Necrotizing (malignant) otitis externa
Eczematoid otitis externa

5. Can allergic conditions cause otitis externa?

Allergic conditions have been associated with pathology involving the outer, middle, and inner ear. Because the clinical manifestations of allergy are not by themselves diagnostic, the history and clinical manifestations on other target organs may assist in making the correct diagnosis and treatment.

6. Who is at risk for serious complications associated with otitis externa?

Patients older than age 50 years and patients with diabetes are at risk for severe complications related to simple otitis externa. The disease may progress rapidly to a life-threatening condition of necrotizing (malignant) otitis externa. This syndrome is characterized by severe pain, purulent discharge, and progressive cellulitis of the ear and the base of the skull. If not adequately treated, otitis externa may be complicated by facial and other cranial nerve palsies, meningitis, mastoiditis, parotitis, osteomyelitis of the temporal bone or base of the skull, and death. It is frequently caused by *Pseudomonas aeruginosa,* and treatment requires specific oral antipseudomonal antibiotics. In the more severe forms complicated by cranial nerve involvement, hospitalization with intravenous antibiotics and surgical intervention may be required.

7. Can otitis externa extend to involve other anatomic sites?

In certain cases of acute otitis externa, the infection may spread to the parotid gland via the foramen of Santorini located in the anterior cartilaginous portion of the external canal. The clinical manifestations include severe pain and swelling in the parotid region.

8. What causes otorrhea?

Otorrhea is a discharge from the ear canal associated with disease of both the middle ear and external canal. Disorders of the middle ear that result in otorrhea include acute otitis media with perforation (or the presence of a tympanostomy tube) and chronic suppurative otitis media. Disorders of the external canal that lead to otorrhea include otitis externa and necrotizing otitis externa.

9. How is otitis media classified?

For purposes of treatment and evaluation, otitis media is classified as acute ($<$ 3 weeks' duration), subacute (3 weeks–3 months), and chronic ($>$ 3 months).

10. Name the four pathogens most commonly identified in acute otitis media.

1. *Streptococcus pneumoniae* (most common)
2. *Haemophilus influenzae*
3. Group A streptococci
4. *Moraxella catarrhalis*

11. Do viruses have a role in the pathogenesis of acute otitis media?

Although acute otitis media is caused by a bacterial infection, numerous studies have demonstrated that respiratory viruses may play a critical role in the cause and pathogenesis of this common condition. For some time, respiratory viruses have been known to have a suppressive effect on the host immune defenses, induce a release of inflammatory mediators in the nasopharynx, and increase bacterial colonization and adherence. Some viruses have been known to actively invade the middle ear, enhancing the inflammatory process.

12. What is the most important factor in the pathogenesis of middle ear disease?
Abnormal function of the eustachian tube appears to be the most important pathogenic factor. The normal eustachian tube serves three functions: (1) it provides protection from nasopharyngeal secretions and sound pressure, (2) it acts to clear middle ear secretions by its mucociliary activity, and (3) it provides a ventilatory function for the middle ear. This function depends on gas absorption and on the characteristics of the mastoid air-cell system of the middle ear.

13. What is the most reasonable treatment approach to an acute episode of otitis media?
Uncomplicated otitis media should be treated with oral antimicrobials. Amoxicillin should be considered the drug of first choice; additional considerations include trimethoprim–sulfamethoxazole, erythromycin, sulfisoxazole, amoxicillin–clavulanate, and cefaclor. Clinical improvement should be evident in 72 hours, and a 10-day course is usually adequate. If no significant improvement is seen with amoxicillin, a beta-lactamase–producing organism should be suspected and antibiotic therapy should be changed. In refractory acute cases, tympanocentesis with or without myringotomy relieves pain, and culture of the middle ear effusion may yield the causative organism.

14. How does otitis media in neonates or young children differ from otitis media in older children or adults?
In neonates and young infants, the incidence of unusual organisms, particularly gram-negative bacilli and *Staphylococcus aureus,* is higher.

15. What is the incidence of persistent middle ear effusion after a 10-day course of antibiotics?
Up to 50% of patients are clinically well but have a persistent middle ear infection after a full course of antibiotics. Several options should be considered because persistent effusions may lead to hearing loss with speech and language delay as well as provide a medium for bacterial growth. These patients should be treated for a longer time with the same antimicrobial agent, and systemic decongestants, antihistamines, or both should be used to encourage evacuation of the eustachian tube. The Valsalva maneuver may be performed in the physician's office to inflate the eustachian tube.
A middle ear effusion may persist for approximately 3 months after an acute episode of otitis media resolves. However, if the patient is asymptomatic, watchful waiting is a reasonable approach. If the patient is continuously symptomatic, a more aggressive approach is necessary. In children with multiple episodes of acute otitis media with or without persistent middle ear effusions, speech and language delays may result from hearing loss.

16. What considerations must be given to adults who fail to resolve otitis media or a middle ear effusion?
In adults, the nasopharynx must be examined carefully and repeatedly for pathology. Nasopharyngeal carcinoma and lymphoma may cause intermittent or persistent middle ear problems.

17. How is recurrent otitis media managed?
The development of recurrent otitis media should be considered an indication for intervention. Initially, diseases that have a role in the cause of recurrent episodes must be considered, including sinusitis, nasal allergy, immune deficiency, nasopharyngeal pathology, cleft palate, and submucosal palate. A child with recurrent episodes of otitis media and persistent middle ear effusion may be treated more aggressively. Chemoprophylaxis with chronic antibiotics may be used. Myringotomy, which may decrease the frequency of episodes and possible complications, should be considered carefully.

18. What are the consequences of untreated or inadequately treated acute otitis media?

Because of the widespread use of antimicrobial therapy, the incidence of complications from acute otitis media has decreased dramatically. However, because of the potential for serious morbidity, complications must be recognized early. Intracranial complications include lateral sinus thrombophlebitis, extradural abscesses, subdural abscesses, brain abscess, and meningitis. Local complications include conductive or sensorineural hearing loss; perforation of the tympanic membrane; chronic suppurative otitis media with or without cholesteatoma; atelectasis with retraction pockets and adhesions of the tympanic membrane; and erosion of the incus with ossicular discontinuity, labyrinthitis, and facial nerve paralysis.

19. What is Gradenigo's syndrome?

Gradenigo's syndrome is the triad of otalgia, otorrhea, and paralysis of the abducens nerve. It occurs as a complication of otitis media and requires immediate referral to an otolaryngologist.

20. What are the signs of coalescent mastoiditis in children?

With the emergence of antibiotic-resistant microorganisms, a slight increase in the number of children presenting with clinical signs and symptoms of acute mastoiditis has been noted. The presenting signs are varied and include any of the following: pain behind the ear, tenderness over the mastoid, persistent aural discharge, displacement of the auricle, fever, leukocytosis, and conductive hearing loss. The auricular displacement is characteristic in that the ear is pointing downward and outward as a result of a subperiosteal abscess that ruptures above the insertion of the sternocleidomastoid muscle. Occasionally, if the abscess breaks through the attachment of the posterior belly of the digastric muscle, the child presents with a neck mass, signifying the presence of a deep neck abscess.

21. How is chronic otitis media manifested?

Chronic otitis media is an indolent inflammatory process that involves the eustachian tube, middle ear, and mastoid air-cell system. Two varieties are commonly recognized: chronic suppurative otitis media (CSOM) and chronic otitis media with effusion (COME). Both conditions begin in childhood, usually in patients with a history of recurrent otitis media. In CSOM, hearing loss, painless otorrhea, and tympanic perforation are common. In COME, the hallmark is a 24- to 40-dB conductive hearing loss.

22. What is the most serious complication of chronic otitis media?

The development of cholesteatoma is the most serious complication of chronic otitis media. In the presence of chronic otitis media, retraction pockets or cysts form in the middle ear and are lined by skin. Desquamation leads to a buildup of keratin. Keratin-containing cysts, called cholesteatomas, invade the surrounding bone, leading to facial nerve paralysis, vertigo, and meningitis. As they grow in the middle ear, the cysts may cause destruction of the incus, stapes, and malleus, leading to severe conductive hearing loss. Cholesteatomas are often visible as a white ball in the middle ear. Their presence is usually an indication for surgery.

BIBLIOGRAPHY

1. Barker RL, Burton JR, Zieve PD, et al (eds): Principles of Ambulatory Medicine, 6th ed. Philadelphia, Lippincott Williams & Wilkins, 2002.
2. Bartoshuk LM, Kveton JF, Karrer T: Taste. In Bailey J, et al (eds): Head and Neck Surgery—Otolaryngology, 3rd ed. Philadelphia, Lippincott Williams & Wilkins, 2002.
3. Bluestone CD, Klein JO: Otitis Media in Infants and Children. Philadelphia, W.B. Saunders, 1995.
4. Boustred N: Practical guide to otitis externa. Austral Fam Phys 28:217–221, 1999.
5. Chandler JR: Malignant external otitis and osteomyelitis of the base of the skull. Am J Otol 10:108–110, 1989.
6. Chartrand SA, Pong A: Acute otitis media in the 1990s: The impact of antibiotic resistance. Pediatr Ann 27:86–95, 1998.

7. Hirsh BE: Infections of the external ear. Am J Otolaryngol 13:145–155, 1992.
8. Heikkinen T, Chonmaitree T: Increasing importance of viruses in acute otitis media. Ann Med 32:157–163, 2000.
9. Jahn AF: Chronic otitis media: Diagnosis and treatment. Med Clin North Am 75:1277–1291, 1991.
10. Kenna MA: Otitis media with effusion. In Bailey BJ, et al (eds): Head and Neck Surgery—Otolaryngology, 3rd ed. Philadelphia, Lippincott Williams & Wilkins, 2002.
11. Klein JO: Review of consensus reports on management of acute otitis media. Pediatr Infect Dis J 18:1152–1155, 1999.
12. Lee KJ: Essential Otolaryngology. New Haven, CT, Medical Examination Publishing, 1995.
13. Paparella MM: Otalgia. In Paparella MM, et al (eds): Otolaryngology, vol 2. Philadelphia, W.B. Saunders, 1980, p 1354.
14. Pelton SI, Klein JO: The draining ear. Otitis media and externa. Infect Dis Clin North Am 2:117–129, 1988.
15. Ramilo O: Role of respiratory viruses in acute otitis media: Implications for management. Pediatr Infect Dis 18:1125–1129, 1999.
16. Rubin J, Yu VL: Malignant external otitis: Insights into pathogenesis, clinical manifestations, diagnosis, and therapy. Am J Med 85:391–398, 1988.
17. Shambaugh GE: Surgery of the Ear, 4th ed. Philadelphia, W.B. Saunders, 1990.

28. SORE THROAT AND HOARSENESS

Robert H. Harris, M.D., and Andy W. Steele, M.D., M.P.H.

1. What are the main causes of sore throat?

Viruses cause about 50% of cases of sore throat. The most common causative viruses include adenovirus, influenzavirus, parainfluenza virus, coxsackievirus, rhinovirus, coronavirus, and respiratory syncytial virus. Acute human immunodeficiency virus (HIV-1) and Epstein-Barr virus (EBV) are less common causes of sore throat, but because both have specific diagnostic or therapeutic implications, providers should consider them in the correct clinical setting. Bacteria cause about 20% of cases. Group A beta-hemolytic streptococcus (GAS) is the most common cause, accounting for about 10–20% of pharyngitis in adults. Other bacterial causes for pharyngitis include non–group A streptococci (C and G), *Mycoplasma pneumoniae, Chlamydia trachomatis, Neisseria gonorrhoeae, Haemophilus influenzae,* and *Corynebacterium diphtheriae.* In about 30% of cases, no cause is found. The causes in such cases are believed to be a combination of environmental factors, allergies, and mouth breathing. Common causes in immunocompromised hosts include *Candida albicans* (thrush), herpes simplex virus, and cytomegalovirus (CMV). Rare noninfectious causes of sore throat include tortuous carotid artery, thyroiditis, spontaneous pneumomediastinum, lymphoma, and leukemia.

2. What three life-threatening infections may present with severe sore throat in adults?

(1) Epiglottitis, (2) peritonsillar abscess, and (3) retropharyngeal abscess are usually accompanied by evidence of pharyngitis, fever, and malaise. In all three cases, clues may be provided by the presence of odynophagia, drooling, and voice changes. Epiglottitis is usually abrupt in onset in children; in adults, it may be less acute, although still complicated by airway obstruction, especially when stridor and erect posture are evident. Peritonsillar and retropharyngeal abscesses may be insidious in nature. *Haemophilus influenzae* type b remains a cause of epiglottitis in adults. Peritonsillar and retropharyngeal abscesses are frequently polymicrobial (especially anaerobes); *Streptococcus pyogenes* is the most commonly isolated pathogen.

3. What presenting clinical features help to distinguish viral from bacterial pharyngitis?

Causes of Pharyngitis

SYMPTOM	VIRAL	BACTERIAL
Cough	Common	Rare
Rhinitis	Common	Occasional
Red throat	Common	Common
Fever (> 38.0°C)	Occasional	Common
Exudate	Occasional	Common
Tender anterior cervical nodes	Occasional	Common
Enlarged tonsils	Occasional	Common

4. Why should the primary care provider treat streptococcal infection?

1. Treatment prevents rheumatic fever.

2. Treatment prevents suppurative complications (peritonsillar and retropharyngeal abscess, cervical lymphadenitis, mastoiditis, sinusitis, and otitis media).

3. Treatment shortens the course of illness with decreased fevers and decreased pain by 24–48 hours.

4. Treatment decreases person-to-person spread of disease.

5. What is the probability that a person with streptococcal pharyngitis will develop acute rheumatic fever?

The probability of developing acute rheumatic fever depends on whether the patient has epidemic or endemic pharyngitis. For epidemic GAS, the probability of developing acute rheumatic fever is about 3%. In endemic areas, the probability is about 0.3%. At least one third of episodes of acute rheumatic fever result from unrecognized streptococcal infections.

6. To what degree does antibiotic treatment lower the risk of developing acute rheumatic fever?

Treatment has been shown to decrease the risk of subsequent acute rheumatic fever by 90%. This effect may occur even if antibiotics are started later than 9 days after the onset of symptoms. To be fully effective, antibiotics should be given for 10 days.

7. How often do patients with acute rheumatic fever develop cardiac disease?

Assuming that patients with acute rheumatic fever receive appropriate prophylactic antibiotic therapy, about 1% subsequently develop severe cardiac disease (class IV rheumatic heart disease) and 4% develop debilitating rheumatic heart disease.

8. What are the main local suppurative complications of GAS?

The main complications are peritonsillar abscess (quinsy) and retropharyngeal abscess. Less common complications include suppurative otitis media and cervical lymphadenitis. It is estimated that antibiotic treatment decreases the suppurative complications from about 5% to < 1%.

9. What is the recommended treatment for acute streptococcal pharyngitis?

The drug of choice is penicillin V with a newly recommended dosage of 500 mg two to three times daily for 10 days. Benzathine penicillin G, given intramuscularly in a dose of 1.2 million units, is also effective. Amoxicillin also may be used but has a higher incidence of associated rashes. For penicillin-allergic patients, the first choice is erythromycin, 250 mg four times daily for 10 days. Azithromycin, clarithromycin, and oral cephalosporins also may be used, although they have not yet been proved in clinical trials to prevent acute rheumatic fever. The length of treatment is crucial; failure rate decreases when treatment is increased from 7 to 10 days. A recent meta-analysis has shown that cephalosporins may have higher eradication rates than penicillin, but concern still exists over higher costs and problems related to using broad-spectrum antibiotics.

10. How quickly do antibiotics reduce the contagion of acute streptococcal pharyngitis?
Recovery of GAS from throat cultures is greatly reduced after 24 hours of antibiotic therapy, and antibiotic treatment is recommended as a way to reduce spread of GAS in schools and institutionalized settings.

11. Is it necessary to reculture after treatment to confirm eradication of GAS?
No. Treatment has been shown to be 85–90% effective in numerous studies. Patients with culture-positive GAS after treatment appear to have strains of streptococcus that are not associated with developing acute rheumatic fever. Follow-up cultures should be considered in patients with persistent or recurring symptoms and in patients who have had rheumatic fever and are at high risk for recurrence.

12. How should a care provider decide when empirical treatment for suspected GAS is appropriate in a patient with sore throat?
1. Determine the clinical probability that the patient has GAS on the basis of the history and physical examination. The probability (%) of GAS pharyngitis based on prevalence and clinical findings is determined by the "strep score," which is derived by giving 1 point for each of the following: tonsillar exudate, anterior cervical lymphadenopathy, absence of cough, and presence of fever.

Prevalence of Group A Streptococcal Pharyngitis

STREP SCORE	IN MOST OFFICE PRACTICES (%)	IN EMERGENCY DEPARTMENT (%)
0	1	3
1	4	8
2	9	18
3	21	38
4	43	63

Adapted from Centor RM, Meier FA, Dalton HP: Throat cultures and rapid tests for diagnosis of group A streptococcal pharyngitis. Ann Intern Med 105:892, 1986.

2. Use the predicted probability of GAS in the following evaluation and treatment algorithm.

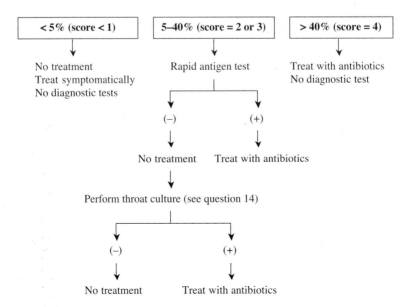

Empirical treatment for group A beta-hemolytic streptococcus based on predicted probability.

13. Should rapid strep test kits be used to guide the treatment of GAS?

Many rapid strep test kits or antigen detection tests (ADTs) are available to help in the diagnosis of GAS. In general, they have a sensitivity of about 80–90% and a specificity of 90–98%. The low sensitivity may be mainly operator dependent, and newer optical immunoassay tests have shown sensitivities close to 95% when studied in pediatric populations. Currently, a positive rapid test result is adequate to initiate treatment; however, in some cases, a negative test result (with sensitivity < 80%) should be followed by a blood agar plate culture.

14. Should throat culture continue to be used in the routine primary evaluation of adults with pharyngitis?

Recently published guidelines recommend that throat cultures should not be used in the routine primary evaluation of adults with pharyngitis or for confirmation of negative ADT results, especially when the test sensitivity exceeds 80%. Using the treatment algorithm in question 12, in a low GAS prevalence population, the additional sensitivity gained by culture verification of a negative ADT identifies only a very small number of additional GAS cases. In high-risk patients (previous acute rheumatic fever) or during investigations of GAS outbreaks, throat culture is more often indicated.

15. What is the correct method for obtaining a pharyngeal swab for GAS culture or ADT?

The posterior pharynx and both tonsils should be swabbed vigorously when obtaining a sample for culture or ADT. Culture and ADT sensitivity correlate with the size of inoculum used. The buccal mucosa, tongue, and hard palate are not adequate sampling sites.

16. What antibiotic regimens are recommended for patients with multiple repeated culture-positive episodes of symptomatic pharyngitis?

Clindamycin and amoxicillin–clavulanate are the antibiotics of choice for previously treated patients with multiple recurrent episode of culture-proven symptomatic pharyngitis. These antibiotics provide higher rates of pharyngeal streptococcal eradication compared with penicillin in circumstances of recurrent pharyngitis.

17. What are the most common causes of hoarseness?

Hoarseness is due to abnormal vibration of the vocal cords, which may result from local disorders or paralysis of the laryngeal nerve. The most common cause of hoarseness is local inflammation of the vocal cords due to upper respiratory tract infection or acute voice strain. Other local causes result from laryngeal carcinoma, papillomas and polyps, trauma, or irritants (gastroesophageal reflux disease, chronic alcohol use, and chronic postnasal drip). The common causes of laryngeal nerve paralysis in adults are carcinoma (20%), nerve injury from cardiomegaly, chest trauma, or other factors (23%); surgical damage (23%); and inflammatory lesions or lesions of the central nervous systems such as from stroke (14%).

18. What is the best medical treatment for hoarseness?

The patient with hoarseness should rest the voice and stop smoking (if this applies). Humidifiers may help. Underlying diseases should be treated when possible (e.g., antibiotics for bacterial infections and thyroid hormone replacement for myxedema).

19. When should a complaint of hoarseness undergo more aggressive evaluation?

Hoarseness that persists for 6–8 weeks, especially in smokers, or that is accompanied by other symptoms suggestive of malignancy (mass, neck or chest pain, weight loss, shortness of breath, and aspiration) should be evaluated immediately.

20. What systemic medical diseases may be associated with hoarseness?

Hypothyroidism, rheumatoid arthritis (cricoarytenoid arthritis), and diabetes mellitus.

21. What is the initial evaluation of hoarseness?

After the history and physical examination, laryngoscopy should be performed to evaluate voice quality, vocal cord mobility, and presence or absence of masses. Because many of the local causes of hoarseness may result from small changes in the laryngeal mucosa, a computed axial tomography (CAT) scan of the neck does not substitute for laryngoscopy.

BIBLIOGRAPHY

1. Bisno AL: Acute pharyngitis. N Engl J Med 344:205–211, 2001.
2. Bisno AL, Gerber MA, Gwaltney JM Jr, et al: Diagnosis and management of group A streptococcal pharyngitis: A practice guideline. Infectious Disease Society of America. Clin Infect Dis 25:574–583, 1997.
3. Blumer JL, Goldfarb J: Meta-analysis in the evaluation of treatment for streptococcal pharyngitis: A review. Clin Ther 16:604–620, 1994.
4. Centor RM, Meier FA: Sore throat. In Dornbrand L, Hoole A, Fletcher R (eds): Manual of Clinical Problems in Adult Ambulatory Care, 3rd ed. Philadelphia, Lippincott-Raven, 1997, pp 76–82.
5. Centor RM, Meier FA, Dalton HP: Throat cultures and rapid tests for diagnosis of group A streptococcal pharyngitis. Ann Intern Med 105:892, 1986.
6. Cooper JC, Hoffman JR, Bartlett JG, et al: Principles of appropriate antibiotic use for acute pharyngitis in adults: Background. Ann Intern Med 134:509–517, 2001.
7. Dajani A, Taubert K, Ferrieri P, et al: Treatment of acute streptococcal pharyngitis and prevention of rheumatic fever: A statement for health professionals. Committee on Rheumatic Fever, Endocarditis, and Kawasaki Disease of the Council on Cardiovascular Disease in the Young, the American Heart Association. Pediatrics 96:758–764, 1995.
8. Frantz TD, Rasgon BM, Quesenberry CP: Acute epiglottitis in adults. JAMA 272:1358–1360, 1994.
9. Gerber MA, Tanz RR, Kabat W, et al: Optical immunoassay test for group A β-hemolytic streptococcal pharyngitis. JAMA 277:899–903, 1997.
10. Goldenberg D, Golz A, Joachims HZ: Retropharyngeal abscess: A clinical review. J Laryngol Otol 3:546–550, 1997.
11. Hillner BE, Centor RM: What a difference a day makes: A decision analysis of adult streptococcal pharyngitis. J Gen Intern Med 2:242, 1987.
12. Kline JA, Runge JW: Streptococcal pharyngitis: A review of pathophysiology, diagnosis, and management. J Emerg Med 12:665–680, 1994.
13. Komaroff AL, Pass TM, Aronson MD, et al: The prediction of streptococcal pharyngitis in adults. J Gen Intern Med 1:1, 1986.
14. Koster F: Respiratory tract infections. In Barker LR, Burton JR, Zieve PD, et al (eds): Principles of Ambulatory Medicine, 6th ed. Philadelphia, Lippincott Williams & Wilkins, 2002.
15. Maragos ND: Hoarseness. Primary Care 17:347, 1990.
16. Mayo-Smith MF, Spinale JW, Konskey CJ, et al: Acute epiglottitis. An 18-year experience in Rhode Island. Chest 108:1640–1647, 1995.
17. Millan SB, Cumming WA: Supraglottic infections. Prim Care 23:741–758, 1996.
18. Randolph MF, Gerber MA, DeMeo KK, Wright L: Effect of antibiotic therapy on the clinical course of streptococcal pharyngitis. J Pediatr 106:870, 1985.
19. Tompkins RK, Burnes DC, Cable BS: An analysis of the cost-effectiveness of pharyngitis management and acute rheumatic fever prevention. Ann Intern Med 86:481, 1977.

29. ORAL LESIONS

Michael L. Lepore, M.D.

1. What is the most common cause of xerostomia (dry mouth)?

Medications are the most common cause of oral dryness, especially in older persons. In fact, increased use of medications in the geriatric population may explain the widely believed myth that salivary gland dysfunction is part of the normal aging process.

2. How do medications cause xerostomia?

The mechanisms by which medications may cause xerostomia include salivary gland hypofunction, mucosal dehydration, total body dehydration, altered sensory function, and cognitive disorders. Medications that frequently decrease salivary flow rates by blocking cholinergic activity are tricyclic antidepressants; antipsychotics; centrally acting antihypertensives such as clonidine; diphenhydramine; and the belladonna alkaloids, such as atropine, scopolamine, and hyoscyamine.

3. What medical conditions are commonly associated with xerostomia?

The two most common medical conditions associated with xerostomia are **Sjögren's syndrome** and **radiation-induced salivary gland dysfunction.** In its primary form, Sjögren's syndrome is characterized by lymphocytic infiltration of the salivary and lacrimal glands, thus leading to dry mouth and dry eyes. It also may occur in association with another major rheumatologic disease, such as rheumatoid arthritis, systemic lupus erythematosus, primary biliary cirrhosis, or scleroderma. The majority of patients with radiation-induced salivary gland dysfunction have received ionizing radiation for head and neck carcinoma. This type of salivary dysfunction is usually more severe during the active radiation, but return to normal salivation almost never occurs. A number of other disorders may lead to dysfunction of one or more of the major salivary glands (parotid, submandibular, and sublingual). Patients are rarely symptomatic because salivary flow must decrease by approximately 50% before xerostomia develops.

4. Are there any complications of salivary gland hypofunction?

Saliva contains various polypeptides and glycoproteins that have antimicrobial activity. In the absence of these elements, the patient is prone to recurrent **oral candidiasis** and **dental decay.**

5. What is the most common cause of recurrent painful mouth sores?

Aphthous ulcers are the most common type of nontraumatic mouth sores. In the general population, the incidence is 10–20%. Among professionals and upper socioeconomic groups, the incidence is higher.

6. What are the causes of aphthous ulcers?

The cause of aphthous ulcers is still unknown. However, the following have been implicated:

Viral agents (herpes simplex virus)	Stress
Bacteria (*Streptococcus sanguis*)	Trauma
Nutritional deficiencies (B_{12}, folate, iron)	Food allergies (nuts, chocolate, gluten)
Hormonal alterations	Immunologic abnormalities

7. Name the three types of aphthous ulcers.

Minor, major, and herpetiform.

8. How do the various types of aphthous ulcers differ?

In the **minor variety,** the patient usually notices a tingling or burning sensation before the ulcer appears. The ulcerations usually measure < 1.0 cm and are localized to the freely movable keratinized gingiva. They are white in the center surrounded by a red border. They are extremely painful and usually resolve in approximately 7–10 days.

The **major variety** may occur on the movable mucosa, soft palate, tongue, and tonsillar pillars. They are much more painful than the minor ulcers and are also much larger, measuring 1–3 cm. One to 10 ulcers may be present at a time.

Herpetiform ulcers are similar to herpetic lesions. Ten to 100 ulcers are usually present, measuring 1–3 mm in diameter. The small ulcers may coalesce, forming larger ulcers. The minor and major types generally do not leave a scar, whereas the herpetiform variety may leave a scar if the ulcerations coalesce.

9. A 27-year-old woman comes to your office with painful mouth sores that began 24 hours ago. On examination, you find several white lesions on her pharynx, soft palate, and tongue. She had similar lesions 3 years ago, which resolved over 1 week. What is the most likely diagnosis?

Most likely, recurrent aphthous stomatis. Aphthous ulcers are the most common type of nontraumatic ulcers. In the general population, the incidence is 10–20%. For reasons that we do not understand, the incidence in professionals and upper socioeconomic groups is higher.

10. What is the current treatment for aphthous stomatitis?

Treatment includes both medical management and cauterization, if necessary. The ulcer bed may be cauterized either chemically or electrically. Silver nitrate is commonly used for chemical cauterization. After the application of silver nitrate, the area should be swabbed with a cotton-tip applicator impregnated with sodium chloride, which converts the silver nitrate to silver chloride, thereby preventing a deep burn.

Medical treatment includes oral antibiotics, anti-inflammatory agents, or immunosuppressants. Local measures include the use of an oral suspension of tetracycline or topical steroids such as 0.5% fluocinonide ointment or a betamethasone solution.

11. A 30-year-old, otherwise healthy man presents with small, creamy white, curdlike lesions on his tongue and buccal mucosa of several weeks' duration. What is your diagnosis?

Creamy white, curdlike lesions are likely caused by oral candidiasis (thrush). *Candida* species are present in normal oral flora in 40–60% of the population. In certain immunocompromised states, candidal overgrowth may lead to thrush. The lesions represent patches of *Candida albicans* with leukocytes and desquamated epithelial cells.

12. How is the diagnosis of thrush made?

The diagnosis can be made easily by scraping the lesions, which are easy to remove and have an erythematous base, and examining the scrapings in potassium hydroxide under the microscope. Characteristic hyphae and blastospores are easily recognized.

13. When thrush is suspected, what should the diagnostic workup include?

Common conditions that lead to thrush include inhaled corticosteroid use for reactive airway disease, debilitating systemic illnesses such as cancer, and other immunocompromised states such as acquired immunodeficiency syndrome (AIDS) and neutropenia. Less common causes include diabetes, pregnancy, adrenal insufficiency, systemic antibiotic and systemic steroid use, nutritional deficiencies, and poor oral hygiene; the differential diagnosis includes leukoplakia and hyperkeratosis. Patients who have thrush for no obvious reason, such as the patient presented in question 11, should be evaluated for human immunodeficiency virus (HIV) infection.

14. What is desquamative gingivitis?

Desquamative gingivitis, which affects women older than age 30 years, is characterized by diffuse erythematous desquamation, ulceration, and sometimes bullae formation involving the free and attached gingiva. Associated conditions include lichen planus, cicatricial pemphigoid, bullous pemphigoid, pemphigus vulgaris, dermatitis herpetiformis, and drug reactions. Incisional biopsy is frequently necessary for diagnosis. Immunofluorescent studies may aid in differentiating between the various entities.

15. How often are white oral lesions malignant?

Acutely, lesions of the oral cavity may be erythematous. However, during the course of the disease, white elements may appear and predominate. White lesions of the mouth are often benign. However, 5–10% of oral malignancies present as white lesions. Thus, examining physicians must always be concerned that a lesion in question is a possible malignancy.

16. How can one differentiate among the various white lesions of the oral cavity?

Lesions of the oral cavity may present acutely as red lesions, but during the course of the disease, white elements appear and may predominate. White lesions of the mouth may be separated into two broad clinical categories: keratotic and nonkeratotic. The most important clinical feature distinguishing the two groups is the ability of the lesion to adhere to the surface epithelium. Leukoplakia, carcinoma, and primary skin disease are usually keratotic. Infectious and bullous skin diseases usually present as nonkeratotic lesions.

Keratotic and Nonkeratotic Factors

KERATOTIC	NONKERATOTIC
Firmly adherent	Removed relatively easily
Usually of long duration	Usually of short duration
Usually change slowly	Frequently change rapidly
Surface is usually elevated and may be smooth, roughened, or even verrucous	Usually erosive or ulcerative

17. What are characteristically premalignant lesions?

Leukoplakia is a white patch or plaque of the mouth that cannot be removed by rubbing and cannot be ascribed to other apparent skin diseases, such as lichen planus. The incidence of malignancy may be as high as 30% in patients with leukoplakia; thus, a biopsy is necessary. Asymptomatic, velvety red lesions of the mouth may be even more suspect for carcinoma *in situ* and should be biopsied.

18. What is "geographic" tongue?

Loss and regrowth of papillae lead to red patches on the tongue. This "geographic" appearance is asymptomatic and results from an idiopathic inflammatory condition.

19. What are the most common locations of squamous cell carcinoma of the mouth?

The most common locations are the lower lip, floor of the mouth, and tongue. Painless ulcers not healing in 1–2 weeks are highly suspect and should be biopsied.

20. What is the major differential diagnosis of an oral pigmented lesion?

The most worrisome diagnosis is malignant melanoma, but other possibilities include nevi and benign macules, lesions of Peutz-Jeghers disease, and Addison's disease. Any new suspicious lesion should be followed and biopsied early.

21. Who develops hairy leukoplakia?

White, painless lesions that appear "hairy" are often found in patients with AIDS, usually on the lateral aspects of the tongue. They are caused by Epstein-Barr virus and may temporarily respond to high-dose acyclovir.

22. What is the difference between loss of taste (ageusia) and loss of flavor?

Smell and taste are separate senses. The combination of both produces the sensation of flavor, which is distinct from either sense alone. If the olfactory neurons are damaged (by head trauma or viral invasion) or if the nasal passages are blocked (by polyps or edema), the only sensation is produced by the taste buds. This loss of flavor is perceived by the patient as loss of taste.

23. How can taste and olfactory problems be differentiated?

If the patient can differentiate between table salt, sugar, the sour taste of lemon juice, or the bitter taste of dark chocolate or coffee, the taste system is intact. Patients who lack the ability to smell state that they can taste the above but nothing else.

24. A 42-year-old woman presents with the chief complaint that sweet beverages taste bitter. Does this dysgeusia (abnormal taste) represent a true pathologic condition?

The effect of taste pleasure and displeasure is present at birth. Sugar produces a pleasurable response, whereas quinine produces a displeasurable response. Some patients may suffer from a chronic bitter taste in the mouth (bitter dysgeusia). To determine the possible origin of the dysgeusia, the mouth may be anesthetized with a topical anesthetic for 60 seconds. If a strong taste solution is given, the patient should not be able to taste. If the dysgeusia is not abolished, it does not originate in the mouth. Most patients usually complain that a sweet beverage, such as cola, tastes bitter. If topographic testing reveals that the patient has lost the ability to taste sweet flavors, the residual taste of the cola is genuinely bitter. Various substances can alter taste because they affect the taste membrane:

1. The **orange juice effect.** Sodium laurel sulfate, the detergent in toothpaste and mouthwash, decreases the intensity of sweet tastes (orange juice) and adds bitter taste to acids.

2. The **artichoke effect.** If the tongue is exposed to artichoke, which contains chlorogenic acid, beverages such as milk, water, or wine taste as if they have been sweetened.

3. **Acetazolamide,** which is used to treat glaucoma, also may make substances taste bitter.

25. A 69-year-old man who drinks and smokes heavily presents with the chief complaints of difficulty tasting food and numbness on the anterior two thirds of his tongue. What are the possible causes and sites of lesions?

Taste sensation in the anterior two thirds of the tongue is supplied by a branch of the facial nerve called the chorda tympani nerve. This nerve travels along the posterior wall of the middle ear to the infratemporal fossa and the submandibular gland region, where it joins the lingual nerve to innervate the ipsilateral anterior two thirds of the tongue. Pathology involving these regions must be carefully ruled out. Possible pathologic processes include neoplastic lesions in the floor of the mouth, submandibular gland region, or infratemporal fossa; acute and chronic otitis media; Bell's palsy; and Lyme disease.

26. During a routine physical examination, a 32-year-old man is noted to have a papillary lesion involving the uvula and anterior tonsillar pillar on the left. What is the significance of this finding?

Squamous papillomas are the most common benign tumors of the oral cavity and pharynx. These papillary growths are locally noninvasive similar to their laryngeal counterparts. Malignant degeneration of this benign tumor is rare. Polymerase chain reaction (PCR) studies of the DNA of the oral papilloma fail to demonstrate any human papillomavirus (HPV) type 6a or 11a, which is normally associated with the more aggressive types found in laryngeal papillomas of children.

27. What are torus mandibularis and torus palatinus?

Torus mandibularis is a benign bony enlargement on the lingual surface of the mandible opposite the cuspid and premolar teeth, above the insertion of the mylohyoid muscle. It is believed that this deformity is caused by an autosomal dominant trait with variable penetrance according to gender. It occurs in 1 in 13 whites, 1 in 9 African-Americans, 1 in 7 American Indians, and 1 in 2.5 Eskimos. **Torus palatinus** is a benign bony enlargement that occurs on the hard palate at the junction of the midpalatal suture. The mass is normally covered by normal oral mucosa. The cause may be related to a dominant trait, but it is questioned whether autosomal dominant or X-linked dominance is a factor. It occurs in females more often than males. In both lesions, surgical removal is indicated only if they interfere with function, particularly if dentures are needed.

28. What are mucoceles of the oral cavity?

A mucous retention cyst, or mucocele, is a lesion of the lower lip or buccal mucosa. Chiefly of cosmetic concern, this benign nodular lesion is either translucent or bluish in color and ranges from 1 to 2 cm in diameter. These cysts result from the retention of saliva and are commonly caused by trauma to the lower lip. The lesions are usually superficial and very thin walled, transparent in nature, and true cysts. If a thin wall is not present with mucoid material, this type of lesion is commonly referred to as a *mucous retention cyst*. Mucoceles located deep in the lip tissue may appear as ill-defined discrete masses.

29. How should severe toothaches be managed by primary care providers?

Toothaches are most commonly a manifestation of inflammation of the pulp (pulpitis). They generally occur in the presence of a large dental caries or large restorations (fillings). Management depends greatly on the clinical presentation.

1. In the absence of fever and intraoral or extraoral swelling, patients can be managed with analgesics (acetaminophen with or without codeine) and a dental referral within 24 hours.

2. In patients with intraoral or extraoral swelling or with a low-grade fever, antibiotics (penicillin or erythromycin for penicillin-allergic patients) also should be given.

3. For patients with a fever > 101°F or with edema that causes facial asymmetry, an urgent dental referral is mandatory. Complications may include full-blown facial cellulitis or destruction of the alveolar bone that supports the teeth.

BIBLIOGRAPHY

1. Allen CM, Blozis CG: Oral mucosal lesions. In Cummings CW, Frederickson JM, Harper LA (eds): Otolaryngology: Head and Neck Surgery, 3rd ed. St. Louis, Mosby, 1998.
2. Aragon SB, Jafek BW: Stomatitis. In Bailey BJ, et al (eds): Head and Neck Surgery—Otolaryngology, 3rd ed. Philadelphia, Lippincott Williams & Wilkins, 2002.
3. Atkinson JC, Fox PC: Salivary gland dysfunction. Clin Geriatr Med 499–508, 1992.
4. Barker RL, Burton JR, Zieve PD, et al (eds): Principles of Ambulatory Medicine, 6th ed. Philadelphia, Lippincott Williams & Wilkins, 2002.
5. Cannon RD, Chaffin WL: Oral colonization by *Candida albicans*. Crit Rev Oral Biol Med 10:359–383, 1999.
6. Epstein JB: The painful mouth: Mucositis, gingivitis, stomatitis. Inf Dis Clin North Am 2:183–200, 1988.
7. Krull EA, Fellman AC, Fabian LA: White lesions of the mouth. Ciba Clin Symp 25:1–32, 1973.
8. Lucente FE: Otolaryngologic aspects of acquired immunodeficiency syndrome. Med Clin North Am 75:1389–1398, 1991.
9. Mandell GL, Bennett JE, Dolin R (eds): Principles and Practice of Infectious Disease, 5th ed. New York, Churchill Livingstone, 2000.
10. Martin W: Oral health and the older diabetic. Clin Geriatr Med 15:339–350, 1999.
11. McBride DR: Management of aphthous ulcers. Am Fam Physician 62:149–154, 160, 2000.
12. Nakamo K: Characteristics of human papillomavirus (HPV) infection in papilloma of the head and neck: Detection of HPV according to clinical features and type specificity. Pippon Jibbinkoka Gakkai Kaiho 97:1381–1392, 1994.
13. Popovsky JL, Camisa C: New and emerging therapies for diseases of the oral cavity. Dermatol Clin 18:113–125, 2000.
14. Rosenthal C, Karthaus M, Ganser A: New strategies in the treatment and prophylaxis of chemo- and radiotherapy-induced oral mucositis. Antibiot Chemother 50:115–132, 2000.
15. Triantos D, Porter SR, Scully C, Teo CG: Oral hairy leukoplakia: Clinicopathologic features, pathogenesis, diagnosis, and clinical significance. Clin Infect Dis 25:1392–1396, 1997.

V. Endocrine and Metabolic Disorders

30. DIABETES MELLITUS

Jonathan P. Castro, M.D., Linda Joseph, M.D., Dawn A. Mellish, M.D., Reba Williams, M.D., and Samy I. McFarlane, M.D.

1. What is diabetes mellitus?

Diabetes mellitus is a disorder of carbohydrate, fat, and protein metabolism characterized by chronic hyperglycemia resulting from defects in insulin secretion, insulin action, or both. Untreated, the metabolic derangement leads to **macrovascular** (myocardial infarction, stroke, peripheral vascular disease) and **microvascular** complications (retinopathy, neuropathy, and nephropathy) and results in early mortality and significant morbidity.

2. What are the classic symptoms of diabetes?

Diabetes mellitus commonly presents with symptoms such as polydipsia, polyuria, blurring of vision, and weight loss. Symptoms are often mild or may even be absent; therefore, hyperglycemia sufficient to cause pathologic changes may be present long before the diagnosis of diabetes mellitus is made. In its most severe form, ketoacidosis or a nonketotic hyperosmolar state may develop and lead to stupor, coma, and, in absence of effective treatment, even death.

3. What criteria are used for diagnosing diabetes?

Three criteria are used to diagnose diabetes in nonpregnant adults, but each diagnosis should be confirmed by repeat testing of glucose on a different day. Because of ease of use, lower cost, and patient acceptability, **fasting plasma glucose (FPG)** is the preferred test (*fasting* is defined as having no caloric intake for at least 8 hours). An **oral glucose tolerance test (OGTT)** is not recommended for routine clinical use but may be required in the evaluation of patients with impaired fasting glucose (IFG) or when diabetes is suspected despite a normal FPG. The criteria for diagnosing diabetes are:

- Symptoms of diabetes such as polyuria, polydipsia, *and* unexplained weight loss and a random plasma glucose of $\geq$ 200 mg/dL *or*
- FPG $\geq$ 126 mg/dL *or*
- 2-hour plasma glucose $\geq$ 200 mg/dL during an OGTT using a glucose load containing the equivalent of 75 g of anhydrous glucose dissolved in water, as described by the World Health Organization

4. How do you screen for diabetes?

Currently, no clear evidence from randomized trials indicates that screening asymptomatic individuals for diabetes is beneficial or improves outcomes. As such, current practice guidelines for screening asymptomatic individuals are based on expert consensus. The American Diabetes Association (ADA) recommends testing of asymptomatic nonpregnant patients by measuring FPG every 3 years beginning at age 45 years. However, testing should be considered at a younger age or carried out more frequently in individuals with any of the following risk factors:

- Being overweight (body mass index [BMI] $\geq$ 25 kg/m^2)
- Having a first-degree relative with diabetes

- Belonging to a high-risk ethnic or racial group (e.g., African American, Latino, Native American, Asian American, Pacific Islander)
- Having delivered a baby weighing > 9 lb or having been diagnosed with gestational diabetes mellitus
- Being hypertensive (≥ 140/90 mmHg)
- Having a high-density lipoprotein (HDL) cholesterol level < 35 mg/dL (0.90 mmol/L) or triglyceride level > 250 mg/dL (2.82 mmol/L)
- Having impaired glucose tolerance (IGT) or IFG
- Having other clinical conditions associated with insulin resistance (e.g., polycystic ovarian syndrome or acanthosis nigricans)
- Having a history of vascular disease

5. What are the three categories defined by the measurement of FPG?
1. **Normal:** < 110 mg/dL (< 6.1 mmol/L)
2. **IFG:** 110–125 mg/dL (6.1–6.9 mmol/L)
3. **Diabetes mellitus:** ≥ 126 mg/dL (> 6.9 mmol/L)

6. What is the difference in risk between patients with diabetes and patients with IFG?
Diabetics are at increased risk for both macrovascular and microvascular complications. Individuals with impaired fasting plasma glucose are at increased risk mainly for macrovascular disease (myocardial infarction, stroke, peripheral vascular disease).

7. Why was the cutoff for the diagnosis of diabetes lowered from 140 mg/dL to 126 mg/dL?
The FPG cutoff for the diagnosis of diabetes mellitus has been lowered from 140 mg/dL (7.8 mmol/L) to 126 mg/dL (7.0 mmol/L) because the latter was found to reflect more accurately the plasma glucose concentration at or above which the risk for microvascular complications is increased. Furthermore, this lower value has been shown to correlate better with the risk for complications associated with a random (or 2-hour post-glucose challenge) plasma glucose concentration of 200 mg/dL (11.1 mmol/L). With the new criterion for diagnosis of diabetes mellitus based on a fasting blood glucose of 126 mg/dL versus 140 mg/dL, the number of diabetics in the United States population has doubled and is estimated to be 18 million persons.

8. What is the new classification scheme for diabetes mellitus?
The Expert Committee on the Diagnosis and Classification of Diabetes Mellitus recommends classifying diabetes according to etiology rather than age at onset or pharmacologic treatment. Terms such as *insulin-dependent, non-insulin-dependent, juvenile-onset, maturity-onset,* and *adult-onset diabetes* have been eliminated from this classification and should be avoided. These terms can be confusing and frequently result in patients being classified on the basis of treatment rather than pathogenesis. The new etiologic classification includes four major types:
- Type 1 diabetes mellitus
- Type 2 diabetes mellitus
- Gestational diabetes mellitus
- Other specific types

9. Describe and characterize the four types of diabetes mellitus.
Type 1 diabetes mellitus is a state of absolute insulin deficiency that results from autoimmune destruction of the insulin-producing cells of the pancreas, the beta cells. Serologically, it can be identified by the presence of antiglutamic acid decarboxylase (GAD) islet cell or insulin antibodies. Insulin deficiency predisposes patients to ketoacidosis, coma, and possibly even death if insulin is not replaced. Hence, exogenous insulin is required for survival. Typically, type 1 diabetes has its onset during childhood and presents with ketoacidosis. Patients with type 1 diabetes are usually lean and comprise less than 10% of the diabetic population. The term *type 1 diabetes*

mellitus does not include those forms of beta-cell destruction or failure to which specific causes can be assigned (e.g., cystic fibrosis, mitochondrial defects).

Type 2 diabetes mellitus is the most common form of diabetes and is characterized by disorders of insulin action (insulin resistance) or insulin secretion. Alterations in the insulin receptor or postreceptor function prevent normal cellular uptake of glucose, resulting in hyperglycemia. The specific reasons for the development of these abnormalities are not yet known. Type 2 diabetes usually presents after the age of 30 years in genetically predisposed people. Patients present with the usual symptoms of hyperglycemia such as polyuria, polydipsia, and blurring of vision. Ketoacidosis is an infrequent presentation. Patients can be treated with diet alone or diet plus oral hypoglycemics, but exogenous insulin may be required in some cases to adequately control hyperglycemia. Patients with type 2 diabetes are usually obese and represent over 90% of the diabetic population.

Gestational diabetes mellitus is a state of insulin resistance and hyperinsulinemia that results from placental production of diabetogenic hormones such as growth hormone, corticotropin-releasing hormone, placental lactogen, and progesterone. The diagnosis and treatment of gestational diabetes are important because of the association of poor glucose control with complications. **Maternal complications** include preeclampsia, higher likelihood of operative delivery, and later development of diabetes mellitus; **fetal complications** include macrosomia, birth trauma, neonatal metabolic complications (e.g., hypoglycemia, hyperbilirubinemia, hypocalcemia, polycythemia vera), perinatal mortality, and development of obesity and diabetes during childhood.

Other specific types of diabetes include maturity-onset diabetes of the young (MODY), drug- and chemical-induced diabetes, and endocrinopathies such as Cushing's, acromegaly, and glucagonoma.

10. Describe the metabolic syndrome. What are the National Cholesterol Education Program (NCEP) diagnostic criteria for metabolic syndrome?

The metabolic syndrome, also known as **syndrome X, insulin resistance syndrome,** and **obesity dyslipidemia syndrome,** is a metabolic disorder characterized by the presence of the "deadly quartet": abdominal obesity, hypertension, diabetes, and dyslipidemia. Abdominal obesity or visceral fat is associated with resistance to the actions of insulin on peripheral glucose utilization, leading to the development of type 2 diabetes. Because of insulin resistance, compensatory hyperinsulinemia develops and leads to hypertension and dyslipidemia, both of which promote atherogenicity and increase the risk for coronary artery disease. Thus, individuals with metabolic syndrome are at increased risk of mortality from cardiovascular causes compared with the general population. The diagnosis of metabolic syndrome is established when three or more of the following five criteria are present:

- FPG ≥ 110 mg/dL
- Blood pressure ≥ 130/85 mmHg
- HDL cholesterol
  Men: < 40 mg/dL
  Women: < 50 mg/dL
- Triglycerides ≥ 150 mg/dL
- Waist circumference
  Men: > 40 inches
  Women: > 35 inches

11. What are the long-term complications of diabetes mellitus?

- Retinopathy (most common cause of blindness)
- Nephropathy (most common cause of renal failure)
- Autonomic dysfunction, including sexual dysfunction
- Cardiovascular disease
- Peripheral vascular disease
- Cerebrovascular disease

12. How do you screen for diabetic retinopathy?

Diabetic retinopathy is the leading cause of adult blindness in the U.S. It accounts for as many as 20% of new cases of blindness per year. By age 20 years, evidence of retinopathy is present in almost all patients with type 1 diabetes and in approximately 50–80% of those with type 2 diabetes. This underlines the importance of screening to preserve vision. **Seven-field stereoscopic photography** through dilated pupils is considered the gold standard for screening but may be impractical in clinical practice. Hence, simple **direct ophthalmoscopy with dilated pupils** is the next best alternative and, in studies, has been shown to be a dependable, practical, and cost-effective method of screening for retinopathy. Postpubertal patients with type 1 diabetes should be screened within 3–5 years after the onset of diabetes. Retinopathy of sufficient severity that necessitates specific ophthalmologic therapy usually develops 5 years after the onset of diabetes. Retinopathy before the age of puberty is rare. Thus, screening for retinopathy in type 1 diabetics is not indicated before puberty.

In contrast, type 2 diabetes has an insidious onset, and, in some cases, retinopathy of significant severity may be present long before diabetes is diagnosed. It is for this reason that type 2 diabetics should be screened at the time of diagnosis. Subsequent examinations and follow-ups are then individualized based on the presence and severity of retinopathy at the initial examination. However, the minimum recommendation is annual examination by an ophthalmologist for those without retinopathy and follow-up visits every 6 months for those with established retinopathy.

13. What measures can be taken to lower the rate of progression of diabetic retinopathy?

Strict control of major risk factors such as hyperglycemia, hypertension, hyperlipidemia, and smoking and the use of angiotensin-converting enzyme (ACE) inhibitors are the most important measures in slowing the rate of progression of retinopathy. **Panretinal photocoagulation** is the mainstay of treatment for proliferative retinopathy or severe nonproliferative retinopathy and has been shown to be effective in reducing the risk of developing severe visual loss among treated diabetics.

14. How do you screen for and monitor diabetic nephropathy?

Diabetic nephropathy is the single most common cause of end-stage renal disease (ESRD) in the U.S. It accounts for as many as 40% of new cases of ESRD per year. All in all, an estimated 20–30% of patients with diabetes will develop some evidence of nephropathy in their lifetime. The earliest clinical evidence of nephropathy is the appearance of low but abnormal levels (30–300 mg/day or 20–200 μg/min) of albumin in the urine, a condition known as **microalbuminuria**. Microalbuminuria, a harbinger of renal failure and cardiovascular complications in diabetes, is an albumin concentration in the urine that is greater than normal (but is not detectable with common urine dipstick assays for protein). Routine screening for microalbumin should be performed yearly in adults with type 2 diabetes. If the screening is positive for microalbumin, a quantitative measure is helpful for developing a treatment plan. After the initial screening and in the absence of previously demonstrated microalbuminuria, a test for the presence of microalbuminuria should be performed annually. Three methods to screen for microalbuminuria are as follows:

- Measurement of the albumin-to-creatinine ratio in a random spot urine collection
- Timed (4-hour or overnight) urine collection
- 24-hour urine collection with creatinine, allowing the simultaneous measurement of creatinine clearance

The random spot urine collection is preferred in an office-based setting and generally provides accurate information. Because of marked day-to-day variability in albumin excretion, at least 2 of 3 samples done in a 3- to 6-month period should show elevated levels before designating a patient as having microalbuminuria. If normal, repeat yearly. Microalbuminuria rarely occurs with short duration of type 1 diabetes; therefore, screening in individuals with type 1 diabetes should begin after 5 years' disease duration.

Screening for microalbumin with dipsticks or reagent tablets may also be done if assays are not readily available. Reagents and tablets show 95% sensitivity when performed by trained personnel.

Several factors may influence the albumin excretion rate. Screening should be postponed in the following situations: short-term hyperglycemia, exercise, marked hypertension, urinary tract infection, acute febrile illness, or heart failure. ACE inhibitors or nonsteroidal anti-inflammatory drugs (NSAIDs) may also influence results. All positive tests by reagent strips or tablets should be confirmed using one of the quantitative urine assays listed in the table below.

Quantitative Urine Assays

	SPOT URINE (μg/mg creatinine)	TIMED URINE COLLECTION (μg/min)	24-HOUR URINE COLLECTION (mg/24 hours)
Normal	< 30	< 20	< 30
Microalbuminuria	30–300	20–200	30–300
Clinical albuminuria	> 300	> 200	> 300

15. What measures lower the rate of progression of diabetic nephropathy?

Improving glycemic control, aggressive antihypertensive treatment, and the use of ACE inhibitors or angiotensin receptor blockers (ARBs) slow the rate of progression of nephropathy. In both hypertensive and nonhypertensive type 1 diabetics with microalbuminuria or clinical albuminuria, ACE inhibitors are the initial agents of choice. In hypertensive type 2 diabetic patients with microalbuminuria or clinical albuminuria, ARBs are the initial agents of choice. If one class is not tolerated, the other should be substituted. In addition, with the onset of overt nephropathy, initiating protein restriction to $\leq$ 0.8 g/kg body weight per day may be useful in slowing the decline of glomerular filtration rate (GFR) in selected patients.

16. What are the different types of diabetic neuropathy?

- **Focal neuropathies**—involve sensory or motor loss of a particular nerve (e.g., wrist drop, foot drop, diplopia)
- **Distal symmetric polyneuropathy** (e.g., stocking or glove paresthesias)
- **Autonomic neuropathy**—manifests as gastrointestinal dysmotility, bladder overfilling with incomplete emptying, impotence, impaired glucose counterregulation, hypoglycemic unawareness, orthostatic hypotension, loss of cardiac rate deceleration, and distal anhydrosis with compensatory increased sweating on face and trunk

17. Describe the macrovascular complications of diabetes. What can be done about them?

Patients with diabetes are at increased risk for macrovascular complications such as myocardial infarction, peripheral vascular disease, and stroke. The presence of atherosclerotic disease should be screened with (1) careful history-taking with emphasis on cardiovascular symptoms such as chest pain, exertional dyspnea, and claudication; (2) physical examination for carotid bruits and peripheral pulses; and (3) electrocardiogram (ECG) if $\geq$ 40 years of age. A fasting lipid profile and a spot urine for microalbumin should also be obtained to further assess cardiovascular risk.

Encouraging weight loss with diet and exercise, controlling blood glucose, treating hypertension, smoking cessation, and optimizing lipids are the most important adjuncts to disease prevention. Feet should be examined annually. To prevent amputation, the high-risk foot should be identified early on. Clinical features associated with increased risk include abnormal gait, neuropathy, peripheral vascular disease, structural deformity, history of foot ulcers, abnormal skin or nails, and history of skin infections.

18. How can the level of glycemic control be determined?

Glycemic control is best measure by using either the hemoglobin A_{1c} (HbA_{1c}) or the fructosamine assay. The HbA_{1c} reflects glucose control over a period of 2–3 months, roughly the life span of an average red blood cell. For patients under good control, HbA_{1c} may be checked every 6–12 months, whereas those with poor control should be checked every 3 months. In contrast, the fructosamine assay, which reflects glucose control over a 3- to 6-week period, is useful in monitoring glycemic control among pregnant women and patients on intensive insulin therapy.

19. Who should be screened for gestational diabetes mellitus?

Screening and risk assessment for gestational diabetes mellitus (GDM) should be undertaken at the first prenatal visit. Patients with high-risk features such as significant obesity, past history of GDM, glycosuria, or a strong family history of diabetes should undergo glucose testing to rule out GDM. An FPG of $\geq$ 126 mg/dL or a random plasma glucose of $\geq$ 200 mg/dL done twice on two different occasions establishes the diagnosis of GDM. However, women at moderate risk for GDM, despite negative screen, should be retested for GDM between 24 and 28 weeks of gestation.

20. What are the goals of diabetic therapy as suggested by the Diabetes Control and Complications Trial (DCCT)?

In the DCCT, 1441 patients with type 1 diabetes were randomized to either standard or intensive care. The standard care group received 1–2 daily insulin injections and routine follow-up. Treatment in this group was aimed at minimizing symptoms. In contrast, the intensive care group was treated with multiple daily injections or continuous insulin infusion and was provided with intensive diabetes self-management education. Furthermore, a health care team with active case management that included monthly visits and weekly phone contacts also followed this group closely. The intensive treatment group achieved a mean HbA_{1c} of approximately 7%, whereas the standard group maintained an approximate HbA_{1c} of 9%. With a mean follow-up of 6.5 years, there was significant reduction in the incidence and rate of microvascular endpoints. Intensive glycemic control reduced the onset of retinopathy by 27%, severe nonproliferative and proliferative retinopathy requiring laser treatment by 45%, progression of clinically meaningful retinopathy by 34–46%, microalbuminuria by 35%, clinical grade albuminuria by 56%, and clinical neuropathy by 60%. Thus, it is clear from the results of the DCCT that intensive glycemic control should be the goal for all type 1 diabetics in an effort to reduce microvascular complications.

21. What are the risks of intensive insulin therapy as determined by DCCT?

Risks attributable to intensive insulin therapy include a threefold increase in severe hypoglycemia and weight gain. However, despite these concerns, the occurrence of major macrovascular events or deterioration of neurobehavioral status has not been observed. Quality of life was not adversely affected by intensive insulin therapy.

22. Which patients may be at greater risk for an adverse outcome during intensive therapy?
- Children younger than 13 years
- Patients with known coronary artery or cerebrovascular disease
- Patients with far-advanced complications (e.g., renal failure)
- Patients with recurrent severe hypoglycemia or hypoglycemic unawareness

23. Which patients have the greatest risk of severe hypoglycemia?

Diabetic patients who have lost the ability to sense and compensate for hypoglycemia are at greatest risk of severe hypoglycemia. This condition is know as **hypoglycemic unawareness.** As a result of autonomic neuropathy, the normal counterregulatory responses that protect against hypoglycemia are lost. The secretion of epinephrine, a counterregulatory hormone that produces sympathetic responses (e.g., sweating, palpitations, anxiety) that warn patients of hypoglycemia, is impaired. In addition, the secretion of hormones that increase hepatic glucose output in response to hypoglycemia such as glucagon and epinephrine have also been impaired. This creates a precarious situation for diabetic patients because not only do they not sense hypoglycemia, but also, more importantly, they have lost the physiologic ability to raise they glucose.

24. What advice should be given to patients about hypoglycemia?

At all times, diabetic persons must carry glucose snacks to treat hypoglycemic symptoms. Identification cards help to direct treatment if the individual is found unconscious. Frequent home glucose monitoring may avoid hypoglycemia by therapeutic alterations.

25. What is included in the annual evaluation of a patient with diabetes?

Morbidity from renal, ocular, neurologic, and cardiovascular causes should be monitored annually. British authorities suggest the following comprehensive list for annual review:

Weight	Proteinuria
HbA_{1c}	Creatinine
Blood pressure	Peripheral neuropathy, vibratory sense, light touch, pain
Smoking	Impotence
Visual acuity and optic fundi	Family planning advice about glycemic control during
Feet	conception
Lipid assessment	Annual review of educational concepts

26. What are the current nutrition recommendations and principles for people with diabetes mellitus as specified by ADA guidelines?

Diet serves to (1) achieve or maintain ideal body weight, (2) improve glycemic control, (3) optimize serum lipids, (4) prevent and treat both acute complications of insulin-treated diabetes (e.g., hypoglycemia, exercise-related problems) and long-term complications (e.g., renal disease, autonomic neuropathy, cardiovascular disease), and (5) improve overall health through optimal nutrition.

In general, caloric requirements should be modified to help the patient reach and maintain ideal body weight. Weight reduction for obese patients may be achieved by moderately reducing caloric intake by 5–15 kcal/kg/day (i.e., down to 20–30 kcal/kg/day), particularly if sedentary. Usual caloric intake, when reduced by 500 calories/day, should result in gradual weight loss of 1 lb per week. Weight maintenance for moderately active individuals may be achieved by restricting caloric intake to 30–35 kcal/kg/day.

Carbohydrates should be maintained at 50–60% of calories, proteins at 10–20%, and fats at < 30%, with saturated fat limited to < 10% of total calories and total cholesterol intake of < 300 mg/day (NCEP step I diet). Diabetics with coexisting lipid abnormalities (e.g., elevated low-density lipoprotein [LDL] cholesterol) should further reduce their fats by reducing saturated fats to < 7% of total calories and dietary cholesterol to < 200 mg/day (NCEP step II diet). In addition, a diet high in fiber (20–35 g/day of soluble and insoluble fiber) should also be emphasized.

Sodium should be restricted to 2400–3000 mg/day. If hypertensive, the patient's sodium intake should be reduced further to < 2400 mg/day and, if nephropathy is present in addition to hypertension, to < 2000 mg/day. Furthermore, in patients with overt diabetic nephropathy, restricting proteins to < 10% or 0.8 g/kg/day may protect against the progression of nephropathy. As for alcohol intake, drinks should be limited to one per day for women and to less than two per day for men. Multivitamins should also be considered. Non-nutritive artificial sweeteners are acceptable when taken in moderate amounts.

27. What are the beneficial effects of exercise? What advice should be given to patients?

In most patients with diabetes, some form of exercise is likely to be beneficial. Exercise promotes cardiovascular fitness, maintains ideal body weight, and, by complementing nutritional goals, improves overall glycemic control. On the whole, exercise decreases the diabetic's risk for macrovascular complications.

However, certain considerations must be emphasized to prevent injury to the exercising diabetic. Before beginning any exercise program, diabetics older than 35 years should have a complete physical examination and an exercise stress test. Myocardial ischemia must be ruled out because sudden exercise, especially in sedentary patients, can precipitate myocardial infarction. Patients with proliferative retinopathy should avoid intense isometric exercise (e.g., weight lifting), which can cause a marked increase in blood pressure that might precipitate intraocular bleeding. On the other hand, patients with neuropathy should avoid traumatic weight-bearing exercise (e.g., long-distance running, prolonged downhill skiing), which may precipitate stress fractures in small bones of the foot and ankle and predispose to the development of pressure ulcers on the toes and feet. Well-fitting protective footwear and comfortable shoes are also needed.

For patients on insulin, blood glucose should be monitored before, during, and after exercise. Exercise can worsen glycemic control, promote ketosis in poorly controlled diabetes, and predispose patients with well-controlled diabetes to hypoglycemia. In general, patients with poorly controlled diabetes whose blood glucose levels consistently exceed 250 mg/dL should be advised against exercise until better glycemic control in achieved. On the other hand, patients with well-controlled diabetes may safely carry out a mild exercise regimen so long as they avoid hypoglycemia by applying the **"15 to 30 rule":** 15–30 g of carbohydrates (e.g., glucose tablets, hard candies, or juice) taken 15–30 minutes before exercise and then approximately every 30 minutes during exercise. Patients also should be advised to ingest slowly absorbed carbohydrates (e.g., dried fruit, fruit jerky, granola bars, trail mix) immediately after exercise to prevent late hypoglycemia as the body replenishes its depleted glycogen stores. Another consideration is to reduce by 30% the insulin dose for that time of the day of the patient's exercise. Runners should be advised to use the abdomen rather than the legs as the injection site because absorption and bioavailability of insulin is increased by exercising muscles and predisposes to hypoglycemia.

28. What is the initial therapy for patients with type 2 diabetes?

Lifestyle modification is essential in the treatment of type 2 diabetes. Mild disease often can be controlled with diet and exercise alone, obviating the need for expensive pharmacologic therapy. Even a modest weight loss of as little as 10 lb can significantly improve metabolic control and, in some cases, induce remissions. Hence, weight reduction must be emphasized in all patients as a therapeutic goal. However, in some cases, hyperglycemia persists despite these lifestyle changes. Pharmacology therapy then becomes necessary. The pharmacologic armamentarium for the treatment of type 2 diabetes includes a variety of oral agents, such as sulfonylureas, meglitinides, biguanides, thiazolidinediones, and alpha-glucosidase inhibitors.

29. Discuss the different oral agents used in the treatment of type 2 diabetes mellitus.

Sulfonylureas are the most widely used drugs for the treatment of type 2 diabetes. They stimulate pancreatic beta cells to secrete insulin and, to a very minor extent, enhance insulin sensitivity. Sulfonylureas can be used as monotherapy or in combination with insulin or other oral hypoglycemic agents. The are effective, well tolerated, and can effectively lower glucose concentrations by as much as 20%. Hypoglycemia is the most common side effect and is more common with the longer acting sulfonylureas such as chlorpropamide and glyburide. Infrequent side effects include nausea, skin sensitivity, and abnormal liver function tests.

Nonsulfonylurea insulin secretagogues, such as repaglinide and nateglinide, are insulin secretagogues and, like sulfonylureas, stimulate pancreatic beta cells to increase insulin secretion. Although structurally different from sulfonylureas, they act in a similar fashion by regulating adenosine triphosphate (ATP)-dependent potassium channels in pancreatic beta cells, thereby increasing insulin secretion. The clinical efficacy of meglitinide is similar to that of sulfonylureas. They can be used either as monotherapy or in combination with metformin. Compared with glyburide, nateglinide has a greater effect on postprandial hyperglycemia, whereas glyburide has a greater effect on fasting plasma glucose.

Thiazolidinediones, such as pioglitazone and rosiglitazone, enhance insulin sensitivity by acting on muscle and liver to improve glucose utilization and decrease glucose production. The exact mechanism by which insulin sensitivity is enhanced is unknown, but thiazolidinediones are known to bind and activate a transcription factor called **peroxisome proliferator-activated receptor gamma** (PPAR-gamma), which is found in adipose tissue, muscle, and liver and is thought to be involved in the transcription of insulin-responsive genes. Both rosiglitazone and pioglitazone can be used as monotherapy or in combination with metformin, insulin, or sulfonylureas.

Thiazolidinedione monotherapy can decrease HbA_{1c} values by as much as 1.0–1.6%. They can also reduce serum triglycerides and raise serum HDL concentrations. Pioglitazone has also been shown to decrease serum total and LDL cholesterol concentrations, an effect not shared by rosiglitazone. Side effects include dose-related weight gain, fluid retention, and heart failure.

Biguanides, such as metformin, act as insulin sensitizers. In the presence of insulin, metformin decreases hepatic glucose production, increases insulin-mediated glucose utilization in peripheral tissues, lowers serum triglycerides and free fatty acid concentrations, promotes modest weight reduction, and reduces FPG concentrations by about 20%. Metformin is less likely to cause hypoglycemia compared with sulfonylureas. Side effects are most commonly gastrointestinal (GI): metallic taste in the mouth, mild anorexia, nausea, bloating, diarrhea, and a reduction of intestinal absorption of vitamin B_{12} in up to 30% of patients. A rare but worrisome problem is lactic acidosis, which can be fatal in as many as 50% of cases. Metformin is contraindicated in the following:

- Renal insufficiency (serum creatinine > 1.5 mg/dL)
- Concurrent liver disease or alcohol abuse
- Heart failure
- History of lactic acidosis
- Severe infection with decreased tissue perfusion
- Hypoxic states
- Serious acute illness or hemodynamic instability
- Age 80 years or older

Alpha glucosidase inhibitors, such as acarbose and miglitol, inhibit upper GI digestive enzymes and prevent the conversion of carbohydrates into monosaccharides. These drugs slow the absorption of glucose and can, therefore, limit postprandial glucose excursions, an effect that can lower HbA_{1c} values by 0.4–0.9%. Furthermore, acarbose may also have beneficial effects on lipids. Acarbose can decrease serum LDL concentrations and increase serum HDL concentrations. Side effects are mainly GI, including flatulence and diarrhea. Acarbose should be started at a low dose and titrated slowly. Acarbose-induced hypoglycemia should be treated with oral glucose (dextrose) instead of sucrose (cane sugar) because the latter can be absorbed in the presence of enzyme inhibition.

Comparison of Oral Hypoglycemic Agents

AGENT	FORMULATION (mg)	DOSE/DAY (mg)	DOSE INTERVAL	PEAK (hrs)	DURATION OF ACTION (hrs)	SIDE EFFECTS
Alpha-glucosidase inhibitors						
Acarbose (Precose)	25, 50, 100	150–300	3 times/day (w/meals)	N/A	2–3	Abdominal pain, gas, diarrhea
Miglitol (Glyset)	25, 50, 100	150–300	3 times/day (w/meals)	N/A	2–3	Abdominal pain, gas, diarrhea
Biguanides						
Metformin (Glucophage)	500, 850, 1000	1000–2550	2–3 times/day	2–3	12–18	
Metformin extended release (Glucophage XR)	500	1000–2000	1–2 times/day	4–8	24	Abdominal pain, gas, diarrhea
Nonsulfonylurea secretagogues						
Repaglinide (Prandin)	0.5, 1.0, 2.0	1.5–16.0	3–4 times/day (w/meals)	1	4–6	Hypoglycemia, weight gain
Nateglinide (Starlix)	60, 120	180–360	3 times/day (w/meals)	0.3	4	Hypoglycemia, weight gain

Table continued on following page.

Comparison of Oral Hypoglycemic Agents (Continued)

AGENT	FORMULATION (mg)	DOSE/DAY (mg)	DOSE INTERVAL	PEAK (hrs)	DURATION OF ACTION (hrs)	SIDE EFFECTS
Sulfonylureas (second-generation)						
Glyburide (Diabeta Micronase)	2.5, 5.0	1.25–20.0	1–2 times/day	4	12–24	Hypoglycemia, weight gain
Micronized glyburide (Glynase)	1.5, 3.0, 6.0	0.75–12.0	1–2 times/day	2	12–24	Hypoglycemia, weight gain
Glipizide (Glucotrol)	5, 10	2.5–40.0	1–2 times/day	1–	12–24	Hypoglycemia, weight gain
Glipizide GITS (Glucotrol XL)	2.5, 5.0, 10.0	2.5–40.0	Daily	6–12	24	Hypoglycemia, weight gain
Glimepiride (Amaryl)	1, 2, 4	1–8	Daily	2–3	24	Hypoglycemia, weight gain
Thiazolidinediones						
Rosiglitazone (Avandia)	2, 4, 8	4–8	1–2 times/day	N/A	Days to weeks	Weight gain, edema
Pioglitazone (Actos)	15, 30, 45	15–45	Daily	N/A	Days to weeks	Weight gain, edema
Combinations						
Metformin-glyburide (Glucovance)	250–1.25, 500–1.25, 500–2.5, 500–5	2–3 tabs	2 times/day	For the peak, duration of action, and side effects, refer to the individual components above		

30. How is insulin therapy initiated in patients with type 2 diabetes?

Type 2 diabetics who require exogenous insulin to achieve better glycemic control may begin with a morning injection that combines neutral protamine Hagedorn (NPH) and regular insulin. A second injection can be added before dinner, if needed. A reasonable starting dose is 0.5 U/kg body weight. It is best to adjust the dose with patients at their usual level of physical activity while consistently following their diet and doing home glucose monitoring. Intervals of 2–4 days between dosage changes are best. The addition of a small dose of sulfonylurea, metformin, or troglitazone may improve glucose control. Liver function tests must be monitored closely in patients treated with troglitazone, because it has been implicated in 26 deaths from liver failure worldwide. Establishing normoglycemia may temporarily improve insulin secretion and insulin action so that the need for exogenous insulin is reduced and the patient's condition improves (glucotoxicity).

31. How should patients with type 1 diabetes mellitus be treated?

An insulin regimen that is both acceptable to the patient and results in long-term glycemic control while minimizing hypoglycemia is the goal of insulin therapy in type 1 diabetics. In general, two insulin regimens are recommended in patients with type 1 diabetes:

1. Two injections (in the morning and before dinner) of combined NPH-regular insulin (starting ratio = 70/30) with a third injection of regular insulin before lunch

2. Ultralente insulin in the morning or evening with semilente insulin before breakfast, lunch, and dinner. When glycemic control is erratic, ultralente combined with three injections of Humalog (LISPRO), a rapid-acting insulin, may give better control.

An arbitrary dose of 24 U/day or an insulin dose calculated at 0.5 U/kg, divided into two separate doses (two thirds of the total dose given before breakfast and one third before dinner) may be used as a starting dose for insulin therapy. Dose adjustments may then be done every 2–4 days on an outpatient basis to achieve better control. Dose adjustments are generally made in 10–20% increments, which usually calculates to 1–5 U at a time.

32. What is the approach to diabetic dyslipidemia?
- (1) Lower LDL, (2) raise HDL, (3) lower triglycerides
- HDL goal: women: > 55 mg/dL; men: > 45 mg/dL
- Drugs for lowering LDL: statins, followed by binding resins (may raise triglycerides) or fenofibrate
- Drugs for lowering triglycerides: fibric acid derivatives, followed by high-dose statins
- No consensus on the use of drug therapy for triglycerides between 200 and 400 mg/dL or on raising HDL cholesterol levels

33. What are the guidelines for lipid management according to the ADA?

American Diabetes Association Lipid Guidelines

LIPID	MONITORING	THERAPEUTIC GOAL	DRUG INITIATION
LDL cholesterol			
With cardiovascular disease	Annually	≤ 100 mg/dL	> 100 mg/dL
No cardiovascular disease*	Annually	≤ 100 mg/dL	> 130 mg/dL
HDL cholesterol	Annually	Men: > 45 mg/dL	?
		Women: > 55 mg/dL	
Triglycerides	Annually	≤ 200 mg/dL	> 400 mg/dL

*Some experts initiate drug therapy at LDL > 100 mg/dL if multiple cardiac risk factors are present (e.g., cigarette smoking, hypertension, known cerebrovascular or peripheral vascular disease, HDL cholesterol < 40 mg/dL, male sex, first-degree family relative with coronary artery disease before age 55 years, severe obesity).

BIBLIOGRAPHY

1. American Diabetes Association: Standards of medical care for patients with diabetes mellitus. Diabetes Care 26(suppl 1):S55–S50, 2003.
2. American Diabetes Association: Screening for type 2 diabetes. Diabetes Care 26(suppl 1):S21–S24, 2003.
3. DeFronzo RA: Pharmacologic therapy for type 2 diabetes mellitus. Ann Intern Med 131:281–303, 1999.
4. Diabetes Control and Complications Trial: The effect of intensive treatment of diabetes on the development and progression of long-term complications in insulin-dependent diabetes mellitus. N Engl J Med 320:977–986, 1993.
5. Expert Panel on Detection, Evaluation, and Treatment of High Blood Cholesterol in Adults: Executive summary of the Third Report of the National Cholesterol Education Program (NCEP) Expert Panel on Detection, Evaluation, and Treatment of High Blood Cholesterol in Adults (Adult Treatment Panel III). JAMA 285:2486–2497, 2001.
6. Kirpichnikov D, McFarlane SI, Sowers JR: Metformin: An update. Ann Intern Med 137:25–33, 2002.
7. Larsen PR, Kronenberg HM, Melmed S, Polonsky KS (eds): Williams Textbook of Endocrinology, 10th ed. Philadelphia, W.B. Saunders, 2003.
8. McFarlane SI, Banerji M, Sowers JR: Insulin resistance and cardiovascular disease. J Clin Endocrinol Metabol 86:713–718, 2001.
9. McFarlane SI, Kumar A, Sowers JR: Mechanism by which angiotensin-converting enzyme inhibitors prevent diabetes and cardiovascular disease. Am J Cardiol 91:30–37, 2003.
10. McFarlane SI, Shin JJ, Rundek T, Bigger JT: Prevention of type 2 diabetes. Curr Diab Rep 3:235–241, 2003.
11. United Kingdom Prospective Diabetes Study (UKPDS): Relative efficacy of randomly allocated diet, sulfonylurea, insulin, or metformin in patients with newly diagnosed non–insulin-dependent diabetes mellitus followed for three years. BMJ 310(6972):83–88, 1995.

31. ABNORMALITIES OF LIPIDS

Alicia L. Wolfert, M.D., and Robert H. Eckel, M.D.

1. What are lipoproteins?

Lipoproteins are carrier proteins that transport lipids, which are insoluble, to various tissues, where they are utilized. All lipoproteins consist of cholesterol (ester and unesterified), triglyceride (TG), phospholipid, and apoprotein (the protein component). The two major classes of lipoproteins are distinguished by a change in the relative proportion of these components as the lipoprotein becomes progressively smaller and more dense:

1. **TG-rich lipoproteins:** chylomicrons and very low-density lipoproteins (VLDLs)
2. **Cholesterol-rich lipoproteins:** low- and high-density lipoproteins (LDLs and HDLs, respectively)

2. Which lipoprotein is most important in the pathogenesis of atherosclerosis?

LDL, remembered as "lethal" cholesterol. Increased levels of LDL cholesterol have been shown in multiple studies to increase the risk of coronary heart disease (CHD). Every 1% decrease in LDL cholesterol is associated with about a 2% decrease in risk of CHD. Current evidence suggests that LDL moves into the subintimal space and becomes oxidized. It is then taken up by macrophages and forms foam cells within the extracellular space. Smooth muscle cells then proliferate around this lipid core, leading to the formation of the atherosclerotic plaque.

3. How is LDL cholesterol calculated?

LDL cholesterol is usually calculated rather than measured. The formula used is:

LDL cholesterol = Total cholesterol − Triglycerides/5 − HDL cholesterol

This formula is accurate unless triglycerides are > 400 mg/dl. LDL cholesterol can also be measured directly, but this is not routinely done in practice.

4. What is the role of HDL in atherosclerosis?

HDL cholesterol, remembered as "healthy" cholesterol, is antiatherogenic because of its role in reverse cholesterol transport, a process that removes excess cholesterol from cells. Low HDL cholesterol has been shown to increase the risk of CHD. For every 5 mg/dL decrement in HDL cholesterol below median levels, there is a 25% increased risk of myocardial infarction (MI). Conversely, high levels of HDL cholesterol have been shown to be cardioprotective. The new National Cholesterol Education Program guidelines list an HDL cholesterol < 40 mg/dL as a risk factor for CHD.

5. What are physical manifestations of hyperlipidemia?

1. **Xanthelasma:** irregularly shaped, slightly raised, yellowish-white lesions on the upper or lower eyelids that are cholesterol deposits in the skin.
2. **Tendinous xanthomas:** deposits of cholesterol in the tendons.
3. **Eruptive xanthomas:** deposits of cholesterol on the trunk and extensor surfaces of the extremities; they appear as painless papules with yellow centers and are seen in patients with severe hypertriglyceridemia.
4. **Arcus cornealis:** whitish ring seen around the cornea caused by lipid deposits in the periphery of the cornea.
5. **Lipemia retinalis:** change in color of the blood vessels in the retina from red to pink or white; this occurs when serum triglyceride levels exceed 1000 mg/dL.

6. Who should be screened for hyperlipidemia?

The recommendations for screening are controversial and variable.

1. **National Cholesterol Education Program (NCEP)/Adult Treatment Panel (ATP) III** guidelines suggest screening all adults age 20 years and older with a fasting lipoprotein profile (total cholesterol, LDL cholesterol, HDL cholesterol, and triglycerides) every 5 years.

2. **US Preventive Health Services** Task Force recommends screening men age 35 years and older and women age 45 years and older (class A). They recommend screening men and women younger than this (age 20 years and older) if they have risk factors for coronary heart disease (class B). The screening test recommended is a total cholesterol and HDL cholesterol.

3. The **American Diabetic Association** recommends yearly screening with a full lipoprotein profile for all adults with diabetes.

7. How important is fasting when screening for hyperlipidemia?

Total cholesterol and HDL cholesterol are affected very little by fasting, but triglycerides can change substantially between fasting and nonfasting states. Because LDL cholesterol is a calculated value derived from levels of triglycerides, HDL cholesterol, and total cholesterol, accurate calculation of LDL cholesterol requires a fasting sample.

8. Name two major primary prevention trials that showed a benefit to lowering cholesterol.

1. The **Air Force/Texas Coronary Atherosclerosis Prevention Study (AFCAPS/Tex-CAPS)** showed that lovastatin decreased the risk of first acute major coronary event in men and women with average total cholesterol and LDL cholesterol levels and below-average HDL cholesterol levels

2. The **West of Scotland Coronary Prevention Study (WOSCOPS)** showed that treatment with pravastatin reduced the incidence of MI and death from cardiovascular causes in men with moderately high total cholesterol and LDL cholesterol levels.

9. Name three major secondary prevention trials that showed a benefit to lowering cholesterol.

1. The **Scandinavian Simvastatin Survival Study (4S)** randomized patients with known CHD and moderately high cholesterol to simvastatin versus placebo and found a 30% decrease in overall death and 42% decrease in cardiovascular death.

2. The **Cholesterol and Recurrent Events (CARE)** study randomized patients with known CHD and average cholesterol levels to pravastatin versus placebo and found a 24% decrease in risk of coronary event.

3. The **Long-Term Intervention with Pravastatin in Ischaemic Disease (LIPID)** study randomized patients with known CHD and broad range of cholesterol levels to pravastatin versus placebo and found a 24% decrease in risk of coronary events.

10. What are the goals of lipid-lowering therapy according to the most recent guidelines?

The National Cholesterol Education Program (NCEP)/Adult Treatment Panel (ATP) III in 2001 came out with its third report on the treatment of high blood cholesterol in adults (NCEP III). This report focuses on LDL cholesterol as the primary goal of therapy and lists different LDL cholesterol goals based on an individual's risk factors.

- 0 or 1 risk factor: LDL cholesterol goal < 160 mg/dL
- ≥ 2 risk factors: LDL cholesterol goal < 130 mg/dL
- Known CHD or CHD equivalents: LDL cholesterol goal < 100 mg/dL

11. Are screening or treatment goals different for elderly patients?

Age should not be a factor in screening and treating older patients provided they have no major comorbidities that affect survival. NECP III/ATP III guidelines recommend no upper age limit for lipid-lowering drug therapy. CHD is much more prevalent in patients older than age 65 years; therefore, the number needed to treat to prevent one death is much smaller in this group.

12. What are cardiac risk factors?
- Cigarette smoking
- Hypertension defined as a blood pressure (BP) = 140/90 mmHg or taking an antihypertensive medication
- Low HDL cholesterol (< 40 mg/dL)
- Family history of premature CHD:
    Age < 55 years in male first-degree relative
    Age < 65 years in female first-degree relative
- Age:
    45 years in men
    55 years in women

13. What are CHD risk equivalents?
Certain patients have diseases that place them at the same risk to have a first coronary event as patients who have already had a coronary event. These diseases include:
- Diabetes
- Aortic aneurysm
- Symptomatic carotid artery disease
- Peripheral vascular disease
- Stroke
- Multiple risk factors that confer a > 20% risk of major coronary events in 10 years (this risk can be calculated using a point system known as Framingham scoring)

14. Are high triglycerides dangerous?
Very high triglyceride levels (> 500 mg/dL) increase the risk of developing acute pancreatitis. It is not completely clear if high triglycerides are an independent risk factor for CHD. High triglycerides are often associated with low HDL cholesterol and insulin resistance.

NCEP/ATP III defines the sum of LDL cholesterol and VLDL cholesterol (non-HDL cholesterol) as a secondary target of therapy in persons with high triglycerides (200–499 mg/dL). Patients who have high triglycerides should have their LDL cholesterol–lowering drug therapy intensified or a triglyceride-lowering agent added. Those with very high triglycerides (> 500 mg/dL) should have triglyceride lowering as the primary goal of therapy. After the triglyceride level has decreased to < 500, the focus of treatment can be changed to LDL cholesterol goals.

15. What factors elevate triglycerides?
- Decreased insulin sensitivity (obesity, type II diabetes)
- Physical inactivity
- Hypothyroidism
- Cigarette smoking
- Alcohol
- Diseases: nephrotic syndrome, Cushing's syndrome
- Medications: estrogens, corticosteroids, retinoids, beta-blockers, cyclosporine, tamoxifen, diuretics, protease inhibitors
- Genetic disorders: familial combined hyperlipidemia, familial dybetalipoproteinemia, familial hypertriglyceridemia

16. What can be done to lower cholesterol?
Therapeutic lifestyle changes (TLC) are recommended for all patients with high cholesterol. Pharmacologic therapy is used when TLC cannot lower cholesterol sufficiently.

17. What are therapeutic lifestyle changes?
1. Diet
    a. Saturated fat: < 7% of total daily calories

    b. Monounsaturated fat: < 20% of total daily calories

    c. Total fat: 25–35% of total daily calories

    d. Total cholesterol: < 200 mg/day

    e. Carbohydrates: 50–60% of total daily calories

    f. Protein: about 15% of total daily calories

    g. Soluble fiber intake: 10–25 g/day

    h. Increased intake of plant stanols and sterols (2 g/day)

2. Weight loss

3. Increased physical activity

18. How does physical activity affect lipids?

Aerobic exercise increases HDL cholesterol levels and decreases triglyceride levels. If exercise results in weight loss, LDL cholesterol levels can also decrease. However, the effect of exercise on LDL cholesterol is highly variable.

19. What drugs are most effective in treating high levels of LDL?

The 3-hydroxy-3-methylglutaryl coenzyme A (HMG CoA) reductase inhibitors, known as "statins," are considered first-line therapy for treating high levels of LDL cholesterol. These drugs bind to HMG CoA, a substrate for cholesterol, and competitively inhibit the rate-limiting step in cholesterol synthesis. The statins currently on the market include atorvastatin (Lipitor), fluvastatin (Lescol), lovastatin (Mevacor), pravastatin (Pravachol), and simvastatin (Zocor). Atorvastatin is the most potent, and fluvastatin is the least potent.

If patients cannot take statins, other options include bile acid sequestrants or nicotinic acids.

20. What are the potential side effects of statins?

Elevation of transaminases (AST, ALT) can occur and need to be monitored. If levels reach above two times normal, the dose needs to be decreased or the medicine discontinued. Fewer than 1% of patients taking statins will have an elevation in transaminases high enough to necessitate discontinuing the drug.

Myopathy can occur, with elevations of creatinine phosphokinase (CPK). Patients who complain of muscle pain should have their CPK level checked, and, if elevated, the medicine should be discontinued. Myopathy is more common when statins are combined with fibrates or other drugs that inhibit or compete for the cytochrome P450 3A4 enzyme (e.g., cyclosporine, macrolide antibiotics).

Other more common side effects include gastrointestinal symptoms and muscle aches.

21. What drugs are most effective in treating high triglyceride levels?

Fibric acid derivatives increase fatty acid oxidation in liver and muscle, decreasing VLDL production. They can also increase the metabolic clearance rate of VLDL. These drugs can lower triglycerides from 20–50% and increase HDL cholesterol ≤ 15%.

Nicotinic acid (niacin) inhibits VLDL production in the liver. It lowers triglycerides by 20–50%.

HMG CoA reductase inhibitors (statins) have a lesser effect, achieving a < 35% reduction in triglycerides.

22. What are potential side effects of fibrates?

Nausea, abdominal pain, and myopathy. There is an increased risk of myopathy when fibrates are combined with statins.

23. What are potential side effects of nicotinic acid?

With crystalline niacin, flushing occurs in > 90% of patients. This can be reduced by taking an aspirin about 30 minutes beforehand or by using NiaSpan, a relatively safe extended-release preparation of nicotinic acid. Nicotinic acid also can elevate blood glucose and uric acid and, rarely, produces severe hepatotoxicity.

BIBLIOGRAPHY

1. Choice of lipid lowering drugs. Med Lett 43:43–48, 2001.
2. Downs JR, Clearfield M, Weis S, et al: Primary prevention of acute coronary events with lovastatin in men and women with average cholesterol levels. Results of AFCAPS/TexCAPS. JAMA 279:1615–1622, 1998.
3. Expert Panel on Detection, Evaluation and Treatment of High Blood Cholesterol in Adults: Executive Summary of the Third Report of the National Cholesterol Education Program (NCEP) Expert Panel on Detection, Evaluation, and Treatment of High Blood Cholesterol in Adults (Adult Treatment Panel III). JAMA 285:2486–2497, 2001.
4. Long-Term Intervention with Pravastatin in Ischaemic Disease (LIPID) Study Group: Prevention of cardiovascular events and death with pravastatin in patients with coronary heart disease and broad range of initial cholesterol levels. N Engl J Med 339:1349–1357, 1998.
5. Mahley RW, Weisgraber KH, Farese RV: Disorders of lipid metabolism. In Larsen PR, Kronenberg HM, Melmed S, Polonsky KS (eds): Williams Textbook of Endocrinology, 10th ed. Philadelphia, W.B. Saunders, 2003, pp 1642–1705.
6. Sacks FM, Pfeffer MA, Moye LA, et al, for the Cholesterol and Recurrent Events Trial Investigators: The effect of pravastatin on coronary events after myocardial infarction in patients with average cholesterol levels. N Engl J Med 355:1001–1009, 1996.
7. Scandinavian Simvastatin Survival Study Group: Randomised trial of cholesterol lowering in 4444 patients with coronary heart disease: The Scandinavian Simvastatin Survival Study (4S). Lancet 344:1383–1389, 1994.
8. Screening for Lipid Disorders in Adults: Recommendations and rationale, U.S. Preventive Services Task Force. Am Fam Physician 65:273–276, 2002.
9. Shepherd J, Cobbe SM, Ford I, et al, for the West of Scotland Coronary Prevention Study Group: Prevention of coronary heart disease with pravastatin in men with hypercholesterolemia. N Engl J Med 333:1301–1307, 1995.

32. PRECONCEPTION COUNSELING AND INFERTILITY

Anne Kastor, M.D.

1. What is preconception counseling?

Preconception counseling provides information and medical care *before* pregnancy in order to increase the likelihood of healthy future pregnancies and births.

2. Who should receive preconception counseling?

Any woman of child-bearing age who is considering pregnancy or who is sexually active with men and might experience an unintended pregnancy.

3. What does preconception counseling involve for healthy women?

Folic acid supplementation. Adequate preconception stores of folic acid decrease the risk of neural tube defects. All women who might become pregnant should be advised to take 400 µg of folic acid each day, as well as a multivitamin.

Infectious disease screening, prevention, and treatment. All reproductive-age women should be screened for **rubella** and **varicella** immunity. Nonimmune women should be vaccinated and should wait at least 3 months after vaccination before becoming pregnant. **Hepatitis B, HIV,** and **sexually transmitted disease** testing should also be encouraged. Women who are not immune to hepatitis B should be offered vaccination. Women diagnosed with HIV should be referred to an experienced provider who can help determine if antiretroviral therapy is indicated and, if so, choose a regimen that will maximally suppress HIV viral load while limiting teratogenicity.

Genetic disease screening. Family history and ethnic background should be evaluated to determine the risk of sickle cell disease, Tay-Sachs disease, thalessemia, hemophilia A, cystic fibrosis, and other genetic disorders. All at-risk patients should be referred to a genetic counselor.

Smoking, alcohol, and drug counseling. Preconception counseling is an ideal time to assist women to stop smoking or using alcohol or drugs that may negatively impact a developing fetus. Nicotine replacement therapy and methadone use appear to be safe for both mother and fetus and are certainly safer than cigarette smoking or heroin use. Physicians can recommend these modalities, along with support groups and other methods, and reassure their patients that they can continue as needed during pregnancy.

Environmental toxin screening. The physician should assess occupational and household exposure to teratogens and abortifacients. Household hazards include lead-based paint, paint thinner, and carbon monoxide. Occupational hazards include solvents used in the dry-cleaning and electronics industries and anesthetic gases used in dental and medical settings. Upon employee request, employers are required to provide the Material Safety Data Sheets for toxic substances used in the workplace.

4. What does preconception counseling involve for women with chronic illnesses?

Women with chronic illnesses such as diabetes, seizure disorders, and rheumatic disorders require special care before and during pregnancy. Family planning is a crucial part of primary care for all patients with chronic illnesses. Tight preconception glucose control has been shown to decrease the risk of congenital anomalies in children of diabetic women. Medications should be closely reviewed for teratogenicity (e.g., tegretol, warfarin) and risk of spontaneous abortion (e.g., methotrexate). Preconception consultation with an obstetrician specializing in high-risk pregnancy may be indicated.

5. How long does it take the average healthy woman to conceive?

Twenty percent of women will become pregnant during 1 month of unprotected intercourse, 50% within 6 months, and 85–90% within 12 months. The likelihood of conception decreases as a woman's age increases, dropping off dramatically in the woman's late 30s.

6. How can a woman determine if and when she ovulates?

1. **Urine luteinizing hormone (LH) level:** Quick and reliable enzyme-linked immunosorbent assays that measure the LH surge are commercially available. Ovulation occurs approximately 36 hours after the onset of the LH surge. The unfertilized egg is viable for only 12–24 hours after ovulation. Sperm may be viable for up to 5 days after intercourse or insemination. Therefore, intercourse or insemination immediately before ovulation optimizes the likelihood of fertilization.

2. **Fertility awareness:** Fertility awareness (charting the menstrual cycle, basal body temperature [BBT], and cervical mucus) can help a women determine if and when she ovulates. Cervical mucus becomes stringy during a woman's fertile period. The BBT decreases slightly and then increases 0.5 mmHg after ovulation. Regular thermometers cannot detect this small increase in temperature, so a more precise basal body thermometer, available at pharmacies, is used. Because the temperature increase occurs after ovluation, BBT is not useful for timing intercourse or insemination. A biphasic pattern, however, does confirm that a woman is ovulatory.

7. What is infertility?

Infertility is defined medically as the inability to conceive after attempting pregnancy for 1 year. It is estimated that 10% of women who try to conceive fall into this category. Half of these women will conceive in the second year.

8. When should a woman or couple be referred to a fertility specialist?

Traditionally, it has been recommended that pregnancy be attempted for 1 year before referral. Many experts now recommend that women in their mid to late 30s or 40s be referred much sooner, given the rapid decline in fertility in the late 30s.

9. How frequently are male or female factors responsible for infertility?

Currently available data on this question are problematic. Most reports are based on patients in infertility clinics and therefore are not representative of the population as a whole. Also, the most frequently cited study was published in 1985. Most studies report that male factors are identified in 20–40% of cases, female factors in 30–40% of cases, and combined factors or unknown etiologies in the remainder.

10. What causes infertility in men?

Testicular disorders (hypergonadotropic hypogonadism) (20% of all infertility cases)

Congenital or developmental

- Varicoceles (most common cause of male infertility)
- Cryptorchidism (particularly if bilateral)
- Chromosomal anomalies (Klinefelter syndrome, Y chromosome microdeletions)
- Genetic disorders (myotonic dystrophy, androgen insensitivity syndromes, cystic fibrosis, immotile cilia syndrome)

Acquired

- Infection (mumps, tuberculosis, gonorrhea, chlamydia)
- Trauma, including prior genital or pelvic surgery
- Drugs (alkylating agents; spironolactone and other antiandrogens)
- History of ionizing radiation
- Environmental toxins (some pesticides, heavy metals)
- Hyperthermia (frequent hot baths or saunas)
- Antisperm antibodies
- Chronic illness, (renal insufficiency, cirrhosis, sickle cell anemia)

Disorders of sperm transport (10–15% of all infertility cases)

- Epididymis or vas deferens obstruction (congenital anomalies, prior trauma or infection)
- Ejaculatory dysfunction (premature or retrograde ejaculation, erectile dysfunction, or spinal cord injury)

Hypothalamic-pituitary disorders (hypogonadotropic hypogonadism)

Congenital

- Prader-Willi syndrome (genetic syndrome characterized by obesity, hypotonia, genital hypoplasia and characteristic facial features; mental retardation may be present)
- Kallmann syndrome (congenital defect in gonadotropin-releasing hormone (GnRH) secretion, associated with anosmia and midline facial anomalies)
- Mutations in LH or follicle-stimulating hormone (FSH) genes (rare)

Acquired

- Hyperprolactinemia
- Pituitary gland compression or infiltration (brain tumor, hemochromatosis)
- Androgen excess (anabolic steroid use, congenital adrenal hyperplasia, testicular or adrenal tumors)
- Estrogen excess
- Chronic illness
- Massive obesity

11. What causes infertility in women?

Ovulatory dysfunction (approximately 20% of all infertility cases)

- Hypothalamic-pituitary anovulation (low body weight, high-intensity exercise, extreme physical or emotional stress)
- Hyperprolactinemia
- Polycystic ovary syndrome
- Other endocrine disorders (thyroid disease, diabetes)
- Age-related or premature ovarian failure
- Luteal phase defect (inadequate progesterone during the luteal phase)

Tubal obstruction (approximately 14% of all cases)
- Endometriosis
- Prior pelvic inflammatory disease or surgical adhesions

Uterine factors
- Asherman's syndrome (scarring of the endometrium during prior instrumentation)
- Fibroids and uterine malformations

12. What aspects of the history help to determine if a woman ovulates regularly?
- Cycle regularity
- Presence of premenstrual symptoms (breast tenderness, bloating) or mittelschmerz (unilateral pelvic pain at the time of ovulation)

13. What aspects of the history suggest endometriosis
Severe and worsening dysmenorrhea
Dyspareunia

14. What is polycystic ovary syndrome (PCOS)?
PCOS is a syndrome of anovulatory menstrual irregularities and hyperandrogenism (hirsutism, male pattern balding). Multiple small ovarian cysts may be present but are not required for the diagnosis. Obesity, insulin insensitivity, and other metabolic disorders may also be present.

15. What testing is performed in an infertility work-up?
Testing is determined by findings on the history and physical examination. Based on the results of the tests listed below, infertility specialists may order additional, more specific tests.

SUSPECTED ETIOLOGY	TEST	COMMENTS
Male Factor	Semen analysis	Semen is collected by masturbation and analyzed for sperm quantity, morphology, and motility and semen volume and viscosity. Results, along with the history and physical, determine the need for additional hormonal testing (testosterone, FSH) to distinguish hypogonadotropic vs. hypergonadotropic hypogonadism.
Ovulatory Dysfunction	BBT	Biphasic BBT pattern confirms ovulation.
	Transvaginal ultrasound	Transvaginal ultrasound documents follicular development.
PCOS	Serum androgens	
Hyperprolactinemia	Serum prolactin level	
Ovarian failure	Day 3 FSH	Elevated FSH indicates poor ovarian reserve.
LPD	Mid-luteal serum progesterone	Fertility experts disagree as to whether and when endometrial biopsies should be performed.
	Late-luteal phase endometrial biopsy	
Tubal Obstruction	Hysterosalpingogram	A hysterosalpingogram is performed during the follicular phase. Radiopaque dye is injected into the uterus. X-rays document its movement into the fallopian tubes, illuminating any obstruction.
	Laparoscopy	Laparoscopy may reveal endometriosis or pelvic adhesions.
Uterine Factor	Pelvic sonogram	
	Hysterosalpingogram	
Cervical Factor	Postcoital test	Performed 1 day after ovulation and 12 hours after intercourse or insemination, the PCT evaluates cervical mucus quality and sperm motility. The test, however, has poor reproducibility, and its value is debatable.

BBT = basal body temperature; FSH = follicle stimulating hormone; LPD = luteal phase defect; PCOS = polycystic ovarian syndrome; PCT = postcoital test.

16. How and when is ovulation induced?

Ovulation induction may be accomplished with clomiphene, a central estrogen antagonist that increases the release of GnRH, or with GnRH agonists. It is used in women with ovulatory dysfunction and to increase oocyte yield during assisted reproduction.

17. What is ovarian hyperstimulation syndrome?

Ovarian hyperstimulation syndrome is a potentially life-threatening side effect of ovulation induction. It is more common with gonadotropin-based regimens than with clomiphene and with higher doses of gonadotropins. Ovarian enlargement, third-spacing of fluids, hypovolemia, and acute respiratory distress syndrome are the most dangerous forms. The pathophysiology is poorly understood.

18. What are sperm banks and who uses them?

Sperm banks are government-regulated facilities that provide frozen sperm for insemination. Donors are screened for infectious diseases, and semen analysis is performed. People who purchase semen from banks include lesbian women, single heterosexual women, and women with azoospermic partners.

19. Describe assisted reproductive techniques (ARTs).

1. **In vitro fertilization (IVF).** Ovulation is induced, and the oocytes are harvested with a transvaginal needle and catheter under ultrasound guidance. They are fertilized and then transferred into the uterus as embryos. IVF-ET is the method of choice for women with tubal obstruction. It is also used in cases of ovarian dysfunction.

2. **Gamete intrafallopian transfer (GIFT).** This method uses IVF protocols to obtain oocytes. The oocytes and spermatozoa are then placed directly into the fallopian tube via laparoscopy. Theoretically, GIFT offers the advantage of fertilization occurring in the natural physiologic environment. However, laparoscopy, an invasive procedure, is required.

3. **Zygote intrafallopian transfer (ZIFT).** This is similar to GIFT, but the oocyte is fertilized and the resulting embryo is placed in the fallopian tube laparoscopically.

4. **Oocyte donation.** This procedure may be considered for women with ovarian failure whose endometrium is capable of responding to gonadal steroids. The patient's endometrium is prepared with a hormonal regimen. The donated oocytes are fertilized and placed into the patient's uterine cavity. Oocyte donation may be the most successful method of achieving pregnancy in older patients.

5. **Intracytoplasmic sperm injection (ICSI).** ICSI was introduced as a therapy for infertility in men with obstructive azoospermia or low sperm counts. Sperm are collected surgically from the epididymis or testicle and directly transferred into the oocyte for fertilization. The embryo is then introduced into the uterine cavity.

20. How is infertility treated in women with PCOS?

In women who are obese, weight loss can induce spontaneous ovulation. Clomiphene is the most common means of inducing ovulation in women with PCOS and has been shown to increase live birth rates. Insulin-sensitizing agents, such as metformin, used either alone or in combination with clomiphene, can improve ovulation rates and probably live births. During the first three cycles, 56% of women treated with clomiphene will become pregnant. After 6 months of treatment, the pregnancy rate decreases dramatically.

21. How is infertility treated in women with endometriosis?

Surgical ablation of endometrial implants has been shown to increase pregnancy rates, particularly in women with moderate-severe endometriosis. Ovulation induction and ART may also be used.

22. How is male factor infertility treated?

Treatment depends on the specific cause.

- **Medical treatment** aimed at the primary disorder is indicated for hyperprolactinemia, Cushing's syndrome, and other endocrine disorders.

- **Gonadotropin therapy** can stimulate spermatogenesis in Kallmann syndrome and other forms of hypogonadotropic hypogonadism.
- **Glucocorticoid therapy** can correct hormonal imbalances of congenital adrenal hyperplasia. Glucocorticoids are also sometimes used to treat antisperm antibodies.
- **Surgical treatment** is indicated for men with varicoceles and cryptorchidism. Ligation of large varicoceles and correction of cryptorchidism improve infertility.
- **ICSI** may be indicated for men with obstructive azoospermia, antisperm antibodies, infectious orchitis, Klinefelter syndrome, Y chromosome microdeletions, and idiopathic infertility.

23. How is unexplained infertility treated?

Intrauterine insemination, ovulation induction with clomiphene or gonadotropins, and ART can all increase pregnancy and live birth rates in cases of unexplained infertility. ART produces the best results, with live birth rates of 20–40% per cycle.

24. How is luteal phase defect treated?

Progesterone support or ART.

25. How successful is ART?

Pregnancy and live birth rates vary depending on the underlying cause of infertility and the woman's age. In 1999, 25% of ART cycles using fresh, non-donor eggs resulted in a live birth.

26. How often does ovulation induction and ART result in multiple births?

In 1999, 37% of IVF deliveries produced multiple births (32% twins, 5% triplets or more). Ovulation induction without IVF is much more likely to result in multiple births because there is no control over the number of embryos transferred into the uterus. Clomiphene-based regimens are less likely to produce multiple births than gonadotropin-based regimens.

27. Does health insurance cover fertility treatments?

Coverage varies. Some states now mandate that insurance companies offer infertility coverage to employers, but most do not require that employers offer it to their employees. Many insurance policies cover only certain types of treatment and only under specific circumstances.

28. When should infertility treatments stop?

Each woman or couple must decide for themselves when to stop treatment. Primary care providers can assist patients by providing realistic information about the possibilities of pregnancy and live birth, providing emotional support, and, when patients are ready, discussing alternatives, including adoption and child-free living.

29. What emotional issues do people with infertility face?

Many reactions, including grief, shame, anger, and depression, may occur. Infertility and its treatments may strain relationships. Financial stress is a major concern. Primary care providers can assist their patients by providing referrals to local and national support groups and by encouraging the patient or couple to use all available means of emotional support (family, close friends, clergy).

BIBLIOGRAPHY

1. American College of Obstetricians and Gynecologists: ACOG practice bulletin no. 34: Management of infertility caused by ovulatory dysfunction. Obstet Gynecol 99:347–358, 2002.
2. Archie C: Methadone in the management of narcotic addiction in pregnancy. Curr Opin Obstet Gynecol 10:435–440, 1998.
3. Brundage S: Preconception health care. Am Family Physician 65:2507–2514, 2002.
4. Buyalos R, Agarwal S: Endometriosis-associated infertility. Curr Opin Obstet Gynecol 12:377–381, 2000.

5. Centers for Disease Control and Prevention, et al: 1999 Assisted Reproductive Technology Success Rates, 2001. Atlanta, CDC, 2001. Available at www.cdc.gov/nccdphp/drh/art.htm.
6. Dempsey D, Benowitz N: Risks and benefits of nicotine to aid smoking cessation in pregnancy. Drug Safety 24: 277–322, 2001.
7. Guzick D: Evaluation of the Infertile Couple. Wellesley, MA, UpToDate, 2003.
8. Hatcher R: Contraceptive Technology, 17th ed. New York, Arden Media, 1998.
9. Hull MGR: Population study of causes, treatment and outcome of infertility. Br Med J 291:1693–1697, 1985.
10. Stotland N: Psychiatric issues related to infertility, reproductive technologies and abortion. Prim Care Clin Office Practice 29:13–25, 2002.
11. Swerdloff R, Wang C: Causes of Male Infertility. Wellesley, MA, UpToDate, 2003.
12. U.S. Preventive Services Task Force: Guide to Clinical Preventive Services, 2nd ed. Baltimore, Williams & Wilkins, 1996. See www.ahcpr.gov for updated recommendations.
13. Wang C, Swerdloff R: Treatment of Male Infertility. Wellesley, MA, UpToDate, 2003.

33. THYROID DISEASE

Samy I. McFarlane, M.D.

1. What is the thyroid gland?

The thyroid gland is a shield-like (in Greek, *thyrus* = shield) endocrine organ located in the neck anterior to the trachea and below the thyroid cartilage. In adults, the thyroid gland weights about 20 g and consists of two lobes (right and left) connected with a thin isthmus. The isthmus is located under the cricoid cartilage (important landmark for palpation).

2. Where does the thyroid gland originate? Why is this information important?

The thyroid gland originates at the foramen cecum located at the base of the tongue. It then descends along the thyroglossal duct tract to its final location in the lower neck. The tract then atrophies and disappears by the tenth week of gestation.

Clinical relevance

- If the gland descent is completely arrested, a lingual thyroid results.
- If the gland partially descends, the result is an ectopic thyroid (e.g., sublingual, prelaryngeal).
- Excessive migration or descent can result in a substernal or retrosternal gland.

About one third of the patients with ectopic thyroid gland are hypothyroid. With thyroid enlargement, local symptoms develop. For example, lingual thyroid may lead to respiratory symptoms, hemoptysis, dysphagia, or dysphonia. Retrosternal goiter, on the other hand, can lead to dysphagia and upper respiratory obstruction.

3. What is the thyroglossal duct cyst?

The thyroglossal duct cyst is the most common form of congenital cyst in the neck. It is a cystic expansion of the thyroglossal duct tract (see question 2). Although it is more common in children, one-third of the cases occur in adults. The cyst usually presents as a midline upper neck mass that moves upward with protrusion of the tongue or with swallowing. It is often brought to the attention after an upper airway infection. It is not clear whether infection leads to cystic formation or simply attracts attention to the neck and leads to the discovery of a preexisting cyst. Although thyroid disorders are generally more common in females, thyroglossal duct cysts affects both sexes equally.

4. What are the unusual features regarding the blood flow to the thyroid ?

The thyroid gland is highly vascular, relative to its weight. The blood flow to the gland exceeds that of most other organs in the body. In cases of hyperthyroidism, the blood flow to the thyroid can be in excess of 1 L/ minute. For this reason, a bruit is audible and a thrill is palpable over the thyroid in Graves' disease. Patients with hyperthyroidism who are treated surgically should be pretreated with antithyroid medications and iodine to decrease the vascularity of the gland and avoid excessive bleeding during surgery.

5. What hormones are secreted by the thyroid gland?

The thyroid gland secretes primarily tetraiodothyronine, which is also known as thyroxine (T_4). It contains four atoms of iodine and is 99.98% protein-bound and 0.02% unbound or free (free T_4). Triiodothyronine (T_3) contains three atoms of iodine and is secreted in much smaller amounts by the thyroid gland itself. T_3 in the serum is produced mainly from T_4 by removal of one iodine atom through monodeiodination. T_3 is the most potent thyroid hormone. It is also highly protein-bound, with a shorter half-life than T_4, which serves as a reservoir for T_3 production.

6. How is thyroid hormone secretion regulated?

The principal regulator of thyroid function is thyroid-stimulating hormone (TSH), which is also known as thyrotropin and is secreted by the pituitary gland. TSH, in turn, is regulated by thyroptopin-releasing hormone (TRH) from the hypothalamus. TSH acutely increases the blood flow to the thyroid and stimulates biosynthesis and secretion of T_4 and T_3, both of which, through a negative feedback loop, inhibit TRH and TSH secretion.

7. What are the effects of prolonged stimulation of the thyroid by TSH?

Prolonged stimulation by TSH, as in primary hypothyroidism, can lead to thyroid enlargement (goiter). TSH stimulation causes hypertrophy and hyperplasia of the gland by stimulating RNA and DNA synthesis. This fact is important in the treatment of thyoid cancer, in which suppresion of TSH by exogenous thyroxine is mandatory after surgery and radioactive iodine ablation therapy to prevent recurrence of the cancer.

8. Describe the biologic effects of thyroid hormone.

Thyroid hormone affects virtually every system in the body through regulation of metabolic rate, gastrointestinal motility, cardiac contractility, heart rate, body temprature, mood, body weight, and skin texure. It is also essential for normal growth and development. Thyroid hormone exerts its biologic actions through binding to a nuclear receptor complex, where protein transcription occurs. A summary of the effects of thyroid hormone on different body systems is provided in the table below. Normal thyroid hormone levels are necessary for the optimal function of the various organ systems. Contrasts between the state of hormone excess (hyperthyroidism) and the state of hormone deficiency (hypothyroidism) are also illustrated in the table.

Effects of Thyroid Hormone on Various Body Systems

BIOLOGIC EFFECT	HYPERTHYROIDISM	HYPOTHYROIDISM
Oxygen consumption and basal metabolic rate	Increased—heat intolerance (fever in thyroid storm)	Decreased—cold intolerance (hypothermia in myxedema coma)
Cardiac contractility	Increased—high cardiac output	Decreased— diastolic dysfunction
Peripheral vascular resistance	Decreased—systolic hypertension with wide pulse pressure	Increased—Diastolic hypertension with narrow pulse pressure
Heart rate	Increased (tachycardia)	Decreased (bradycardia)
Gastrointestinal motility	Increased (hyperdefecation)	Decreased (constipation)
Body weight	Weight loss	Weight gain
Skin texture	Warm and moist	Cold and dry
Lipid metabolism	Increased cholesterol hepatobiliary excretion	Decreased hepatobiliary excretion of cholesterol—hypercholesterolemia
Deep tendon reflexes	Hyperreflexia	Delayed relaxation phase
Psychiatric	Anxiety, irritability, and nervous	Depression
Skeletal system	Increased bone turnover; may lead to osteoporosis	Decreased bone turnover

Table continues on following page.

Effects of Thyroid Hormone on Various Body Systems (Continued)

BIOLOGIC EFFECT	HYPERTHYROIDISM	HYPOTHYROIDISM
Muscular system	Myopathy, with normal creatinine phosphokinase (CPK) Hypokalemic periodic paralysis (in Asians)	Myopathy, usually with increased CPK

9. How do I interpret thyroid function tests (TFTs)?

TFTs are one of the most common endocrine investigations requested by primary care physicians; therefore, accurate interpretation is very important. The table below should assist interpretation. However, there are a few "secrets" that you need to know:

In hyperthyroidism:
- TSH is suppressed (i.e., less than the lower limit detectable by the laboratory). Thus, once you see TSH reported as "less than," you are probably dealing with thyroid hormone excess, whether endogenously secreted or exogenously administered.
- T_4 and T_3 resin uptake (T_3RU) go in the same direction; they are increased.

In hypothyroidism:
- TSH is elevated in primary hypothyroidism, but in central hypothyroidism (pituitary or hypothalamic), TSH is either low or normal (measurable but biologically inactive).
- T_4 and T_3RU go in the same direction; they will be decreased.
- Because the body does not want to be hypothyroid, initially conversion of T_4 to T_3 is increased in order to keep T_3 at normal or near-normal levels (see question 5).

Assessment of Thyroid Function

CONDITION	TSH	T_4 (TOTAL)	T_3RU (T_3 RESIN UPTAKE)	T_3 (TOTAL)
Hyperthyroidism	Suppressed	Increased	Increased	Increased
Subclinical hyperthyroidism	Low or suppressed	Normal	Normal	Normal
Hypothyroidism				
Primary	Increased	Decreased	Decreased	Decreased (or borderline normal)
Central (pituitary or hypothalamic)	Decreased (or normal)	Decreased	Decreased	Decreased (or borderline normal)
Subclinical hypothyroidism	Increased	Normal	Normal	Normal
Increased binding protein	Normal	Increased	Decreased	Normal (or increased)
Decreased binding protein	Normal	Decreased	Increased	Normal (or decreased)
Euthyroid sick syndrome	Normal (or decreased)	Decreased	Normal	Decreased

10. What causes increase in protein binding?

Both T_4 and T_3 are highly ($> 99.9\%$) bound to thyroid-binding protein (TBG), albumin, and prealbumin (transthyretin). Only the free portion of the hormone is biologically active. Conditions that cause increased TBG production from the liver include acute liver disease (e.g., hepatitis), estrogen therapy, and pregnancy. The typical patient is a woman presenting with nonspecific symptoms of irritability and nervousness that lead to clinical suspicion of hyperthyroidism. TFT measurement shows increased total T_4 and normal TSH. You need to take a medication history (e.g., contraceptive pills) and to check for pregnancy. Also make sure that the disorder is not common in the patient's family (familial dysalbuminimic hyperthyroxinemia) and that her liver functions are normal. One secret to remember is that T_4 and T_3RU go in the opposite direction: T_4 is high, and T_3RU is low. There are no clinical consequences of increased binding protein because the free portion of thyroid hormone is normal. You need to know this information only to make the correct diagnosis and to avoid treating the patient for hyperthyroidism.

11. Discuss the causes of decreased thyroid-binding protein.

Androgen therapy, protein malnutrition, nephrotic syndrome, and congenital abnormalities in protein binding are causes. Again, the same rules apply as in question 10; T_4 is low, and T_3RU is high (see table in question 9). TSH and free T_4 are normal; therefore, there are no clinical consequences.

12. Why do we not simply measure free T_4 to avoid confusion?

Some thyroidologists advocate the use of free T_4 to avoid the confusion related to binding protein abnormalities. However, none of the currently available methods actually measure the free hormone; they provide only an estimate of the unbound T_4. Correct free T_4 values for all binding protein with the method and laboratory used. The most commonly used and standardized tests of thyroid function are listed in the table in question 9.

13. What are the thyroid autoantibodies? How are they useful?

The most commonly used thyroid autoantibodies include **antithyroid peroxidase (antimicrosomal)** antibodies and **antithyroglobulin** antibodies, both of which are common in Hashimoto's thyroiditis and may help confirm the diagnosis. In addition, antimicrosomal antibody concentrations have a predictive value in patients with subclinical hypothyroidism. In one study of patients with subclinical hypothyroidism, one third of those older than 60 years developed overt hypothyroidism in 4 years. Eighty percent of those who developed overt hypothyroidism had serum antimicrosomal antibody titers of 1:1600 or higher, but none of those with titers less than 1:1600 developed the disease. **Anti-TSH receptor** antibody and **thyroid-stimulating antibodies** (TSI) may be used in Graves' disease—for example, euthyroid Graves' ophthalmopathy.

14. What is the difference between thyroid scan and thyroid uptake?

Both thyroid scan and thyroid uptake exploit the high affinity of the thyroid gland for iodine. Using radioactive iodine (RAI), **thyroid scan** gives an actual image taken by the gamma camera and placed onto a film (like an x-ray film). The film gives anatomic information (e.g., retrosternal goiter or ectopic thyroid gland). Thyroid scan also helps distinguish functional from nonfunctional tissues—for example, cold vs. hot nodules. **Thyroid uptake,** on the other hand, is useful in assessing the ability of the thyroid to trap iodine; it gives a percentage of the total amount of the radioactive iodine that is trapped by the thyroid over a period of time (e.g., 20% at 24 hours). This information is important for RAI dose calculation, as in the treatment of Graves' disease or the ablation of thyroid cancer.

15. When should you order a thyroid sonogram?

Simply speaking, the thyroid sonogram offers a good and reliable physical exam of the thyroid. For example, when you are not sure whether a nodule is present or how big it is, the sonogram can delineate the structure of the thyroid. It can distinguish between cystic and solid masses in the thyroid. It also provides measurements of different structures (e.g., size of a nodule). A thyroid sonogram is particularly helpful for follow-up to determine the interval changes in the size of a given structure.

16. What are the major causes of primary hypothyroidism?

Hashimoto's thyroiditis is the most common cause of primary hypothyroidism. It results from autoimmune destruction of the thyroid gland, followed by lymphocytic infiltration and usually goiter. In older patients, goiter might not be present but rather atrophy of the gland. Other causes of hypothyroidism include thyroidectomy, previous neck irradiation, and radioactive iodine treatment for hyperthyroidism.

17. Discuss the medications that alter thyroid function.

Various medications that contain iodine, such as amiodarone, can cause hypothyroidism. In addition, medications that mimic iodine, such as lithium, can also cause hypothyroidism. Iodine itself can cause hypothyroidism (e.g., in radiocontrast or foods that contain excessive amounts of iodine, such as kelp and seaweed). Iodine can also cause hyperthyroidism, especially after repletion of a patient who had chronic iodine deficiency. Amiodarone also causes hyperthyroidism through hypersecretion or drug-induced thyroiditis. Some medications increase the rate of metabolism of thyroxine by the liver. Examples include rifampin and antiseizure medications such as phenytoin, carbamazepine, and phenobarbital. Increasing the dose of thyroxine is often necessary to keep the patient euthyroid.

18. What are the major clinical manifestations of hypothyroidism?

The major manifestations are mentioned in the table in question 8. Delayed relaxation phase of the deep tendon reflexes is a highly specific physical finding. Other manifestations of hypothyroidism include slowed mentation, menstrual irregularities, and yellowish discoloration of the skin (carotenemia).

19. Define subclinical hypothyroidism.

Subclinical hypothyroidism is defined as mildly elevated serum TSH level with normal T_4 and T_3 concentrations in the absence of symptoms. The causes are the same as for overt hypothyroidism. Subclinical hypothyroidism occurs in about 15% of women older than age 60 years. Progression to clinical hypothyroidism can be predicted by high antimicrosomal antibody concentrations (see question 13). There is no consensus on whether or not to treat patients with subclinical hypothyroidism. The American College of Physicians questioned whether enough data are available to recommend treatment. However, given the link between subclinical hypothyroidism and atherosclerosis and myocardial infarction, some thyroidologists elect to treat patients until normal TSH values are achieved. In addition, thyroxine therapy may be useful for patients with subclinical hypothyroidism and abnormal myocardial contractility, as shown in a randomized, double-blind, placebo-controlled trial.

20. Discuss the management of hypothyroidism.

T_4 (thyroxine) replacement is the mainstay of therapy. In elderly patients and patients with coronary artery disease, the rule is to "start low and go slow." The goal of therapy in primary hypothyroidism is to normalize TSH. Check TSH every 6 weeks in the initial (dose titration) period. In central hypothyroidism, we cannot monitor TSH (the pituitary is gone); therefore, we rely on clinical assessment and maintenance of T_4 levels in the mid-normal range. There are two important secrets to remember:

1. Avoid excessive thyroid hormone replacement, which can lead to atrial fibrillation and osteoporosis.

2. In central hypothyroidism, check adrenal function prior to thyroid replacement, because T_4 may accelerate cortisol metabolism and precipitate adrenal crisis.

21. What may happen if a patient with hypothyroidism is left untreated?

The most feared consequence is myxedema coma, which carries a mortality rate of over 60%, even if treated early. It is usually precipitated by an acute event such as myocardial infarction, stroke, sepsis, or trauma. Myxedema coma is manifested by stupor, hypothermia, hypoventilation, and cardiovascular failure. Patients with myxedema coma should be treated in an intensive care unit with intravenous thyroxine, pulmonary and cardiovascular support, and management of the precipitating event.

22. Name the major causes of hyperthyroidism.

The most common causes of overproduction of endogenous thyroid hormone are Graves' disease (diffuse toxic goiter), toxic multinodular goiter, and toxic adenoma. Thyroiditis can also cause hyperthyroidism by releasing the preformed thyroid hormone from the gland. The other common cause of biochemical hyperthyroidism is the use of thyroid-hormone medication, as in excessive thyroid hormone replacement in hypothyroidism (see question 20).

23. Describe the clinical features of hyperthyroidism.

Hyperthyroidism from any cause can lead to the signs and symptoms mentioned in the table in question 8. The exception is subacute thyroiditis, which also causes neck tenderness that may radiate to the jaw, arm, or chest. In general, hyperthyroidism represents increased sensitivity to catecholamine; therefore, most of the signs and symptoms are sympathomimetic. In addition, Graves' disease is associated with specific signs such as exophthalmos and (in rare cases) pretibial myxedema. Examination of the thyroid in Graves' disease shows diffuse enlargement, sometimes associated with a bruit due to high vascularity (see also question 4)

24. Discuss geriatric (apathetic) hyperthyroidism.

Hyperthyroidism in elderly patients may be apathetic rather than show hyperactivity and other symptoms of sympathetic overactivity. The placid or even depressed presentation may be more suggestive of hypothyroidism than hyperthyroidism. Weight loss is often a striking feature, as are cardiovascular manifestations such as atrial fibrillation and congestive heart failure. Many patients also manifest a proximal myopathy. Elderly patients with hyperthyroidism are less likely to have a goiter. Diagnosis is usually made during work-up of other diseases, such as new-onset atrial fibrillation.

25. What is subclinical hyperthyroidism?

Subclinical hyperthyroidism is defined as low serum TSH cocentration with normal T_4 and T_3 levels. Patients have few or no symptoms or signs of hyperthyroidism. Therefore, the diagnosis is a biochemical one. Causes of subclinical hyperthyroidism are the same as those of overt hyperthyroidism. The skeleton and cardiovascular systems are the major target organs. Both osteoporosis and atrial fibrillation can lead to substantial morbidity in older patients. However, few data are available to guide clinical decision-making; therefore, management is somewhat controversial. A trial of antithyroid medications may be undertaken with the goal of normalizing the TSH for a period of 3–6 months. At the end of that time, the clinician and patient can decide whether more definitive therapy with I^{131} would be beneficial. If the patient refuses therapy for subclinical hyperthyroidism, periodic assessment of bone density should be considered to ensure that osteoporosis does not develop.

26. What is subacute thyroiditis?

As the name implies, it is an inflammatory process of the thyroid. It usually follows a viral illness and presents with neck tenderness (see question 23). Nearly all patients are hyperthyroid, and the diagnosis is essentially a clinical one. Characteristically, erythrocyte sedimentation rate is highly elevated, usually more than 50 mm/hour. Because it is a destructive process with the release of preformed thyroid hormones, thyroid uptake is low (less than 1%) and treatment is only symptomatic. Aspirin or other nonsteroidal anti-inflammatory agents should be given. If no response is seen, a short course of prednisone will provide relief of pain and inflammation. We do not treat with antithyroid medications, as in Graves' disease, because the increase is in the release rather than the production of the preformed thyroid hormones. If the patient is highly symptomatic (e.g., palpitations, anxiety, or tremors), beta blocker therapy may be helpful until the disease resolves spontaneously.

27. Discuss the treatment options for Graves' disease.

Since most of the signs and symptoms of hyperthyroidism are due to enhanced catecholamine sensitivity (see question 22), symptomatic treatment is provided with beta blockers (e.g., propranolol, metoprolol, atenolol) to reduce tremulousness and tachycardia. Antithyroid medications (thionamides), radioactive iodine (RAI), and surgery are the available treatment options. In general, a thionamide such as propylthiouracil (PTU) or methimazole (tapazole) is usually started until a definitive therapy is decided upon. In the United States, RAI (I^{131}) is the most common form of treatment. It is highly effective and relatively safe (no evidence of increased cancer). Dosage is based on thyroid uptake (see question 14): the higher the uptake, the lower the dose. I^{131} usually takes about 2 months to work, and over 90% of patients become hypothyroid, mostly within 1.5 years, requiring long-term thyroid hormone replacement. In the U.S. surgery is unpopular and is indicated only in patients who have a large goiter with obstructive symptoms or patients who refuse RAI treatment and cannot tolerate antithyroid medications.

28. How do the antithyroid medications work? What are their side effects?

The thionamides, PTU and methimazole, inhibit thyroid hormone production. In addition, PTU inhibits conversion of T_4 to T_3. Methimazole has a longer duration of action and can be given once daily. PTU is the preferred therapy during pregnancy, because it crosses the placenta to a lesser degree than methimazole. The most common side effects of thionamides is rash. Less common side effects include arthralgia, hepatitis, and neuritis. Agranulocytosis is a rare but serious complication of thionamide therapy, with a prevalence of 0.2–0.5%. The value of monitoring white blood cell (WBC) counts in patients taking a thionamide is controversial. However, patients should be advised to have a WBC count with differential if they develop fever, sore throat, or any other sign of infection and to discontinue the drug. Agranulocytosis usually resolves in a few days, but serious infections and death can occur. Granulocyte-colony stimulating factor (G-CSF) has been used as adjunctive therapy, but no evidence supports its efficacy.

29. Which hyperthyroid patients should be admitted to the hospital?

Patients with hyperthyroidism who have (or are at risk for) thyroid storm. Thyroid storm is defined as exacerbated manifestations of hyperthyroidism and fever, central nervous system manifestations (e.g., mental status change or seizure), cardiovascular manifestations (e.g., congestive heart failure), and gastrointestinal manifestations (e.g., abdominal pain, liver tenderness, elevated liver enzymes). Thyroid storm has a high mortality rate that approaches 100% if not recognized and treated early. In addition, patients with hyperthyroidism and new-onset atrial fibrillation should be admitted and anticoagulated due to the high risk of systemic embolization.

30. Which patients with thyroid nodules are more likely to have cancer?

About 5% of thyroid nodules are cancerous. The incidence of thyroid cancer is higher among children, patients younger than 30 or older than 60 years, and patients with prior head and neck radiation.

31. How do you work up a thyroid nodule?

Obtain a TSH level. If the level is normal, fine-needle aspiration (FNA) is the next step. For benign macrofollicular lesions, follow the patient clinically. For cancer, refer the patient for surgery, followed by RAI remnant ablation therapy and TSH suppression with exogenous thyroxine. For intermediate or suspicious lesions, obtain a radionuclide scan. If the nodule is cold (low uptake on the scan), refer the patient to surgery because of the higher risk of malignancy. If the nodule is hot (high uptake on the scan), follow the patient. If the patient is hyperthyroid (TSH is suppressed), treat with antithyroid medications, RAI, or surgery. In general, hot nodules (autonomously secreting T_4) and simple, thin-walled cysts are usually benign. If the report of the FNA specifies follicular neoplasm, the patient must be referred to surgery because the only way to differentiate follicular adenoma from follicular carcinoma is to determine whether invasion of the capsule of the nodule has occurred. If so, the entire nodule must be removed and examined.

BIBLIOGRAPHY

1. Charib H: Changing concepts in the diagnosis and management of thyroid nodules. Endocrinol Metab Clin North Am 26:777–800, 1997.
2. Cooper DS, Halpern R, Wood LC, et al: L-Thyroxine therapy in subclinical hypothyroidism: A double-blind, placebo-controlled trial. Ann Intern Med 101:18–24, 1984.
3. Fukata S, Kuma K, Sugawara M: Granulocyte colony-stimulating factor (G-CSF) does not improve recovery from antithyroid drug-induced agranulocytosis: A prospective study. Thyroid 9:29–31, 1999.
4. Hak AE, Pols HA, Visser TJ, et al: Subclinical hypothyroidism is an independent risk factor for atherosclerosis and myocardial infarction in elderly women: The Rotterdam Study. Ann Intern Med 132:270–278, 2000.
5. Harjal KJ, Licata AA: Effects of amiodarone on thyroid function. Ann Intern Med 126:63–73, 1997.
6. Helfland M, Redfern CC: American College of Physicians Clinical Guideline. Part 2: Screening for thyroid disease: An update. Ann Intern Med 129:144–158, 1998.
7. Klee GG, Hay ID: Biochemical thyroid function testing. Endocrinol Metab Clin North Am 26:763–776, 1997.

8. Klein I: Clinical, metabolic, and organ-specific indices of thyroid function. Endocrinol Metab Clin North Am 30:415–427, 2001.
9. Klein I, Becker DV, Levey OS: Treatment of hyperthyroid disease. Ann Intern Med 121:281–288, 1994.
10. Mallette LE: Solitary thyroid nodules. N Engl J Med 32:361, 1993.
11. Swain CT, Geller A, Wolf PA, et al: Low serum thyrotropin concentrations as a risk factor for atrial fibrillation in older persons. N Engl J Med 331:1249, 1994.
12. Toft AD: Clinical practice: Subclinical hyperthyroidism. N Engl J Med 345:512–516, 2001.

34. OSTEOPOROSIS

Alicia L. Wolfert, M.D., and Philip S. Mehler, M.D.

1. Why is osteoporosis a major public health problem?

Osteoporosis affects 25 million Americans. It is responsible for 1.5 million fractures annually. The total health care expenditures are more than $13 billion annually. Currently, it is estimated to be the twelfth leading cause of death in adults because of the 20% mortality rate associated with medical complications from hip fractures. Of those who survive hip fractures, fewer than 50% are able to continue living independently.

A 50-year-old white woman has a 40% lifetime risk of having an osteoporotic fracture. The National Osteoporotic Association estimates that the number of postmenopausal women in the United States will double over the next 20 years, leading to a threefold increase in osteoporotic fractures by the year 2040.

Osteoporosis also occurs in men. In the United States, 1.5 million men older than age 65 years are affected. By age 90 years, 1 of every 6 men will suffer a hip fracture, and the mortality rate of hip fractures is higher in men than women.

2. What is osteoporosis?

Osteoporosis is a systemic metabolic skeletal disease characterized by low bone mass and microarchitectural deterioration of bone tissue, which results in increased bone fragility and fracture susceptibility. This process may involve loss of cortical or trabecular bone.

Primary osteoporosis is defined as a loss of bone mass not associated with other chronic illness or medication. **Secondary osteoporosis** occurs as a result of chronic conditions or medications that accelerate bone loss. Osteoporosis can occur in association with high or low turnover states.

3. What is osteomalacia?

Osteomalacia is abnormal bone mineralization that is frequently caused by defects in substrate availability (e.g., calcium or phosphate). It also may be caused by alterations in vitamin D metabolism or certain drugs that cause abnormal mineralization (e.g., sodium fluoride or bisphosphonates).

4. What does osteopenia mean in a radiologist's report?

Osteopenia is a descriptive radiologic diagnosis suggesting that the bone mass is reduced by standard radiographic techniques. This interpretation usually is based on radiographs of the chest or lumbar spine. When bone loss is evident radiographically, approximately 30–40% of the skeleton has demineralized.

5. How is osteoporosis detected?

Osteoporosis is diagnosed based on bone mineral density (BMD). Different methods are used to measure bone density, but the gold standard test currently used is dual-energy x-ray absorptiometry (DEXA). DEXA scans measure bone density at the hip and spine and express the results as T-scores and Z-scores. A T-score is defined as the number of standard deviations above or below the average BMD value for young, healthy, white women. The Z-score is defined as the number of standard deviations above or below the average BMD for age- and sex-matched control subjects.

Osteoporosis is defined as a T-score < -2.5. Osteopenia is defined as a T-score between -1 and -2.5. A T-score of < -2.5 is thought to represent the fracture threshold. However, recent studies have evaluated other risk factors for fracture, and in the future, a combination of these other risk factors plus BMD may be used to decide on treatment. Plain radiographs can suggest osteopenia, but a DEXA is needed to diagnose osteoporosis.

One disadvantage to DEXA scanning is the high cost of the scanners and their large size. Other forms of testing, such as single x-ray absorptiometry (SXA) and quantitative ultrasonography (QUS), are gaining popularity because of the low cost per test, low cost of the equipment, and easy mobility of the equipment. These tests are used to measure bone density at peripheral sites such as the heel, forearm, and calcaneus. However, the predictive value of these measures in determining fracture risk at the hip or spine is not yet clear.

6. When are bone density measurements clinically indicated?

The appropriate use of bone densitometry is somewhat controversial. Currently, mass screening for osteoporosis in all postmenopausal women is not recommended.

The American Association of Clinical Endocrinologists (AACE) Clinical Practice Guidelines recommends screening concerned perimenopausal women willing to start drug therapy, patients with radiographic evidence of bone loss, patients on long-term glucocorticoid therapy, patients with asymptomatic hyperparathyroidism in whom osteoporosis would suggest parathyroidectomy, and women already on treatment for osteoporosis to monitor the effect of therapy.

The National Osteoporosis Foundation recommends screening all postmenopausal women who present with fractures, postmenopausal women younger than 65 years who have one more risk factors for osteoporosis, and all women 65 years and older regardless of risk factors.

7. What are the most common causes of osteoporosis?

Idiopathic age-related osteoporosis (most common)
1. Juvenile
2. Young adults
3. Postmenopausal (type I)
4. Senile (type II)

Osteoporosis secondary to disease states

1. Metabolic conditions
   Calcium deficiency
   Vitamin D–deficient states
   Malnutrition
   Idiopathic hypercalciuria
   Renal tubular acidosis and other
     systemic acidosis
   Scurvy
2. Endocrine conditions
   Thyrotoxicosis
   Cushing's syndrome
   Male and female hypogonadal states
   Hypoamenorrheic female runners
   Prolactinoma
   Hyperparathyroidism
3. Renal disease
4. Gastrointestinal–liver disease
5. Hereditary connective tissue disease
   Osteogenesis imperfecta
   Homocystinuria
   Ehlers-Danlos syndrome
   Marfan syndrome

6. Bone marrow infiltrations
   Multiple myeloma
   Lymphoma
   Leukemia
7. Drugs
   Diphenylhydantoin
   Phenobarbital
   Thyroid hormone
   Corticosteroids
   Chronic heparin therapy
8. Lifestyle
   Nutrition
   Alcohol use
   Smoking
   Inactivity
   Immobilization
   Excessive caffeine intake
   Excessive phosphate intake (e.g., soft
     drinks, red meat)
9. Miscellaneous
   Rheumatoid arteritis
   Systemic mastocytosis
   Anorexia nervosa

8. What are the risk factors for osteoporosis?

- Family history
- Lifelong poor calcium intake, especially during the adolescent years
- Physical inactivity or immobilization
- Smoking
- Malnutrition or eating disorders (e.g., anorexia nervosa)
- Hypogonadal states (e.g., primary and secondary amenorrhea)
- Low weight and body mass index
- Ingestion of substances with high phosphate content (e.g., soft drinks, large portions of red meat)
- High intake of caffeinated or alcoholic beverages
- White race
- Increased age

9. What laboratory tests help to evaluate osteopenic patients?

The initial tests are a complete blood count and routine chemistry panel that includes assessment of electrolytes, calcium, phosphate, and alkaline phosphatase as well as liver and renal function tests. A 24-hour urine collection is analyzed for calcium, phosphate, and creatinine levels. Calcium and phosphate measurements help to assess the calcium–phosphate balance. In osteopenic patients with anemia and an elevated sedimentation rate, multiple myeloma should be considered, and serum protein electrophoresis, urine protein electrophoresis, or both should be performed.

Abnormalities of liver and kidney function define secondary causes of osteopenia. Electrolytes are helpful in identifying patients with renal tubular acidosis. Serum alkaline phosphatase is a marker of bone osteoblast function and helps identify patients with high-turnover osteoporosis or osteomalacia. A 24-hour urine collection for measurement of calcium excretion identifies patients with renal hypercalciuria (i.e., urinary calcium > 4 mg calcium/kg body weight) or hypocalciuria, which suggests a calcium-deficient state. An extremely low urine phosphate level value may identify a patient who is phosphate depleted, consuming phosphate-binding antacids, or vegetarian.

Other more specific but expensive laboratory tests may be selectively indicated, including measurement of parathyroid hormone, serum osteocalcin, vitamin D metabolites [$25(OH)D_3$ and $1,25(OH)_2D_3$], urinary hydroxyproline, pyridinoline, or n-telopeptide. Osteocalcin is a marker of osteoblast function, whereas urinary hydroxyproline, pyridinoline, and n-telopeptide reflect osteoclast function. These tests are generally reserved for patients followed by specialists in a metabolic bone clinic.

10. What preventive measures should be recommended to patients at risk for osteoporosis?

An adequate calcium intake of at least 1000–1500 mg of elemental calcium per day can be ingested in food substances; however, because of hypercholesterolemic issues and the recommendation to avoid foods high in saturated fats, patients may need calcium supplements. If calcium supplements are prescribed, they are best taken with meals. Because peak bone mass is the primary determinant of fracture risk, simple dietary interventions must be encouraged in adolescents and adults in their twenties and thirties. Outdoor activities should be encouraged; minimal erythemic sunlight exposure provides 400–1200 U of vitamin D from synthesis in the skin. The recommended daily intake of vitamin D is 400–600 IU/day for adults. This can be obtained from a multivitamin or from a combined calcium–vitamin D supplement. Foods high in vitamin D include cod liver oil, salmon, sardines, and milk. Weight-bearing exercises stimulate bone remodeling and inhibit osteolysis. Risk factor modification is important, including cessation of smoking and alcohol abuse as well as participation in a regular exercise program.

11. What drugs are used to prevent osteoporosis?

Adequate calcium (1500 mg/day) and vitamin D (800 IU/day) intake is essential in both the treatment and prevention of osteoporosis. Many combination supplements are available for women who do not get enough of these nutrients through diet alone.

Estrogen replacement therapy prevents postmenopausal bone loss through its antiresorptive effect. This therapy can be in the form of a pill or a transdermal patch. Addition of a progestational agent does not impair the skeletal response to estrogen. Estrogen replacement therapy is most effective when started at the time of menopause and continued for life. However, estrogen replacement therapy has become increasingly controversial because of its increase in the risk of breast cancer and questionable cardiac benefits. Estrogen replacement therapy should not be used in women with a history of breast cancer, history of or active thromboembolic disorder, or abnormal uterine bleeding.

For women with breast cancer or other contraindications to estrogen therapy, bisphosphonates are an alternative. At 5 mg/day, alendronate is effective at preventing osteoporosis in early postmenopausal women.

12. How is glucocorticoid-induced osteoporosis prevented?

Prednisone therapy at doses of 7.5 mg/day or more for $\geq$ 6 months often causes rapid bone loss. Calcium and vitamin D have been shown to be effective for preventing bone loss in patients treated with corticosteroids. Estrogen replacement therapy should be initiated in all postmenopausal women without contraindications. Bisphosphonates should be used if ongoing bone loss occurs despite treatment or if estrogen is contraindicated.

13. What drugs are used to treat established osteoporosis?

Estrogen replacement therapy, **vitamin D**, and **calcium** are all used to treat established osteoporosis as well as prevent osteoporosis.

Bisphosphonates, through inhibition of osteoclastic activity, have also been found to be very effective in the treatment of osteoporosis. Alendronate, at 10 mg/day or 70 mg/week, is the most commonly used drug of this class. The drug is not well absorbed orally and, therefore, has to be taken on an empty stomach with water only. The most worrisome, albeit rare, side effect of alendronate is esophagitis. For this reason, patients are advised to remain upright for at least 30 minutes after taking their doses. Risedronate is the newest oral bisphosphonate approved by the Food and Drug Administration (FDA) for the treatment and prevention of osteoporosis. Alendronate and risedronate have both been shown to reduce the risk of vertebral fractures by 30–50% and reduce the risk of nonvertebral fractures in women with osteoporosis. Their effect on preventing nonvertebral fractures in patients without osteoporosis is unclear.

Selective estrogen receptor modulators (SERMs), which are used to treat estrogen-positive breast cancer, have been shown to have an antiresorptive effect on bone. Raloxifene, a SERM approved by the FDA for the treatment and prevention of osteoporosis, has been shown in large clinical trials to decrease the risk of vertebral fractures by 36%.

Calcitonin decreases bone loss at vertebral and femoral sites, but very few studies have examined its effect on fracture risk. Its effects on BMD are less than that of estrogen or alendronate, and for these reasons, it is not commonly used. It does have a unique property compared with other osteoporosis medications, in that is has an analgesic effect on bone pain and is therefore useful in the symptomatic treatment of patients who have had an acute osteoporotic fracture.

14. How should young amenorrheic female athletes or patients with anorexia nervosa be treated to prevent osteoporosis?

Because peak bone density is a major predictor of subsequent fracture risk, the amenorrhea associated with competitive female athletes and patients with anorexia nervosa can have profoundly deleterious effects on osteoporosis risk. Although restoration of weight and resumption of normal eating habits are the mainstays of treatment, vigilant attention to calcium and vitamin D intake, together with hormone replacement therapy and alendronate, may be needed to prevent further bone loss.

BIBLIOGRAPHY

1. NIH Consensus Panel on Osteoporosis Prevention, Diagnosis, and Therapy: Osteoporosis prevention, diagnosis, and therapy. JAMA 285:785–795, 2001.

2. Rose HL, Basow DS: Screening for osteoporosis. In Rose BD (ed): UpToDate. Wellesley, MA, UpTo-Date, 2001.
3. Rose HL, Basow DS: Overview of osteoporosis in men. In Rose BD (ed): UpToDate. Wellesley, MA, Up-ToDate, 2001.
4. Scheiber LB, Torregrosa L: Postmenopausal osteoporosis: When—and how—to measure bone mineral density. Consultant (Apr):781–789, 2000.
5. Scheiber LB, Torregrosa L: Osteoporosis: What to tell postmenopausal women about prevention and therapy. Consultant (May):1021–1028, 2000.
6. South-Paul J: Osteoporosis: Part I. Evaluation and assessment. Am Fam Physician 63:897–904, 908, 2001.
7. South-Paul J: Osteoporosis: Part II. Nonpharmacologic and pharmacologic treatment. Am Fam Physician 63:1121–1128, 2001.
8. Watts NB: Treatment of osteoporosis with bisphosphonates. Rheumat Dis Clin North Am 27:197–214, 2001.

VI. Problems of the Gastrointestinal Tract

35. HEARTBURN AND DYSPHAGIA

Kevin T. White, M.D., and Stephen E. Steinberg, M.D.

1. What are the symptoms of gastroesophageal reflux disease (GERD)?

GERD is the spectrum of signs and symptoms related to the reflux of acid or alkaline secretions from the stomach into the esophagus. Common symptoms include heartburn (pyrosis) and noncardiac chest pain that often occurs after meals and is made worse by bending or recumbency. These symptoms are often relieved by antacids. Physicians also should suspect GERD when patients complain of dysphagia; recurrent nausea; atypical chest pain; or extraesophageal symptoms such as nocturnal wheezing, chronic cough, sore throat, or hoarseness. Bleeding may result from chronic injury, leading to inflammation and ulceration (erosive esophagitis). Symptoms often occur in the absence of even histologic evidence of inflammation; conversely, even severe esophagitis and its complications may be present without associated symptoms.

2. What warning symptoms suggest complicated GERD?

Warning symptoms include dysphagia, weight loss, and bleeding, all of which warrant an expeditious evaluation, usually with upper endoscopy.

3. What is waterbrash?

It is the spontaneous and abrupt onset of salivary secretions followed by a bitter or acidic taste in the mouth. This symptom is believed to be initiated by esophageal acid and, therefore, may represent a symptom of GERD.

4. What impact does GERD have on the health of the population?

More than one third of healthy Americans experience heartburn at least once a month, and an estimated 7% experience heartburn daily. Two to three billion dollars are spent each year on over-the-counter and prescription medications to treat symptoms of acid reflux. Furthermore, reflux esophagitis may lead to complications, such as strictures, bleeding, ulceration, and perforation, that require hospitalization or invasive interventions.

5. How are diagnostic tools useful in the evaluation of patients with GERD?

For the majority of cases, the history combined with response to an antireflux regimen is sufficient to establish the diagnosis of GERD. In instances in which the symptoms are unusual or do not respond as expected, additional tests may be helpful:

1. **Esophagoscopy** is the gold standard for evaluating esophageal mucosal and structural abnormalities that result from GERD. Upper endoscopy can demonstrate obvious evidence of acid injury to the esophagus (e.g., erosions, ulceration). Biopsies are taken at the esophagogastric (EG) junction to look for microscopic evidence of inflammation. Endoscopy cannot, however, quantitate the frequency or duration of esophageal reflux.

2. A **barium esophagogram** is useful in defining intraluminal lesions that may result as complications of acid reflux. It is poor overall in evaluating mucosal inflammation and, similar to

endoscopy, does not aid in the quantitation of reflux episodes. Reflux demonstrated at esophagogram does not correlate well with symptoms of GERD.

3. **Esophageal manometry** is helpful in evaluating the resting pressure of the lower esophageal sphincter (LES) and esophageal peristalsis (acid clearing) but provides little information about the actual extent of reflux. It is helpful as a preoperative evaluation to confirm that a procedure to tighten the LES (e.g., Nissen fundoplication) is likely to be helpful and that peristalsis is adequate to overcome the surgically increased pressures. It is also useful in evaluating noncardiac chest pain, which is occasionally related to motility abnormalities.

4. **Twenty-four–hour esophageal pH testing** is the gold standard for documenting and quantitating the number and extent of reflux episodes. It also helps to define which episodes are symptomatic. A probe is passed through the nose and positioned 5 cm from the LES. The pH of the esophagus is measured over 24 hours, and any symptoms are noted (similar to a Holter monitor for cardiac events). The total time the pH is < 4 and the number of episodes lasting longer than 5 minutes are tabulated and correlated to the patient's symptom diary. In patients whose symptoms do not respond to empiric therapy and in whom endoscopy does not demonstrate evidence of inflammation, 24-hour esophageal pH testing is the best test to confirm that reflux is indeed present and that symptoms are associated. It is particularly helpful for patients with atypical chest pain and asthma that may be related to GERD.

5. The **acid perfusion test,** also known as the Bernstein test, involves dripping 0.1-N solution of hydrochloric acid alternated (unknown to the patient) with normal saline into the distal esophagus. A positive test reproduces the patient's symptoms with the acid infusion phase of the test. This qualitative test is rarely used today.

6. What pathophysiologic factors influence GERD?

- Decreased resting amplitude of the LES results in reflux of gastric contents, including acid, into the esophagus.
- Impaired esophageal luminal clearance of acid caused by ineffective peristaltic activity (low-amplitude, aperistaltic, retrograde, or spastic esophageal contractions) allows a greater period of exposure to acid for any given episode of reflux.
- Rarely, decreased salivation (a source of bicarbonate) may contribute to impaired acid neutralization.
- A decrease in the mucosal protective mechanisms, such as the unstirred mucus layer and epithelial bicarbonate secretion, often occurs.
- Increased pain sensitivity of the esophageal mucosal receptors to acid may cause some patients more symptoms than others for the same degree of acid exposure.

7. How are patients with GERD managed?

When patients have symptoms of reflux more than three times a week, medical intervention is warranted. Mechanical measures should be implemented first, along with proton pump inhibitors (PPIs). PPIs are so effective that most patients experience relief with medication alone. Because gravity is one of the most important factors in the reduction of esophageal reflux, elevating the head of the bed 4–6 inches is especially useful for patients with nocturnal reflux symptoms. It has been shown that the efficacy of this maneuver alone is equivalent to using H_2 blockers. Other mechanical measures include the avoidance of tight-fitting clothing and weight loss for obese patients. Dietary alterations also should be implemented, such as not eating 3–4 hours before bedtime, not lying down after meals, avoiding excessive alcohol consumption, and smoking cessation. Avoiding offending foods or medications when possible may decrease the frequency and duration of reflux episodes.

If a patient does not respond to initial measures in 6–8 weeks, acid suppression therapy with a PPI is indicated. Increased doses may be required. Finally, in patients who are refractory to the above measures or who may require extended pharmacologic therapy (e.g., young patients), aggressive evaluation by a gastroenterologist and antireflux surgery should be considered.

8. What are the risks of prolonged therapy with PPIs?

Early data on omeprazole in rodents suggested the possibility of increased risk of gastrinomas with prolonged PPI ingestion. Subsequent studies have demonstrated no increased risk, and these agents now have approval by the Food and Drug Administration for prolonged treatment regimens.

9. What foods and medications may contribute to GERD?

The following foods and medications have been shown to increase esophageal reflux by diminishing LES pressure or diminishing peristaltic activity:

Foods	Medications
Citrus fruits and juices	Theophylline
Caffeinated products (e.g., coffee, tea, soda)	Progesterone (oral contraceptives)
	Xanthines (including caffeine)
Fatty or fried foods	Beta-adrenergic antagonists
Oils (including peppermint, onion, and garlic)	Calcium channel blockers (CCBs)
	Sedatives and tranquilizers
Chocolate, alcohol, and nicotine	Nitrates
Tomato products	Anticholinergics

10. What can be done if a patient with GERD does not want to take lifelong antisecretory therapy?

Endoscopic and surgical options are available for the treatment of GERD. Several novel endoscopic treatments are now available, although experience is limited and long-term outcomes are lacking. Options include plication of the gastric cardia folds with an endoscopic suturing device; the Stretta procedure, which uses focal radiofrequency thermal current to induce local injury, thereby tightening the LES; and injection of bulking agents, such as collagen or polymer, in the LES. Surgical options include the Nissen (full 360° wrap) or Toupet (partial wrap) fundoplication. These procedures can be performed laparoscopically by experienced surgeons.

11. Which esophageal disorders are associated with an increased incidence of cancer?

1. **Barrett's esophagus,** also known as intestinal metaplasia of the mucosa. Columnar epithelium replaces the normal squamous epithelium, possibly as a result of continuous irritation and inflammation. Because 10–15% of patients with Barrett's epithelium may develop adenocarcinoma of the esophagus, frequent endoscopic surveillance with mucosal biopsy and brushings is warranted.

2. **Plummer-Vinson syndrome.** This syndrome, which consists of intermittent solid food dysphagia (from a cervical esophageal web) and iron deficiency anemia, may be associated with glossitis, stomatitis, and achlorhydria as well as an increased incidence of squamous cell carcinoma of the esophagus.

3. **Caustic ingestion.** In addition to the immediate injury and subsequent complications resulting from alkaline and acid substances, the risk of malignancy is significantly increased in subsequent years.

4. **Achalasia and a history of oral cancer** also increase the risk for the development of esophageal carcinoma.

12. Who is at risk for developing Barrett's esophagus, and what should be done if it is detected?

Risk factors include male gender, white race, age > 50 years, and a history of GERD for > 5 years, although the risk in patients with chronic GERD is low (< 0.5% per year). One percent of the general population has Barrett's esophagus, and 5–15% of patients with a long history of GERD develop a Barrett's esophagus that is fairly long, often > 3 cm. An area of affected columnar epithelium in the esophagus that is < 3 cm is defined as short-segment Barrett's esophagus. Both long- and short-segment Barrett's esophagus carry a 10–15% increased risk of developing adenocarcinoma, which appears to progress through degrees of dysplasia before the development of malignancy.

After Barrett's esophagus is detected, surveillance endoscopy with four-quadrant biopsies every 1 cm should be performed every 2–3 years. If low-grade dysplasia is found, surveillance is increased to every year. If high-grade dysplasia is found, surgery (or other ablative therapy) is recommended, although recent studies suggest that intense screening every 3–6 months may be an alternative in certain patients.

13. List the major types of dysphagia and their common causes.

Dysphagia is the subjective sensation of impairment in the transit of a food bolus through the esophagus. A history of greater impairment to solids than to liquids generally implies a mechanical obstruction such as a stricture, whereas equal impairment or impairment to liquids implies a functional abnormality. Dysphagia can be subdivided into three categories:

1. **Oropharyngeal disorders of the neuromuscular components** of the proximal esophagus and distal pharynx may be caused by cerebrovascular accidents, multiple sclerosis, amyotrophic lateral sclerosis, Parkinson's disease, and myasthenia gravis.

2. **Mechanical obstruction** is caused by a structural abnormality that results in obstruction of food bolus transport. It may occur with strictures (benign and malignant), rings, webs, and Zenker's diverticulum.

3. **Esophageal motility disorder** is caused by motor dysfunction of the peristaltic mechanism of the esophagus. Causes include achalasia, scleroderma, diabetic neuropathy, amyloidosis, and various medications.

14. What causes the "steakhouse" syndrome?

Meat impaction of the lower tubular esophagus caused by a distal esophageal mucosal ring (B ring) or Schatzky's ring is referred to as steakhouse syndrome. Symptomatic dysphagia occurs when the diameter of the ring is $\leq$ 13 mm; mucosal rings are often asymptomatic until challenged with a large bolus of food. Rings are usually amenable to dilatation treatment.

15. A patient presents to the emergency department with symptoms consistent with esophageal food impaction. The patient is unable to handle secretions and is drooling. What should or should not be done to resolve the impaction?

Medications that may help to relax the esophageal obstruction and thus relieve the impaction may be administered, including intravenous glucagon, sublingual nitroglycerin, or a CCB (e.g., nifedipine). Meat tenderizers such as papain should be avoided because they may injure the esophageal wall. Endoscopy should be used if conservative measures fail. Endoscopy is both diagnostic and therapeutic; the offending object may be removed and the type of esophageal obstruction identified. A barium swallow should be avoided because it provides no therapy; pulmonary aspiration of barium may result, and barium mixed with food and secretions in the esophagus makes subsequent endoscopy more difficult.

16. What diagnosis should be considered in a patient who complains of halitosis associated with dysphagia and regurgitation of undigested food?

Zenker's diverticulum is a mucosal herniation formed by the protrusion of the posterior hypopharyngeal mucosa between the oblique fibers of the inferior pharyngeal constrictor and the transverse fibers of the cricopharynx. Zenker's diverticulum is proximal to the esophagus and is not a true diverticulum because it has no muscular wall. The typical history includes dysphagia and occasional regurgitation of undigested food. It is often associated with bad breath from putrefaction of food remaining in the pouch. An upper gastrointestinal series (cine swallow) is the best way to establish the diagnosis. Surgical resection, the definitive treatment, is usually reserved for markedly symptomatic cases.

17. On chest radiograph, a patient experiencing progressive dysphagia and weight loss over 1 year is found to have an air–fluid level midway up the esophagus. What is the most likely diagnosis?

Achalasia is a disorder of the esophagus in which peristalsis is absent and the sphincter between the esophagus and the stomach fails to relax in response to a swallow. As a result, food is not propelled down the esophagus through the sphincter and into the stomach. The chest radiograph often shows a dilated esophagus with an air–fluid level. Esophagram reveals a dilated, tortuous esophagus with distal tapering ("bird's beak" appearance). Patients find that remaining upright allows gravity to assist in emptying the esophagus. Medications such as nitrates and CCBs can be used to aid in relaxation of the LES, but they are often unsuccessful. Achalasia can also be treated endoscopically with pneumatic dilatation or botulinum toxin injection in the LES or surgically with a Heller myotomy performed laparoscopically or openly.

18. What swallowing problems do patients with scleroderma or CREST syndrome experience?

Progressive systemic sclerosis (scleroderma) and CREST syndrome (subcutaneous **c**alcinosis, **R**aynaud's phenomenon, **e**sophageal dysmotility, **s**clerodactyly, and **t**elangiectasia) are associated with impaired or absent LES function and esophageal peristalsis caused by involvement of esophageal smooth muscle. The result is often free reflux of acid into the esophagus, the effect of which is worsened by the inability to clear the acid (absent peristalsis). Reflux symptoms are often severe, and complications such as Barrett's esophagus, ulcerative esophagitis, and strictures are frequent.

19. What options are available for palliation of dysphagia related to malignant obstruction of the esophagus?

Options include surgical excision and bypass, laser and alcohol ablation of the tumor, and placement of esophageal stents. Surgery has been shown to be effective palliation for cancers of the distal esophagus. Tumor ablation, which requires multiple sessions and follow-ups, had been the mainstay of endoscopic management because repeated dilatation is generally ineffective in malignant disease. It has largely been replaced by the use of expandable metal stents. The stents are placed across a narrowing, after which their self-expanding property dilates the stricture. This outpatient procedure provides good palliation and may replace surgery.

20. Do all complaints of dysphagia warrant evaluation?

Single episodes of dysphagia may be followed if the event is minor (e.g., having a pill stuck in the esophagus); all others should be explained. Weight loss is the most significant associated finding. The following tests can be used to evaluate the cause of dysphagia, each with its own diagnostic and therapeutic strengths and weaknesses:

1. **Endoscopy** is the gold standard for evaluating esophageal lesions such as rings, webs, strictures, masses, and esophagitis. Biopsy can be performed to establish benignity of the lesion. Dilatation of the obstruction with balloon dilators or esophageal bougienage also may be performed.

2. The **cine-esophagogram** is useful in investigating the swallowing mechanism and evaluating patients with oropharyngeal dysphagia. A tailored barium study also may be performed, in which barium "foods" with various consistencies are administered to evaluate the patient's ability to initiate swallowing.

3. An **esophageal motility** study helps to determine the general contraction profile of the esophagus. It provides amplitude and duration of the esophageal contraction wave and sphincter pressure.

21. What is the most common cause of dysphagia or odynophagia in patients with AIDS?

Candidal esophagitis is the most frequent cause of difficult or painful swallowing in patients with AIDS. Thus, an appropriate anticandidal agent should be initiated empirically early in the course of symptoms. Common agents include nystatin, ketoconazole, and fluconazole. Keto-conazole, however, needs an acidic environment for optimal absorption. Many patients with AIDS are achlorhydric or take acid-suppressing medications that may reduce the effectiveness of ketoconazole. Anticandidal therapy relieves symptoms in > 50% of patients. However, if the pa-tient's symptoms persist or progress after several days of anticandidal therapy, endoscopy with biopsy and brushing should be performed to evaluate the esophagus for lesions from cy-tomegalovirus, herpes simplex virus, or idiopathic ulceration caused by human immunodefi-ciency virus (HIV). Barium studies miss a significant number of lesions, and definitive diagnosis is difficult to obtain from esophageal contrast studies.

BIBLIOGRAPHY

1. Baron TH: Expandable metal stents for the treatment of cancerous obstruction of the gastrointestinal tract. N Engl J Med 344:1681–1687, 2001.
2. DeVault KR, Castell DO: Updated guidelines for the diagnosis and treatment of gastroesophageal reflux disease. Am J Gastroenterol 94:1434–1442, 1999.
3. Koop H: Gastroesophageal reflux disease and Barrett's esophagus. Endoscopy 34:97–103, 2002.
4. Lehman GA: Endoscopic therapy for GERD. ASGE Clin Update 9:1–4, 2001.
5. Owen W: Dysphagia. Br Med J 323:850–853, 2001.
6. Shaheen N, Ransohoff D: Gastroesophageal reflux, Barrett's esophagus, and esophageal cancer: Scientific review. JAMA 287:1972–1981, 2002.
7. Spechler SJ: AGA technical review on treatment of patients with dysphagia caused by benign disorders of the distal esophagus. Gastroenterology 117:223–254, 1999.
8. Spechler SJ: Barrett's esophagus. N Engl J Med 346:836–842, 2002.
9. Wilcox CM, Schwartz DA, Clark WS: Esophageal ulceration in human immunodeficiency virus infection. Causes, response to therapy, and long-term outcome. Ann Intern Med 123:143–149, 1995.

36. DYSPEPSIA AND PEPTIC ULCER DISEASE

Thomas E. Trouillot, M.D., and Stephen E. Steinberg, M.D.

1. What is dyspepsia? How is it treated?

Dyspepsia refers to pain or discomfort focused in the epigastrium or upper abdomen. Symp-toms include abdominal pain, fullness, bloating, gas, belching, nausea, vomiting, and early satiety. These symptoms are often confused with gastroesophageal reflux disease (GERD), esophagitis, pep-tic ulcer disease (PUD), or irritable bowel syndrome (IBS). Patients with true nonulcer dyspepsia have the above constellation of findings in the absence of peptic ulcers or other mucosal pathology (i.e., after a negative endoscopy). When mucosal lesions are present, treatment is directed at their cause. Nonulcer dyspepsia accounts for 2–3% of office visits to primary care physicians.

2. Should an extensive workup be performed on patients with dyspepsia?

Often, it is difficult to identify patients that need further evaluation given the overlap of dys-peptic symptoms with those of GERD, PUD, or possibly gastrointestinal (GI) malignancy. Upper endoscopy should be reserved for patients who are older than 45 years presenting with new-onset dyspeptic symptoms and those with alarming symptoms such as dysphagia, weight loss, persis-tent vomiting, GI bleeding, or anemia.

3. How should dyspepsia be treated?

Management of dyspepsia is difficult, but a useful approach is focusing treatment toward the predominant symptom. This includes antisecretory (histamine receptor blockers, proton pump inhibitors [PPIs]) for ulcer or refluxlike symptoms, or prokinetics for dysmotility-like symptoms. Antiserotoninergic agents have been shown to be helpful in select patients, possibly related to improving postprandial relaxation of the proximal stomach.

4. What symptoms do patients with PUD commonly exhibit?

Abdominal pain, primarily in the epigastrium, that radiates to the back is suggestive of PUD. Although the pain is not continuous, it usually occurs on a daily basis. Ingestion of food (an excellent antacid) or antacids may relieve the pain of patients with duodenal ulcers, although pain may recur 1–3 hours after meals and often awakens patients at night. PUD may be asymptomatic in 15–44% of cases, especially in elderly individuals, and the presence or absence of symptoms does not correlate with the risk of complications.

5. How is the diagnosis of PUD best made?

Endoscopy provides a safe means of diagnosis as well as an opportunity to obtain mucosal biopsies to confirm or eliminate the presence of *Helicobacter pylori* or malignancy. Endoscopic inspection of the mucosa also identifies esophagitis, gastritis, or duodenitis, which often are missed radiographically. In cases complicated by acute bleeding, endoscopy provides therapeutic intervention by various modalities that may result in hemostasis. The major complications from endoscopy, although rare (0.001–0.01%), include perforation, bleeding, aspiration, and complications associated with the anesthetics used for conscious sedation. Compared with endoscopy, an upper GI series has lower morbidity; is less expensive; and with an air contrast study, may have a sensitivity approaching 80–90%. However, direct comparisons between an upper GI series and endoscopy reveal a sensitivity of 54% versus 92%, respectively, when other gastroduodenal lesions are included.

6. What is the role of *H. pylori* in PUD?

H. pylori infection has been associated with antral (type B) gastritis, duodenal ulcers (> 85%), and, to a lesser degree, gastric ulcers (> 65%). It should now be considered the most common cause of nonrelated peptic ulcers. Successful treatment of *H. pylori* infection reduces the risk of recurrent ulcers from 75% to 2–5%.

7. What tests are available for *H. pylori*? When is each used?

Invasive tests to determine presence of *H.* pylori can only be performed with endoscopy and biopsy. Histology can detect bacteria with hematoxylin and eosin stain, but more often, special stains are needed. A rapid urease or CLO test can be done on an antral biopsy specimen as well. Noninvasive tests for *H. pylori* include serologic tests for IgG antibody, a urea breath test (UBT), and stool antigen test. The serologic test is not useful after treatment because titers may remain elevated for years. The best utilization of the UBT is after therapy to determine eradication. The stool antigen test has been recently developed, has a similar role as the UBT, and is less expensive.

8. What are the risk factors for developing *H. pylori* infection?

Risk factors include low socioeconomic status, geographic location, and ethnic background. There is a higher incidence of *H. pylori* infection in developing countries compared with the United States and Europe. In developed countries, the annual infection rate of *H. pylori* increases at a rate of 1% per year.

9. What other diseases may be related to *H. pylori* infection?

H. pylori is associated with adenocarcinoma of the antrum and body of the stomach. There is also evidence that *H. pylori* is associated with an unusual non-Hodgkin's lymphoma of the stomach, mucosa-associated lymphoid tissue (MALT) lymphoma, which often regresses after eradication of *H. pylori*.

10. How is *H. pylori* infection treated?

The best treatment includes a combination of PPI, clarithromycin, and amoxicillin or metronidazole given twice a day for 14 days; this has approximately 90% efficacy. Side effects include nausea, diarrhea, and taste disturbances. Successful clearance is often confirmed with a UBT or stool antigen.

11. What pertinent history should be obtained from a patient with PUD?

1. *Does the patient have a history of PUD?* Previous PUD that has not been adequately treated (i.e., eradication of *H. pylori*) has a high recurrence rate.

2. *Does the patient use aspirin or nonsteroidal anti-inflammatory drugs (NSAIDs)?* These agents interfere with normal mucosal defense mechanisms, which utilize prostaglandins. NSAIDs also may cause a topical irritation that directly damages the mucosa. Symptoms correlate poorly with NSAID-induced ulceration.

3. *Does the patient smoke cigarettes?* Smokers have an increased incidence of ulcer recurrence as well as impaired healing and require higher doses of histamine (H_2) blockers to achieve the same degree of acid suppression.

4. *Are other risk factors present?* Although the evidence is controversial, psychological stress, alcohol consumption, and caffeine use have been implicated in ulcer formation and impaired healing.

12. Is there a difference between NSAIDs and cyclooxygenase inhibitors (COXIBs) with respect to their GI side effects?

COX-1 is responsible for many of the gastroprotective effects, whereas COX-2 is important in inflammatory lesions. Given the toxicity of NSAIDs, COXIBs were developed for patients with chronic inflammatory disease (arthritis) who are at risk of developing ulcer disease. COXIBs have less ulcerogenic potential and a much decreased risk in the development of ulcer disease and its complications. Given their high cost, COXIBs should be reserved for high-risk patients.

13. Describe the relationship between upper GI bleeding and PUD.

Significant bleeding occurs in approximately 25% of patients with PUD. Patients may present acutely with orthostatic hypotension, hematemesis, and melena. When the bleeding is sudden, the hematocrit may be normal and the indices normocytic. Chronic blood loss from PUD may present more subtly with minimal peptic symptoms and microcytic anemia that, on further evaluation, is found to be related to iron deficiency and associated with hemoccult positive stools.

14. Why is careful observation necessary after an upper GI bleed?

Careful observation is necessary because the rebleed rate in the first 48 hours may be as high as 50%, depending on the endoscopic findings.

15. What complications other than GI bleeding may occur with PUD?

Scarring may result in obstruction, most often at the pylorus or in the duodenal bulb. This scarring usually is associated with recurrent vomiting and weight loss. Severe esophagitis may result from impaired emptying of gastric contents. Perforation of an ulcer into the peritoneal cavity or penetration of the ulcer into adjacent structures, most commonly the pancreas, also may occur. In either instance, pain often is accompanied with an elevated level of amylase or lipase. Surgical repair is recommended when such complications occur.

16. How can benign and malignant ulcers be distinguished?

A benign-appearing ulcer has a smooth, regular rim with a smooth, flat base when evaluated endoscopically or radiographically. Folds radiating from the edge of the ulcer crater are usually symmetrical. In contrast, malignant ulcers may have an irregular raised margin surrounded by clubbed gastric folds that suggest local tumor invasion. Large (> 2 cm), recurrent, or malignant-appearing gastric ulcers should be biopsied and brushed for cytologic evaluation to rule out cancer. Follow-up endoscopy may be required after 4–6 weeks.

17. What are the pharmacologic options in treating PUD?

First, medications or habits that impair ulcer healing, including aspirin, NSAIDs, cigarettes, and alcohol, should be discontinued. H_2 antagonists, the mainstay of PUD treatment before recognition of the role of *H. pylori,* bind to histamine receptors on the basolateral membrane of parietal cells and thus diminish gastric acid secretion. PPIs (omeprazole, lansoprazole, esomeprazole, pantoprazole, and rabeprazole) can essentially eliminate acid secretion by inhibiting the hydrogen-potassium adenosine triphosphatase pump on the luminal surface of parietal cells. Compared with H_2 antagonists, omeprazole shortens the healing rates of duodenal ulcers, although it is more costly when used longer than 8 weeks. Sucralfate provides local cytoprotection by enhancing mucosal defenses and has healing rates similar to those of H_2 blockers, although the relapse rate was lower in one study. Misoprostol inhibits acid secretion by blocking histamine-stimulated cyclic adenosine monophosphate in the parietal cell. Misoprostol and H_2 antagonists are the only agents with proven efficacy in preventing NSAID-induced mucosal injury.

18. How does treatment affect the natural history of duodenal ulcer disease?

Although the complete healing rates for antacids ($> 80\%$), H_2 blockers (85–90%), and omeprazole ($> 90\%$) are high, each has a high recurrence rate after therapy is discontinued ($> 50\%$ in the first year). Studies have shown that eradication of *H. pylori* appears to alter the natural history and markedly reduces the relapse rate.

19. What are the indications for surgical management of PUD?

The primary indication for surgery is an ulcer that fails to heal, although with currently available agents this indication is uncommon. Recurrent disease is a more common indication, particularly when the cost of long-term medical management is considered. Ulcer disease complicated by bleeding, perforation, penetration, and gastric outlet obstruction is usually managed surgically. Lastly, giant duodenal ulcers (> 5 cm) are often resected because of the high complication rate.

20. What are the surgical options for treatment of PUD?

Vagotomy is the basis of all peptic ulcer operations. Proximal gastric vagotomy (highly selective vagotomy, parietal cell vagotomy) has become the most popular routine surgical procedure for the management of duodenal ulcer disease. The operation is designed to denervate the parietal (acid-secreting) cells in the stomach while preserving vagal innervation to the antropyloric region to allow near-normal gastric emptying of solids. The recurrence rate is 5–20%. Truncal vagotomy or antrectomy is the best operation in terms of ulcer recurrence (10–20%); however, the incidence of postoperative problems is greater.

21. What is the difference between a Billroth I and a Billroth II operation?

In a Billroth I operation, after resection of a portion of the stomach and the duodenal bulb, the cut ends are reanastomosed. After a similar resection, a Billroth II operation is completed by oversewing the duodenal remnant and anastomosing the cut edge of the stomach to the jejunum.

22. What problems result from ulcer surgery?

Virtually all ulcer operations result in the more rapid emptying of liquids from the stomach or gastric remnant and delayed emptying of solids. This delay may be so severe as to result in formation of a bezoar, a mass of fiber and food material that does not leave the stomach. The rapid movement of hypertonic liquid nutrients from the stomach into the small intestine may result in large volumes of intestinal fluid secretion (at the expense of blood volume) as well as elevation of various hormones (e.g., serotonin, bradykinin, substance P, vasoactive intestinal peptide). The patient may experience flushing, lightheadedness, diaphoresis, tachycardia, and postural hypotension as well as cramping and diarrhea. This constellation is referred to as "dumping syndrome." Other problems include alkaline gastritis, in which bile refluxes into the stomach and injures the gastric mucosa; ulcers at the gastrointestinal anastomosis; weight loss; and iron deficiency, particularly with Billroth II anatomy, in which blood loss at the anastomosis (small ulcers) is common.

23. In a patient with recurrent peptic ulcers, routine screening tests reveal an elevated level of serum calcium. In addition, the patient reveals a family history of pituitary tumor. What is the suspected cause of her PUD?

Zollinger-Ellison syndrome is due to an endocrine tumor that secrets gastrin, which results in gastric acid hypersecretion. Such gastrinomas result in recurrent PUD that is refractory to conventional therapy. Gastrinomas, which are usually found in the duodenum or pancreas, are diagnosed most specifically by an elevated gastrin level, which paradoxically increases after an infusion of secretin. Approximately 25% of patients with gastrinomas have the multiple endocrine neoplasia (MEN I) syndrome, like the above patient. MEN I syndrome includes gastrinoma, hyperparathyroidism, and pituitary gland hyperplasia or tumor. The gastrinomas are often difficult to identify when they are solitary and are rarely resectable when associated with the MEN I syndrome because such tumors are frequently multifocal.

BIBLIOGRAPHY

1. Bytzer P, Talley NJ: Dyspepsia. Ann Intern Med 134:815–822, 2001.
2. Du M, Isaacson PG: Gastric MALT lymphoma: From etiology to treatment. Lancet Oncol 3:97–104, 2002.
3. Fennerty MB: NSAID-related gastrointestinal injury: Evidence-based approach to a preventable complication. Postgrad Med 110:87–94, 2001.
4. Gisbert JP, Pajares JM: Diagnosis of *Helicobacter pylori* infection by stool antigen determination: A systematic review. Am J Gastroenterol 96:2829–2838, 2001.
5. Hawkey CJ: Gastrointestinal safety of COX-2 specific inhibitors. Gastroenterol Clin North Am 30:921–935, 2001.
6. McNamara DA, Buckley M, O'Morain CA: Nonulcer dyspepsia, current concepts and management. Gastroenterol Clin North Am 29:807–818, 2000.
7. Meurer LN, Bower DJ: Management of *Helicobacter pylori* infection. Am Fam Physician 65:1327–1336, 1339, 2002.
8. Peterson WL, Fendrick AM, Cave DR, et al: *Helicobacter pylori*-related disease: Guidelines for testing and treatment. Arch Intern Med 160:1285–1291, 2000.
9. Tack J, Bisschops R, DeMarchi B: Causes and treatment of functional dyspepsia. Curr Gastroenterol Rep 3:503–508, 2001.
10. Vaira D, Gatta L, Ricci C, Migioli M: Diagnosis of *Helicobacter pylori* infection. Aliment Pharmacol Ther 16(suppl 1):16–23, 2002.
11. Wu JC, Jung JJ: Ulcer and gastritis. Endoscopy 34:104–110, 2002.

37. ABDOMINAL PAIN

Stephen E. Steinberg, M.D.

1. What are the four types of processes that cause abdominal pain?
1. Inflammation: serosal or parietal irritation
2. Ischemia
3. Nerve involvement (i.e., due to neoplasm)
4. Distention, stretching

2. Distinguish between visceral (splanchnic) and parietal pain.

Visceral pain is associated with tension or stretching of a hollow viscus such as the intestine. Pain is diffuse and tends to be poorly localized because innervation to most viscera is multisegmental. This type of pain is frequently associated with autonomic responses such as vomiting, tachycardia, bradycardia, diarrhea, hypotension, and muscle rigidity. Uncomplicated small bowel obstruction is an example of visceral pain.

Parietal pain results from irritation or inflammation of a parietal surface. As a result, the pain is sharp and more localized. It is associated with voluntary muscular rigidity called *guarding* and is likely to be aggravated by coughing or movement.

Parietal pain also may be associated with cutaneous hypesthesia. Severe acute appendicitis and peritonitis, in which parietal surfaces are inflamed and irritated, provide examples of parietal pain.

3. What is the difference between rebound and referred pain?

Both types of pain are caused by irritation of serosal surface. **Rebound tenderness** occurs when the palpating hand pushes into the abdomen and is rapidly withdrawn. The inflamed surfaces of the peritoneum rub against each other, and the patient experiences sharp pain. The presence of rebound pain supports the diagnosis of disorders falling under the category of "surgical abdomen."

Referred pain occurs at a site distant from the location of the inciting process. Some examples include irritation of the diaphragm resulting from pancreatitis; subphrenic abscess after splenectomy; and a bile leak after laparoscopic cholecystectomy, resulting in pain referred to the shoulder. In the latter instance, the pain is referred to the shoulder as a result of irritation of a branch of the phrenic nerve in the diaphragm.

4. What is the significance of involuntary guarding?

Guarding is said to be present when the abdominal musculature becomes tense or rigid as a result of peritoneal irritation. It is one of the most important indicators of a surgical abdomen.

5. What physical examination maneuvers are helpful in assessing the retroperitoneal area?

1. The **psoas sign** is right or left lower quadrant pain resulting from psoas muscle irritation. To evaluate the right psoas, the patient lies on the left side and the right leg is passively extended at the hip. The test is positive if extension produces pain, suggesting a focal inflammatory process on the psoas muscle. The test result is frequently positive in retroperitoneal (psoas muscle) abscesses, which usually occur on the right side and are related to Crohn's disease; it may be positive with acute appendicitis, particularly when the appendix is in the retrocecal location.

2. The **obturator test** involves passive internal rotation of a flexed thigh with the patient in the supine position. A positive obturator sign indicates irritation at that site, often related to an abscess.

In addition, **percussion of the paravertebral areas** may elicit pain in patients with renal inflammation, particularly pyelonephritis or perinephric abscess. Auscultation of the abdomen such as a complete lack of bowel sounds may be found in advanced peritonitis or adynamic ileus resulting from a retroperitoneal lesion.

6. List the medical and surgical differential diagnosis of acute abdominal pain.

Surgical	Medical
Perforated viscus (stomach, duodenum, colon)	Biliary disease
	Pancreatitis pseudocyst
Ruptured spleen	Crohn's disease
Dissecting or ruptured abdominal aortic aneurysm	Intermittent small bowel obstruction
	Endometriosis
Bowel obstruction	Mesenteric lymphadenitis
Appendicitis	Vasculitis
Ischemic bowel disease	
Volvulus	

Nongastrointestinal causes

Ruptured ovarian cyst   Ovarian tumor
Strangulated hernia   Pneumonia
Acute cholecystitis   Diabetic ketoacidosis
Ruptured pancreatic pseudocyst   Sickle cell crisis
Ectopic pregnancy   Porphyria

7. Does the chest radiograph have value in the assessment of patients with acute abdominal pain?

The technique used for a chest radiograph may be helpful in the identification of free air under the diaphragm, which is not as easily seen with an abdominal series. Occasionally, pleural effusions may be associated with subdiaphragmatic processes such as pancreatitis. Lastly, pneumococcal pneumonia may present as abdominal pain in the absence of abdominal pathology.

8. What is a sentinel loop?

In the setting of a localized inflammatory process such as pancreatitis, a loop of bowel adjacent to the lesion may become distended with gas, thus becoming more apparent on radiographs. It occurs most often with the small bowel and is described as a sentinel loop because it heralds an underlying process.

9. What is McBurney's point?

The pain of acute appendicitis typically originates as poorly localized periumbilical visceral pain; it then changes to a more localized right lower quadrant (RLQ) parietal pain that is frequently associated with guarding and rebound. The location in the RLQ midway between the symphysis pubis and the iliac crest where the pain settles is referred to as McBurney's point. Tenderness at McBurney's point is said to be pathognomonic of appendicitis; however, it may occur with inflammation related to Crohn's disease, Meckel's diverticulum, or of the right ovary.

10. How is the location of abdominal pain helpful in the diagnosis?

Visceral pain tends to be poorly localized and diffuse. When visceral pain originates from the upper gastrointestinal (GI) tract, it tends to occur above the umbilicus; pain of colonic origin is more likely to be suprapubic. Pain produced by irritation of parietal peritoneum is confined to the area involved by the disease. Pain resulting from biliary tract disease, duodenal ulcers, or pancreatic disease is often described as radiating to the back. The anatomic location of the pain is also helpful but not definitive.

Right upper quadrant
  Hepatitis
  Cholecystitis
  Cholangitis
  Pancreatitis
  Budd-Chiari syndrome
  Pneumonia or empyema pleurisy
  Subdiaphragmatic abscess
Right lower quadrant
  Appendicitis
  Salpingitis
  Endometriosis
  Ectopic pregnancy
  Inguinal hernia
  Inflammatory bowel disease
  Mesenteric adenitis
Epigastric
  Peptic ulcer disease

Left upper quadrant
  Splenic abscess or splenic infarct
  Gastritis
  Gastric ulcer
  Pancreatitis
Left lower quadrant
  Diverticulitis
  Salpingitis
  Ectopic pregnancy
  Inguinal hernia
  Irritable bowel disease
  Inflammatory bowel disease
  Colon cancer
Diffuse
  Gastroenteritis
  Mesenteric ischemia
  Metabolic (e.g., diabetic ketoacidosis
    [DKA], porphyria)

Epigastric (*continued*)
    Gastroesophageal reflux
    Gastritis
    Pancreatitis
    Myocardial infarction
    Pericarditis
    Ruptured aortic aneurysm
Periumbilical
    Early appendicitis
    Gastroenteritis

Diffuse (*continued*)
    Malaria
    Familial Mediterranean fever
    Bowel obstruction
    Peritonitis

    Bowel obstruction
    Ruptured aortic aneurysm

11. How does the duration of abdominal pain help in the assessment of etiology?
Pain that is persistent and lasts 6 hours or longer suggests a problem requiring surgery.

12. Why is biliary colic a misnomer?
Whereas colicky pain usually means intermittent crampy pain, biliary colic is most often constant, lasting from a few minutes to several hours. Of note, it is impossible to distinguish gallbladder pain from stones that intermittently obstruct the common bile duct.

13. What is postcholecystectomy syndrome?
Ten percent to 15% of cholecystectomy patients continue to experience the same pain for which they underwent the operation. It is then referred to as the postcholecystectomy syndrome. Some patients have biliary tract disease (e.g., retained common duct stones) or sphincter of Oddi dysfunction (the muscle at the opening of the bile and pancreatic ducts into the small intestine is found to be hypertensive). Such patients usually have intermittent elevations of liver function tests or amylase levels, which may be associated with progressive dilation of the bile duct. Other patients with this syndrome have irritable bowel syndrome, esophagitis, or peptic ulcer disease. For many patients, no explanation will be uncovered. Most patients with postcholecystectomy syndrome had a cholecystectomy for symptoms not originating with the gallbladder.

14. Which is more dangerous, ischemic disease of the colon or small intestines?
Because of its blood supply (the superior mesenteric artery), small bowel ischemia frequently involves the entire bowel from the ligament of Treitz (proximal jejunum) to the caecum, with dire consequences. In contrast, the collateral circulation to the large bowel usually means that vascular compromise resulting in ischemic colitis with pain and bloody diarrhea is usually self-limited. It does not often progress to full-thickness injury and perforation, although strictures may ultimately occur. The duodenum is less likely to develop ischemia secondary to additional blood supply from the gastroduodenal artery

15. When should ischemic small bowel be considered a cause of abdominal pain?
Mesenteric ischemia is one of the most difficult and dangerous entities to be considered in patients with acute abdominal pain. It is most difficult because the clinical and laboratory findings often do not reflect the significance of the problem. The abdomen may be tender and bowel signs diminished, but early in the process, the examination is not impressive. Likewise, the radiographs show a nonspecific bowel gas pattern. Only when injury has progressed to bowel necrosis and the likelihood of patient survival is markedly diminished does the seriousness of the situation become apparent. The diagnosis of ischemic bowel should be considered when prolonged mid or migratory abdominal pain occurs in a patient with risk factors, such as previous embolic events, atrial fibrillation, atherosclerotic cardiovascular disease, or diabetes. Nonthrombotic (vasospastic) mesenteric ischemia is even more difficult to diagnose because it may occur in patients with few, if any, risk factors. An elevated white blood cell count or acidosis may be clues that a significant process is involved, even when patients are relatively asymptomatic. When mesenteric ischemia is suspected, an angiogram should be performed. Even when mesenteric ischemia is diagnosed early, mortality exceeds 60%.

16. What test proves that chronic pancreatitis is the cause of a patient's abdominal pain?

No proof is possible. Such patients frequently have exacerbation with no change in amylase or lipase level and no evidence of acute disease activity by radiographic studies. This difficulty frequently results in the labeling of patients as "drug seeking."

17. How does abstinence from alcohol affect the pain of chronic pancreatitis?

Abstinence from alcohol may diminish acute exacerbations in patients with chronic pancreatitis. Unfortunately, chronic pancreatitis is a process that, once initiated by chronic alcohol ingestion, progresses even in the absence of continued alcohol intake.

18. Describe the treatment options for the pain of chronic pancreatitis.

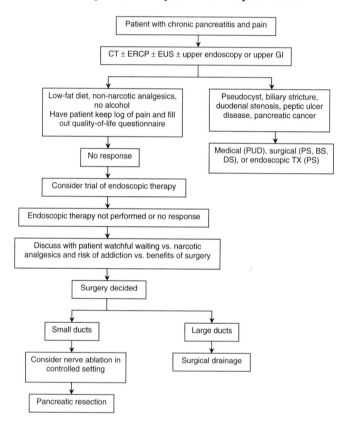

Guideline for treatment of pain in chronic pancreatitis. (Adapted from Warshaw AL, Banks PA, Fernandez-del Castillo C: AGA technical review: Treatment of pain in chronic pancreatitis. Gastroenterology 115:765–776, 1998.)

1. An empirical trial of pancreatic enzyme supplementation is usually the first option. An early study suggested that it may be effective, and there are few, if any, side effects. However, results are often disappointing.

2. Patients frequently require narcotic analgesics; regimens are best managed in the setting of a formal pain clinic.

3. Percutaneous or endoscopic celiac axis block may be beneficial and, in addition, may predict a favorable response to surgical ablation of the celiac axis.

4. Endoscopic retrograde cholangiopancreatography (ERCP) may be helpful in identifying a mechanical lesion (stone or stricture) that can be managed endoscopically or surgically.

5. The most radical step, surgical pancreatectomy, improves pain in 70–90% of patients.

6. Lastly, the pain of chronic pancreatitis burns out in many patients over years.

19. How should patients with chronic undefined abdominal pain be managed?

Serious or identifiable processes are eliminated by negative endoscopic, radiographic, and laboratory studies; absence of constitutional findings (especially weight loss); and passage of time (the most important test). Patients should not be told that nothing is wrong or that they are not having pain; rather, they should be advised that by the means available today, it is not possible to identify the cause of their pain. They should be reassured that under such circumstances, an undiscovered serious problem is unlikely. Attention should be turned to addressing quality-of-life issues. Patients may be better managed by referral to a pain clinic.

20. What is the most common cause of abdominal pain for which patients seek treatment?

Irritable bowel syndrome is characterized by chronic abdominal pain and altered bowel habits in the absence of any organic explanation. It is the most commonly diagnosed GI condition. Treatment consists of:

Education and reassurance

Treatment of symptoms:

- Pain and bloating—antispasmodics (anticholinergics), tricyclic antidepressants, or selective serotonin reuptake inhibitors
- Constipation—dietary fiber
- Diarrhea—loperamide

Psychological treatment

Antidepressants

BIBLIOGRAPHY

1. Abdu RA, Zakhour BJ, Dallis DJ: Mesenteric venous thrombosis 1911 to 1984. Surgery 101:383–388, 1987.
2. Drossman DA, Whitehead WE, Camilleri M: Irritable bowel syndrome: A technical review for practice guideline development. Gastroenterology 112:2120–2137, 1997.
3. Kaleya RN, Boley SJ: Acute mesenteric ischemia. Crit Care Clin 11:479–511, 1995.
4. Malfertheiner P, Buchler M: Indications for endoscopic or surgical therapy in chronic pancreatitis. Endoscopy 23:185–190, 1991.
5. Rolny P, Geenen JE, Hogan WJ: Post-cholecystectomy patients with objective signs of partial bile outflow obstruction: Clinical characteristics, sphincter of oddimanometry findings and results of therapy. Gastrointest Endosc 39:778–780, 1993.
6. Toskes PP: Medical therapy of chronic pancreatitis. Semin Gastrointest Dis 2:188, 1991.
7. Vozkurt T, Orth KH: Long-term clinical outcome of post-cholecystectomy patients with biliary-type pain: Results of manometry, non-invasive techniques and endoscopic sphincterotomy. Eur J Gastroenterol Hepatol 8:245–249, 1996.
8. Warshaw AL, Banks PA, Fernandez-del Castillo C. AGA technical review: Treatment of pain in chronic pancreatitis. Gastroenterology 115:765–776, 1998.
9. Yamada T, Alpers DH, Laine L, et al (eds): Textbook of Gastroenterology, 4th ed. Philadelphia, Lippincott Williams & Wilkins, 2003.
10. Yamamoto W, Kono H, Maekawa H, Fukui T: The relationship between abdominal pain regions and specific diseases: An epidemiologic approach to clinical practice. J Epidemiol 7:27–32, 1997.

38. CONSTIPATION

James Goff, M.D., and Stephen E. Steinberg, M.D.

1. How does a caregiver determine whether a patient is constipated?

Constipation is diagnosed by the patient, not the physician; it is a subjective symptom, particularly in American culture. Most surveys suggest that a daily stool is common in healthy populations, but the frequency is quite variable and related to dietary intake. Of healthy persons, 5% report two or fewer stools per week. Consistency is another aspect of constipation; hard, pellet-like stools, even if defecation occurs daily, often are considered to represent constipation. It is often best to use the patient's baseline pattern and to consider a decrease in frequency or an increase in hardness as constipation.

2. Can any test objectively assess constipation?

In addition to the history and a rectal examination that provides information about stool consistency, a test of colonic transit time may be helpful. The patient ingests radiopaque markers ("sitzmarks"), and daily flat plates are used to evaluate transit through the colon. This technique provides an objective test for a symptom that is often highly subjective. In normal people without a diet excessively high in fiber, stool transit time is about 3 days, with a great deal of variability.

3. Is constipation more common with increasing age?

Depending on the definition, the prevalence of constipation is 5–20%. With increasing age, three to five times more women than men have complaints of constipation. Although elderly persons often complain of constipation (23% in one study), 50% of the same individuals report daily bowel movements and > 90% report at least three bowel movements per week.

4. What is the most common gastrointestinal (GI) condition that causes patients to visit a health care provider?

Irritable bowel syndrome (IBS) is characterized by bowel habits that alternate between constipation and diarrhea, accompanied by abdominal pain. It is the most common GI condition for which help is sought. It appears to be a motor disorder that is affected by stress and food intake. Concomitant psychiatric illness is more common in patients with IBS.

5. How are patients with IBS managed?

The management of IBS usually consists of eliminating other significant pathology (chronicity with absence of weight loss, fever, other constitutional signs); high-fiber diet or supplements; identification of specific dietary intolerances; antispasmodic, antidiarrheal, antiflatulent, and analgesic medications; and attention to contributing psychological factors.

6. What mechanical problems should be considered with new-onset constipation?

- Strictures related to tumors, inflammation (e.g., diverticulitis, ischemic colitis), or surgery
- Perianal disease (e.g., fissures, abscesses)
- Volvulus
- Hernias

7. Which metabolic and endocrine disorders may be associated with constipation?

Diabetes (acidosis, neuropathy)	Hypokalemia
Hypothyroidism	Pheochromocytoma
Uremia	Hypercalcemia (of any cause)
Panhypopituitarism	

8. List the classes of drugs that may be associated with constipation.

Analgesics	Barium sulfate	Iron
Anesthetic agents	Bismuth	Antihypertensives
Antacids (calcium,	Diuretics	Laxative addiction
aluminum)	Antiparkinsonian	Monoamine oxidase
Anticholinergics	agents	inhibitors
Anticonvulsants	Heavy metals	Opiates
Antidepressants	Ganglionic blockers	Psychotropic agents

9. How is constipation managed?

After eliminating mechanical, metabolic, endocrine, systemic, and drug causes, attention is turned to symptomatic management; reassurance is perhaps most important. Many patients are unaware that "normal" encompasses a wide variety of bowel patterns. Furthermore, bowel patterns may vary for any individual as a result of change in dietary intake, illness, travel, change in emotional state, and a variety of other factors. If intervention is required, the initial approach is to recommend increased fiber and fluid intake and increased exercise to the degree possible. Medication should be tried only after these are ineffective.

Deficiency of dietary bulk is probably the most common cause of constipation in Western countries. This problem is addressed by an increase in dietary fiber (wheat bran, oatmeal, fruits, root vegetables) and supplementation with psyllium-containing compounds. Behavioral modification may be helpful in varying degrees for patients who frequently suppress the urge to defecate because of busy lifestyle or lack of facilities. Exercise also appears to enhance colonic motility.

10. What disorder should be considered in young adults with a history of chronic constipation and a dilated sigmoid on flat-plate radiography of the abdomen?

In addition to considering the above factors, the patient should be evaluated for Hirschsprung's disease, which is the absence of neurons in the diseased segment of the internal anal sphincter that results in failure of reflex relaxation during defecation. The result is chronic constipation. Although more common in children, it is occasionally seen in young adults. Anal manometry documenting the sphincter disorder and biopsies showing the absence of neurons suggest the need for surgical correction.

11. What other neurologic problems are associated with constipation?

Peripheral: autonomic neuropathies; various disorders that affect the ganglions.

Central: medulla and cord lesions and injuries (e.g., cauda equina tumor, tabes dorsalis, multiple sclerosis); cerebral lesions such as cerebrovascular accidents, parkinsonism, and tumors

12. Describe the six different types of laxatives.

1. Bulk-forming agents are high in fiber (natural foods, psyllium). They increase stool volume by absorbing water and require water ingestion (without water, obstruction has been reported).

2. Emollient laxatives (dioctyl potassium sulfosuccinate) are surfactants that may increase water secretion into the gut and facilitate the mixture of water and fatty substances into the stool, thus softening it.

3. The most common lubricant laxative is mineral oil, which decreases the colonic removal of water from the stool and lubricates it for easier passage.

4. Magnesium, sulfate, phosphate, and citrate-based laxatives exert an osmotic effect to draw water into the colon; they also promote motility.

5. Stimulant laxatives (anthraquinone derivatives such as cascara and phenolphthalein) enhance motility by neurologic stimulation and may alter fluid secretion and absorption as well.

6. Hyperosmotic laxatives include glycerin and lactulose.

13. When should laxative abuse be suspected?

The patient may complain of abdominal pain, nausea, vomiting, weight loss, muscle weakness, and lassitude. Hypokalemia and abnormalities on barium enema and rectal biopsy may be noted. Diagnosis of laxative abuse may be supported by the finding of alkalization of the stool (and urine) or a change in the color of phenolphthalein from colorless (pH < 8.5) to pink or red (pH > 9.0).

14. Are there any potential risks for patients who experience chronic constipation?

Yes. The frequency of urinary tract infections appears to increase in women with constipation. Several controlled studies have also shown a link between colorectal cancer and constipation, particularly in women. This association may be related to low dietary fiber intake, which leads to smaller stool volumes and slower colonic transit time. Potential carcinogens may spend more time in contact with the colonic mucosa.

15. What is Ogilvie's syndrome?

Acute colonic pseudo-obstruction (Ogilvie's syndrome) is a disorder characterized by progressive dilatation of the cecum and right hemicolon (occasionally extending to the rectum) in the absence of an anatomic lesion causing obstruction. Most patients have had recent surgery and ventilatory support, multiorgan system failure, metabolic derangements, and polypharmacy. Constitutional findings such as fever and elevated white blood count or peritoneal signs should prompt an investigation of other causes (e.g., toxic megacolon) or evidence of perforation. One study correlated cecal perforation with a cecal diameter > 14 cm; however, experience varies greatly, and perforation appears to depend as much on the rate of increase and the duration. Management consists of:

- Daily radiographs to assess progression and response
- Confirmation that there is no mechanical obstruction
- Supportive care: fluids
- Placement of a nasogastric tube, rectal tube, or both
- Correction or removal of possible precipitants (e.g., metabolic or electrolyte abnormalities, medications)
- Pharmacologic agents (e.g., neostigmine)
- Colonoscopic decompression
- Surgery

The majority (85–90%) of patients recover with a decrease in colonic diameter after conservative management.

BIBLIOGRAPHY

1. Abyad A, Mourad F: Constipation: Common-sense care of the older patient. Geriatrics 51:28–34, 36, 1996.
2. Brandt LJ, Bjorkman D, Fennerty MB, et al: Systematic review on the management of irritable bowel syndrome in North America. Am J Gastroenterol 97:S7–S26, 2002.
3. Dalton CB, Drossman DA: Diagnosis and treatment of irritable bowel syndrome. Am Fam Phys 55:875–880, 883–885, 1997.
4. Locke GR 3d, Pemberton JH, Phillips SF: AGA technical review on constipation. Gastroenterology 119:1766–1778, 2000.
5. Mellgren A: Diagnosis and treatment of constipation. Eur J Surg 161:623–634, 1995.
6. Mollen RM, Claasen AT, Kuijpars JH: Evaluation and treatment of constipation. Scand J Gastrol 223(suppl):8–17, 1997.
7. Romero Y, Evans JM, Fleming KC, Phillips SF: Constipation and fecal incontinence in the elderly population. Mayo Clin Proc 71:81–92, 1996.
8. Turegano-Fuentes F, Munoz-Jimenez F, Del Valle-Hernandez E, et al: Early resolution of Ogilvie's syndrome with intravenous neostigmine: A simple, effective treatment. Dis Colon Rectum 40:1353–1357, 1997.
9. Vanek VW, Al Salti M: Acute pseudoobstruction of the colon (Ogilvie's syndrome). An analysis of 400 cases. Dis Colon Rectum 29:203–210, 1986.
10. Velio P, Bassotti G: Chronic idiopathic constipation: Pathophysiology and treatment. J Clin Gastrol 22:190–196, 1996.

11. Verne GN, Cerda JJ: Irritable bowel syndrome: Streamlining the diagnosis. Postgrad Med 102:197–198, 201–204, 207–208, 1997.
12. Wofford SA, Verne GN: Approach to patients with refractory constipation. Curr Gastroenterol Rep 2:389–394, 2000.

39. DIARRHEA

Terry Linn, D.O., and Stephen E. Steinberg, M.D.

1. Is diarrhea defined by the frequency of bowel movements?

No. Diarrhea is defined as daily stool weight > 200 g, regardless of the consistency or frequency of the stool. It is important to make this distinction, because many patients complain of diarrhea when they experience loose stools, increased frequency of small amounts of stool, fecal incontinence, or urgency (tenesmus), all of which have distinct differential diagnoses. It should be differentiated from incontinence, which is the involuntary release of rectal contents often caused by abnormal neuromuscular function or pelvic problems.

2. What elements should be included in the history of patients with diarrhea?

Character of the stool	Medical and surgical history
Weight loss	Travel history
Timing of bowel movements	Fever
Medications	Relationship of diarrhea to food
Duration of symptoms	

3. What is the difference between diarrhea and dysentery? What organisms most often cause infectious dysentery?

Dysentery is a subgroup of diarrhea in which the stool is bloody and contains polymorphonuclear leukocytes and mucus. It implies an inflammatory process that has affected the mucosal lining of the colon or the ileum. Organisms cause dysentery by invading the mucosa or producing a toxin that injures the epithelium. In the United States, dysentery is most often caused by *Campylobacter* and *Salmonella* species and less commonly by *Shigella* species and *Escherichia coli* (strain 0157H).

4. What is the significance of nocturnal diarrhea?

Nocturnal occurrence suggests that the diarrhea is likely to have an identifiable pathologic cause. For example, patients with irritable bowel syndrome (IBS) frequently complain of diarrhea, but it occurs most often early in the morning and rarely awakens the patient from sleep. On the other hand, patients with diarrhea associated with diabetes frequently are awakened from sleep. The absence of nocturnal occurrence, however, does not exclude an organic cause and is even typical of diarrhea related to malabsorption.

5. What food history is helpful in the evaluation of diarrhea?

Diarrhea may be caused by milk (lactose deficiency), soft drinks (sucrose intolerance), food allergies, or gluten-containing foods (celiac sprue). In addition, heavy alcohol consumption, through its effect on the intestinal mucosa, may lead to episodes of diarrhea.

6. How does the duration of diarrheal symptoms affect the evaluation and management?

The differential diagnosis for diarrhea varies by the duration of symptoms. **Acute diarrhea,** with a typical duration < 2 weeks, is most commonly caused by infections. **Chronic diarrhea,** with a duration of > 2–3 weeks, is more difficult to characterize and may be caused by either structural or functional diseases.

7. How does the symptom of weight loss help with the differential diagnosis of diarrhea?

Not all patients with diarrhea have weight loss. When present, weight loss is suggestive of malabsorption, inflammation (enteritis or colitis), hyperthyroidism, or malignancy.

8. Which historical features suggest that a patient may be at increased risk for infectious diarrhea?

- Recent travel (developing nations, camping, Peace Corps)
- Ingestion of unusual food (seafood, raw foods, food at picnics)
- Institutional care (hospitals, nursing homes, day care centers)
- Homosexual behavior (male)
- Prostitution
- Injection drug use

9. What is the most important consideration in managing patients with acute diarrhea?

The cardinal principle in the management of acute diarrhea is the assessment of the degree of dehydration and replacement of fluid and electrolyte deficits. For patients who have had symptoms for less than 3 days and are not toxic, symptomatic therapies (i.e., anxiolytics or antiemetics; antimotility agents are not recommended) and oral hydration are usually sufficient. In general, antibiotics are not appropriate.

For patients who are toxic and cannot tolerate oral intake, intravenous hydration, stool studies, and antibiotic therapy are indicated. In patients who have persistent symptoms for more than 3 days, stool specimen for leukocytes, culture, and sensitivity may be considered along with empiric antibiotic therapy (e.g., quinolones). Flexible sigmoidoscopy is indicated if symptoms persist, stool study results are negative, or therapeutic trial of antibiotics fails.

10. What can patients do to prevent traveler's diarrhea?

Traveler's diarrhea generally occurs in people who have traveled from an industrialized to a developing country. Most cases of traveler's diarrhea are caused by bacterial pathogens, most commonly enterotoxigenic *E. coli*. Prevention can be attempted in two ways. First, travelers should avoid eating and drinking risky foods such as unpeeled fruits, tap water, and salads. Second, when the risk is high, pharmacologic agents may be taken to reduce the incidence of traveler's diarrhea, although the risk of adverse side effects, the potential emergence of drug resistance, and the relative cost should be recognized. In immunosuppressed patients (e.g., HIV/AIDS, elderly patients), antibiotic prophylaxis is generally recommended. Appropriate antimicrobial agents include bismuth subsalicylate, trimethoprim-sulfamethoxazole, trimethoprim alone, norfloxacin, and ciprofloxacin. Protective efficacy is variable, correlating with site of travel, length of stay, and choice of antimicrobial agent.

11. What is the significance of bloody diarrhea? What is the most common cause in an otherwise healthy patient?

Bloody diarrhea indicates mucosal damage or invasion. It may be caused by infections (dysentery), inflammatory bowel disease (IBD), ischemic colitis, or malignancy (colon cancer with tissue necrosis and postobstructive diarrhea). Aggressive workup is indicated. In otherwise healthy persons, the most common cause is infection by *Campylobacter jejuni*. In most cases, the disease is self-limited, and no treatment is required.

12. What does the symptom of tenesmus indicate?

Tenesmus is the sensation of incomplete rectal emptying. Tenesmus indicates rectal involvement in the pathologic process. Examples include proctitis from IBD or infections, anorectal fissures, and anorectal cancer.

13. Name six noninfectious causes of hospital-acquired diarrhea.
1. Fecal impaction (postobstructive diarrhea)
2. Medications (e.g., omeprazole, magnesium-containing antacids)
3. Radiographic studies using osmotically active agents such as Gastrografin
4. Elixirs (high content of sorbitol)
5. Enteral feedings
6. Cancer treatment (chemotherapy, radiation-induced colitis)

14. What are the causes of noninfectious chronic diarrhea?
The causes are usually divided into four categories based on their predominant underlying pathophysiology:
1. **Osmotic**
   Malabsorption
      Pancreatic insufficiency
      Sprue
      Lactose or fructose intolerance
   Bacterial overgrowth
   Dumping syndrome (i.e., after Billroth I or II, Roux-en-Y gastroenterostomy)
   Laxatives (magnesium containing)
2. **Secretory**
   Tumors (carcinoid syndrome, gastrinoma, glucagonoma, VIPoma, villous adenoma)
   Bile acid diarrhea (post partial ileal resection)
   Systemic mastocytosis
   Laxatives (Na_2SO_4, Na_2PO_4)
3. **Inflammatory**
   IBD
   Microscopic and collagenous colitis
   Eosinophilic gastroenteritis
   Radiation colitis
4. **Functional** (e.g., IBS)
Note that causes may overlap. For example, the Billroth II procedure may cause dumping and bacterial growth.

15. What clinical clues may help to distinguish functional from organic causes of chronic diarrhea?
Symptoms and signs suggestive of functional disease include diarrhea that occurs only during the day, absence of substantial weight loss, alternating constipation, and a long history of bowel problems dating back to adolescence or childhood.

16. What routine examinations should be done in the evaluation of diarrhea?
1. **Stool for leukocytes.** Unless the cause of diarrhea is obvious, stool should be examined for white blood cells (WBCs) and blood (occult or gross), which suggest inflammatory disease (usually colonic). Leukocytes are not normally present in the stool. They are found in instances of infectious dysentery (e.g., *Campylobacter, Salmonella, Shigella, Yersinia, C. difficile,* hemorrhagic and invasive *E. coli*), ischemic colitis, and IBD. Diarrhea resulting from toxigenic bacteria (cholera), *Giardia,* and viruses do not contain WBCs.
2. **Fecal fat.** Further evaluation for stool malabsorption may be useful. A sample of stool for assessment of fat content may suggest fat malabsorption. Although 24-hour fecal fat values that are abnormal in the range of 7–14 g may result for diarrheal processes themselves, values > 14 g indicate a primary process of fat malabsorption (e.g., pancreatic insufficiency).
3. **Stool osmolality.** Sodium and potassium concentrations in stool water may be measured so that the fecal osmotic gap can be calculated. The fecal osmotic gap is best calculated as 290 −

$2([Na^+] + [K^+])$. Osmotic diarrheas are characterized by osmotic gaps > 125 mOsm/kg, whereas secretory diarrheas typically have osmotic gaps < 50 mOsm/kg.

4. **Stool pH.** Stool pH may be assessed. Values of < 5.6 are consistent with carbohydrate malabsorption (e.g., lactose, sorbitol).

5. **Laxative screening.** This should be done in any patient with chronic diarrhea that has defied diagnosis. Stool water can be analyzed specifically for phenolphthalein, emetine (one component of ipecac syrup), and bisacodyl and its metabolites using chromatographic or chemical tests. If stool electrolyte analysis suggests osmotic diarrhea (osmotic gap > 125 mOsm/kg), magnesium laxatives may have been ingested. A soluble fecal magnesium concentration > 45 mmol/L (90 mEq/L) or a daily fecal magnesium output much above 15 mmol/day (30 mEq/day) strongly suggests magnesium-induced diarrhea. Urine can be analyzed for anthraquinone derivatives. It should be remembered that sporadic use may result in negative test results in patients with surreptitious laxative use.

6. **Serologic test for celiac sprue.** Antigliadin IgA antibodies are more specific but less sensitive for a diagnosis of celiac sprue than the IgG fraction percent. Antiendomysial antibodies are the most specific of the serologic tests for celiac sprue, with a specificity in villous atrophic disease of nearly 100%. However, their sensitivity has ranged from 74% to 100%.

7. **Sigmoidoscopy.** Most patients with chronic diarrhea also should undergo flexible sigmoidoscopy for evidence of colitis or tumors. Biopsies should be considered for histologic changes (e.g., IBD; microscopic, collagenous colitis) even if the mucosa appears normal on endoscopic examination. The value of the additional information obtained at colonoscopy (examination of the entire colon and often the terminal ileum) has yet to be determined.

8. **Upper endoscopy.** Standard upper endoscopy (EGD) is the preferred way to obtain biopsy and culture samples of the small intestine. Steatorrhea or fecal occult blood increases the likelihood of a diagnosis at EGD. Small bowel biopsy may be useful in establishing the diagnosis of Crohn's disease, giardiasis, celiac sprue, intestinal lymphoma with or without villous atrophy, and a variety of relatively uncommon disorders (e.g., Whipple's disease). It is useful in the setting of mycobacterial, fungal, protozoal, and parasitic infections.

17. What parasitic infections are most likely to cause diarrhea?

Amebiasis and giardiasis. However, their epidemiology in the United States is different. Amebiasis is usually asymptomatic and is found in individuals who have come from endemic countries (e.g., Mexico, South American countries) or individuals who are institutionalized in the United States. It may become apparent as extraintestinal disease (e.g., liver cysts). Giardiasis may occur in individuals who have had a prolonged visit to an endemic area of the world (areas of poor sanitary conditions) or, in the United States, in those who have been camping and have been exposed to contaminated water. The clinical disease of giardiasis is highly variable on presentation, from acute giardiasis (50% of patients), to asymptomatic carriers, to chronic disease with or without malabsorption or extraintestinal complications.

18. How should a physician evaluate a patient with potential giardiasis?

When giardiasis is symptomatic, examining three separate fresh stool specimens on three separate days for *Giardia* will yield a positive diagnosis in as many as 90% of patients with diarrhea. Examination of small bowel fluid (duodenal aspirate) or small bowel biopsy may be necessary for diagnosis of giardiasis. Serology is not useful, but enzyme-linked immunosorbent assay (ELISA) may also make the diagnosis. In the appropriate clinical setting, empiric treatment with metronidazole (albeit not approved by the Food and Drug Administration [FDA] for *Giardia* spp.) is often undertaken.

19. Which infectious enterocolitis is associated with hemolytic uremic syndrome (HUS)?

Patients with diarrheal disease caused by *E. coli* strain O157:H7 are at risk for HUS. This form of dysentery is caused by a Shiga toxin produced by this strain of *E. coli,* which targets intestinal endothelial cells. Receptors are also found on renal endothelial cells. The clinical manifestations of HUS include renal failure, microangiopathic hemolytic anemia, and thrombocytopenia. This strain is found in the intestines of beef cattle. The initial reports of infection were related to undercooked hamburger. Outbreaks have also been associated with contamination of raw milk, lake water, or drinking water and even freshly pressed apple cider contaminated by cattle feces.

20. How is the diagnosis of pseudomembranous colitis established?
Pseudomembranous (antibiotic-associated) colitis is caused by a toxin produced by *Clostridium difficile*, which colonizes the human intestinal tract after the normal gut flora has been altered by antibiotic or chemotherapy. After colonization, *C. difficile* releases two protein exotoxins that bind to receptors on intestinal epithelial cells, leading to secretory diarrhea and an acute inflammatory response. Diagnosis is most often made by identification of *C. difficile* toxin in the stool. There are also characteristic finding at sigmoidoscopy or colonoscopy. The distal colon is involved in most cases of pseudomembranous colitis, but up to one third of patients have findings limited to the right colon and thus require colonoscopy for diagnosis. Typical lesions seen at endoscopy are multiple elevated yellowish-white plaques of varying sizes; adjacent mucosa either is normal or exhibits hyperemia and edema.
The most important step in the treatment of diarrhea induced by *C. difficile* is cessation of the inciting antibiotic. Oral *metronidazole* at a dose of 500 mg three times daily (10–14 days) is the recommended choice for the treatment. Oral *vancomycin,* 125 mg four times daily, is offered to treatment failures.

21. Name the potential pathogens associated with AIDS diarrhea.
- Parasitic infections: *Cryptosporidium* species, microsporidians, *Isospora belli, Entamoeba histolytica,* and *Giardia lamblia*
- Viral infections: cytomegalovirus, herpes simplex virus, and adenovirus
- Bacterial infection: *Mycobacterium avium* complex, *Salmonella* species, *Shigella flexneri, Campylobacter jejuni,* and *C. difficile*

22. What are the causes of hospital-acquired diarrhea?
C. difficile is the most commonly acquired infectious organism. Hyperosmolar feeding preparations and elixirs (sorbitol) are often at fault as are commonly used medications (e.g., antacids, magnesium-containing preparations, chemotherapeutic agents, cholinergics, theophylline).

23. Which viral pathogen most commonly causes diarrhea?
Rotavirus is the single most common viral cause of severe gastroenteritis in children worldwide. It occurs primarily in children between the ages of 6 months and 2 years. Severe infections with volume losses leading to dehydration are a leading cause of death in malnourished children. Adults usually contract the infection from affected children. Rotavirus may cause traveler's diarrhea and enteritis in elderly and immunosuppressed individuals.
The clinical manifestations are similar but usually less severe than those seen in children, with frequent vomiting and diarrhea. In otherwise healthy adults, the disease is self-limited and usually passes without specific diagnosis.

24. When do symptoms of food poisoning occur in relationship to ingestion?
The timing of the onset of symptoms is dependent on the mechanism involved:
- **Mucosal invasion:** Organisms that damage the epithelial cell surface or invade the intestinal epithelial cell barrier produce a clinical presentations ranging from watery diarrhea (e.g., *Cryptosporidium parvum,* enteric viruses) to inflammatory diarrhea (e.g., *Salmonella, Campylobacter,* or *Shigella* spp.) to systemic disease (e.g., *L. monocytogenes*). Transmission in these individuals is vertical, separated by 1–3 days, as the disease is passed from person to person usually by the fecal–oral route.
- **Toxin produced during incubation:** When organisms produce toxin in the food before

the food is ingested, consumption of the toxin-contaminated food will usually lead to the rapid onset of symptoms (6–12 hours) that are predominantly upper intestinal (i.e., nausea, vomiting, and diarrhea). Examples of this are *Staphylococcus aureus, Bacillus cereus,* and botulism. Case identification is *horizontal* (i.e., affected individuals ingested the source at the same time and become sick at the same time).

- **Toxin produced in the host:** Pathogens that make toxin after ingestion usually take longer to induce symptoms (approximately 24 hours or longer) and cause diarrhea that may be watery (e.g., enterotoxigenic *E. coli*) or bloody (e.g., Shiga toxin–producing *E. coli*). Transmission in these individuals is also *vertical,* separated by 1 to 3 days, as the disease is passed from person to person usually by the fecal–oral route.

BIBLIOGRAPHY

1. Blaser MJ: Epidemiologic and clinical features of *Campylobacter jejuni* infections. J Infect Dis 176(suppl 2):S103–S105, 1997.
2. Camilleri M: Gastrointestinal problems in diabetes. Endocrinol Metab Clin North Am 25:361–378, 1996.
3. Donowitz M, Kokke FT, Saidi R: Evaluation of patients with chronic diarrhea. N Engl J Med 332:725–729, 1995.
4. DuPont DL: Guidelines on acute infectious diarrhea in adults. The Practice Parameters Committee of the American College of Gastroenterology. Am J Gastroenterol 92:1962–1975, 1997.
5. Farthing M, Feldman R, Finch R, et al: The management of infective gastroenteritis in adults. A consensus statement by an expert panel convened by the British Society for the Study of Infection. J Infect 33:143–152, 1996.
6. Fekety R: Guidelines for the diagnosis and management of *Clostridium difficile*-associated diarrhea and colitis. American College of Gastroenterology, Practice Parameters Committee. Am J Gastroenterol 92:739–750, 1997.
7. Fine KD, Seidel RH, Do K: The prevalence, anatomic distribution, and diagnosis of colonic causes of chronic diarrhea. Gastrointest Endosc 51:318–326, 2000.
8. Framm SR, Soave R: Agents of diarrhea. Med Clin North Am 81:427–447, 1997.
9. Herbert ME: Medical myth: Measuring white blood cells in the stools is useful in the management of acute diarrhea. West J Med 172:414, 2000.
10. Kroser JA, Metz DC: Evaluation of the adult patient with diarrhea. Primary Care 23:629–647, 1996.
11. Larson SC: Travelers' diarrhea. Emerg Med Clin North Am 15:179–189, 1997.
12. Lew EA, Poles MA, Dieterich DT: Diarrheal diseases associated with HIV infection. Gastroenterol Clin North Am 26:259–290, 1997.
13. Marousis CG, Cerda JJ: Malabsorption: A clinical update. Comprehens Ther 23:672–678, 1997.
14. Mead PS, Slutsker L, Dietz V, et al: Food-related illness and death in the United States. Emerg Infect Dis 5:607–625, 1999.
15. Nataro JP, Kaper JB: Diarrheagenic *Escherichia coli.* Clin Microbiol Rev 11:142–201, 1998.
16. Neild RJ, Nelson MR: Management of HIV-related diarrhoea. Int J STD AIDS 8:286–296, 1997.
17. Wolfe MS: Protection of travelers. Clin Infect Dis 25:177–184, 1997.

40. ANORECTAL DISEASES

Iqbal S. Sandhu, M.D., and Stephen E. Steinberg, M.D.

1. What is the difference between internal and external hemorrhoids?
Internal hemorrhoids, which arise from the superior hemorrhoidal cushion above (internal to) the dentate line and occur in the right anterior, right posterior, and left lateral positions, are lined with columnar rectal mucosa. External hemorrhoids, which occur below (external to) the dentate line and arise from the inferior hemorrhoidal venous plexus, are lined by perianal squamous epithelium. Because of the many pain receptors in the squamous epithelium, thrombosis of external hemorrhoids causes a significant amount of pain.

2. Are hemorrhoids more common in patients with portal hypertension?

The incidence of hemorrhoids is not increased in patients with portal hypertension. Hemorrhoidal bleeding may be a significant problem in patients with liver disease because of accompanying thrombocytopenia and coagulopathy. Hemorrhoids and anorectal varices, however, are separate entities. Hemorrhoids have no connection to the portal system; although the distinction may be difficult, anorectal varices span the dentate line and may bleed from either the squamous or rectal side.

3. What are the usual presenting complaints of internal hemorrhoids?

Internal hemorrhoids may be associated with discomfort, pruritus, prolapse, fecal soiling, and (most commonly) hematochezia. Bright red blood usually is seen on toilet paper or dripping into toilet water at the end of defecation. Blood may coat the stool.

4. When is it appropriate to attribute occult bleeding to hemorrhoids?

Hemorrhoids should not be presumed to be the source of bright red or occult bleeding until flexible sigmoidoscopy or colonoscopy has excluded other more significant sources.

5. What are the choices in the treatment of internal hemorrhoids?

Treatment is based on the severity of the hemorrhoids. Internal hemorrhoids are classified by the degree of protrusion. First-degree hemorrhoids bulge into the rectal lumen but not out of the anus; second-degree hemorrhoids protrude into the anal canal with straining but reduce easily; third-degree hemorrhoids require manual reduction; and fourth-degree hemorrhoids are not reducible and are at risk to strangulate. Treatment of first- and second-degree hemorrhoids is usually conservative, consisting of a high-fiber diet, sitz baths, and anal hygiene. Definitive therapies, which result in thrombosis of the hemorrhoidal vessels, include photocoagulation, electrocoagulation, rubber band ligation, and cryosurgery. For third- and fourth-degree hemorrhoids, the treatment of choice is hemorrhoidectomy, in which both the vessel and redundant tissue are removed. Sclerotherapy and laser or infrared coagulation are other definitive therapies.

6. What triad of findings occurs with anal fissures?

Anal fissures are linear ulcers in the anal canal that cause pain and bleeding. The classic triad of a chronic anal fissure comprises the fissure, a proximal hypertrophic anal papilla, and the sentinel pile, a fibrotic piece of skin just distal to the fissure.

7. When should a search for a secondary cause of anal fissures be undertaken?

Ninety percent of anal fissures are located in the posterior midline. If a fissure is found in the lateral position, a search for a secondary cause, such as Crohn's disease, tuberculosis, carcinoma, or syphilis, should be undertaken. A history of anal intercourse also should be sought.

8. What is the treatment for anal fissures?

1. Medical therapy
   High-fiber diet
   Stool softeners
   Topical nitroglycerin
   Botulinum toxin
   Calcium channel blockers (topical diltiazem or bethanechol)
2. Surgery (for fissures that do not heal despite adequate medical therapy)

9. How are anorectal abscesses related to the development of anorectal fistula?

The anal glands arise from the anal canal at the level of the crypts of Morgagni. Both anorectal abscesses and fistulas appear to begin with an infection in an occluded gland. Acutely infected anal glands result in anorectal abscess, whereas chronically infected glands give rise to anorectal fistulas. Approximately two thirds of perirectal abscesses evolve into anal fistulas or recurrent abscesses.

10. Which patients should avoid surgical treatment for rectal fistulas?

In the majority of patients without underlying problems, fistulas should be managed surgically. However, the fistulas that develop in patients with Crohn's disease present a difficult problem. A rectal ulcer may give rise to fistulas that open into the perianal skin, scrotum, vulva, or groin. The management of such fistulas requires optimal treatment of the underlying Crohn's disease. Asymptomatic fistulas do not require treatment. A commonly used medical regimen is metronidazole, 20 mg/kg/day. Partial and complete healing is seen in up to 68% of patients, but therapy with metronidazole is hampered by a high rate of paresthesias with prolonged use and recurrence of fistulas after discontinuation of the antibiotic. Ciprofloxacin (Cipro), 500 mg twice a day, can also be used as an alternative for patients who are intolerant to metronidazole. Immunomodulator therapy with 6-mercaptopurine, azathioprine, cyclosporine, and infliximab can be used for patients with severe or refractory disease under the guidance of a gastroenterologist. Surgical management is considered only after medical treatments have failed.

11. Who is at risk for rectal prolapse?

Rectal prolapse is more common in women than men and is associated with straining while defecating, fecal incontinence, poor pelvic muscle tone, and pelvic trauma (including childbirth). The three types of rectal prolapse are *complete, occult,* and *mucosal.* Complete rectal prolapse occurs when all layers of the rectum descend through the anal canal. Clinically, one sees red, concentric folds that protrude with double thickness with straining. In occult rectal prolapse, no protrusion is visible; the intussusception occurs internally and is best seen with defecography. Mucosal rectal prolapse occurs when a short segment of rectum, not circumferential, protrudes through the anus. Instead of concentric rings, as in complete rectal prolapse, radial folds are present.

12. What causes pruritus ani?

Pruritus ani (chronic perianal itching) most often occurs without obvious explanation. Toilet papers with perfumes, dyes, or cleansing agents may be identified as the irritant. Patients are advised to cleanse the area fastidiously with water only and to use absorbent cotton or plain white facial tissue for wipes.

13. What is the differential diagnosis of anorectal pain?

The various causes of anorectal pain include acute proctitis, tumor (e.g., cauda equina and pelvic tumors), anal fissure, intersphincteric abscess, prostatitis, endometriosis, trauma or arthritis of the coccyx, and idiopathic factors such as proctalgia fugax and levator syndrome. Proctalgia fugax is characterized by severe, short-lived (< 1 minute) attacks of rectal pain that occur infrequently. Most patients do not seek medical attention. Although the cause is unknown, it appears to be associated with irritable bowel syndrome. Levator syndrome is a chronic aching pain of the levator ani muscles, usually precipitated by defecation or prolonged sitting. Rectal examination reveals tenderness and spasm of the levator ani muscles, usually left sided, as the examining finger sweeps forward from the coccyx.

14. What is the differential diagnosis of acute proctitis (rectal pain, discharge) in immunocompetent gay men?

The differential diagnosis includes four major causative organisms: *Neisseria gonorrhoeae, Chlamydia trachomatis,* herpes simplex virus (HSV), and *Treponema pallidum.* The symptoms of gonorrhea include rectal discharge, bleeding, and anal dyspareunia. Asymptomatic infections are quite common. Constipation is more common than diarrhea. Acute chlamydial infection may cause bloody diarrhea, tenesmus, discharge, and (on rare occasions) fistula formation. It is associated with tender, enlarged inguinal lymph nodes that harbor the intracellular organism. Infection with HSV causes anal pain, constipation, urinary symptoms (e.g., retention), sacral paresthesias, and buttock and thigh pain. Many patients have no visible mucocutaneous lesions. Finally, anorectal syphilis may be associated with pain, discharge, and tenesmus. The chancre of primary syphilis is present on the squamous epithelium of the anal canal, and inguinal adenopathy is often present.

15. What are the risk factors for the development of anal carcinoma?
Anal carcinoma is associated with male homosexual behavior and a history of genital warts, which suggests a role for human papillomavirus as a causal agent. Other factors associated with increased risk include smoking, other sexually transmitted diseases, Crohn's disease, and renal transplantation. Recent studies suggest that radiation therapy and combination chemotherapy provide improved results over wide surgical excision for noninfiltrating anal carcinoma. Tumor regression occurs in most cases, and normal anal function is retained.

Other risk factors for anal carcinoma include injection drug use, vulvar and cervical cancer, and high-grade cervical or vulvar lesion in women.

BIBLIOGRAPHY

1. Banerjee S, Peppercorn MA: Inflammatory bowel disease: Medical therapy of specific clinical presentations. Gastroenterol Clin North Am 31:185–202, 2002.
2. Berkelhammer C, Moosvi SB: Retroflexed endoscopic band ligation of bleeding internal hemorrhoids. Gastroint Endosc 55:532–537, 2002.
3. Chawla AK, Willett CG: Squamous cell carcinoma of anal canal and anal margin. Hematol Oncol Clin North Am 15:321–344, 2001.
4. Hulme-Moir M, Bartolo DC: Hemorrhoids. Gastroenterol Clin North Am 30:183–197, 2001.
5. Jonas M, Scholefield JH: Anal fissure. Gastroenterol Clin North Am 30:167–181, 2001.
6. Pfenninger JL, Zainea GG: Common anorectal conditions: Part I: Symptoms and complaints. Am Fam Physician 63:2391–2398, 2001.
7. Pfenninger JL, Zainea GG: Common anorectal conditions: Part II: Lesions. Am Fam Physician 64:77–88, 2001.
8. Schwartz DA, Pemberton JH, Sandborn WJ: Diagnosis and treatment of perianal fistulas in Crohn disease. Ann Intern Med 135:906–918, 2001.

41. ACUTE LIVER DISEASE

Priya Grewal, M.D., and Kevin T. White, M.D.

1. What do elevated levels on liver chemistry tests indicate?
Elevation of aspartate aminotransferase (AST) and alanine aminotransferase (ALT) levels is significant for hepatocellular injury, whereas elevation of bilirubin and alkaline phosphatase levels is more consistent with a cholestatic pattern of liver injury, although frequent overlap occurs. The albumin and prothrombin time (PT) are markers of liver synthetic function and are altered in patients with cirrhosis.

2. How is the level of elevation of transaminases helpful in differentiating the cause?
The highest transaminase levels (> 800–1000) can be caused by acute viral hepatitis (hepatitis A–E, herpes), ischemia, or various medications and toxins. Mild elevations of transaminases can be induced by a variety of causes, including chronic viral hepatitis, alcohol, fatty liver, autoimmune hepatitis, or hemochromatosis.

3. How is the ratio of the hepatic transaminases AST to ALT useful in differentiating alcoholic hepatitis from viral and stone-related liver disease?
Alcohol represses the synthesis of ALT more than the synthesis of AST. With hepatic injury (alcoholic hepatitis), the released enzymes reflect this effect. Thus, a serum AST/ALT ratio > 2

is characteristic of acute alcoholic hepatitis. Elevations in AST are modest, rarely exceeding 300 IU/L, regardless of the severity of hepatic injury. In contrast, patients with acute common duct obstruction (e.g., gallstones) may have a transient (sharp) increase in transaminases, occasionally to very high levels and usually with associated elevation of alkaline phosphatase; however, the AST/ALT ratio is < 1 in these patients. In acute viral or drug-induced hepatitis, enzymes typically exceed 1000 if the injury is moderate or severe; the AST/ALT ratio is again < 1.

4. What liver diseases are associated with pregnancy?

Preeclampsia with hepatic involvement, HELLP (hemolysis, elevated liver enzymes, low platelets) syndrome, and acute fatty liver of pregnancy (AFLP) are three conditions that occur in late pregnancy that may lead to severe hepatic dysfunction and acute liver failure. Preeclampsia is characterized by hypertension, proteinuria, and edema and occurs in 5–7% of all pregnancies in the late second or third trimester. Complications include subcapsular hematoma, hepatic rupture, infarction, or fulminant liver failure. HELLP syndrome is a severe form of preeclampsia that occurs in 0.1–0.6% of pregnancies as early as the 27th week, although a third of cases are postpartum. Symptoms include right upper quadrant pain, malaise, and (rarely) jaundice. Complications are similar to those of preeclampsia.

AFLP is a rare disease of the third trimester with a mortality rate of 10–20%. AFLP can be differentiated from HELLP syndrome by the presence of leukocytosis, transaminitis, hyperbilirubinemia, hypoglycemia, and an elevated prothrombin time with a low fibrinogen level. Intrahepatic cholestasis of pregnancy and hyperemesis gravidarum may lead to premature birth or low birth weight but not acute liver failure. Hepatitis E, endemic to parts of Africa, Asia, and South America, has a high mortality rate (15–25%) in pregnant women, especially during the third trimester.

5. Which serologic tests are useful in evaluating acute hepatitis of possible viral etiology?

IgM antibodies to hepatitis A virus are the best test for diagnosing acute hepatitis A. For acute hepatitis B, the appropriate tests are hepatitis B surface antigen (HbsAg) and IgM-antibody to hepatitis B core antigen. For hepatitis C, the first screening test is the enzyme-linked immunosorbent assay (ELISA) for the hepatitis C antibody. In the acute phase (and occasionally in the chronic phase) of hepatitis C infection, the antibody may not be positive despite active viral infection. In this case, detection of hepatitis C virus RNA by polymerase chain reaction (PCR) is the most sensitive test.

6. What is the range of incubation periods for hepatitis A, B, and C viruses?

It is easiest to remember the incubation periods by the "2 to 6 rule": hepatitis A, 2–6 weeks; hepatitis B, 2–6 months; and hepatitis C, 2 weeks to 6 months.

7. Which hepatitis viruses are spread by sexual contact?

Hepatitis B can be transmitted by sexual contact, but this route has not been clearly established for hepatitis C virus. Hepatitis A and E viruses are spread by the fecal–oral route. Hepatitis B, C, and D viruses are spread by serum. Hepatitis G virus is a recently described virus transmitted parenterally. It may, however, not be a pathogen. In addition, another non–A through G hepatitis virus appears to be transmitted by the fecal–oral route.

8. What is the mode of transmission of hepatitis C?

Hepatitis C is primarily transmitted through exposure to infected blood. Intravenous drug use and sharing of needles is the most common route of infection. In many cases now being diagnosed in the United States, patients may have experimented with drugs in the distant past for only a short period of time. Many persons may not be forthcoming with such information, accounting for some of the cases of unknown transmission. Blood transfusion before 1992 was a common means of transmission of hepatitis C, but it is now extremely rare because all blood donors are screened.

Of the 50 million people worldwide believed to be infected with hepatitis C, only 25% give a history of blood transfusion, and the mode of infection is uncertain in 40%. Likewise, the route of infection in community-acquired cases is unknown. Body secretions from patients who test positive for RNA of the hepatitis C virus seem to contain the virus, although at very low levels. The virus may be passed in blood product concentrates, but this method of transmission is now extremely rare. All studies indicate that sexual transmission occurs infrequently.

9. What recommendations should you give to persons traveling to areas endemic for hepatitis?
- For **hepatitis A:** strict sanitation (handwashing, avoiding local water, peeling fruit); avoiding known vectors (e.g., oysters). Immunoglobulin (there is no "hyperimmune" globulin), and vaccination is indicated when prolonged stays are planned.
- For **hepatitis B:** vaccination and avoidance of high-risk activities (any activity that provides exposure to blood or body fluids). Endemic areas include Southeast Asia.
- For **hepatitis C:** no current recommendations.

10. What advice should you give to casual, household, and sexual contacts of patients with hepatitis A, B, and C?

HEPATITIS TYPE	CASUAL/HOUSEHOLD CONTACTS	SEXUAL CONTACTS
A	Strict sanitation practice Immunoglobulin is preferred	Strict sanitation practice Immunoglobulin is preferred
B	Avoid contact with blood and body secretions; vaccination	Hepatitis B immunoglobulin is preferred; vaccination
C	Simple hygiene principles	Controversial (transmission rate is very low)

11. Who should be vaccinated for hepatitis B?
It is recommended that everyone 18 years of age and younger and adults older than 18 years who are at risk should be vaccinated against hepatitis B. Adults at risk include heterosexuals with more than one sex partner in the past 6 months, homosexual men, intravenous drug users, hemodialysis patients, household and sexual contacts of persons with chronic hepatitis B, and persons at occupational risk (including health-care workers and staff at prisons and institutions). The vaccine is given at 0, 1, and 6 months; it does not contain any live virus and may be given with other vaccines. Common side effects include mild fever and soreness at the injection site. Anaphylactic reactions are extremely rare. There is currently no scientific evidence to support an association between the hepatitis B vaccine and the development of autoimmune diseases, transverse myelitis, or multiple sclerosis.

12. Who should receive hyperimmune globulin to prevent hepatitis?
Hyperimmune globulin is used only in the prophylaxis of hepatitis B infection. It should be given in the following situations:
1. After homosexual or heterosexual contact with an HBsAg-positive partner
2. After a percutaneous puncture (e.g., in health care workers or drug abusers sharing needles)
3. In neonates who are born to HBsAg-positive mothers. Such offspring (after the neonatal period) also should be started on hepatitis B vaccine.
4. Patients with cirrhosis caused by HBV received after transplantation

13. Can patients be reinfected with hepatitis viruses?
It is extremely unlikely for HAV and HBV. Patients with chronic hepatitis C often have exacerbations that should not be confused with reinfection. However, infection with different genotypes of HCV is possible.

14. Which patients with viral hepatitis should be considered for treatment with interferon?

Interferon does not have a proven role in the treatment of acute viral hepatitis. Chronic hepatitis caused by B, C, or D viruses may be treated with interferon. Preliminary results from the treatment of acute hepatitis C exposure (e.g., needlesticks) with interferon are encouraging.

15. What are the treatment options for viral hepatitis?

Hepatitis A is generally a self-limited disease, although fulminant hepatic failure may occur in < 1% of cases. Treatment is supportive, and liver transplant is needed in fulminant disease. Chronic hepatitis B can be treated with interferon, lamivudine, or adefovir. Interferon must be given as a subcutaneous injection and is expensive, but mutants rarely develop. Lamivudine is more economical and well tolerated, but resistant mutants may result from therapy. Adefovir, which has been recently approved, has similar efficacy to lamivudine without the development of mutant strains. Hepatitis C is treated with a combination of pegylated interferon injection given once a week and ribavirin taken twice daily. Response rates range from 45% to 90% depending on genotype, although side effects may limit the tolerability to therapy. Acute hepatitis C, although rare, has been successfully treated with interferon monotherapy.

16. When should a patient with acute viral hepatitis be hospitalized?

Patients who are severely debilitated and, in particular, unable to maintain adequate oral intake because of nausea and vomiting should be hospitalized. In addition, any patient whose clinical features suggest the possible development of acute liver failure (encephalopathy and coagulopathy) should be hospitalized immediately and referred to the nearest liver transplant center.

17. What syndromes other than liver disease are associated with viral hepatitis?

Atypical manifestations of **hepatitis A** include immune complex deposition, which causes leukocytoclastic vasculitis; cryoglobulinemia; arthritis; and acute oliguric renal failure. All resolve spontaneously. An acute illness that resembles serum sickness—with symptoms of fever, rash, urticaria, arthralgias, and (on occasion) acute arthritis—occurs in 10–20% of patients during the incubation period of **hepatitis B**. HBsAg–HBs complexes apparently play a role in the pathogenesis. With persistent hepatitis B infection, immune complex glomerulonephritis may occur, and 30–50% of patients with polyarteritis nodosa have evidence of hepatitis B infections. **Hepatitis C** appears to be causal in some cases of aplastic anemia. Viral antibodies are highly prevalent in the serum and cryoprecipitate of patients with essential mixed cryoglobulinemia. Hepatitis C also has been associated with Sjögren's syndrome and glomerulonephritis.

18. What is the clinical course of acute liver failure?

Initially, nonspecific symptoms such as malaise and nausea develop in a previously healthy person; jaundice develops shortly thereafter, followed by the rapid onset and progression of altered mental status (hepatic encephalopathy) and coagulopathy. Death occurs within 2–10 weeks in 80% of patients unless they undergo orthotopic liver transplantation.

19. How often is acute liver failure of viral etiology?

Viral hepatitis accounts for about 40–70% of all cases, including hepatitis A (rare), B (most commonly identified virus), C (rare), D (common with B), and E (rare) but occurs in epidemics with a high incidence of fulminant hepatitis, particularly in pregnant women. Cytomegalovirus, Epstein-Barr virus, and herpes viruses are occasionally implicated; herpes viruses affect immunosuppressed patients and, at times, pregnant women. The remaining cases are accounted for by (1) drugs and toxins, including fluorinated hydrocarbons (trichloroethylene and tetrachloroethane), *Amanita phalloides* (death-cap mushroom), and acetaminophen; (2) vascular causes (low flow states); and (3) various other disorders, including Wilson's disease, acute fatty liver of pregnancy, and Reye's syndrome. In 40% of all cases of acute liver failure, the cause is unclear and attributed to an unknown hepatitis virus (non-A, non-B, non-C).

20. What drugs are implicated in acute liver failure?

Acetaminophen is the most common drug causing acute liver failure. Liver injury is dose dependent and may occur at lower doses with alcohol ingestion through induction of the cytochrome P450 system and depletion of glutathione. Treatment with *N*-acetylcysteine is highly effective in repleting glutathione stores and preventing significant hepatotoxicity when administered within 16 hours of ingestion. Many other medications have been implicated in acute liver failure, including nonsteroidal anti-inflammatory drugs (NSAIDs), antibiotics, antituberculosis drugs, antifungals, anesthetics (halothane), anticonvulsants (valproic acid, phenytoin), antidepressants, antipsychotics, lipid-lowering agents, thiazolidinediones, and drugs of abuse (cocaine, PCP, ecstasy).

21. What is the significance of a "flap" in acute liver disease?

A flap, or asterixis, is a manifestation of progressive hepatic encephalopathy, but it is not specific to liver disease. It also may be seen with other instances of metabolic toxicity, such as uremia and carbon dioxide narcosis, as well as after cerebrovascular events. Evaluation for a flap consists of having the patient extend the arms and pronate the hands (with fingers spread and extended). Patients with asterixis are unable to maintain tonic extension. The sudden relaxation results in a quick drop of the hand and slower restoration to the extended position.

22. What causes death in patients with fulminant liver failure?

Cerebral edema is the usual cause of death. Less commonly, sepsis and metabolic complications, including hypoglycemia and multiorgan failure, are responsible.

23. What is the treatment of fulminant liver failure?

The most effective treatment is liver transplantation. Although some patients with acute liver failure recover spontaneously with supportive therapy, the mortality rate without transplantation approaches 80%. A progressive increase in PT, development of encephalopathy, and progressive renal failure are indications for transplantation. Such patients are best cared for in an intensive care setting by specialists with access to liver transplantation. Because the transport of patients with advancing encephalopathy is hazardous, consideration should be given to early transfer of any patient with altered mentation; bleeding, decrease in liver size, or precipitous decrease in transaminase level predicts a poor prognosis. In addition, several liver support systems, including the Molecular Adsorbent Recycling System (MARS), which removes toxins in a method similar to hemodialysis, have been used in patients as a bridge to transplant while waiting for a donor organ.

24. What is the success rate of orthotopic liver transplantation in acute liver failure?

The 1-year survival rate of liver transplant for fulminant hepatic failure ranges from 50% to 75%. This rate is lower than liver transplant for all other causes in which the 1-year survival is > 85% in some centers. Given the shortage of donor organs, living-related liver donation is becoming increasingly common. The criteria for donation are stringent given the high risk of potential donor complications, and its use is restricted to specialized transplant centers.

BIBLIOGRAPHY

1. Bernstein D, Tripodi J: Fulminant hepatic failure. Crit Care Clin 14:181–197, 1998.
2. Broughan TA, Soloway RD: Acetaminophen hepatotoxicity. Dig Dis Sci 45:1553–1558, 2000.
3. Carithers RL: Liver transplantation. Liver Transplant 6:122–135, 2000.
4. Gill RQ, Sterling RK: Acute liver failure. J Clin Gastroenterol 33:191–198, 2001.
5. Green RM, Flamm S: AGA technical review on evaluation of liver chemistry tests. Gastroenterology 123:1367–1384, 2002.
6. Lewis JH: Drug-induced liver disease. Med Clin 84:1275–1311, 2000.
7. Rahman T, Hodgson H: Clinical management of acute hepatic failure. Intensive Care Med 27:467–476, 2001.

8. Rahman TM, Wendon J: Severe hepatic dysfunction in pregnancy. Q J Med 95:343–357, 2002.
9. Rajvanshi P, Larson AM, Kowdley KV: Temporary support for acute liver failure. J Clin Gastroenterol 35:335–344, 2002.
10. Regev A, Schiff ER: Viral hepatitis A, B, C. Clin Liver Dis 4:47–71, 2000.
11. Riordan SM, Williams R: Fulminant hepatic failure. Clin Liver Dis 4:25–45, 2000.
12. Trotter JF, Wachs M, Everson GT, Kam I: Adult-to-adult transplantation of the right hepatic lobe from a living donor. N Engl J Med 346:1074–1082, 2002.

42. CHRONIC LIVER DISEASE

Priya Grewal, M.D., and Kevin T. White, M.D.

1. When is chronic hepatitis diagnosed?

Chronic hepatitis is defined as persistence of elevated transaminases for at least 6 months. Because enzyme levels may fluctuate (particularly with hepatitis C), occasional normal values do not exclude the diagnosis of chronic hepatitis.

2. What disorders should be considered in patients with chronic hepatitis?

The differential diagnosis includes viral hepatitis (B, C, and D), drug-induced hepatitis, autoimmune hepatitis, hemochromatosis, Wilson's disease, and alpha$_1$ antitrypsin deficiency. Alcoholic hepatitis, nonalcoholic steatohepatitis (NASH), and primary biliary cirrhosis should also be considered.

3. What laboratory tests should be ordered in the initial evaluation of chronic liver disease?

- For **hepatitis C:** hepatitis C antibody
- For **hepatitis B:** hepatitis B surface antigen (HBsAg), hepatitis B surface antibody (HbsAb), and hepatitis B core antibody (HbcAb)
- For **hemochromatosis:** serum iron and total iron binding capacity (TIBC)
- For **autoimmune hepatitis:** antinuclear antibody (ANA), anti–smooth muscle antibody (ASMA), quantitative immunoglobulins (IgG, IgM)
- For **primary biliary cirrhosis:** antimitochondrial antibody (AMA)
  Less common causes and screening tests include:
- For **Wilson's disease:** ceruloplasmin
- For **alpha$_1$-antitrypsin deficiency:** alpha$_1$-antitrypsin level

If serologic workup results are negative, alcohol use and medications should be investigated.

4. Describe the proper use and interpretation of hepatitis B serology.

Of the widely available serologic tests, HBsAg is the most useful marker of chronic infection and carrier state. Antibody to surface antigen is found in patients who have cleared the infection or who have been immunized. Core antibody can be useful in identifying early hepatitis B infections (before test results for surface antigen become positive). Because it is long lived, core antibody is also useful in epidemiologic studies to identify people infected with hepatitis B in the past. The HBV DNA test, similar to hepatitis B early antigen (HBeAg), is indicative of a high replicative, highly infectious state.

5. What is the best way to diagnosis hepatitis C (HCV)?

Hepatitis C antibody identifies patients whose chronic hepatitis may be caused by HCV. The third-generation enzyme-linked immunosorbent assay (ELISA) is > 95% sensitive and specific in diagnosing HCV. Because of the 5–10% false-negative rate, antibody-negative patients in whom there is high clinical suspicion for HCV should be evaluated with an HCV RNA polymerase chain reaction (HCV RNA PCR) qualitative test, which will confirm the presence of virus. Alternatively, 10–15% of patients spontaneously clear HCV and remain hepatitis C antibody positive. The HCV RNA PCR qualitative test is useful in this instance as well to confirm lack of viremia.

6. What is the likelihood of chronicity for hepatitis B and C?

Of acute hepatitis B infections, 10–15% ultimately progress to chronicity; for hepatitis C infections, the rate is at least 80–85%.

7. What tests should be ordered to screen for hereditary hemochromatosis (HHC)?

HCC, an autosomal recessive disorder, is the most common genetic disorder of caucasians, with a prevalence of close to 1 per 200. Screening tests include standard iron markers of serum iron and TIBC to calculate the transferrin saturation (serum iron/TIBC). Elevations > 50% are suspicious for HHC and need further workup by checking serum ferritin level. If both transferrin saturation and ferritin are elevated, patients should undergo genetic testing. The HFE gene for HCC has been isolated to the short arm of chromosome 6. Two mutations (C282Y, H63D) have been found in 85–90% of patients with HHC. Diagnosis is confirmed by an elevated hepatic iron index on liver biopsy.

8. When should a diagnosis of NASH be considered?

NASH is a form of chronic liver disease characterized by fatty infiltration and inflammation within the liver. It should be considered in patients with diabetes, hyperlipidemia, and obesity who have chronically elevated transaminases with negative serologic workup results and an intake of < 20 g of alcohol per day. Liver biopsy is often needed for definitive diagnosis in order to determine the degree of fibrosis.

9. When should a diagnosis of Wilson's disease be considered?

The diagnosis should be considered in children or young adults with chronic elevation of transaminases. The disease is almost always diagnosed before age 30 years. Patients with classic Wilson's disease show both liver and neurologic involvement and a positive family history; often, however, only one organ is affected initially. Initial tests include serum copper (high), 24-hour urine copper (high), ophthalmologic examination (for Kayser-Fleischer rings), and ceruloplasmin levels (low). If the screening test results are abnormal, the diagnosis is established by quantitation of copper in liver biopsy specimen.

10. How are patients screened for alpha₁-antitrypsin deficiency?

Alpha$_1$-antitrypsin is a protease inhibitor synthesized by the liver. People who are homozygous for a variant of the normal protein are predisposed to the early onset of chronic active hepatitis, liver cirrhosis, and emphysema. Screening for the alpha$_1$ peak on serum protein electrophoresis helps to rule out alpha$_1$-antitrypsin deficiency. The diagnosis is established by measuring the serum alpha$_1$-antitrypsin level and phenotyping. Because expression is variable, some patients with the deficiency may not develop hepatitis or may do so only with additional insults (e.g., alcohol, hepatitis C).

11. What are the autoimmune liver diseases, and how are they distinguished?

Autoimmune hepatitis (AIH) is primarily a disease of young women with elevated transaminases, positive ANA, positive ASMA, and gammaglobulinemia. Primary biliary cirrhosis (PBC) is a cholestatic hepatitis affecting middle-aged women with an elevated alkaline phosphatase level and a positive AMA. Primary sclerosing cholangitis (PSC) is also a cholestatic liver disease mainly found in men with an elevated alkaline phosphatase and stricturing and beading of the biliary tree on endoscopic retrograde cholangiopancreatography (ERCP). Seventy percent of cases of PSC are associated with ulcerative colitis, most often diagnosed before the onset of liver disease.

12. Which patients are at risk for the development of hepatocellular carcinoma?

Chronic hepatitis that results in cirrhosis is a significant risk factor for the development of hepatoma; chronic hepatitis B and C infection confers an additional risk, independent of cirrhosis. Hepatic ultrasonography and alpha-fetoprotein have been used as screening modalities in high-risk patients.

13. What three laboratory findings suggest the diagnosis of primary biliary cirrhosis?

Increased levels of alkaline phosphatase, gammaglobulins (mostly IgM type), and antimitochondrial antibody titers are highly suggestive of primary biliary cirrhosis. Bilirubin is elevated late in the disease, which occurs with greatest frequency in middle-aged women.

14. List five findings in the extremities that are associated with chronic liver disease.

Palmar erythema	Dupuytren's contracture (most often seen in alcoholic cirrhosis)
Spider angiomata	Thenar and hypothenar atrophy
White nails	

15. When is a caput medusae seen?

Caput medusae is the name given to engorged veins surrounding the umbilicus; normally, venous filling is away from the umbilicus. This physical finding is most commonly seen in patients with portal hypertension caused by cirrhosis, but it may occur with thrombosis of the inferior or superior vena cava.

16. Should asymptomatic esophageal varices be treated prophylactically to prevent bleeding?

Prophylactic eradication of incidentally discovered varices by sclerotherapy or variceal ligation banding is not indicated. Sclerotherapy has proven ineffective, and ligation has not yet been evaluated. However, recent data suggest that one can delay the time to initial bleeding by treating nonbleeding varices with nonselective beta-adrenergic blockers and nitrates.

17. What is the role of endoscopy in the initial management of acute variceal hemorrhage?

After resuscitation, patients should undergo endoscopic evaluation with sclerosis or banding of varices. This approach controls the initial bleeding in > 90% of patients. Pharmacologic therapy, with a continuous infusion of octeotide, should be started empirically in patients with suspected variceal bleeding, even before endoscopy. Banding of varices has become the procedure of choice over sclerotherapy because it is equally effective with fewer side effects and complications. If bleeding continues despite banding, the next treatment option is placement of a transjugular intrahepatic portosystemic shunt (TIPS). Also, prophylactic antibiotics should be initiated in all cirrhotics with gastrointestinal bleeding of any cause.

18. Why should acetaminophen be avoided in patients with alcoholic liver disease?

Chronic alcohol intake increases the activity of the cytochrome P450 system, normally a minor pathway of acetaminophen metabolism. In this setting, a larger fraction of the acetaminophen is metabolized through the P450 system, resulting in increased amounts of toxic metabolites that need to be detoxified by glutathione. Alcoholics also have low amounts of glutathione in the liver because of concomitant poor nutrition. As a result, the increased levels of toxic metabolites cannot be detoxified, and hepatocyte necrosis results, occasionally even with modest amounts of acetaminophen (3–6 g/day).

19. Describe the management of the patient with moderate ascites.

Most patients with mild ascites can be managed with salt restriction (< 2 g/day). Moderate ascites (visible but not tense) usually requires a potassium-sparing diuretic (spironolactone or amiloride), occasionally in combination with a loop diuretic (furosemide or bumetanide). The combination is synergistic in patients with liver disease and should be given together as a single morning dose. If ascites is still refractory, large-volume paracentesis, placement of a LeVeen shunt, or TIPS may provide alternatives.

BIBLIOGRAPHY

1. Befeler AS, Di Bisceglie AM: Hepatocellular carcinoma: Diagnosis and treatment. 122:1609–1619, 2002.
2. Czaja AJ, Freese DK: Diagnosis and treatment of autoimmune hepatitis. Hepatology 36:479–497, 2002.
3. Harrison SA, Kadakia S, Lang KA, Schenker S: Nonalcoholic steatohepatitis: What we know in the new millennium. Am J Gastroenterol 97:2714–2724, 2002.
4. Lauer GM, Walker BD: Hepatitis C virus infection. N Engl J Med 345:41–52, 2001.
5. Menon KVN, Gores GJ, Shah VH: Pathogenesis, diagnosis and treatment of alcoholic liver disease. Mayo Clin Proc 76:1021–1029, 2001.
6. Pratt DS, Kaplan MM: Evaluation of abnormal liver-enzyme results in asymptomatic patients. N Engl J Med 342:1266–1271, 2000.
7. Riley TR, Bhatti AM: Preventive strategies in chronic liver disease: Part II. Cirrhosis. Am Fam Physician 64:1555–1560, 2001.
8. Sharara AI, Rockey DC: Gastroesophageal variceal hemorrhage. N Engl J Med 345:669–681, 2001.
9. Tavill AS: Diagnosis and management of hemochromatosis. Hepatology 33:1321–1328, 2001.
10. Wongcharatrawee S, Garcia-Tsao G: Clinical management of ascites and its complications. Clin Liver Dis 5:833–850, 2001.

43. BILIARY TRACT DISEASE

Henry Chun, M.D., and Stephen E. Steinberg, M.D.

1. Distinguish among cholelithiasis, choledocholithiasis, and biliary colic.

Cholelithiasis and *choledocholithiasis* are simply the descriptions for stones in the gallbladder and bile duct, respectively. Both often occur without symptoms. *Biliary colic*, however, is the term used to refer to pain caused by gallstones or other abnormalities of the gallbladder. In reality, biliary pain is not colicky but rather a steady (not fluctuating) pain localized to the epigastrium or the right upper quadrant. It may last from 1 to 6 hours and often occurs at random with no relation to meals. Pain frequently radiates to the right scapula or shoulder or into the back. Because it is related to obstruction rather than infection, it usually occurs without constitutional signs (e.g., fever, chills). The biliary colic of a typical "gallbladder attack" is indistinguishable from that of transient obstruction of the bile duct with a stone.

2. What are the clinical manifestations of acute cholecystitis?

- Right upper quadrant abdominal pain
- Nausea and vomiting
- Fever
- Mild jaundice ($\sim$20% of cases)
- Positive Murphy's sign (right subcostal tenderness with inspiratory arrest during palpation)
- Laboratory results of leukocytosis and mild elevation of transaminases

3. What radiologic studies are useful in the diagnosis of patients with suspected gallstones?

Ultrasonography has high specificity and sensitivity for the diagnosis of gallstones and is usually the first test. The false-negative rate is approximately 5%. Ultrasound is also useful in detecting thickening of the gallbladder wall (chronic cholecystitis), fluid around the gallbladder (acute cholecystitis), and dilation of the biliary tree (choledocholithiasis). However, it is not helpful in excluding stones in the common bile duct; the false-negative rate is high unless the bile duct is markedly dilated. Oral cholecystography may identify stones that are not picked up by ultrasonography.

4. What is the best test to order when acute cholecystitis is suspected?

When the clinical findings are not definitive, hepatobiliary scintigraphy (HIDA scan) is useful in the diagnosis of acute cholecystitis. After a 2-hour fast, the patient is given a radiolabeled agent, which is taken up by the liver and excreted into the biliary system. Images of the gallbladder, common bile duct, and small bowel should appear within 45 minutes. Failure to image the gallbladder by 90 minutes is strongly suggestive of cystic duct obstruction. False-positive scans may result from prolonged fasting or in the presence of total parenteral nutrition (TPN). The false-negative rate of this test is < 5%.

5. Can cholecystitis develop without gallbladder stones?

Acalculous cholecystitis accounts for 5–10% of the patients presenting with acute cholecystitis. It usually occurs in the setting of major surgery, critical illness, intensive trauma, or burn-related injury. Hypotension and sympathetic vasoconstriction may predispose patients to ischemic injury. The patients are predominantly men older than 50 years. Many are on TPN. The pathogenesis probably involves a combination of stasis, chemical inflammation, and ischemia. Acalculous cholecystitis is a more fulminant disorder than calculus cholecystitis, possibly because the patients are older and sicker.

6. Is fatty food intolerance related to gallstone disease?

It is commonly believed that fatty foods cause increased biliary pain; however, studies using test meals in a blinded fashion have shown no correlation between fat content and symptoms. In addition, gallbladder contractility does not change significantly when fatty or nonfatty foods are ingested. Symptoms such as belching, bloating, and fatty food intolerance are not statistically related to gallstones.

7. A 49-year-old obese woman on estrogen replacement therapy has gallstones. What is the most likely composition of the stones?

In the United States, 80% of gallstones are composed of cholesterol. Cholesterol stones are extremely common and occur more frequently in women and with advancing age. By age 75 years, 20% of men and 35% of women have gallstones.

8. List the risk factors for cholesterol gallstones.

Age: ≥ 50 years	Obesity: > 20% above ideal body
Gender: female	Ethnic group: Native American
Diet: high fat	Pregnancy
Drugs: clofibrate, oral estrogens	Rapid weight loss
Genetics: siblings	TPN

9. What is biliary sludge?

Biochemically, sludge is composed of calcium bilirubinate and cholesterol monohydrate crystals embedded within a mucous gel. It has been called by many names including bile gravel, microcrystal disease, microlithes, and bile sand. Sludge is best diagnosed by microscopic examination of a fresh sample of gallbladder bile; it can be seen ultrasonographically as echogenic material that layers in the dependent portion of the gallbladder. In certain conditions, sludge is a risk factor for the subsequent development of cholelithiasis. It is quite common in patients receiving prolonged TPN. By 4–6 weeks, 50% of TPN recipients usually have sludge, and after 6 weeks, its appearance is universal. Significantly, the reinstitution of oral feedings results in sludge resolution. Ceftriaxone also may contribute to sludge formation because it precipitates as a calcium salt.

10. A 30-year-old African-American man with sickle cell anemia has gallstones. What type of gallstone is the patient most likely to have?

The patient most likely has pigment stones, which are formed in the presence of unconjugated bilirubin and precipitate with calcium to form calcium bilirubinate stones. Amounts of unconjugated bilirubin are increased in hemolytic anemia and cirrhosis. Pigment stones come in two varieties: brown and black. Black stones are radiopaque and hard, whereas brown stones are soft and radiolucent. Brown stones are common in Asia as a result of infections by bacteria and parasites that deconjugate bilirubin.

11. What is the current recommendation for patients with an incidental finding of gallstones?

Most patients with gallstones (60–80%) are asymptomatic. Several studies have followed patients with initially asymptomatic stones and recorded the incidence of symptoms or complications. In a study of 123 faculty members of the University of Michigan who were followed for 24 years, the rate of development of biliary pain was 1.3% per year. At 20 years of follow-up, only 18% were symptomatic. Other studies have confirmed the development of symptoms at 1–2% per year. These studies show that most patients with gallstones have a benign course; therefore, prophylactic therapy is not warranted. In certain subsets of patients, it may be prudent to make exceptions, including children with gallstones, patients with sickle cell disease and gallstones, and morbidly obese patients. In the last group, cholecystectomy is recommended at the time of other abdominal surgery if indicated.

12. After symptoms develop, does the natural history of gallstones change?

After a patient develops biliary pain, recurrent attacks are likely, although ≤ 30% of patients have no further episodes. The rate of recurrence may be as high as 30–50% per year in the first few years. Acute complications in patients who present with biliary pain occur at a rate of approximately 1.0–1.5% per year.

13. What are Charcot's triad and Reynolds' pentad?

Stones within the common bile duct are usually associated with infected bile, and cholangitis results if obstruction occurs. **Charcot's triad** consists of upper abdominal pain, fever secondary to bacteremia, and jaundice from extrahepatic obstruction. **Reynolds' pentad** is the addition of hypotension and mental confusion in more severe suppurative cases. The most common organisms include *Escherichia coli*, *Klebsiella* species, *Pseudomonas* species, enterococci, and anaerobes.

14. Which tests provide the strongest clues to the presence of a common duct stone?

Serial liver function tests, including assessment of direct bilirubin, transaminases, and alkaline phosphatase, provide the strongest evidence for or against the diagnosis of choledocholithiasis. When a stone obstructs the duct, the transaminases increase abruptly, occasionally to very high levels. Within a few hours, they begin to decrease (even if the obstruction persists), and the levels of direct bilirubin and alkaline phosphatase increase at a moderate pace. When the obstruction is alleviated (by passage, movement of the stone back into the duct, or removal), all abnormalities rapidly return toward normal. Cholecystitis is associated with only minimal changes in liver function tests. In hepatitis, the liver may be tender, but pain is not a common feature, and liver function tests do not fluctuate dramatically. Although the finding of a dilated common duct on ultrasound or computed tomographic (CT) scan suggest biliary pathology, both modalities often fail to find common duct stones, especially when the duct is of normal caliber. Neither test is required to make or act on the diagnosis of common bile duct stone. If the clinical features and liver function tests suggest biliary obstruction, endoscopic retrograde cholangiopancreatography (ERCP) should be performed for diagnosis and treatment.

15. What is the most common cause of pancreatitis in nondrinkers?

Gallstone-related (biliary) pancreatitis is the most frequent type in nondrinkers. It typically occurs in patients with smaller rather than larger stones, presumably because small stones are able to migrate to the end of the bile duct at its junction with the pancreatic duct. The mechanisms by which the stones cause pancreatitis are unclear. Biliary sludge and crystals are also associated with pancreatitis. Biliary sludge occurs when cholesterol or calcium bilirubinate precipitates in bile and may be a precursor to gallstone formation. Studies have shown that after gallstones and alcohol, biliary sludge is the third most common cause of acute pancreatitis. Sphincter of Oddi dysfunction, pancreas divisum, and unsuspected stones are less common causes of pancreatitis. Ceftriaxone, a third-generation cephalosporin, has been implicated as a cause of biliary sludge; it may precipitate with calcium to form crystals and sludge. The crystals and sludge dissolve when the drug is discontinued; thus, symptoms rarely require surgical intervention.

16. What percentage of patients with pancreatitis secondary to gallstones will pass the gallstone?

It is postulated that the lodging of a gallstone at the duodenal papilla is the precipitant of an attack of acute gallstone pancreatitis. In approximately 80–90% of patients with gallstone pancreatitis, the stone will pass without intervention.

17. What is the risk of cholelithiasis during pregnancy?

The risk is related to both number and frequency of pregnancies. For example, a woman who has four pregnancies before age 25 years has a 4–12-fold increased risk of cholesterol cholelithiasis. Certain changes in hepatobiliary physiology during pregnancy promote gallstone formation. This period is characterized by stimulation of cholesterol synthesis, decreased secretion of the bile acids, and hypomotility of the gallbladder.

18. What is the appropriate treatment for gallstones in diabetic patients?

Early autopsy studies purported to show an increased risk for gallstones in diabetic patients, but the studies were not controlled for confounding risk factors such as obesity and hyperlipidemia, disorders that are common in the diabetic population. Studies that controlled for these factors have not shown an increased risk of gallstone formation. In addition, previous studies appeared to show significantly greater morbidity and mortality for cholecystectomy in diabetic patients than in the general population. More recent data indicate that biliary surgery in diabetic patients is not associated with increased morbidity and mortality. Therefore, diabetic patients should be managed no differently from other patients.

19. What is the role of ERCP in acute gallstone pancreatitis?

A recent study found that ERCP with papillotomy performed within 24 hours of the onset of symptoms resulted in a decrease in incidence of biliary sepsis. There was no change in mortality or other complications, such as pseudocyst. ERCP is indicated in episodes of gallstone pancreatitis that are deemed to be severe, that do not resolve with conservative measures, or that are associated with possible acute cholangitis.

20. What are the causes of acute cholecystitis in immunocompromised patients?

Cytomegalovirus and cryptosporidia can infect the biliary system and produce symptoms in patients with AIDS or after bone marrow transplantation.

21. What are the manifestations of the bile duct injury?

Bile duct injury leads to two clinical manifestations: bile leakage into the peritoneum, with resulting bile peritonitis and abdominal pain, and biliary obstruction caused by partial or complete hepatic or common duct ligation or to late-onset stricture. Patients may present 3–7 days after surgery with fever, abdominal pain, anorexia, nausea, jaundice, ileus, and ascites. Cholescintography with 99m technetium-1DA may be used to diagnose bile leakage and may show activity in the right paracolic gutter. ERCP can be used for diagnosis as well as treatment (stricture dilation, stent placement). Surgical repair may be necessary in some patients.

22. What is the role of magnetic resonance cholangiopancreatography (MRCP)?

MRCP represents a noninvasive method of obtaining cholangiography and pancreatography. It is based on imaging capabilities of MR combined with powerful computers, which can subtract unwanted portions of the image and reconstruct them in three dimensions. It can be performed without administration of contrast agents and with any degree of obstruction. There are several disadvantages, however: MRCP cannot currently distinguish stones from tissues, and there is no potential for interventions such as biopsy or brushings.

A number of studies have compared MRCP with ERCP. In general, the correlation of findings has been high. However, in most cases, MRCP ultimately was an additional procedure and did not replace ERCP, resulting in additional cost rather than more efficient evaluation.

23. Which procedure is associated with more complications, laparoscopic or open cholecystectomy?

Laparoscopic cholecystectomy. Open cholecystectomy is one of the safest surgical procedures, with mortality rates of $< 1\%$, although the rate increases with age and for urgent procedures. The incidence of bile duct injury is 0.1–0.2%. Recovery time after open cholecystectomy may take months because of the extensive abdominal incision. Laparoscopic cholecystectomy has gained popularity since its introduction in 1989. The advantages include minimal incisions, decreased postoperative pain, improved recovery time with discharge from the hospital in 1–2 days, and unrestricted activity at 8 days. The disadvantages of laparoscopic cholecystectomy include longer anesthesia time and an increased rate of complications, which is likely to improve as experience with the procedure increases. The rate of bile duct injury is approximately 0.5%; 5% of patients require conversion to open cholecystectomy.

24. What are the contraindications to laparoscopic cholecystectomy?

Contraindications to laparoscopic cholecystectomy include generalized peritonitis, severe acute pancreatitis, cirrhosis with portal hypertension, unresponsive coagulopathy, and carcinoma of the gallbladder. Pregnancy in the third trimester is a contraindication because of potential injury to the uterus. Patients with chronic obstructive pulmonary disease need to be monitored carefully because the CO_2 used to insufflate the abdominal cavity may cause hypercarbia and acidosis. Obesity is generally not a problem unless the abdominal wall is so large that the instruments cannot reach the gallbladder.

25. What are alternatives to surgery for acute and chronic cholecystitis?

Patients with acute cholecystitis who are high risk for surgery can often be managed initially by percutaneous drainage, usually under ultrasound guidance. For patients in need of a longer term solution, cannulation of the cystic duct at ERCP can be done fairly predictably, and stents or nasobiliary tubes can be passed into the gallbladder with resolution of cholecystitis in most cases. This procedure is indicated in high-risk patients in whom an operation is to be avoided (e.g., before liver transplantation). Elective dissolution of gallbladder stones with a nasobiliary tube also has received limited application.

26. What is the treatment for gallstones during pregnancy, and what are its complications?

Initial management is conservative medical treatment with intravenous fluids, bowel rest, and antibiotics. Surgical intervention is needed after failure of conservative medical treatment in patients with recurrent episodes of biliary colic and complications of cholecystitis, choledocholithiasis, and pancreatitis. Cholecystectomy is standard of care for surgical treatment of gallstone disease. The second trimester is the best time because of completion of fetal organogenesis; the presence of a relatively small uterus, allowing a technically easier operation; and a lower rate of spontaneous abortion. ERCP with biliary sphincterotomy may also be used safely to treat choledocholithiasis and gallstone pancreatitis in pregnant women if proper precautions are implemented.

27. What are the risk factors for gallbladder cancer?

The incidence of gallbladder cancer in the United States is low even though it is the most common biliary tract malignancy and the fifth most common cancer of the gastrointestinal tract. The incidence of gallbladder cancer is increasing, however, with approximately 6000–7000 new case per year. Factors that increase risk are:

Gallstones (threefold increase in cancer and stronger among certain ethnic groups)
Obesity
Reproductive and hormonal factors
Certain dietary factors
Biliary tract infections
Cholecystitis
Family history of gallbladder cancer
Porcelain gallbladder
Choledochal cyst
Gallbladder polyps

Despite a definite association with gallstones (70–90% of patients with gallbladder cancer have gallstones), the incidence of gallbladder cancer in patients with gallstones is low (0.5–3.0%), and a causal role has not been proven. In general, cholecystectomy is not recommended for the prevention of gallbladder carcinoma with the possible exception of very large stones (> 3 cm).

28. What is a "porcelain gallbladder"?

This term originated because of the intramural calcifications of the gallbladder wall that made it visible on plain film of the abdomen and, later, CT. Carcinoma is a late complication of this condition (about 20% of cases). Prophylactic cholecystectomy is indicated.

BIBLIOGRAPHY

1. Ahrendt S, Nakeeb A, Pitt H: Liver tumors. Clin Liver Dis 5:191–218, 2001.
2. Ahuja V, Garg PK, Kumar, et al: Presence of white bile associated with lower survival in malignant biliary obstruction. Gastrointest Endosc 55:186–191, 2002.
3. Aucott JN, Cooper GS, Bloom AD, et al: Management of gallstones in diabetic patients. Arch Intern Med 153:1053–1058, 1993.
4. Borum ML: Hepatobiliary diseases in women. Med Clin North Am 82:51–75, 1998.
5. Custis K, Brown C, El Younis C: Hepatobiliary disease. Clin Fam Practice 2:141–154, 2000.
6. Fan ST, Lai ECS, Mok FPT, et al: Early treatment of acute biliary pancreatitis by endoscopic papillotomy. N Engl J Med 328:228–232, 1993.
7. Fenster LF, Lonborg R, Thirlby RC, Traverso LW: What symptoms does cholecystectomy cure? Insights from an outcomes measurement project and review of the literature. Am J Surg 169:533–538, 1995.
8. Fulcher A: MRCP and ERCP in the diagnosis of common bile duct stones. Gastrointest Endosc 56:S175–S177, 2002.
9. Kalloo A, Kantsevoy S: Gallstones and biliary diseases. Prim Care Clin Office Practice 28:591–606, 2001.
10. Ko CW: Epidemiology and natural history of common bile stones and prediction of disease. Gastrointest Endosc 56:S165–S169, 2002.
11. Michaud D: The epidemiology of pancreatic, gallbladder, and other biliary tract cancers. Gastrointest Endosc 56:S195–S200, 2002.
12. Motohara T, Semelka RC, Bader TR: MR cholangiopancreatography. Radiol Clin North Am 41:89–96, 2003.
13. Nash JA, Cohen SA: Gallbladder and biliary tract disease in AIDS. Gastroenterol Clin North Am 26:323–335, 1997.
14. Opatrny L: Porcelain gallbladder. Can Med Assoc J 166:933, 2002.
15. Siegel JH, Kasmin FE: Biliary tract diseases in the elderly: Management and outcomes. Gut 41:433–435, 1997.
16. Schwesinger WH, Diehl AK: Changing indications for laparoscopic cholecystectomy. Stones without symptoms and symptoms without stones. Surg Clin North Am 76:493–504, 1996.

17. Sheth S: Primary gallbladder cancer: Recognition of risk factors and the role of prophylactic cholecys-tectomy. Am J Gastroenterol 95:1402–1410, 2000.
18. Sivak M: EUS for bile duct stones: How does it compare with ERCP? Gastrointest Endosc 56:S175–S177, 2002.
19. Soto JA, Barish MA, Yucel EK, et al: Magnetic resonance cholangiography comparison with endoscopic retrograde cholangiopancreatography. Gastroenterology 110:589–597, 1996.
20. Yates M, Baron T: Pregnancy and liver disease. Clin Liver Dis 3:131–146, 1999.

44. ENDOSCOPY: INDICATIONS AND OUTCOMES

Stephen E. Steinberg, M.D.

1. What is the diagnostic accuracy of colonoscopy, double-contrast barium enema (DCBE), and virtual colonoscopy?

The sensitivity of colonoscopy varies with the size of the lesion. Colonoscopy has a detection rate $> 95\%$ for lesions larger than 1.0 cm, 85–90% for lesions 0.5–1.0 cm, and 70–80% for lesions smaller than 0.5 cm in diameter. DCBE detects 50–80% for polyps < 1 cm, 70–90% for polyps > 1 cm, and 55–85% for Dukes' stage A and B cancers. DCBE, although it has a lower sensitivity than colonoscopy, is sufficient to detect the majority of clinically important lesions. Virtual colonoscopy is still finding its niche. Sensitivities for detecting polyps are $> 90\%$ for polyps larger than 1.0 cm and 70–80% for polyps smaller than 1.0 cm.[4,6,7] Although the accuracy of virtual colonoscopy is comparable to "standard" colonoscopy, its role in colon cancer screening has yet to be determined. Insensitivity for all of these procedures is mainly related to inadequate visualization caused by poor bowel preparation or cleansing.

2. Distinguish between colonoscopy for screening and colonoscopy for surveillance.

Screening involves the search for a finding (malignant or premalignant lesion) in a group of **asymptomatic** individuals based on some demographic feature (e.g., age). Surveillance colonoscopy is performed repeatedly at intervals in individuals with a known risk (e.g., ulcerative colitis, previous polyp, or colon cancer).

3. Which patients fall into the category of increased risk when considering screening for colorectal cancer (CRC)?

All men and women aged 50 years and older should be considered for screening in the category of average risk. Patients at increased risk include those who have the following:

- A personal history of CRC or adenomatous polyps
- A family history in one or more first-degree relatives (parents, brothers, sisters, or children) of CRC or adenomatous polyps
- A family history of multiple cancers involving the breast, ovary, uterus, and other organs
- A personal history of inflammatory bowel disease, such as ulcerative colitis or Crohn's disease

4. What are the recommendations for CRC screening in asymptomatic patients older than 50 years at average risk (i.e., no family history of colorectal cancer or history of polyps)?

There are now several recommendations:

1. **Fecal occult blood test (FOBT)** annually and flexible sigmoidoscopy every 3–5 years. With the above combination screening tests, one can achieve 50% risk reduction in preventing cancer development. If the FOBT result is positive or adenomatous polyps are found on sigmoi-

doscopy, a colonoscopy is recommended to assess the proximal colon. This is the strategy that has been most intensely studied.

2. **Colonoscopy.** No studies have evaluated whether screening colonoscopy alone reduces the incidence or mortality from CRC in people at average risk of the disease. Colonoscopy has been shown to reduce the incidence of CRC in a cohort of people with adenomatous polyps. Because colonoscopy permits visualization of the entire colon directly, detection and removal of polyps, and biopsy of cancers throughout the colon, it can be considered for screening average-risk individuals. An interval of 10 years was chosen for asymptomatic, average-risk people because of strong direct evidence that few clinically important lesions are missed by this examination and there is a low incidence of advanced lesions on follow-up colonoscopy. Attention in the lay media has made this the procedure of choice among patients.

3. **DCBE.** No studies have evaluated whether screening DCBE alone reduces the incidence or mortality from CRC in people at average risk of the disease. It allows visualization of the entire colon, although small polyps may be missed. Adding flexible sigmoidoscopy to DCBE increases sensitivity but is also more difficult to accomplish. It is suggested that this be performed every 5–10 years.

4. **Virtual colonoscopy** offers the potential for visualizing the entire colon with accuracy approaching that of colonoscopy. It is still evolving as a technology, and no studies have yet defined its role in screening

Screening tests should be continued until patients reach age 80 years because further screening is not cost effective.

5. What is the recommended surveillance interval after colonoscopic removal of a few benign adenomatous polyps?

According to data from the National Polyps Study, after an initial high-quality colonoscopy during which all synchronous adenomas are removed, a follow-up colonoscopy should be performed in 1–2 years. The purpose of this surveillance is to check for adenomas that may have been missed on the first colonoscopy (synchronous lesions) or that may have formed in the interim (metachronous lesions). If this 1- to 2-year examination is unremarkable, the subsequent intervals may be extended to 5 years. Patients with large sessile adenomas should have a subsequent colonoscopy at 3–6 months to confirm complete removal. In general, it takes 3–6 years for a polyp to grow to visibility and another 4–6 years for the small proportion that will become malignant to do so; therefore, a relatively long surveillance window is possible.

6. When should colonoscopy be performed instead of a DCBE or virtual colonoscopy?

Colonoscopy is the preferred method for evaluation of symptoms of hematochezia, surveillance after resection of colon cancer or polyps, and surveillance of inflammatory bowel disease. For these indications, the ability to perform hemostasis therapy, obtain biopsies, and remove polyps during colonoscopy outweighs the cost savings of the purely diagnostic DCBE and of virtual colonoscopy. Although colonoscopy has become the gold standard for colon cancer screening, DCBE, combined with flexible sigmoidoscopy, represents an effective strategy. The role of virtual colonoscopy for colon cancer screening is currently being evaluated.

7. What are the usual indications for esophagogastroduodenoscopy (EGD)?

EGD is usually indicated to evaluate upper abdominal symptoms that have not responded to an appropriate trial of therapy or that are associated with anorexia and weight loss, complaints of dysphagia or odynophagia, or persistent nausea and vomiting. Additionally, EGD is indicated to biopsy lesions detected by radiographs, treat upper gastrointestinal (GI) bleeding, and assess mucosal injury after ingestion of a corrosive agent.

8. How effective is endoscopic therapy of bleeding peptic ulcers?

Endoscopic therapy with thermal probe, bipolar electrical probe, or epinephrine injection induces acute hemostasis in an actively bleeding peptic ulcer in approximately 90% of patients.

Compared with conservative medical therapy, endoscopic hemostasis significantly reduces the cost of hospitalization, need for transfusions, and requirement for emergency surgery.

9. What are the advantages of early upper endoscopy for acute GI bleeding?

In addition to controlling hemorrhage in many situations, early endoscopy can be used to assess the risk of ongoing or additional bleeding. This assessment may allow a decision for early discharge in patients with a Mallory-Weiss tear (low risk of rebleed), esophagitis, or low-risk ulcer disease; it also affects decisions about which patients need monitoring in an intensive care setting and for how long.

10. When should EGD be performed for a complaint of bright red blood per rectum (BRBPR)?

Melena, or black, tarry stools and "coffee grounds," results from bleeding in the stomach or proximal small bowel. In patients with massive upper GI bleeding, there may not be enough time (or acid) for the conversion to melena because of rapid intestinal transit. Any patient who is hemodynamically unstable or who has an uncertain source of BRBPR should undergo upper endoscopy. A nasogastric tube, even if it returns bile, does not exclude an upper GI source.

11. Why is EGD essential in the evaluation of patients who may have swallowed a corrosive substance?

EGD offers a better assessment of the extent and severity of the chemical burn than the history and physical examination or an upper GI barium radiograph and thus allows better therapeutic decisions. Minor mucosal burns may be managed conservatively. Severe mucosal burns should prompt consideration of urgent surgical resection before perforation develops. Small-caliber, flexible endoscopes do not increase the risk of perforation.

12. What are the usual indications for endoscopic retrograde cholangiopancreatography (ERCP)?

ERCP is usually indicated to evaluate and treat symptoms that suggest disorders of the biliary system and pancreas. Examples include jaundice that is possibly obstructive; cholangitis; acute or recurrent pancreatitis; recurrent upper abdominal pain associated with transient liver function test abnormalities; and, less commonly, steatorrhea. Specific disorders that may be diagnosed and treated by ERCP include choledocholithiasis, benign or malignant bile duct stricture, bile duct leak, pancreatic pseudocyst, and pancreatic duct disruption.

13. What is the role of ERCP in suspected acute cholangitis?

Acute cholangitis is caused by infection in the setting of biliary obstruction from a gallstone or, less often, a stricture. When severe, it is associated with a high mortality rate ($> 30\%$), whether managed conservatively or surgically. Endoscopic drainage is safe and reduces mortality. It should be used as early as possible in the course of the disease.

14. What is the role of ERCP in the evaluation of recurrent acute pancreatitis?

In approximately 30% of patients with recurrent pancreatitis of uncertain cause, ERCP yields an explanation. Findings include previously unsuspected common duct stones; anatomic abnormalities (pancreas divisum, choledochocele); sphincter of Oddi dysfunction; and, rarely, pancreatic malignancy.

15. When is magnetic resonance cholangiopancreatography (MRCP) preferable to ERCP in the evaluation of biliary tract disease?

MRCP has been shown to have a high degree of accuracy in defining the anatomy of the pancreatobiliary system and for identifying abnormalities (e.g., stones). Its noninvasive nature makes it a useful test to exclude disease in patients who are unable to undergo ECRP (e.g., some patients with Billroth II anatomy) or those in whom the index of suspicion is low and disease is to be excluded. The ability to perform therapeutic intervention makes ERCP the preferred test when the clinical data make it likely that therapy will be necessary. "Diagnostic" ERCP should be relatively infrequent and limited to situations in which the radiologic detail provided by ERCP is important (e.g., the identification of the subtle changes of primary sclerosing cholangitis). With good patient selection, only 10–15% of ERCPs should turn out to be "diagnostic."

16. What are the indications for placement of a percutaneous endoscopic gastrostomy (PEG) tube?

A PEG tube should be considered when a patient with a functional GI tract is not expected to ingest orally for 3 or more weeks. Examples include patients with altered mental status after neurologic injury or trauma, oropharyngeal dysphagia caused by neurologic injury, and oropharyngeal and esophageal obstruction during treatment of oropharyngeal and esophageal tumors. In addition, a PEG tube provides effective decompression for patients with chronic bowel obstruction caused by peritoneal carcinomatosis.

17. Describe the management of suspected esophageal foreign body impactions.

If the suspected foreign body is radiopaque, it is helpful to search for it with a plain radiograph of the neck and chest. Endoscopy is the primary modality for evaluation and removal. The prior performance of a barium study makes endoscopy more difficult and is contraindicated. Meat tenderizer may be harmful to the esophagus and should be avoided. For sharp objects (e.g., chicken or fish bones) lodged near the cricopharangeus, rigid endoscopy under general anesthesia is often the safest option.

18. When is an endoscopic ultrasound (EUS) helpful in esophageal malignancy?

EUS detects mediastinal lymph node involvement with an accuracy of 70–80%, whereas computed tomography (CT) detects only 20–50% of such lesions. EUS with fine-needle aspirate (FNA) combined with CT provides the most sensitive approach to defining malignant invasion into the diaphragm, aorta, and pericardium. Mounting data suggest that EUS examinations should be performed in all candidates for curative resection of esophageal carcinoma. EUS does not accurately distinguish benign from malignant strictures, so it is not useful in the primary diagnosis of esophageal carcinoma.

19. How may endoscopy help palliate an unresectable esophageal cancer?

When surgical resection is not possible, several options are available, most of which require endoscopic manipulation. These include:

    Metal stent placement
    Chemical injection (i.e., ethanol polidocanol, sodium morrhuate)
    Laser treatment (Nd:YAG)
    Esophageal dilation
    Photodynamic therapy
    Intracavitary irradiation
    Thermal or bipolar electrocoagulation

20. How does endoscopic management of obstructive biliary tract lesions compare with surgical or percutaneous palliation?

The endoscopic placement of biliary stents is safer and more effective than percutaneous placement of similar stents and allows shorter hospital stays than surgical decompression. Surgery has been preferred when the tumor threatens to obstruct the bowel, although endoscopic techniques are now available to stent bowel lesions as well.

21. What are the alternatives for the management of pseudocysts?

Endoscopic drainage of pseudocysts has been shown to be as effective as traditionally preferred surgical drainages (i.e., cystogastrostomy, cystoduodenostomy, cystojejunostomy) and has, in general, less morbidity and fewer complications. When the pseudocyst is immediately adjacent to the stomach or duodenum and bulges into the lumen or communicates with pancreatic duct, endoscopic drainage can be performed by placing a stent (or stents) into the pseudocyst to drain cystic fluid into GI tract. The limiting factor is the favorable anatomic relationship. CT- or ultrasound-guided drainage has been accompanied with relatively high recurrence rates. For more complicated pancreatic collections (e.g., infected pseudocysts, pancreatic necrosis), a combined approach can often avoid the need for surgical intervention.

22. What is the primary indication for small bowel enteroscopy?
When a patient has recurrent bleeding of obscure origin (i.e., failure to identify the source of bleeding by both EGD and colonoscopy), push enteroscopy may be indicated. The 240-cm endoscope can reach as far as 40–60 cm beyond the ligament of Treitz. It has a success rate of up to 50% in identifying the source of bleeding. Most cases result from arteriovenous malformations.

23. What are the indications for wireless video capsule enteroscopy?
Capsule endoscopy is a novel technology that allows visualization of areas not easily reachable by conventional endoscopy (e.g., the small bowel). In addition, its high magnification (8:1) provides unique views of the small bowel mucosa. Studies are currently in progress to define the role of this technology. Current indications are:

- The evaluation of occult GI bleeding in the absence of findings by conventional endoscopy
- The evaluation of the extent and severity of disorders primarily affecting the small bowel (e.g., Crohn's disease and celiac disease)
- Identifying small bowel tumors and premalignant conditions (Gardener's syndrome)
- The evaluation of diarrheal and malabsortive disorders

BIBLIOGRAPHY

1. Breen N, Wagener DK, Brown ML, et al: Progress in cancer screening over a decade: Results of cancer screening from the 1987, 1992, and 1998 National Health Interview Surveys. J Natl Cancer Inst 93:1704–1713, 2001.
2. Cohen, S, Bacon, BR, Berlin, JA, et al: National Institutes of Health state-of-the-science conference statement: ERCP for diagnosis and therapy, January 14–16, 2002. Gastrointest Endosc 56:803, 2002.
3. Fenlon HM, Nunes DP, Schroy PC 3rd, et al: A comparison of virtual and conventional colonoscopy for the detection of colorectal polyps. N Engl J Med 341:1496–1503, 1999.
4. Jemal A, Murray T, Samuels A, et al: Cancer statistics, 2003. CA Cancer J Clin 53:5–26, 2003.
5. Jiranek GC, Kozarek RA: A cost-effective approach to the patient with peptic ulcer bleeding. Surg Clin North Am 76:83–103, 1996.
6. Kobayashi K, Cooper GS, Chak A, et al: A prospective evaluation of outcome in patients referred for PEG placement. Gastrointest Endosc 55:500, 2002.
7. Scapa E, Jacob H, Lewkowicz S, et al: Initial experience of wireless-capsule endoscopy for evaluating occult gastrointestinal bleeding and suspected small bowel pathology. Am J Gastroenterol 97:2776–2779, 2002.
8. Troisi RJ, Freedman AN, Devesa SS: Incidence of colorectal carcinoma in the U.S.: An update of trends by gender, race, age, subsite, and stage, 1975–1994. Cancer 85:1670, 1999.
9. Tytgat GN (ed): Precancerous Conditions and Endoscopic Screening. Gastrointestinal and Endoscopy Clinics of North America, vol. 7, no. 1. Philadelphia, W.B. Saunders, 1997.
10. Vidyarthi G, Steinberg SE: Endoscopic management of pancreatic pseudocysts. Surg Clin North Am 81:405–411, 2001.
11. Yamada T, Alpers DH, Laine L (eds): Textbook of Gastroenterology, 4th ed. Philadelphia, Lippincott Williams & Wilkins, 2003.

VII. Gender-Specific Care

45. BREAST MASSES AND PAIN

Anne Kastor, M.D.

1. What is the differential diagnosis of a palpable breast mass?

Fibroadenomas are benign masses that occur most commonly among women in their teens and 20s. They are usually firm, rubbery, and mobile with clearly demarcated edges. Even though fibroadenomas are benign, they do confer an increased risk of future breast cancer.

Cysts are benign masses that usually occur in women in their late 30s and 40s. They are usually smooth and mobile with well-demarcated edges. They may feel soft or taut, depending on how much fluid they contain and how rapidly it accumulated.

Fibrocystic changes occur normally as women approach menopause. They often present as rubbery or firm plaques, most commonly in the upper, outer quadrants, with areas of granularity or individual cysts. The changes are usually present in both breasts.

Masses suggestive of **malignancy** are hard, irregular, immobile, fixed to skin or deep fascial attachments, have indistinct borders, or have grown. Skin dimpling, nipple retraction, bloody nipple discharge, and palpably enlarged lymph nodes are also suspicious for malignancy. Although most breast cancers are nontender, the presence of pain does not rule out malignancy.

2. How good are clinicians at distinguishing benign from malignant breast masses?

Studies among experienced clinicians report correct diagnoses in 58–85% of cases. These numbers increase to 90% when the examiner determines the mass to be "clearly benign" or "clearly malignant." However, given the risk of false negatives, almost all palpable masses require additional diagnostic work-up.

3. How should a palpable breast mass be evaluated?

Although the majority of breast masses are benign, all palpable breast masses must be evaluated carefully. The work-up will depend on the patient's age and the characteristics of the mass itself. Although risk factors for breast cancer should be elicited, they should not influence the diagnostic work-up. Most breast cancers occur in women whose only risk factor is age. A breast mass in a woman with no family or personal history of breast cancer should be pursued as aggressively as a mass in a high-risk woman. The evaluation may include:
- Mammography
- Ultrasonography
- Fine needle aspiration (FNA)
- Core needle biopsy
- Open biopsy (lumpectomy)

4. Can any breast masses be followed clinically?

Tender, mobile, clearly demarcated lumps in the breast of a young woman in the luteal phase of her menstrual cycle can be reevaluated during the first week after her next menstrual period. If the mass is still present, additional work-up is required.

5. When should mammography be used in the evaluation of a palpable breast mass?

In women 35 years old and younger, mammography has limited utility. One retrospective analysis of 1908 women in this age group showed that the mammogram did not contribute to the diagnostic work-up. Of the 23 invasive cancers diagnosed, all were palpable and were diagnosed by FNA (i.e., all were diagnosed by means other than the mammogram).

Mammography should be a routine part of the evaluation of women older than 35 years. However, normal mammograms do not rule out malignancy and must be interpreted in the context of other findings.

6. What role does ultrasound play in the evaluation of a palpable breast mass?

Until recently, breast ultrasound was used only to evaluate nonpalpable mammographic abnormalities. Recent technologic advances allow experienced operators to differentiate cystic from solid or mixed cystic and solid masses.

7. What is the role of FNA in evaluation of a palpable breast mass?

FNA is an office-based procedure that can be both diagnostic and therapeutic. Aspiration may result in one of four results:

- Aspiration of nonbloody fluid and disappearance of the mass. These findings confirm the diagnosis of a cyst. The fluid can be discarded. The patient should be reassured and reexamined in 4–6 weeks to ensure the mass has not reappeared.
- Aspiration of nonbloody fluid without disappearance of the mass. The fluid should be sent for cytology and the mass removed.
- Aspiration of bloody fluid with or without disappearance of the mass. The fluid should be sent for cytology. If the mass remains, lumpectomy may be indicated.
- No fluid aspirated. The mass is solid. Any aspirated material should be sent for cytology and the mass removed.

8. What is the triple test?

The triple test refers to the combination of a clinical breast examination, mammogram, and FNA. Recently, ultrasound has begun replacing the FNA. When all three tests results suggest a benign etiology (a "negative triple test") the likelihood of malignancy is < 1% and further evaluation is unnecessary.

9. When is a breast biopsy indicated?

A biopsy should be performed whenever the diagnosis is in question (i.e., the mass is not clearly cystic by FNA or ultrasound or does not meet the criteria for a negative triple test). A core needle or open biopsy may be performed. An open biopsy (lumpectomy) should remove the entire mass with surrounding tissue so that further surgery will not be required should the mass be malignant.

10. What causes breast pain or tenderness?

- **Cyclic mastalgia** (premenstrual breast tenderness) may last for 2 days to 2 weeks per month. Women frequently describe this pain as bilateral aching or burning pain that may radiate to the shoulder.
- **Mastitis,** a bacterial infection that occurs most commonly in the lactating breast
- **Breast abscess**
- **Inflammatory breast cancer**
- **Breast masses,** including cysts, fibroadenomas, and malignancies

11. What treatments are useful in relieving cyclic mastalgia?

- Firm brassiere support
- Local heat application

- Nonsteroidal anti-inflammatory drugs (NSAIDs)
- Evening primrose oil
- Oral contraceptives
- Danazol—prescribed only in severe cases due to its many side effects
- Abstinence from caffeine—many women report it reduces their symptoms

12. What causes mastitis? How is it treated?

Staphylococci and anaerobic organisms (peptostreptococci) are the usual pathogens. It is important for women to continue to empty the breast completely even though it is painful. A breast pump may be helpful. Improvement should be noted in 24–48 hours after starting an oral penicillin derivative. If symptoms worsen, a breast abscess, which requires incision and drainage, should be suspected.

13. What clue suggests inflammatory breast carcinoma as opposed to infection?

Erythema completely surrounding the areola or symptoms of mastitis in a nonlactating breast suggests malignancy and mandates a rapid evaluation.

BIBLIOGRAPHY

1. Ciatto S, Carriaggi P, Bulgaresi P: The value of routine cytologic examination for breast cysts fluids. Acta Cytol 31:301–304, 1987.
2. Dennis MA, Parker SH, Klaus AJ, et al: Breast biopsy avoidance: The value of normal mammograms and normal sonograms in the setting of palpable lumps. Radiology 219:186–191, 2001.
3. Dupont W, Page DL, Parl FF, et al: Long-term risk of breast cancer in women with fibroadenoma. N Engl J Med 331:10–15, 1994.
3. Hindle WH, Davis L, Wright D: Clinical value of mammography for symptomatic women 35 years of age and younger. Am J Obstet Gynecol 180:1484–1490, 1999.
4. Reinikainen HT, Rissanen TJ, Piippo UK, Paivansalo MJ: Contribution of ultrasonography and fine-needle aspiration cytology to the differential diagnosis of palpable solid breast lesion. Acta Radiol 40:383–389, 1999.
5. Soo M, Rosen EL, Baker JA, et al: Negative predictive value of sonography with mammography in patients with palpable breast lesions. AJR Am J Roentgenol 177:1167–1170, 2001.
7. Steering Committee on Clinical Practice Guidelines for the Care and Treatment of Breast Cancer: The palpable breast lump: Information and recommendations to assist decision-making when a breast lump is detected. Can Med Assoc J 158(3 suppl):S3-S8, 1998.
6. Vetto JT, Pommier RF, Schmidt WA, et al: Diagnosis of palpable breast lesions in younger women by the modified triple test is accurate and cost-effective. Arch Surg 131:967–974, 1996.

46. MENSTRUAL DISORDERS

Anne Kastor, M.D.

1. Describe the menstrual cycle.

The term *menstrual cycle* refers to the period from the first day of bleeding (called day 1), through the menses and the intermenstrual days. The hypothalamic-pituitary-ovarian (HPO) axis controls the cycle. Pituitary hormones act on the ovaries and ovarian hormones act on the endometrium. The function of the menstrual cycle is:

- To prepare an oocyte for fertilization
- To prepare the endometrium for implantation

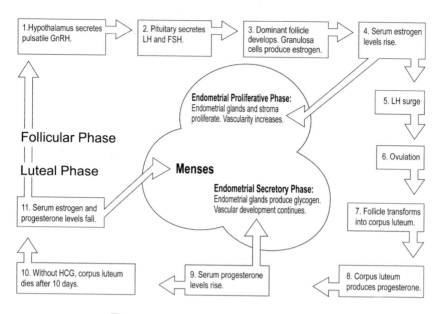

The menstrual cycle. (Designed by Kennia Riekert.)

2. What is a "normal" menstrual cycle?

The average menstrual cycle is 28 days, but cycle lengths of 21–40 days may be considered normal provided they are regular (i.e., the number of days from day 1 of one cycle to day 1 of the next cycle should vary by no more than 1–2 days per month). Flow may last 2–8 days. The average blood loss is 30 ml per cycle. Blood loss of more than 80 ml is abnormal and can cause anemia. Because it is difficult to assess volume of blood loss by history, a complete blood count (CBC) should be sent whenever heavy bleeding is suspected.

3. Define primary and secondary dysmenorrhea. How can they be distinguished?

TERM	DEFINITION
Dysmenorrhea	Painful or difficult menses
Primary dysmenorrhea	Dysmenorrhea with *no underlying pathology*
Secondary dysmenorrhea	Dysmenorrhea *caused by an underlying pathology*

Dysmenorrhea is extremely common, affecting up to 75% of menstruating women. It can be debilitating. **Primary dysmenorrhea** occurs during ovulatory cycles and therefore usually presents in the first 1–2 years after menarche. The pathophysiology is poorly understood, but the prevailing theory holds that high levels of endometrial prostaglandins result in strong, painful uterine contractions, which reduce myometrial blood flow, causing ischemia and further pain. Associated symptoms may include nausea, vomiting, diarrhea, bloating, fatigue, and headaches.

4. What are the common causes of secondary dysmenorrhea?
- Endometriosis
- Uterine leiomyomas (fibroids)
- Pelvic inflammatory disease (PID)
- Adenomyosis (endometrial glands infiltrating the myometrial wall)
- Postsurgical adhesions

- Endometrial polyps
- Uterine outflow tract obstruction

5. When should you suspect secondary dysmenorrhea?

Characteristics suggesting secondary dysmenorrhea include:

- Onset within the first 1–2 menstrual cycles (suggests outflow obstruction)
- Associated menorrhagia (suggests adenomyosis or fibroids)
- Associated abdominal pain or dyspareunia (suggest fibroids, PID or endometriosis)
- New onset or worsening pain after years of regular cycles
- Premenstrual or intermenstrual pain
- History of sexually transmitted diseases (STDs), pelvic surgery, or infertility
- Symptoms not relieved by nonsteroidal anti-inflammatory drugs (NSAIDs) or oral contraceptives

6. How is primary dysmenorrhea treated?

Symptom severity, treatment side effects, and the woman's desire for fertility guide the choice of treatment. Treatments may include:

TREATMENT	MECHANISM OF ACTION	COMMENTS
NSAIDs (e.g. ibuprofen, naproxen, celecoxib)	Decrease endometrial prostaglandins	COX-2 inhibitors (celecoxib, rofecoxib) cause fewer GI side effects but are more expensive and require prescription.
Oral contraceptives	Decrease endometrial thickness	Usually effective; may take up to 3 months to work.
Depo-Provera	Prevents ovulation	Frequently causes amenorrhea.
Thiamine, 100 mg daily		Taken throughout the menstrual cycle, thiamine has been shown to reduce pain.
Transcutaneous electrical nerve stimulation (TENS)	May alter pain reception or perception	Several studies suggest both high-dose TENS and acupuncture are superior to placebo. However, neither has been compared head-to-head with currently available pharmacologic treatments.
Acupuncture	May block pain impulses by stimulating nerve fibers or receptors	Compares head to head with currently available pharmacologic treatments.
Local therapies		Hot baths or compresses and lower back massage can relieve symptoms.
GnRH agonists	Prevent ovulation	Due to side effects, these agents are only prescribed when first and second-line agents fail.

7. When should patients with dysmenorrhea be referred to a gynecologist?

- If secondary dysmenorrhea is suspected
- If the patient does not respond to NSAIDs or oral contraceptives

8. Define the most common terms related to menstrual disorders.

TERM	DEFINITIONS
Menorrhagia	Regular menstrual cycles with increased flow volume or duration
Metrorrhagia	Irregular cycles with normal or reduced flow
Menometrorrhagia	Irregular cycles with increased flow
Hypermenorrhea	Long menses. Sometimes defined as > 8 days

Table continues on following page.

TERM	DEFINITIONS
Hypomenorrhea	Short menses. Sometimes defined as < 3 days
Oligomenorrhea	Long cycles. Sometimes defined as > 45 days or < 10 menses in 12 months
Polymenorrhea	Short cycles. Sometimes defined as < 23 days
Intermenstrual bleeding	Bleeding in between menses
Mid-cycle spotting	Bleeding during ovulation. Triggered by physiologic decrease in estrogen.
Dysfunctional uterine bleeding (DUB)	Heavy or irregular bleeding unrelated to a structural lesion, pregnancy, coagulopathy, systemic disease, or medication.
Primary amenorrhea	No menses by age 16 years *or* No menses 2 years after completing sexual maturation *or* No menses by age 14 years in the absence of any pubertal development
Secondary amenorrhea	No menses for 3 consecutive months in a woman with established regular cycles
Postmenopausal bleeding	Any vaginal bleeding 12 months after menopause

9. **What causes increased or irregular menses in reproductive age women?**
   Pregnancy
   - Ectopic pregnancy
   - Spontaneous abortion
   - Gestational trophoblastic disease
   - Normal pregnancy

   Infection
   - Cervicitis (may cause postcoital bleeding)
   - PID
   - Endometritis (occurs after uterine instrumentation, cesarean section, or complicated vaginal delivery)

   Bleeding diathesis
   - Congenital (e.g., von Willebrand's disease)
   - Acquired (e.g., idiopathic thrombocytopenic purpura, advanced liver disease)

   Medications and devices
   - Hormonal contraceptives
   - Intrauterine devices
   - Anticoagulants
   - Drugs with antiandrogen effects (e.g., aldactone)
   - High-dose corticosteroids
   - Antipsychotic medications

   Benign growths
   - Leiomyomas (fibroids)
   - Endometrial polyps (incidence increases with age)
   - Adenomyosis (seen primarily in parous women)

   Malignancy and premalignant changes
   - Cervical cancer
   - Endometrial cancer (extremely rare in women younger than 35 years)
   - Endometrial hyperplasia
   - Hormone-secreting tumors
   - Vaginal and vulvar cancers (extremely rare)

   Trauma
   - Sexual assault
   - Saddle injuries

Endocrine disorders
- Thyroid disease
- Cushing's syndrome
- Hyperprolactinemia

Dysfunctional uterine bleeding (a diagnosis of exclusion)

Rectal, urinary, and dermatologic bleeding can be mistaken for genital tract bleeding.

10. What are uterine fibroids and how are they diagnosed and treated?

Fibroids are benign uterine tumors composed of smooth muscle and connective tissue. They can cause pelvic pain, menorrhagia, hypermenorrhia, and infertility. They are extremely common, particularly among African-American women. Most women with fibroids, however, are asymptomatic. Diagnosis is made by transvaginal ultrasound. For symptomatic fibroids, treatment may include medical therapy (e.g., oral contraceptives, GnRH-agonists), surgery (myomectomy or hysterectomy), or newer, less-invasive procedures, such as uterine fibroid embolization. Complementary therapies, such as traditional Chinese medicine and vitamin supplementation, may help in some cases.

11. What is polycystic ovary syndrome (PCOS) and how is it evaluated and treated?

PCOS is a syndrome of anovulatory menstrual irregularities and hyperandrogenism. It may be detected clinically (hirsutism, male pattern balding) or biochemically (elevated serum androgens). Multiple small ovarian cysts may be present but are not required for diagnosis. Obesity, insulin resistance, and other metabolic disorders may also be present. Infertility is common. Treatment may include:

- Oral contraceptives or cyclic progesterone for endometrial protection. (Anovulation causes chronic endometrial estrogen exposure, which increases the risk of endometrial cancer.)
- Weight loss, which can stimulate ovulation
- Insulin-sensitizing agents (e.g., metformin) as needed
- Ovulation induction with clomiphene or insulin-sensitizing agents if fertility is desired.

12. What causes irregular or heavy bleeding in adolescents?

Anovulation due to an immature HPO axis is the most common cause. Irregular menses are common during the first post-menarchal year. Menstrual irregularities may be the first sign of several systemic disorders, including PCOS and thyroid disease. Menorrhagia may be the first indication of a coagulopathy (e.g., von Willebrand's disease), thrombocytopenia, or leukemia. Pregnancy and sexual assault must always be considered.

13. How should you address the issues of sexual abuse or sexual activity in adolescents?

Adolescent girls may be hesitant to acknowledge consensual sex or to report sexual assault or abuse. These topics should be discussed in private, without parents or guardians present. Use concrete and specific language. You may want to ask the patient what terminology she uses for her genitals and then use that language or ensure the patient understands the terminology you use. Questions such as "Are you sexually active?" may be too vague. "Has a man or boy ever put his penis in your vagina, even for a moment?" may reveal more information. Ask straightforward, non-judgmental questions. It may help to preface them with statements such as, "Many girls your age are having sex" or "Sometimes people get forced or pressured to do things they don't want to do. Has that ever happened to you?"

14. What is the acute management of heavy vaginal bleeding?

First, make sure the patient is **hemodymanically stable** and determine if she is **pregnant**.

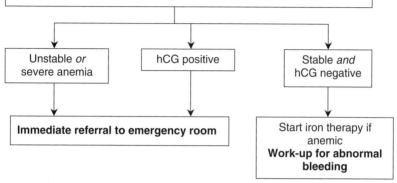

Acute management of heavy vaginal bleeding.

15. How should heavy or irregular bleeding in a stable, nonpregnant patient be evaluated?

A focused history should include:

- The nature of the bleeding (duration, volume, frequency)
- Associated symptoms (intermenstrual pain or pressure, dyspareunia)
- Menstrual history, including evidence of ovulation (menstrual regularity, premenstrual symptoms)
- Reproductive and sexual history
- Pelvic trauma, surgery, or instrumentation history
- Sexual assault history
- Coagulopathies, endocrine disorders, STDs, or abnormal Pap smears
- All medications, including over-the-counter medications, hormonal contraceptives, IUDs, herbs, and supplements
- Review of systems focused on symptoms of a coagulopathy, thyroid disease, Cushing's syndrome, or prolactinoma

The physical examination should include visual inspection for signs of a coagulopathy or Cushing's syndrome, palpation of the thyroid, pelvic examination for cervical polyps, abrasions, or discharge, and a bimanual examination to detect uterine or adnexal masses or tenderness.

A CBC and pregnancy test are mandatory. Gonorrhea and chlamydia tests, as well as thyroid function tests, are usually indicated. Coagulation studies, prolactin levels, transvaginal ultrasound, endometrial biopsy, and dilatation and curettage or hysteroscopy may be indicated based on the history and examination.

16. What if this entire work-up is negative?

The patient has DUB.

17. What is DUB?

DUB is a diagnosis of exclusion. It refers to heavy or irregular bleeding unrelated to a structural lesion, pregnancy, coagulopathy, systemic disease, or medication. It may be ovulatory (10–20% of cases) or anovulatory (80–90% of cases). PCOS is the most common cause of anovulatory DUB.

18. What is the differential diagnosis of postmenopausal bleeding? How is it evaluated?

Post-menopausal bleeding is endometrial cancer until proven otherwise. Diagnostic tests include transvaginal ultrasound to measure endometrial thickness, dilatation and curettage, and endometrial biopsy. Other causes of post-menopausal bleeding include atrophic or infectious vaginitis, cervicitis, endometrial or cervical polyps, endometrial hyperplasia, and breakthrough bleeding in women on hormone replacement therapy.

19. What causes secondary amenorrhea?

Pregnancy is the most common cause of secondary amenorrhea and must be ruled out first. Other causes of secondary amenorrhea can be classified according to their location on the hypothalamic-pituitary-ovarian-endometrial axis.

AXIS LOCATION	CAUSE	EXAMPLE/EXPLANATION
Hypothalamic-pituitary	Hypothalamic anovulation	Eating disorders, hyper intense exercise, profound weight loss or gain
		Severe physical or emotional stress
	Medications/drugs	Antipsychotic medications, prochlorperazine, metoclopramide, and other medications that inhibit dopamine
		Heroin, methadone
		Progestins (e.g., Depo-Provera)
	Hypothalamic or pituitary destruction	Pituitary infarction (Sheehan's syndrome), compression or infiltration (e.g., sarcoidosis)
		History of brain irradiation, trauma, or hemorrhage
		Empty sella syndrome
		Pituitary or other brain tumor
	Endocrinopathies	Hyperprolactinemia (prolactinoma is the most common cause)
		Thyroid disease
		Cushing's syndrome
		Androgen-secreting tumors
Ovarian	PCOS (most common ovarian cause)	
	Spontaneous or surgical menopause	
	Premature ovarian failure	Autoimmune (may be accompanied by adrenal insufficiency, thyroid disease, pancreatic dysfunction, myasthenia gravis, or pernicious anemia)
		History of high-dose alkylating chemotherapy or pelvic irradiation
		Chromosomal abnormalities (e.g., Turner syndrome with mosaicism)
		Infectious oopheritis (mumps, tuberculosis)
Endometrial	Asherman's syndrome (endometrial scarring from aggressive surgical instrumentation)	

20. How is secondary amenorrhea evaluated?

Secondary amenorrhea is pregnancy until proven otherwise. Once pregnancy has been ruled out, the history and physical examination are similar to that for irregular menses. In addition, the history should include questions about:

- Head trauma, radiation, or chemotherapy
- Diet, exercise, and recent weight loss
- Drug use, particularly opiates
- Recent emotional stress, travel, or change in schedule
- Symptoms of menopause or hyperandrogenism

A pregnancy test, thyroid function tests, prolactin level, and follicle-stimulating hormone (FSH) levels are usually indicated. A high FSH indicates ovarian failure. A measure of androgen levels should be ordered for all women with signs of virilization or PCOS. Further evaluation is beyond the scope of this chapter and is usually conducted by a gynecologist or reproductive endocrinologist.

21. What if this entire work-up is negative?
Then the woman has either Asherman's syndrome or hypothalamic amenorrhea.

22. What is Asherman's syndrome and how is it diagnosed?
Asherman's syndrome is endometrial scarring caused by aggressive instrumentation. A progesterone or estrogen–progesterone challenge will determine if the patient bleeds in response to ovarian hormones. Failure to bleed after 21 days of estrogen and 5 days of progesterone administration strongly suggests Asherman's syndrome.

23. What is hypothalamic amenorrhea?
Hypothalamic amenorrhea is a poorly understood entity. It may result from stress-related changes in GnRH pulsation. Precipitating factors include intense athletic training, weight loss, eating disorders, and severe physical or emotional stress. Gonadotropin levels may be normal or low. Estrogen levels are usually low. Brain imaging is indicated for any woman suspected of having hypothalamic amenorrhea to rule out a mass compressing the hypothalamus.

BIBLIOGRAPHY

1. Barbieri R, Ryan K: The menstrual cycle. In Ryan K (ed): Kistner's Gynecology and Women's Health, 7th ed. St. Louis, Mosby, 1999.
2. Coco A: Primary dysmenorrhea. Am Fam Physician 60:489–496, 1999.
3. Miran L, Slap G: Adolescent menstrual disorders: Update. Med Clin North Am 84:851–868, 2000.
4. Namnoum AB, Hatcher R: The menstrual cycle. In Hatcher R (ed): Contraceptive Technology, 17th ed. New York, Arden Media, 1998.
5. Oriel K, Schrager S: Abnormal uterine bleeding. Am Fam Physician 60:1371–1382, 1999.
6. Prentice A: Medical management of menorrhagia. West J Med 172:253–255, 2000.
7. Proctor ML, Smith CA, Farquhar CM, Stones RW: Transcutaneous electrical nerve stimulation and acupuncture for primary dysmenorrhea. Cochrane Database Syst Rev 1:CD002123, 2002.
8. Wilson ML, Murphy PA: Herbal and dietary therapies for primary and secondary dysmenorrhoea. Cochrane Database Syst Rev 3:CD002124, 2001.

47. MENOPAUSE

Anne Kastor, M.D.

1. What is menopause?
Menopause is the cessation of menstrual periods. It may result from the normal age-related decline in ovarian estrogen production, surgical removal of the ovaries, or autoimmune, radiation, or chemotherapy-induced ovarian failure. A serum follicle-stimulating hormone (FSH) level > 40 IU/L is diagnostic. The average age of menopause in the United States is 51 years, with 95% of women experiencing menopause between the ages of 45 and 55 years old.

2. What is perimenopause (also known as the climacteric)?
Perimenopause is the period during which a woman's ovaries gradually stop producing estrogen. With each menstrual cycle, fewer follicles are recruited in the estrogen-producing phase

of folliculogenesis. Menstrual irregularity is common and may include oligomenorrhea or hypermenorrhea. Fertility during this time is unpredictable, because not all cycles are ovulatory.

3. What symptoms are associated with perimenopause?

Hot flashes (also called vasomotor symptoms) are the most common perimenopausal symptom, occurring in up to 85% of women. Women describe a feeling of warmth followed by sweating and chills that lasts from 30 seconds to 5 minutes. Symptoms may begin several years before the cessation of menses. Twenty percent of women will experience hot flashes for less than 1 year, and up to 50% will have symptoms for 5 years.

Headaches, insomnia, depression, and decreased libido may also accompany perimenopause. Urogenital symptoms, resulting from thinning of the vaginal and vulvar epithelium, include recurrent urinary tract infections, dyspareunia, and pruritus and persist into the postmenopausal years.

4. What treatments are available for vasomotor symptoms (hot flashes)?

Many women do not feel the need for treatment. For those who do, a variety of options are available:

- **Behavioral therapy,** including paced respiration and relaxation response techniques, can decrease the number and intensity of hot flashes.
- **Selective serotonin reuptake inhibitors,** including paroxetine and venlafaxine, have been shown to reduce hot flashes.
- **Black cohosh,** an estrogenic herbal treatment marketed as Remifenim, has shown beneficial effect. However, long-term studies have not been completed, and safety concerns remain about black cohosh's estrogenic effects on the breast and endometrium.
- **Clonidine** has been shown to be effective in some, but not all, trials.
- **Hormone replacement therapy** (HRT) was the cornerstone of treatment for menopausal symptoms until recent studies clarified the serious risks of HRT (see question 6). It may be prescribed for a limited period for vasomotor symptoms and is extremely effective. The lowest dose that effectively treats the symptoms should be prescribed. Because continuous estrogen exposure increases the risk of endometrial cancer, a progestin should be prescribed as well to women with a uterus.
- **Soy products,** which contain phytoestrogens, have been proposed as treatment for vasomotor symptoms. Studies of soy supplements and high-soy diets have shown mixed results.
- **Wild yam** and **over-the-counter progesterone creams** can reduce hot flashes, but further study is needed to determine their safety.

5. What treatments are available for urogenital symptoms?

- **Low-dose vaginal estrogen,** delivered either as a cream or through a vaginal ring, improves vaginal dryness and reduces the number of urinary tract infections. Systemic absorption is minimal.
- **Vaginal moisturizers** and water-based lubricants can relieve symptoms of dryness and dyspareunia.

6. What are the indications for HRT?

The treatment of vasomotor symptoms is the only indication for HRT. Until recently, HRT was also prescribed for the prevention of osteoporosis and coronary artery disease. However, recent randomized clinical trials, including the Women's Health Initiative and the HERS trial, have demonstrated an increased risk of stroke, thromboembolic disease, and invasive breast cancer among women using combined estrogen-progestin HRT. In addition, HRT appears to increase, rather than decrease, the risk of cardiac events.

7. How does menopause affect sexual function and libido?

Most menopausal women have normal sexual responses and frequently report improved sexual function. Some women, however, report decreased libido unrelated to the urogenital symptoms mentioned above. Loss of ovarian testosterone production may be responsible. Recent studies of women who have undergone oophorectomy suggest that treatment with testosterone may improve libido.

8. What is the work-up of postmenopausal vaginal bleeding?

Postmenopausal bleeding is endometrial cancer until proven otherwise. Work-up may include an endometrial biopsy, dilatation and curettage, or transvaginal ultrasound to evaluate the endometrial thickness.

9. Who should be screened for osteoporosis?

All women aged 65 years and older should be offered screening for osteoporosis. In the years following menopause, bone strength decreases, increasing the risk of fracture. African-American women have lower osteoporosis rates than white or Mexican-American women, but the rate of osteoporosis and associated fracture is high enough to justify screening. Dual-energy x-ray absorptiometry (DEXA) of the femoral neck is the most accurate method of predicting fracture risk, but a number of less expensive and more readily available modalities appear to produce acceptable results.

10. What can be done to prevent osteoporosis and osteoporotic fractures in postmenopausal women?

- **Calcium and vitamin D supplementation.** All postmenopausal women should be advised to take 1500 mg of calcium and 800 IU of vitamin D daily.
- **Exercise.** Weight-bearing exercise for 30 minutes three times per week has been shown to improve bone mineral density and reduce the risk of hip fracture. Increased muscle strength and improved balance are probably responsible for much of this improvement.
- **Smoking cessation.** All women at risk for osteoporosis should be encouraged to stop smoking because smoking can decrease bone mineral density. Smoking cessation support groups, nicotine replacement products, and bupropion can improve quit rates.
- **Bisphosphonates.** Treatment with alendronate or risedronate has been shown to reduce vertebral, forearm, and hip fracture rates in women with osteoporosis.
- **Selective estrogen receptor modulators.** Raloxifene has been shown to increase bone mineral density and decrease vertebral fractures.

A variety of other treatments, including nasal calcitonin and parathyroid hormone, may be helpful but are rarely prescribed because of adverse reactions. Because of the risks mentioned in question 6 and the availability of other safer agents, HRT is no longer recommended for treatment of osteoporosis.

BIBLIOGRAPHY

1. Kronenberg F, Fugh-Bewrman A: Complementary and alternative medicine for menopausal symptoms: A review of randomized, controlled trials. Ann Intern Med 137:805–814, 2002.
2. Raz R, Stamm W: A controlled trial of intravaginal estriol in postmenopausal women with recurrent urinary tract infections. N Engl J Med 329:753–756, 1993.
3. Shifren JL, Braunstein GD, Simon JA, et al: Transdermal testosterone treatment in women with impaired sexual function after oophorectomy. N Engl J Med 343:682–688, 2000.
4. Srivastava M, Deal C: Osteoporosis in elderly: Prevention and treatment. Clin Geriatr Med 18:529–555, 2002.
5. U.S. Preventive Services Task Force: Hormone Replacement Therapy for Primary Prevention of Chronic Conditions. Rockville, MD, Agency for Healthcare Research and Quality, 2003. Available at http://www.ahrq.gov/clinic/cps3dix.htm.
6. U.S. Preventive Services Task Force: Screening for Osteoporosis in Postmenopausal Women. Rockville, MD, Agency for Healthcare Research and Quality, 2003. Available at http://www.ahrq.gov/clinic/cps3dix.htm.

48. CONTRACEPTION AND ABORTION

Anne Kastor, M.D.

1. What contraceptive methods are available? How effective are they?

A variety of hormonal, barrier, and surgical methods are available. Contraceptive effectiveness is frequently reported as "perfect use" or "typical use." "Perfect use" refers to the number of pregnancies in 100 women who correctly use the method every time they have intercourse for 1 year. "Typical use" reports the number of pregnancies that actually occur. "Typical use" provides a better "real world" picture of the method's effectiveness because it reflects how difficult it can be to use a method consistently.

Contraceptive Efficacy*

METHOD	TYPICAL USE (%)	PERFECT USE (%)
Chance	85	
Barrier methods		
Condoms (male)	14	3
Condoms (female)	21	5
Diaphragm	20	6
Cervical cap		
Nulliparous women	20	9
Parous women	40	26
Hormonal methods		
Oral contraceptives		
Combined oral contraceptives	3	0.1
Progestin oral contraceptives	3	0.5
Contraceptive patch (Ortho-Evra)	Not available	1.0
Contraceptive vaginal ring (NuvaRing)	Not available	0.7
Progestin injection (Depo-Provera)	0.3	0.3
Progestin implants (Norplant)	0.3	0.3
Emergency contraception	Not available	1–3
Surgical methods		
Vasectomy		0.1
Tubal ligation		0.5
Other		
Fertility awareness	25	1–3
IUD		0.1–1.5

*Percentages in this table are based on a variety of sources referenced in the bibliography.

2. How can I help patients to choose a method and use it effectively?

Method efficacy and safety, as well as the user's health conditions, risk factors for sexually transmitted diseases (STDs), and future childbearing plans influence the choice of method. As a primary care provider, you should:

1. Determine if the patient has medical contraindications to a particular method:
   - Does she have a history of or risk factors (i.e., smoking, diabetes, hypertension, age > 35 years or a hypercoagulable state) for thromboembolic or cardiovascular disease?
   - Does she have a history of or risk factors for pelvic inflammatory disease (PID)?

2. Help the patient and her partner to determine which method will be easiest to adhere to. Some questions that will help are:
   - How do you feel about taking pills? Could you remember to take a pill every day?
   - How comfortable are you touching your vagina or putting your fingers inside it?
   - How involved is your partner(s) in this process?
   - Do you want to have (more) children?

3. Invite women to bring their male partners to contraceptive-related visits. Success is more likely if both partners are committed to the method and understand how to use it correctly.

4. Provide clear, concrete instructions about how to use the method and ask the patient to repeat them back to you. See the appendix of this chapter for helpful instructions for your patients.

3. Are condoms effective contraception?

When used consistently and correctly, latex and plastic condoms are 95–97% effective. Latex condoms provide the best protection against STDs, including HIV. Plastic (polyurethane) condoms are an alternative for people with latex allergies and are equally effective as contraception. They likely protect against other STDs, but they have not been studied as well as latex condoms. Other types of condoms (e.g., lambskin) do not protect against HIV. Condoms may be used alone or with other barrier or hormonal methods. Oil-based lubricants (e.g., petroleum jelly) can cause deterioration of latex condoms, so they should not be used with them.

4. Should spermicides be used with male condoms?

No. In the past, the spermicide nonoxynol-9 was recommended to improve the contraceptive efficacy of condoms. However, recent research suggests that nonoxynol-9 may actually increase the risk of HIV transmission and probably does not improve contraceptive efficacy.

5. What is the female condom?

The female condom (Reality) provides a physical barrier for the vagina and part of the perineum. It looks like a male condom with a flexible ring inserted at each end. It is made of polyurethane, so people with latex allergies can use it and is not susceptible to oil-based products. It is the only female-controlled contraceptive method that protects against HIV.

6. What is the difference between a cervical cap and a diaphragm?

Both are prescription barrier methods that cover the cervix. They reduce the risk of some STDs but provide no significant protection against HIV. The cervical cap is a soft thimble-shaped cup that fits directly over the cervix and is held in place by suction. It is much more effective in nulliparous women than in parous women. The diaphragm is a dome-shaped rubber cup with a flexible rim. The dome covers the cervix, and the rim tucks behind the symphysis pubis and fits snugly in the posterior vaginal fornix.

7. What is the status of the contraceptive sponge?

Marketing of the Today Contraceptive Sponge, a disposable, over-the-counter spermicidal barrier method, stopped in the United States in 1994. The manufacturer recently reapplied for Food and Drug Administration (FDA) approval to re-market this product.

8. How do hormonal contraceptives work?

Hormonal contraceptives (pills, patches, injections, implants, and vaginal rings) contain a synthetic progestin alone or in combination with a synthetic estrogen. They prevent fertilization by making cervical mucus inhospitable to sperm, prevent ovulation by suppressing pituitary and hypothalamic hormones, and prevent implantation by altering the endometrial lining.

9. What oral contraceptives are available, and how do you choose among them?

Combination oral contraceptives (COCs), which contain an estrogen and a progestin, may be monophasic or multiphasic. **Monophasic** COCs contain the same estrogen and progestin dose each day, whereas **multiphasic** pills vary the dose of one or both components. **Progestin-only pills** (or the mini-pill) are reserved primarily for women who have contraindications to taking estrogen. They are slightly less effective and result in more breakthrough bleeding.

In typical users, all COCs are equally effective. Side effect profiles, previous history of oral contraceptive use, and patient risk factors usually guide selection. Most women younger than age 35 years can start on a COC containing $\leq$ 35 µg of ethinyl estradiol and $\leq$ 0.5 mg of the progestin norethindrone or its equivalent. Women older than age 35 years should receive a low-estrogen pill. Some pills may be chosen for their beneficial effects, such as menstrual regulation or reduction in acne.

10. What complications are associated with the use of oral contraceptives?

Severe complications are rare. They include pulmonary embolism, stroke, myocardial infarction, hypertension, hepatic adenoma, gallbladder disease, and depression. Common side effects include nausea, weight gain, breast tenderness, and menstrual irregularities. These side effects result from the variable estrogenic, progestogenic, and androgenic activities of different pills. Nausea and spotting frequently resolve after three cycles. Other side effects may necessitate a change to another pill.

11. What are the absolute contraindications to estrogen-based contraceptive use?

1. History of or high risk for thromboembolic disease:
   - History of deep vein thrombosis or pulmonary embolism
   - Upcoming major surgery with expected prolonged immobilization
   - Complicated valvular disease
2. History of or high risk for cardiovascular disease:
   - History of ischemic heart disease
   - History of stroke
   - Age 35 years or older *and* smokes 15 or more cigarettes/day
   - Current hypertension (systolic blood pressure [BP] $\geq$ 160 mmHg, diastolic BP $\geq$ 100 mmHg)
   - Multiple cardiovascular risk factors
   - Migraine headaches with focal neurological symptoms (increased risk of stroke, particularly in the presence of COCs)
3. Breast cancer
4. Lactating women, particularly during the first 6 weeks postpartum

12. Do oral contraceptive users need to be concerned about efficacy when other medications are prescribed?

Yes. Some medications, including phenytoin (Dilantin) and rifampin, may reduce the efficacy of oral contraceptives, and oral contraceptives may alter the activity of other drugs.

13. Do combination oral contraceptives increase the risk of cancer?

It is unlikely that oral contraceptives increase the risk of breast cancer among average-risk women. High-risk women (i.e., those with a first-degree relative with breast cancer or at least three relatives with breast or ovarian cancer; women with documented *BRCA-1* or *BRCA-2* mutations) who took the older, high-dose oral contraceptives do appear to be at higher risk of developing breast cancer than similar women who did not take oral contraceptives. Whether the current lower dose oral contraceptives pose the same risk for high-risk women is not yet determined. Women who have taken an oral contraceptive for more than 5 years do have a slightly increased risk of cervical cancer, but this is likely because of their increased exposure to human papilloma virus compared with women who use barrier methods.

14. What are the "birth control patch" and the "birth control ring"?

The contraceptive patch (Ortho Evra) and vaginal ring (NuvaRing) both contain estrogen and progestin. The patch is changed weekly for 3 weeks, followed by a patch-free week. The ring is changed every 4 weeks. They are as effective as COCs and do not require daily adherence, but the wearer must remember to change them. Both methods result in more stable blood hormonal levels than oral contraceptives, which may reduce breakthrough bleeding.

15. What is the "birth control shot"?

Depo-Provera, a progestin, is injected every 12 weeks. Many women appreciate how easy this method is to use, requiring only four injections per year. Side effects include amenorrhea, weight gain, breast tenderness, and depression. The most troublesome aspect of these side effects is that the patient must simply wait until the drug leaves her body, which can take 6–8 months.

16. What is Norplant?

The Norplant system consists of six progestin-containing capsules that are placed under the skin of the upper arm. It is effective for 5 years. Norplant's benefits include long-term efficacy and lack of daily adherence requirements. However, a minor surgical procedure is required for capsule insertion and removal, and the capsules are visible beneath the skin. The system's popularity has been limited by reports of difficult capsule removal soon after the system was introduced. Women choosing the method should make sure their providers are experienced in both insertion and removal of the capsules.

17. Is a pelvic examination required before prescribing hormonal contraception?

No. Only a medical history and BP measurement are required. However, a contraceptive visit is often a good opportunity to perform a pap smear and test for STDs.

18. What is the status of the intrauterine device (IUD)?

Three IUDs are available in the United States. The copper-T380A (Paragard) is effective for up to 10 years. Minera, a progesterone-releasing IUD, is effective for 5 years. Progestasert, which also releases progesterone, is slightly less effective and must be replaced annually.

The IUD's mechanism of action is poorly understood, but contrary to some patients' concerns, it is not an abortifacient. The copper-T prevents fertilization. The progesterone-releasing IUDs act primarily through hormonal mechanisms. Side effects include spotting, bleeding, anemia, cramping, and pain.

The Dalkon Shield was removed from the market in 1975 because of its association with high rates of pelvic inflammatory disease (PID) and an increased incidence of septic abortion. A large settlement was paid to more than 100,000 women who had claims of problems related to the shield. Current IUDs are much safer than the Dalkon Shield, but they do increase the risk of PID after a woman has contracted an STD. Therefore, they are contraindicated in women at risk for STDs.

19. What are fertility awareness and periodic abstinence?

By tracking basal body temperature (BBT) and changes in cervical mucus, consistency, and position, women can identify their fertile days and abstain or use barrier methods when fertile. BBT, measured with a special thermometer available at most drug stores, decreases with the LH surge and then increases 0.2–0.5°C as progesterone levels increase. Unprotected intercourse should be avoided from the menses until the third day of elevated temperature. Fertility awareness is most effective when both partners are committed to the method and have learned how to use it correctly. This method of periodic abstinence is much more effective than the "rhythm method," an unpredictable system of predicting fertile days based only on the calendar.

20. Is withdrawal an effective contraceptive method?

No. Up to 20% of couples using this method become pregnant in the first year.

21. What is emergency contraception (EC)?

EC, previously called the "morning-after pill," prevents pregnancy after an episode of unprotected intercourse. Two products, the combined estrogen/progestin Preven and the progestin-only Plan B, are FDA-approved for this purpose. In addition, several oral contraceptives are approved for use as emergency contraception when taken in high doses. All formulations consist of two doses taken 12 hours apart. If taken within 72 hours of intercourse, only 1–3% of women using EC will become pregnant. The exact mechanism by which EC works has not been determined, but it may involve prevention of ovulation, interference with ova or sperm transport, or prevention of implantation.

22. What are the side effects of emergency contraception?

Side effects, including nausea, vomiting, fatigue, dizziness, and breast tenderness, are more common with estrogen-containing compounds. Serious side effects, such as thromboembolism, are extremely rare, but women with risk factors or a history of thromboembolism or stroke should receive a progestin-only compound. Many providers prescribe an antiemetic to take 30–60 minutes before each dose.

23. Is a pregnancy test necessary before taking EC?

A pregnancy test should be performed before taking EC because EC is not effective if a woman is already pregnant.

24. Is a prescription required for EC?

In most states, a prescription is required. However, in several states, pharmacists working with a collaborating physician may dispense EC.

25. How is sterilization accomplished?

Male sterilization (vasectomy) involves occlusion or partial resection of both vas deferens. Female sterilization (tubal ligation) involves occlusion, ligation, and/or partial resection of both fallopian tubes. Vasectomy is an ambulatory surgical procedure. Tubal ligation may be performed via laparoscopy or laparotomy. Both are equally effective. Vasectomy is a quicker and easier procedure than tubal ligation and has fewer risks associated with it.

26. Can vasectomy or tubal ligation be reversed?

The prospects for reversal depend on the surgical technique used at time of sterilization, the skill of the surgeon, the time since sterilization, and a number of other factors. Because of the risks associated with any surgical procedure and the possibility that reversal may not be possible, sterilization should be considered permanent and should not be performed on any patients who are unsure about their desire for future fertility.

27. What long-term risks are associated with surgical sterilization?

The most serious concern for women is an increased risk of ectopic pregnancy. Long-term postvasectomy risks are negligible. Contrary to prior concerns, vasectomy does not appear to increase the risk of prostate or testicular cancer.

28. Why is a 30-day waiting period required for sterilization procedures?

In the 1930s through the 1970s, thousands of women, particularly poor women, women of color, and women with mental disabilities, were sterilized without their consent. This practice took many forms, including presenting women with consent forms while they were in active labor, using English-language consent forms with patients who did not speak English, and failing to inform women that tubal ligation was a permanent procedure. As a result of lawsuits, political organizing, and an expose written by an obstetrics/gynecology intern, regulations were developed to protect Medicaid recipients from unwanted sterilization. These guidelines, which include the waiting period, a prohibition against sterilization of people younger than age 21 years, and a standardized consent form, are now used in almost all cases, regardless of payer source.

29. Can adolescents obtain contraception without parental permission?

Yes. Adolescents are guaranteed confidential care for contraception.

30. Does insurance pay for contraception?

Coverage depends on the insurance plan and the state. Some states require private insurers or insurers of state employees to offer contraception coverage. Most state Medicaid programs cover contraception, and many pay for condoms when prescribed.

31. How is surgical abortion accomplished?

In the first trimester, vacuum aspiration is the most common method of surgical abortion. It can be performed in a medical office or clinic. Between 13 and 16 weeks, dilatation and evacuation is the most common procedure.

32. Is surgical abortion safe?

Surgical abortion is extremely safe, particularly if performed before 13 weeks' gestation. Two percent to 3% of patients experience a minor complication that can be addressed in the physician's office. Fewer than 1% of patients experience a serious complication requiring hospitalization or another procedure.

33. What is medical abortion?

Medical abortion can be effectively accomplished up to 49 days from the last menstrual period. Two regimens are approved for pregnancy termination. Both cause a complete abortion in 96% of cases if used before day 49. Mifepristone (RU-486), followed by the prostaglandin misoprostol 48 hours later, causes a complete abortion within 4 hours of the misoprostol dose. Methotrexate (intramuscularly or orally) followed by patient-administered vaginal misoprostol is equally effective, but complete abortion may not occur for 3–4 weeks. Side effects for both regimens may include heavy bleeding, nausea, vomiting, abdominal pain, and fatigue.

34. Do adolescents need parental permission to obtain an abortion?

Most states require some form of parental involvement. The majority of these states allow for a judicial bypass, which allows the minor to present her case to a judge in lieu of informing her parents.

35. Does insurance cover abortion?

Insurance coverage varies. Most state Medicaid programs do not cover abortion.

APPENDIX: CONTRACEPTIVE INSTRUCTIONS AND PATIENT EDUCATION

Male Condoms
- Roll the condom onto the erect penis before intercourse.
- Hold the tip of the condom between your fingers when rolling it on. This will create a pocket for the ejaculate and prevent breakage.
- Hold onto the base of the condom when pulling out. Otherwise, the condom may fall off inside the vagina and allow ejaculate to escape.
- Use only water-based lubricants with latex condoms.
- Carry condoms with you at all times. Keep them by the bed and anywhere you might have sex.

Female Condoms
- Squeeze the inner ring (closed end) and insert it into the vagina as far as you can. The outer ring (open end) will hang outside the vagina.
- After intercourse, remove the condom before standing up. Squeeze and twist the outer ring and pull gently.
- Throw away after one use.

Cervical Cap
- Fill it one third the way up with spermicidal jelly or cream.
- Locate your cervix with you finger and guide the cap onto your cervix. Pinch the cap rim and twist. Run your finger around the rim to make sure it fits snugly.
- Leave in place for at least 8 hours after intercourse.
- To remove, pull down on the rim to break the suction and pull the cap out.
- You can leave the cap in for up to 48 hours and can have intercourse multiple times.

Diaphragm
- Place a teaspoon of spermicidal jelly or cream in the diaphragm and smear a little around the rim.
- Hold the diaphragm with the dome facing down and bend the ring. In a standing, squatting or lying position, separate your labia and insert the diaphragm into your vagina. Slide it along the back wall of your vagina until it will not go any further. Run your finger all the way around the edge of the diaphragm to make sure it covers your cervix.
- You can insert the diaphragm up to 6 hours before intercourse. If it has been more than 6 hours since you inserted it or you are having intercourse a second time, insert an applicatorful of spermicide into your vagina
- Leave the diaphragm in place for at least 6 hours after intercourse.

Oral Contraceptives
- Start the pills during the first 5 days of your period. Some pill packs recommend starting on a Sunday, but you can choose any day that you will remember.
- Use a backup method for the first cycle.
- Take your pills at the same time every day.
- If you miss one pill, take it as soon as you remember.
- If you miss two pills during the first 2 weeks of your cycle, take two pills/day for 2 days and use a backup method for the rest of that cycle. If you miss two pills during the third week of your cycle, take two pills daily until your active pills are gone and start your next cycle within 7 days. Use a backup method through the first 7 days of your next cycle.

Contraceptive Patch
- Apply the patch to the abdomen, buttocks, upper torso (except breasts), or upper outer arm.
- Change the patch every week on the same day for 3 weeks; then wear no patch for 1 week.
- Do not use any lotions or oils in the area of the patch. It is fine to shower, swim, or get the patch wet.
- If the patch comes off, immediately put on a replacement patch and wear it for the rest of that week.

Contraceptive Ring
- Insert the first ring between the first and fifth days of your period.
- Leave it in place for 21 days and then remove it for 7 days.
- Insert a new ring exactly 28 days after you inserted the first one. Try to insert it as close to the same time as possible.
- The ring can be removed for 3 hours. If it is out of the vagina for more than 3 hours, use a back up method for the rest of the month.

Emergency Contraception
- Take the first dose as soon as possible.
- Take the second dose in exactly 12 hours.
- If you throw up within 1 hour of taking a dose, take another dose.
- If you do not get your period in 3 weeks, take a pregnancy test.

BIBLIOGRAPHY

1. American College of Obstetricians and Gynecologists: ACOG Practice Bulletin. Clinical management guidelines for obstetrician-gynecologists. Medical management of abortion. Obstet Gynecol 97:1–13, 2001.
2. Ballagh S: NuvaRing Vaginal Contraceptive Ring. Slide presentation in Contraception Online at www.contraceptiononline.org/slides/index.cfm.
3. Baylor College of Medicine: Contraception Online at www.contraceptiononline.org.
4. Dickey R: Managing Contraceptive Pill Patients, 11th ed. New Orleans, EMIS Medical Publishers, 2002.
5. Grabrick D: Risk of breast cancer with oral contraceptive use in women with a family history of breast cancer. JAMA 284:1791–1798, 2000.
6. Grimes D, Raymond R: Emergency contraception. Ann Intern Med 137:180–189, 2002.
7. Hatcher RA, Stewart F, et al: Contraceptive Technology, 17th ed. New York, Ardent Media, 1998.

8. Lieberman D, Feierman J: Legal issues in the reproductive health care of adolescents. J Am Med Womens Assoc 54:109–114, 1999.
9. Marchbanks P: Oral contraceptives and the risk of breast cancer. N Engl J Med 346:2025–2032, 2002.
10. Poindexter A, et al: The Ortho Evra/Evra Transdermal Contraceptive System [slide presentation]. Available online at Contraception Online: www.contraceptiononline.org/slides/index.cfm.
11. Seibert C, Barbouche E, Fagan J, et al: Prescribing oral contraceptives for women older than 35 years of age. Ann Intern Med 138:54–64, 2003.
12. World Health Organization/Reproductive Health and Research: Improving Access to Quality Care in Family Planning. Medical Eligibility Criteria for Contraceptive Use, 2nd ed. Geneva, WHO, 2000.

49. VAGINAL DISCHARGE AND PELVIC INFLAMMATORY DISEASE

Simona Bratu, M.D., Michael Augenbraun, M.D.,
Kavita Nanda, M.D., M.H.S., and Susan J. Diem, M.D., M.P.H.

1. Characterize the normal and abnormal vaginal secretions.

Some degree of vaginal secretion is normal. It consist of desquamated vaginal epithelial cells and secretions from cervical glands, sebaceous glands, sweat glands, Bartholin's glands, and Skene's glands. Transudate through the vaginal wall also contributes to the composition of normal secretions. Normal secretions are usually clear or white, odorless, and viscous. Polymorphonuclear leukocytes are rare. The amount of normal vaginal secretion varies with the menstrual cycle, age, sexual arousal, pregnancy, and use of oral contraceptives. An abnormal discharge is usually accompanied by a change in odor, a change in color, or an increase in the amount of discharge. In addition, the patient may note pruritus, dysuria, or staining of underwear.

2. What causes an abnormal vaginal discharge?

- Infections of the vagina, vulva, cervix, or upper genital tract
- Atrophic vaginitis caused by estrogen deficiency, which causes thinning and fragility of the vaginal and vulvar epithelium. Hence, the epithelium is more vulnerable to injury and inflammation, producing desquamation of cells and stimulation of glandular secretions from the cervical area. In addition, such changes may elevate the pH in the vagina and result in a change in the bacteria.
- Foreign bodies, such as tampons or diaphragms, if left in the vagina for a prolonged period
- Irritation from frequent douching
- Neoplasms of the cervix and uterus

3. List the six most common infectious causes of a vaginal discharge.

1. Bacterial vaginosis (BV)
2. Trichomonal vaginitis
3. Vulvovaginal candidiasis
4. Chlamydia cervicitis
5. Gonococcal cervicitis
6. Pelvic inflammatory disease (PID)

4. Which of the infectious causes of a vaginal discharge are sexually transmitted?

Trichomoniasis, chlamydial infection, and gonococcal infection are sexually transmitted. Bacterial vaginosis and candidal vulvovaginitis are not generally thought to be sexually transmitted.

5. What is bacterial vaginosis (BV)?

Also known as *nonspecific vaginitis,* BV is the most common cause of vaginal discharge. Although its cause has been debated for years, it is believed to represent an alteration in the microbial flora of the vagina, with an increase in anaerobes and gram-negative bacilli and a decrease in the endogenous lactobacillus flora. *Gardnerella vaginalis* also has been noted in BV, but its role in pathogenesis is not clear. It is cultured commonly in patients with BV but may be found in up to 50% of healthy, asymptomatic women. Most authors believe that *G. vaginalis* may be necessary but not sufficient alone to cause BV. Patients with BV often present with a vaginal discharge associated with a change in odor, described as musty or fishy. The odor is caused by the production of aromatic amines by the bacteria. The discharge is usually thin, white-yellow, homogeneous, and moderately increased in volume over the patient's normal vaginal secretions.

6. How is the diagnosis of BV made?

The diagnosis of BV requires three of the following four findings:

1. The pH of the vaginal discharge should be > 4.5. The normal pH of vaginal secretions, ranging from 3.8–4.4, is raised by the production of aromatic amines in the altered microbial environment.

2. "Clue" cells are seen on wet mount. Clue cells are epithelial cells with a granulated surface due to adherence of bacteria. They can be seen under high-dry magnification after a drop of the discharge is mixed with a drop of saline.

3. The "whiff" test is positive. A fishy odor is often produced when a drop of discharge is mixed with 10% potassium hydroxide. The alkalinization is thought to volatize amines, producing the characteristic fishy odor.

4. The discharge is consistent with BV.

7. Is BV associated with serious complications?

Yes. BV has been associated with several complications of pregnancy, including preterm delivery, premature rupture of membranes, amnionitis, chorioamnionitis, and postpartum endometritis. For this reason, it is important to treat BV in pregnant patients. It has also been associated with PID and posthysterectomy vaginal cuff cellulitis.

8. Describe the treatment of BV.

Metronidazole is the drug of choice for the treatment of BV. The standard regimen is 500 mg twice daily for 7 days. Patients should be warned to avoid alcohol because of a disulfiram-like reaction. Other options include intravaginal clindamycin cream and metronidazole vaginal gel. Alternative regimens have lower efficacy for BV and include metronidazole, 2 g orally in a single dose; clindamycin, 300 mg orally twice a day for 7 days; or clindamycin ovules intravaginally at bedtime for 3 days. BV should be treated during pregnancy if the patient is symptomatic or has a high risk for premature labor. The regimens in pregnancy include metronidazole, 250 mg orally three times a day for 7 days, or clindamycin, 300 mg orally twice a day for 7 days. Multiple studies have not demonstrated a consistent association between metronidazole use during pregnancy and teratogenic or mutagenic effects in newborns.

9. Why is it important to diagnose and treat trichomonal vaginitis?

Trichomonal vaginitis is caused by *Trichomonas vaginalis,* a protozoan usually transmitted by sexual contact. Infection with *T. vaginalis* is associated with an abnormal discharge that ranges in color from white to yellow, gray, or green. Other manifestations may include vaginal itching, dysuria, and dyspareunia. As many as 50% of infected women are asymptomatic, as are the majority of infected men. Microscopic examination of a drop of the vaginal discharge mixed with saline reveals motile flagellated trichomonads that are approximately twice the size of white blood cells (WBCs). The sensitivity of this procedure in symptomatic women is approximately 50–75%, and the specificity approaches 100%. Additional tests, including direct fluorescent antibody staining, latex agglutination, enzyme-linked immunosorbent assay (ELISA) techniques, DNA probe, and polymerase chain reaction (PCR), may increase the sensitivity of the direct microscopic examination.

Cultures for *T. vaginalis* have a sensitivity of approximately 90% and remain the gold standard for diagnosis of trichomoniasis. The standard treatment for trichomoniasis is a single dose of 2 g of metronidazole. Sexual partners also should be treated. Metronidazole, 500 mg twice daily for 7 days, may be tried for treatment failures. A 2-g single oral dose, once daily for 3–5 days, is recommended for patients who fail repeated treatment courses. Topical metronidazole is not effective.

10. What infection is suggested by a "strawberry cervix"?

Cervicitis caused by *T. vaginalis.*

11. What infection is suggested by a white, cheesy discharge?

Candidal vulvovaginitis is caused by *Candida* species of fungi, most commonly *C. albicans.* Candidal infection may cause vulvar and vaginal irritation and inflammation, resulting in burning, itching, dyspareunia, and dysuria. Many women have an abnormal discharge, often thick and clumpy. *Candida* may be a part of the normal flora in approximately 30% of women. The diagnosis is made by examining the discharge with a Gram stain or a wet preparation (saline or 10% potassium hydroxide solution) for the fungal forms. Culture is a more sensitive method for detecting the yeast, but because many women without symptoms have positive yeast culture findings, routine cultures are not recommended. Culture for *Candida* species is indicated for chronic or recurrent infections to confirm the clinical diagnosis and to identify unusual or resistant strains.

12. What factors predispose women to candidal vaginitis?

Predisposing factors for candidiasis include diabetes, recent antibiotic use, pregnancy, corticosteroids, immunosuppressants, and oral contraceptives with high estrogen content. HIV-infected women have higher vaginal *Candida* colonization rates and more frequent symptomatic *Candida* vulvovaginitis. Prior systemic azoles treatment is associated in HIV-positive women with isolation of non–*C. albicans* species from the vagina.

13. How is vulvovaginal candidiasis treated?

Candidiasis can be treated with any of several topical agents, including miconazole or clotrimazole; all have cure rates of 85% or higher. Fluconazole in a single dose of 150 mg orally is also effective. Only topical azole therapy is recommended for pregnant women with vulvovaginal candidiasis.

14. What is chlamydial cervicitis? How is it treated?

One common cause of cervicitis, *Chlamydia trachomatis,* is transmitted through sexual contact. Symptoms include a mucopurulent discharge, lower abdominal discomfort, fever, and dysuria. However, many patients infected with *C. trachomatis* are asymptomatic. On examination, the cervix may be erythematous, edematous, and friable. The diagnosis can be made by culture, a technique that is expensive and technically difficult. Fluorescent antibody testing and ELISA are easier to perform and have a sensitivity of 60–75% and specificity of > 99% with confirmatory testing. Newer techniques include nucleic acid amplification tests such as PCR and transcription-mediated amplification (TMA). These tests are more sensitive than cultures and are nearly as specific.

The mainstay of treatment for chlamydial infection is doxycycline, 100 mg twice daily for 7 days, or azithromycin, 1 g orally in a single dose. Alternatives include ofloxacin, 300 mg orally twice daily for 7 days; levofloxacin, 500 mg orally for 7 days; erythromycin base, 500 mg orally four times a day for 7 days; or erythromycin ethylsuccinate, 800 mg orally four times a day for 7 days. Erythromycin or azithromycin should be used in pregnant patients, and fluoroquinolones should not be used in adolescents under age 18 years. Erythromycin is not as effective. Sexual partners should also be referred for treatment.

15. When else should patients be treated for chlamydial infection? Why?

Patients should be treated for presumed chlamydial infection in the presence of gonococcal cervicitis. Up to 40% of patients with gonorrhea are also infected with chlamydia.

16. What infection is caused by *Neisseria gonorrhoeae*?

Infection with *N. gonorrhoeae* causes gonorrhea, a sexually transmitted disease. Gynecologic manifestations in women include a purulent vaginal discharge caused by cervicitis and PID. The discharge may be accompanied by pruritus, dyspareunia, dysuria, and lower abdominal discomfort. The diagnosis of gonococcal cervicitis is made by Gram stain of the discharge demonstrating gram-negative intracellular diplococci. Culture with a variety of selective media, including Thayer Martin, is used to confirm the diagnosis. Nucleic acid amplification techniques may also be used.

First-line treatment of gonococcal cervicitis consists of ceftriaxone, 125 mg intramuscularly (IM) in a single dose, or cefixime, 400 mg orally, followed by a 7-day course of doxycycline, 100 mg twice daily, or azithromycin, 1 g orally, to treat undiagnosed coexistent chlamydial infection. Single-dose ciprofloxacin, 500 mg orally; ofloxacin, 400 mg orally; or levofloxacin, 250 mg orally, are safe and equally effective for treatment of uncomplicated gonococcal infections; also, they may be used for patients allergic to cephalosporins. Clinically significant fluoroquinolone resistance has been reported among *N. gonorrhoeae* isolates. Quinolones are no longer recommended for the treatment of gonorrhoeae in the State of Hawaii for infections that may have been acquired in the Far East and are inadvisable for use in California.

Partners also should be treated.

17. Describe the approach to a patient with a vaginal discharge.

History, physical examination, and a few simple laboratory tests identify the cause of many cases of vaginal discharge. The history should focus on the nature of the discharge, associated symptoms, sexual and contraceptive history, and other medical conditions. The physical examination should include inspection of the vulva, vagina, and cervix, noting any erythema, edema, atrophy, abnormal lesions, trauma, or foreign bodies. Characteristics of the discharge, such as color and consistency, also should be noted. A bimanual examination should be performed to evaluate cervical motion tenderness, adnexal masses, and uterine masses or tenderness.

Laboratory studies should include a saline wet-mount preparation to look for clue cells and trichomonads. A 10% solution of potassium hydroxide added to a sample of discharge facilitates identification of *Candida* species. A Gram stain of the discharge should be performed if gonococcal infection is suspected. In addition, pH testing of the discharge may be helpful. Cultures of the discharge for *N. gonorrhoeae* should be performed if mucopurulent cervicitis is seen on physical examination. Infections with *N. gonorrhoeae* or *C. trachomatis* can be evaluated using nucleic acid amplification techniques. Other tests to consider include a urinalysis, particularly if dysuria is present, and a complete blood count if PID is a diagnostic consideration.

18. Define PID.

PID is an infection of the upper genital tract in women and may include salpingitis, tuboovarian abscess, endometritis, and pelvic peritonitis. An estimated 1 million American women per year are diagnosed with PID; the direct and indirect costs of the disease and its complications are estimated to be more than $5.5 billion annually.

19. Which organisms are responsible for PID?

PID is caused by a variety of bacteria, most importantly *N. gonorrhoeae* and *C. trachomatis*, both of which are sexually transmitted. Other organisms that may play a role either in the initial development of PID or as secondary pathogens include aerobes, such as *Streptococcus* species, *Escherichia coli*, and *Haemophilus influenzae*, and anaerobes, such as *Bacteroides* species, *Prevotella* species, *Peptostreptococcus* species, *Peptococcus* species, *G. vaginalis*, cytomegalovirus (CMV), *Mycoplasma hominis*, and *Ureaplasma urealyticum*. *Actinomyces israelii*, a gram-positive anaerobic organism, is seen in PID related to the use of intrauterine devices.

20. Describe the pathogenesis of PID.

C. trachomatis and *N. gonorrhoeae* initially affect the endocervical canal and cause cervicitis. The infection ascends the cervix and spreads into the uterus and fallopian tubes and then to the ovaries and peritoneal cavity. Factors that promote ascension include damage to the endocervical canal by the bacteria, extension of the endocervical columnar epithelium beyond the endocervix, and hormonal changes during the menstrual cycle that affect characteristics of the cervical mucus.

21. List risk factors for PID.

Young age	Previous PID
Multiple sex partners	Menses
Vaginal douching	Risk-taking behavior (e.g., cigarette smoking or
Bacterial vaginosis	substance abuse)
Intrauterine device use	

22. How is the diagnosis of PID made?

The minimal criteria for diagnosis of PID are cervical motion tenderness, lower abdominal tenderness, and adnexal tenderness. Additional criteria used to increase the specificity of the diagnosis include fever > 100.9°F, abnormal cervical or vaginal discharge, elevated erythrocyte sedimentation rate, elevated C-reactive protein, or laboratory confirmation of infection with *N. gonorrhoeae* or *C. trachomatis*. Further testing is warranted if the diagnosis remains in question. Pregnancy should be excluded. The most specific modalities for diagnosis of PID include endometrial biopsy with histopathologic evidence of endometritis; transvaginal sonography or magnetic resonance imaging showing thickened, fluid-filled tubes with or without free pelvic fluid or tubo-ovarian complex; and laparoscopic abnormalities consistent with PID. These specific diagnostic modalities are not commonly performed.

23. What should be considered in the differential diagnoses of PID?

Acute appendicitis	Ectopic pregnancy
Endometriosis	Inflammatory bowel disease
Ruptured ovarian cyst	Spontaneous abortion

24. What are the three principal complications of PID?

(1) Infertility caused by tubal occlusion, which occurs in 8–40% of patients after PID; (2) chronic pelvic pain, which develops in up to 18% of women after acute PID; and (3) ectopic pregnancy, which occurs in approximately 9% of women who have had PID.

25. What is Fitz-Hugh–Curtis syndrome?

Fitz-Hugh–Curtis syndrome is the acute perihepatitis seen with the spread of *N. gonorrhoeae* or *C. trachomatis* from the fallopian tube through the peritoneal cavity to the liver capsule. Patients usually present with right upper quadrant pain and often have clinical evidence of PID.

26. What is the recommended treatment for PID? When should patients with PID be hospitalized?

Empirical broad-spectrum treatment is essential. The Centers for Disease Control and Prevention (CDC) recommends outpatient treatment for mild PID with ceftriaxone, 250 mg intramuscularly (IM), along with doxycycline, 100 mg orally twice daily for 14 days, *or* cefoxitin, 2 g IM in a single dose, and probenecid 1 g orally administered concurrently in a single dose, along with doxycycline, 100 mg orally twice a day for 14 days. An alternative regimen is ofloxacin, 400 mg orally twice a day for 14 days, or levofloxacin, 500 mg orally once a day for 14 days, with or without metronidazole, 500 mg orally twice daily for 14 days. If surgical emergencies such as appendicitis and ectopic pregnancy cannot be excluded; if a pelvic abscess is suspected; if the patient does not respond clinically to oral antibiotic therapy; if the patient is severely ill with nausea, vomiting, and high fever; if the patient cannot take oral medications; or if the patient is pregnant, hospitalization should be considered. Also, hospitalization is recommended if the patient is not able to follow up or a high risk of poor compliance is suspected. No data support the recommendation for hospitalization and more aggressive treatment of adolescent females or HIV-positive patients. Treatments recommended for severe PID include intravenous (IV) cefoxitin, 2 g every 6 hours or cefotetan 2 g every 12 hours, along with doxycycline, 100 mg orally or IV twice daily. Alternative regimens include clindamycin, 900 mg IV every 8 hours, accompanied by gentamicin intravenously; ofloxacin or levofloxacin IV with or without metronidazole; or ampicillin-sulbactam 3 g IV every 6 hours along with doxycycline 100 mg orally or IV every 12 hours. IV treatment should be continued for at least 48 hours after the patient shows clinical improvement. If the patient does not improve in 72 hours, further investigations are necessary to reassess the diagnosis and the possible indication for surgery.

BIBLIOGRAPHY

1. American College of Obstetrics and Gynecologists: Vaginitis. ACOG Technical Bulletin 226, 1996.
2. Centers for Disease Control and Prevention: Sexually transmitted diseases treatment guidelines 2002. MMWR Recomm Rep 51(RR-6):1–78, 2002.
3. Goode MA, Grauer K, Gums JG: Infectious vaginitis: Selecting therapy and preventing recurrence. Postgrad Med 96:85–88, 1994.
4. Hillis SD, Wasserheit JN: Screening for chlamydia—a key to the prevention of pelvic inflammatory disease. N Engl J Med 334:1399–1401, 1996.
5. Holmes KK, Mardh PA, Sparling PF, et al (eds): Sexually Transmitted Diseases, 3rd ed. New York, McGraw-Hill, 1999.
6. Knapp JS, Fox KK, Trees DL, Whittington WL: Fluoroquinolone resistance in *Neisseria gonorrhoeae*. Emerg Infect Dis 3:33–39, 1997.
7. Mandell GL, Bennett JE, Dolin R (eds): Principles and Practice of Infectious Diseases, 5th ed. New York, Churchill Livingstone, 2000.
8. McCormack WM: Current concepts: Pelvic inflammatory disease. N Engl J Med 330:115–119, 1994.
9. McCoy MC, Katz VL, Kuller JA, et al: Bacterial vaginosis in pregnancy: An approach for the 1990s. Obstet Gynecol Surv 50:482–488, 1995.
10. Pumpradit W, Augenbraun M: Bacterial vaginosis complicating pregnancy and gynecologic surgery. Curr Infect Dis Rep 4:141–143, 2002.
11. Reed BD, Eyler A: Vaginal infections: Diagnosis and management. Am Fam Physician 47:1805–1818, 1993.
12. Sweet RL: Role of bacterial vaginosis in pelvic inflammatory disease. Clin Infect Dis 20:S271–S275, 1995.

50. DISEASES OF THE PROSTATE

Iván Colón, M.D.

1. What are the most common disorders affecting the prostate?
Benign prostatic hypertrophy (BPH)
Prostatic cancer (CaP)
Prostatitis

2. What are the typical clinical manifestations of BPH?
BPH is manifested by any combination of the following symptoms: slowing of the size and force of the urinary stream, urinary frequency or urgency, sensation of incomplete bladder emptying, and nocturia. Symptoms usually are gradually progressive and, therefore, may be tolerated until they become severe. Examination may reveal varying levels of residual urine. Digital rectal examination (DRE) typically discloses homogeneous, symmetric enlargement of the prostate. Urodynamic evaluation may demonstrate uninhibited detrusor contractions, which may be relieved by anticholinergic medication or corrected by surgical means. Symptoms of prostate ob-

struction (prostatism) may be exaggerated by coexisting urinary infection or disorders that deleteriously influence bladder function, such as diabetes or chronic vesicle overdistention.

3. Name the complications of BPH.

Obstruction of urine flow may culminate in acute urinary retention that requires catheter relief. Less common complications include urinary incontinence, infection, stone formation, hematuria, and hydronephrosis leading to renal insufficiency or failure.

4. Can patients present with prostatism and a gland of normal size?

Yes. It has been well established that size of the prostate does not correlate with symptomatology. Younger patients (early 50s) presenting with prostatism frequently demonstrate an unenlarged, clinically benign gland. Incongruously severe voiding dysfunction is produced by a small fibrous prostate or median bar hypertrophy of the posterior vesicle neck. Management is similar to that for BPH, although prostatism is less likely to respond to medical management and may warrant surgical incision rather than resection.

5. What is the recommended approach to the patient with BPH?

In the initial evaluation of all patients presenting with lower urinary tract symptoms (LUTS) suggestive of BPH, the following steps are recommended:
- Medical history should be taken to identify other causes of voiding dysfunction or comorbidities that may complicate treatment.
- Physical examination, including DRE and a focused neurologic examination, should be performed.
- Urinalysis should be performed by dipstick testing or microscopic examination of the sediment to screen for hematuria and urinary tract infection (UTI).
- Serum prostate-specific antigen (PSA) measurement is recommended in select patients.
- Urine cytology is recommended as an option in men who predominantly have LUTS.

A serum creatinine measurement is no longer recommended on initial evaluation in the standard patient.

6. What is the American Urological Association (AUA) Symptom Score (also known as the International Prostate Symptom Score [I-PSS])?

This patient self-assessment questionnaire evaluates the patient's symptoms during the last month of symptoms (see Table). It helps to guide treatment options and to monitor the response to such treatments. A total score of 0–7 is classified as **mildly** symptomatic; 8–19 indicates **moderately** symptomatic; and 20–35 indicates **severely** symptomatic.

International Prostate Symptom Score (IPSS)

	NOT AT ALL	LESS THAN 1 TIME IN 5	LESS THAN HALF THE TIME	ABOUT HALF THE TIME	MORE THAN HALF THE TIME	ALMOST ALWAYS	**YOUR SCORE**
Incomplete emptying							
Over the past month, how often have you had a sensation of not emptying your bladder completely after you finish urinating?	0	1	2	3	4	5	
Frequency							
Over the past month, how often have you had to urinate again less than two hours after you finished urinating?	0	1	2	3	4	5	

Table continues on following page.

International Prostate Symptom Score (IPSS) (Continued)

	NOT AT ALL	LESS THAN 1 TIME IN 5	LESS THAN HALF THE TIME	ABOUT HALF THE TIME	MORE THAN HALF THE TIME	ALMOST ALWAYS	YOUR SCORE
Intermittency Over the past month, how often have you found you stopped and started again several times when you urinated?	0	1	2	3	4	5	
Urgency Over the last month, how difficult have you found it to postpone urination?	0	1	2	3	4	5	
Weak stream Over the past month, how often have you had a weak urinary stream?	0	1	2	3	4	5	
Straining Over the past month, how often have you had to push or strain to begin urination?	0	1	2	3	4	5	
Nocturia Over the past month, many times did you most typically get up to urinate from the time you went to bed until the time you got up in the morning?	0	1	2	3	4	5	
Total IPSS score							

QUALITY OF LIFE DUE TO URINARY SYMPTOMS							
	DELIGHTED	PLEASED	MOSTLY SATISFIED	MIXED: ABOUT EQUALLY SATISFIED AND DISSATISFIED	MOSTLY DISSATISFIED	UNHAPPY	TERRIBLE
If you were to spend the rest of your life with your urinary condition the way it is now, how would you feel about that?	0	1	2	3	4	5	6

Total score: 0–7 = mildly symptomatic; 8–19 = moderately symptomatic; 20–35 = severely symptomatic.

7. What is the initial management of patients with symptoms of BPH?

Patients with mild symptoms of BPH (AUA Symptom Score < 7) and patients with moderate or severe symptoms (AUA Symptom Score > 8) who are not bothered by their symptoms (i.e., symptoms do not interfere with activities of daily living) should be managed using a strategy of **watchful waiting.**

Management of patients with bothersome moderate to severe symptoms (AUA Symptom Score > 8) includes watchful waiting and medical, minimally invasive, or surgical therapies. Patients who are bothered enough to consider some form of therapy should be counseled on the risks and benefits of all the BPH treatment options (including watchful waiting).

8. Describe the medical management of BPH.

Two types of medications may help relieve the symptoms of BPH. The most popular form of medical therapy is with **alpha-blocker** type drugs (e.g., alfuzosin, terazosin, doxazosin, and tamsulosin). Other alpha-blockers have been phased out because of their serious side effect (e.g., prazosin, phenoxybenzamine-dibenzyline). Alpha-blockers are sometimes called the "drugs that help relax the muscles of the prostate." These drugs usually provide moderate relief of symptoms. Selective alpha$_1$-antagonists relax smooth muscle fibers at the vesicle outlet, reducing outlet resistance and improving urinary flow. Nonselective alpha-antagonists (phenoxybenzamine-dibenzyline) may reduce voiding symptoms but also have adverse side effects. Selective alpha$_1$-antagonists include prazosin (Minipress), terazosin (Hytrin), doxazosin (Cardura), and tamsulosin (Flomax). The last three are the most common medications prescribed currently.

Another type of medication commonly, the **5α-reductase inhibitors,** helps to shrink the size of the prostate. Examples include finasteride and dutasteride. Improvement in symptoms may take up to 3–6 months.

Recently, a combination of both alpha-blockers and 5α-reductase inhibitors has been advocated.

9. What are common side effects with medical therapy?

- **Alpha-blockers:** Common side effects are stomach or intestinal problems, a stuffy nose, headache, dizziness, and tiredness. A smaller number of patients may have low blood pressure.
- **5α-Reductase inhibitors:** Symptoms may not begin to be relieved until the medication has been taken for 3–6 months. Compared with the alpha-blockers, fewer side effects are seen. Some reported side effects are erectile dysfunction, decreased libido, and a reduced amount of semen. Two medications are available on the market: finasteride (Proscar) and dutasteride (Avodart). Dutasteride may need to be discontinued 6 months before blood transfusion. These medications must be placed out of the reach of children.

10. What are the minimally invasive options for BPH treatment?

- Transurethral microwave heat treatments (e.g., CoreTherm, Prostatron [various versions], Targis, TherMatrx)
- Transurethral needle ablation (TUNA)
- Urethral stents (e.g., UroLume stent)

11. What surgical options are available for treating BPH?

1. **Transurethral procedures**
    Transurethral resection of the prostate (TURP)
    Transurethral electrovaporization (TUEVAP)
    Transurethral incision of the prostate (TUIP)
    Transurethral holmium laser resection or enucleation
    Transurethral laser vaporization
    Transurethral laser coagulation (e.g., visual laser ablation)
2. **Open prostatectomy**

12. Describe the clinical utility of the three most frequently used hormonal therapies for reducing prostatic volume.

1. **Agonists of luteinizing hormone-releasing hormone** (LHRH), which include leuprolide and nafarelin acetate, produce significant benefits but require permanent uninterrupted therapy. Side effects include decreased libido, impotence, gynecomastia, hot flushes, and decreased levels of serum prostate-specific antigen (PSA). Therapy, therefore, is ideally restricted to impotent patients. An additional disadvantage is the requirement for intramuscular or subcutaneous administration. Depot forms permit administration every 3 months.

2. The primary **antiandrogen medication** is **flutamide,** which has advantages similar to LHRH agonists but also alters PSA levels. Side effects include gastrointestinal upset and gy-

necomastia or nipple tenderness. Sustained serum testosterone levels produce the advantage of undiminished libido, potency, and ejaculation. Flutamide is administered orally but may require up to 6 months to achieve maximal benefit. Uninterrupted maintenance therapy is necessary. Observance for hepatotoxicity is advised.

3. **Finasteride (Proscar)** and **dutasteride (Avodart)**, 5α-reductase inhibitors, are once-daily medications that have no significant side effects and may reduce prostatic volume and modestly improve symptoms in 30–50% of patients. Use for up to 6 months may be required for maximal benefit, and permanent maintenance therapy is required. PSA levels typically decrease by 50%, and this effect must be considered during monitoring for prostate cancer. An added advantage is the potential for halting disease progression due to suppressed androgen stimulation of the prostate.

All three agents appear equally effective in reducing prostatic volume by approximately 25% and improving obstructive symptoms and urinary flow rate. However, adrenergic inhibition is commonly preferred as initial therapy.

13. What is the preferred management of acute injury retention?

The obvious answer is catheter decompression of the bladder. Decisions about removal or maintenance of catheter drainage relate to the level of bladder overdistention. Retained volumes exceeding 500 mL are probably best treated by 2 days of catheter decompression to permit recovery of detrusor tonus. Smaller volumes are usually amenable to immediate drainage, with prompt restoration of preretention voiding dynamics. When urethral catheterization is unsuccessful, urologic referral is advised.

14. When urethral catheterization cannot be performed and consultation with a urologist is unavailable, what can be done to relieve urethral obstruction?

Temporary relief is obtainable by suprapubic trocar cystostomy or suprapubic insertion of a large-bore needle into the bladder through which a polyethylene drainage tube is passed. Commercial products are available for these purposes. Suprapubic maneuvers require a distended bladder and the absence of previous surgical scars. Surgical scars adjacent to the small bowel and colon put these organs at increased risk of injury.

15. What is the recommended practice for improving early diagnosis of prostate cancer?

Screening for prostate cancer is recommended for all men aged 50–70 years. Earlier screening (age 40–45 years) is advised for African-American patients and patients with familial (father, brother, uncle) incidence of prostate cancer. PSA elevation without abnormalities at DRE or transrectal ultrasonography (TRUS) warrants referral for sextant needle biopsy. A PSA level less than 20 ng/mL is statistically unassociated with identifiable metastatic dissemination; metastasis is more likely as levels progressively exceed 20 ng/mL. Elevation of the serum prostatic acid phosphatase is associated in most cases with cancer that escapes the confines of the prostate gland.

16. What conditions other than prostatic carcinoma may elevate the PSA to intermediate levels?

Prostatitis, prostate infarction, large BPH, and trauma (including biopsy or surgery).

17. Describe the staging of prostatic cancer.

Whitmore-Jewett Staging Systems for Prostate Cancer

STAGE	DEFINITION
A1–A2	No palpable tumor; incidental finding in operative specimen; positive random biopsy
B1–B3	Palpable tumor confined to the gland or small nodule confined to one lobe
C1–C2	Extension beyond prostatic capsule with or without involvement of lateral sulci or seminal vesicles
D1–D2	Metastases to any site, often including elevated prostatic acid phosphatase

TNM Prostate Cancer Staging

TNM STAGE	DEFINITION
TX	Primary tumor cannot be assessed
T0	No evidence of primary tumor
T1 (A)	Tumor not clinically apparent
T1a (A1)	Tumor incidentally found in $\leq$ 5% of prostate sample
T1b (A2)	Tumor incidentally found in > 5% of prostate sample
T1c	Tumor identified at needle biopsy performed to investigate PSA elevation
T2 (B)	Tumor palpable and confined to prostate
T2a (B1)	Tumor involves one prostate lobe
T2b (B2)	Tumor involves both prostate lobes
T3 (C)	Tumor palpable and extends beyond prostate capsule
T3a (C1)	Tumor extends beyond prostate capsule, either on one side (unilaterally) or both sides (bilaterally)
T3b (C1)	Tumor invades seminal vesicles
T4 (C2)	Tumor is fixed or invades adjacent anatomy other than seminal vesicles: bladder neck, external sphincter, rectum, levator muscles, and/or pelvic wall
NX	Regional lymph nodes cannot be assessed
N0	No regional lymph node metastasis
N1 (D1)	Metastasis in regional lymph node or nodes
MX	Presence of distant metastasis cannot be assessed
M0	No distant metastasis
M1 (D2)	Distant metastasis
M1a (D2)	Metastasis to nonregional lymph nodes
M1b (D2)	Metastasis to bone
M1c (D2)	Metastasis to other distant sites

18. What are the options for management of prostate cancer?
1. **Watchful waiting**
2. For **disease confined to the prostate:**
   - Surgical extirpation
     Open radical prostatectomy
     Perineal prostatectomy
     Laparoscopic radical prostatectomy
     Robotics radical prostatectomy
   - Radiotherapy
     External beam radiation
     Interstitial seed implant
     Combination seed with internal therapy
   - Targeted cryosurgical ablation of the prostate (TCAP; "freezing of the prostate")
3. For **metatastic or advanced disease:**
   - Pharmacologic or surgical hormone suppression—for treatment failure, usually dictated by elevating PSA level
   - Chemotherapy—reserved for advanced metastatic disease, especially hormone refractory cases (i.e., cancer stops responding to hormones)

19. How is pain from bony metastases controlled?
It is important to manage the pain with adequate analgesia. In patients with prostate cancer with symptomatic bone metastases, palliation can be achieved with either selective external beam irradiation therapy to the metastases or hemibody irradiation.

Another option for treatment of bone metastases is the use of strontium 89. Strontium 89 is a pure beta emitter that is taken up in the bones like calcium. Administration of strontium 89 has demonstrated a 20% complete symptomatic response in patients with metastatic prostate cancer.

20. **List potential complications or side effects seen with therapy for prostatic carcinoma.**

Surgery	**Estrogen therapy (rarely used)**
Impotence	Breast enlargement and tenderness
Incontinence	Increased incidence of cardiovascular events
Anastomotic stricture	**Isolated leuprolide therapy**
Rectal injury	Testosterone flare (temporary increase in
External radiotherapy	bone pain and other symptoms
Cystitis	suppressible with antiandrogen therapy)
Bladder contracture	Testicular atrophy
Urethral stricture	Loss of libido
Incontinence	Impotence
Impotence	Flutamide therapy
Cryosurgery	Gynecomastia
Impotence	Nausea and vomiting
Incontinence	
Penile pain	
Fistula between prostate and rectum	
Rectal injury	

21. **What is prostatitis?**

A misdiagnosis of prostatitis is often applied to nonspecific complaints of low back pain, perineal pain or discomfort, constipation, premature ejaculation, or vague voiding discomfort or dysfunction. The correct diagnosis of prostatitis must follow one of the two classification schemes:

1. **Traditional classification.** The traditional classification system is based on the landmark paper by Meares and Stamey (1968) describing the differential diagnosis of the prostatitis syndromes. With the traditional system, prostatitis is described in four categories depending on the analysis of prostatic fluid, which includes microscopy (white blood cells [WBCs] or inflammatory cells) and cultures.

- **Acute bacterial prostatitis** is diagnosed when prostatic fluid is purulent, cultures from seminal fluid are positive for bacteria, and systemic signs of infection are present.
- **Chronic bacterial prostatitis** is diagnosed with positive bacteria cultures from prostatic fluid in the absence of a concomitant UTI or signs of systemic infection.
- **Nonbacterial prostatitis** is diagnosed when significant purulence is still present (presence of WBCs) with negative bacterial cultures.
- **Prostatodynia** is diagnosed in the remaining patients who have persistent pain and voiding complaints as in the previous two categories but with absence of bacteria or WBCs in the prostatic fluid.

2. **National Institutes of Health (NIH) Classification.** The limitations of the traditional diagnostic algorithm and classification system led to the NIH classification:

- **Category I** is identical to the acute bacterial prostatitis category of the traditional classification system.
- **Category II** is identical to the traditional chronic bacterial prostatitis classification.
- **Category III** is defined as the presence of genitourinary pain in the absence of uropathogenic bacteria detected by cultures. It is subcategorized into **category IIIA,** or inflammatory chronic pelvic pain syndrome (CPPS), which is based on the presence of excessive WBCs in expressed prostatic secretion (EPS) or postprostatic massage urine or semen, and **category IIIB,** noninflammatory CPPS (no significant leukocytes in similar specimens).
- **Category IV,** or asymptomatic inflammatory prostatitis, is diagnosed by the presence of significant WBCs (or bacteria or both) in prostate-specific specimens (EPS, semen, and tissue biopsies) in the absence of typical chronic pelvic pain.

The NIH classification differs from the traditional system in two main areas: the descriptions of category III and IV prostatitis.

22. Describe the presentation and management of patients with acute prostatitis.

Acute bacterial prostatitis presents as a florid clinical disorder characterized by toxic systemic symptoms, extreme dysuria with increased frequency, urgency and strangury, severely tender prostate, and rusty urine containing red blood cells, WBCs, and bacteria. The prostatic barrier to antibiotic penetration is destroyed by the acute inflammatory process; therefore, any effective antibiotic suffices. Potentially severe local and systemic symptoms may necessitate hospitalization for parenteral antibiotics, fluid repletion, pain control, and urethral catheter drainage. Recovery is usually prompt.

23. Why should chronic bacterial prostatitis be distinguished from nonbacterial prostatitis?

Prolonged, uninterrupted antibacterial therapy is required for cure of chronic bacterial prostatitis. Diagnosis depends on culture positivity of prostatic secretions (after prostatic massage) or semen in the presence of sterile urine. Clinical manifestations are dominated by recurrent episodes of bacterial cystitis. Effective therapy is usually provided by trimethoprim-sulfamethoxazole (published cure rates of 30%) or quinolone (70%). Recommended duration of therapy is 4–12 weeks, thereby underscoring the importance of accurate diagnosis.

24. How is nonbacterial prostatitis managed?

Nonbacterial prostatitis is manifested as vague, nonspecific symptoms. Prostatic secretions contain inflammatory cells but no bacteria or culture positivity. Antibiotic therapy is the first-line treatment for a period of 4 weeks; if that fails, prostatic congestion may benefit from prostatic massage to express accumulated secretions. Other modalities include pharmacologic relaxation with alpha-blockers, anti-inflammatory agents, phytotherapy, 5α-reductase inhibition, and surgery or microwave of the prostate as last resort.

25. Define prostatodynia.

Prostatodynia is a term intended to incorporate the nonspecific symptoms often misinterpreted as prostatitis. Prostatic secretions are devoid of inflammatory cells. Management involves analgesics (anti-inflammatory agents) with or without muscle relaxants (alpha-blockers, diazepam). Physical therapy may be instituted with biofeedback, perineal or pelvic floor massage, and release of trigger points. If indicated, surgery may be the last resort. In severe cases reassurance and psychological support may be the only therapy available.

26. What is the significance of a diagnosis of prostatic abscess?

Prostatic abscess is uncommon. Contributing factors, therefore, should be considered, including diabetes, AIDS, and other immunosuppressive states. Specific bacterial diagnosis is warranted to identify atypical opportunistic infections. A prostatic abscess may present as either an acute systemic toxic event or a chronic low-grade, nonspecific disorder. Urethral obstruction may result from the abscess mass. DRE reveals asymmetry and nonhomogeneity; the involved lobe may be bulging, fluctuant, and variably sensitive. Prostatic abscess frequently ruptures into the rectum or urethra with resolution of the acute clinical status. Interventional drainage may be accomplished by transurethral resection or transrectal needle aspiration.

BIBLIOGRAPHY

1. Barry MJ, Fowler FJ Jr, O'Leary MP, et al: Measuring disease-specific health status in men with benign prostatic hyperplasia. Measurement Committee of the American Urological Association. Med Care 33:AS145-AS155, 1995.
2. Beduschi MC, Oesterling JE: Percent free-PSA and the early diagnosis of prostate cancer. Urol Grand Rounds 2:1–8, 1997.
3. Childs SJ: Ultrasound-guided laser-assisted transurethral resection of the prostate. Surg Techn Urol 7:2–8, 1994.
4. Denis L, McConnell J, Khoury S, et al: Recommendations of the International Scientific Committee: The evaluation and treatment of lower urinary tract symptoms (LUTS) suggestive of benign prostatic ob-

struction. In Denis L, Griffiths K, Khoury S, et al (eds): Proceedings of the Fourth International Consultation on Benign Prostatic Hyperplasia. United Kingdom, Health Publications, Ltd, 1998, pp 669–684.
5. Falagas ME, Gorbach SL: Practice guidelines: Prostatitis, epididymitis, and urethritis. Infect Dis Clin Pract 4:325–333, 1995.
6. Kabalin JN: Invasive therapies for BPH. Monogr Urol 18:17–47, 1997.
7. Keetch DW, Andriole GL: Prostate cancer screening. Monogr Urol 17:31–48, 1996.
8. Lee C, Cockett A, Cussenot K, et al: Regulation of prostate growth. In Chatelain C, Denis L, Foo KT, et al (eds): Proceedings of the Fifth International Consultation on Benign Prostatic Hyperplasia. UK, Health Publications, Ltd., 2001, pp 79–106.
9. McConnell JD, Barry MJ, Bruskewitz RC, et al: Benign prostatic hyperplasia: Diagnosis and treatment. In Agency for Health Care Policy and Research: Clinical Practice Guideline. Rockville, MD, AHCPR, 1994.
10. Meares EM Jr: Acute and chronic prostatitis: Diagnosis and treatment. Infect Dis Clin North Am 1:855–873, 1987.
11. Nickel JC: Rational management of nonbacterial prostatitis and prostatodynia. Curr Opin Urol 6:53–58, 1996.
12. Nickel JC: The Pre and Post Massage Test (PPMT): A simple screen for prostatitis. Tech Urol 3:38–43, 1997.
13. Nickel JC: Effective office management of chronic prostatitis. Urol Clin North Am 25:677–684, 1998.
14. Nickel JC: Prostatitis: Evolving management strategies. Urol Clin North Am 26:743–751, 1999.
15. Nickel JC, Sorensen R: Transurethral microwave thermotherapy for nonbacterial prostatitis: A randomized double-blind sham controlled study using new prostatitis specific assessment questionnaires. J Urol 155:1950–1954, 1996.
16. Peterson NE: Primary care treatment of prostatic disorders. Prim Care Rep 2:19–26, 1996.
17. Peterson NE: Urinary incontinence and retention. In Harwood-Nuss A, et al (eds): The Clinical Practice of Emergency Medicine, 2nd ed. Philadelphia, Lippincott-Raven, 1996, pp 258–263.
18. Raghavan D, Cooney G, Rosen M, et al: Management of hormone resistant prostate cancer. Semin Oncol 23:20–23, 1996.
19. Roehrborn CG, McConnell JD: Etiology, pathophysiology, epidemiology and natural history of benign prostatic hyperplasia. In Walsh PC, Retik AB, Vaughan ED, Wein AJ (eds): Campbell's Urology, 8th ed. Philadelphia, W.B. Saunders, 2002, pp 1297–1330.
20. Roehrborn CG, Girman CJ, Rhodes T, et al: Correlation between prostate size estimated by digital rectal examination and measured by transrectal ultrasound. Urology 49:548, 1997.
21. Stamey TA: Prostate cancer: Who should be treated? Monogr Urol 16:1–16, 1995.

51. DISEASES OF THE SCROTUM

Iván Colón, M.D., and Rosalia Misseri, M.D.

1. What is the basic workup of a patient who presents with scrotal pathology?

History   Physical examination (ensure transillumination)
Urinalysis   Imaging studies (ultrasound, testicular scan)

2. What is the recommended clinical reaction to the discovery of an intrascrotal mass?

A good history and physical examination, coupled with urinalysis, culture, and scrotal ultrasound. A testicular scan has been used and described in the literature, but its usefulness is still debated. It is important to differentiate between acute versus chronic and painful versus asymptomatic presentations. Be sure to ask about trauma, urinary tract infections (UTIs), sexually transmitted diseases (STDs), acute onset, associated voiding symptoms, and previous scrotal or inguinal surgery. Ultrasound characteristics usually will dictate the next step. Solid masses are considered malignant until proven otherwise.

PATHOLOGY		PAIN	TRANSILLUMINATION	U/A	U/S	TESTICULAR SCAN
Testicular torsion	Insidious Usually young boys, but seen in all ages.	Yes	No	+/−	No mass, decreased to no blood flow	Cold
Testicular tumor	Incidental (may be acute*) Males 20–40 yrs	No (yes*)	No	−	Solid mass	
Testicular rupture	Trauma	Yes	No	+/−	Complex mass	
Epididymitis	Previous STDs History unprotected intercourse Bladder outlet obstruction (BPH)	Yes	No	+	Complex mass, increased blood flow	Hot
Inguinal hernia	History of inguinal hernias	+/−	+/−	−	Complex mass, bowel may be seen	
Hydrocele	Incidental Previous trauma or infection	No	Yes	−	Cystic mass, testis normal	
Spermatocele		No	Yes	−	Cystic mass	

U/A = urinalysis; U/S = ultrasound.

3. List the masses that may involve intrascrotal contents, and specify the presence or absence of pain as a distinguishing feature.

PAINFUL SCROTAL MASSES	PAINLESS SCROTAL MASSES
Testicular or spermatic cord torsion	Testicular tumor
Torsion, testis appendage	Inguinal hernia
Epididymitis/orchitis	Hydrocele
Inguinal hernia (incarcerated/strangulated)	Spermatocele
Testicular tumor (rapidly growing/hemorrhage)	Varicocele
Hematocele	Para testicular tumor
Abscess	

Hydrocele and varicocele may present with pain, but palpation discomfort is uncommon, and symptoms may be exaggerated by anxiety and apprehension. Spermatocele may be painful only in its earliest and smallest manifestations. As the spermatocele enlarges, the fibers of its capsule separate, thereby relieving the pain of capsular distension. Testis tumors are characteristically painless, although intralesional hemorrhage (rare) may be painful. Chronic discomfort also may result from the weight and mass of larger lesions.

4. What is the significance of acute versus chronic scrotal pain?

Scrotal pain of acute onset characterizes torsion of the spermatic cord or testicular appendages and acute epididymitis. Acute pain also may result from hemorrhage into a tumor or traumatic rupture of the testicular capsule (tunica albuginea). Doppler ultrasound scanning is often effective in diagnosis, but contradictory studies impose the requirement for surgical exploration.

Chronic scrotal pain may occur with any subacute inflammatory disorder, including epididymitis, orchitis, or abscess. It also may result from the weight and mass of larger testis tumors. Chronic testicular pain is often claimed with hydrocele, varicocele, and spermatocele but may result from anxiety. Chronic pain associated with testicular elevation may represent chronic cremaster muscle spasm, which is usually self-limited but requires operative intervention in extreme cases.

5. Why is orchiectomy maintained as a last resort for patients with chronic orchidynia?

Debilitating, incapacitating testicular pain resistant to myriad analgesic and psychogenic relief efforts is termed *orchidynia* or *orchalgia*. Postoperative complaints of ipsilateral or contralateral testis pain often follow removal of the symptomatic testis. Referral to pain management consultants or psychotherapy is advised.

6. What diagnostic adjuncts are available for evaluation of intrascrotal pathology?

- Urinalysis (to exclude infection)
- Color Doppler ultrasound (for blood flow)
- Isotope scintigraphy
- Plain radiographs (for evidence of calcification)
- Ultrasound scanning
- Serum tumor marker evaluation (human chorionic gonadotropin [hCG], alpha fetoprotein)
- Drainage cultures
- Surgical exploration

7. What clinical features are helpful for distinguishing spermatic cord torsion from epididymitis?

Epididymitis may present in any age group (although uncommon in young children) as sudden onset of pain and swelling in the scrotum. Physical examination reveals testicular tenderness and a positive Prehn's sign (pain improvement with the testis support or elevation); cremasteric reflexes may or may not be present, and temperature elevation may also be seen. Purulent discharge can be expressed from the urethra, and the urinalysis is usually positive for inflammatory cells.

Spermatic cord torsion usually presents with transverse orientation of testis or epididymis, elevation of the scrotum will not relive the pain, high-riding testis, and cutaneous erythema.

The most reliable clinical feature is rate of onset of pain; pain is instantaneous with torsion and occurs over several hours with epididymitis. Emesis is frequent in pediatric patients. Diagnosis of epididymitis may be supported by pain and induration limited to the posterior aspect of the testis or to one pole.

8. Is spermatic cord torsion restricted to young patients?

No.

9. What is the recommended management of spermatic cord torsion?

If spermatic cord or testicular torsion is suspected, urgent urology consultation is indicated. The recommended management is immediate detorsion. An emergent surgical exploration is the best diagnostic test, and it should not be delayed if the diagnosis of testicular or spermatic cord torsion is highly suspected. Prompt detorsion is required within 6 hours of onset of pain; a delay of more than 12 hours results in poor testicular salvage (< 20%). Manual detorsion can be attempted at first, and, if successful, an elective (nonemergent) testicular orchidopexy or fixation of both testicles must follow.

10. What is the presentation and significance of torsion of a testicular appendage?

Torsion of a testicular appendage presents with symptoms of spermatic cord torsion, but they are much less intense. Vomiting is unlikely. Less extreme pain and swelling contribute to delayed presentation, which is provoked more often by chronicity than intensity of symptoms. Therefore, emergency operative intervention is avoided in favor of adjunctive diagnostic maneuvers (color Doppler ultrasound, isotope scanning). The natural history of a twisted appendage is symptomatic resolution and regression of the tender mass (which may appear blue through the skin, producing the "blue dot" sign). Such lesions may calcify and become separated, accounting for intrascrotal "foreign bodies" occasionally discovered at routine physical examination.

11. Describe the management of acute epididymitis.

Always obtain a urinalysis and urine culture with sensitivities. If an STD is suspected, urethral cultures for gonorrhea and *Chlamydia* must be sent. Acute epididymitis localized to the testis or epididymis must be treated with the appropriate oral antibiotic, anti-inflammatory agents (e.g., ibuprofen), scrotal elevation, and reassessment in 3 weeks. Systemic toxicity must be managed with admission to the hospital for intravenous antibiotics, antipyretics, fluid hydration, scrotal elevation, and anti-inflammatory agents (pain control). In selected patients, severe epididymitis may be managed in an outpatient basis.

12. What is the anticipated response to therapy for acute epididymitis?

Epididymitis that does not respond to therapy within 24–48 hours implies inappropriate antibiotic treatment, inaccurate diagnosis, or abscess formation. Abscess may be identified by ultrasound scanning, and orchiectomy should be considered. Pain is the first symptom that will resolve. Size of the testis or epididymis is the last symptom to disappear. If the patient has persistent scrotal mass after appropriate antibiotic therapy for 3 weeks, suspect testicular tumor and repeat the scrotal ultrasound.

13. What is the potential significance of recurrent epididymitis in an adult?

Recurrent epididymitis suggests lower urinary tract obstruction (e.g., benign prostatic hypertrophy [BPH], urethral stricture disease). An alternative possibility in patients engaged in vigorous work or exercise is retrograde reflux of urine into the vas deferens with straining, producing a chemical epididymitis that tends to be recurrent.

14. What is the potential significance of an episode of epididymitis in a child?

UTI, especially epididymitis, is uncommon in children and, therefore, suggests the possibility of an obstructive urinary defects or voiding dysfunction. Bacteriuria or history of urinary tract infections increases suspicion. UTIs in children must be investigated with an antegrade radiographic study (intravenous pyelogram [IVP]) and a retrograde radiographic study (voiding cystourethrogram).

15. What should be considered in the management of indurated testicular enlargement in a neonate?

Intrauterine testicular torsion presents as an apparently painless, smooth, homogeneously enlarged testis that may appear blue through the scrotal integument and may be distinguished from hydrocele or other lesions by testicular ultrasound. Orchiectomy is usually not necessary.

16. What is the potential significance of varicocele to a child? To an adult?

Varicoceles usually become manifest in early or mid-adolescence and often regress spontaneously during the fourth decade of life. Thus, the published incidence of varicocele among military inductees is 12–15% compared with a nominal incidence of varicocele among older men. Pathologic etiologies such as intra-abdominal or retroperitoneal masses that produce venous obstruction and collateral venous drainage should be considered in preadolescent or presenile patients. Nonpathologic varicoceles in preadolescent boys are significant because of possible deleterious influences on testicular growth and maturation. Therefore, varicocelectomy is recommended to reverse suppressive influences in a testis that is noticeably smaller than its mate. Semen analysis of infertile patients with varicocele may include reduced sperm motility and increased numbers of immature and abnormal forms. Semen characteristics and fertility potential may improve after varicocelectomy, although absolute sperm counts and densities are rarely improved.

17. What is the usual presentation of a testicular tumor?

Testicular tumors usually present as an incidental finding of a painless nodule or "lump" in the scrotum of a man aged 20–40 years. A heavy sensation or dull ache may be experienced in the lower abdomen. A rapidly growing tumor or an acute bleed (hemorrhage) into the tumor may cause acute testicular pain. Physical examination usually reveals hard, nontender nodule (or mass) localized to the testis without transillumination. A hydrocele may be associated with testicular tumors. Epididymitis may be the presenting symptoms in up to 10% of testicular tumors.

18. Should needle aspiration of a painless testicular mass be undertaken for diagnosis?

No, because of the potential of tumor seeding and the inaccuracy of the biopsy. The diagnosis should be performed via inguinal exploration and orchiectomy. Prior to orchiectomy, serum tumor markers must be drawn. Markers include alpha-fetoprotein, β-HCG, lactate dehydrogenase, and placental alkaline phosphatase (PLAP) as an index of tumor volume, aggressiveness, and histology and later as a measure of response to therapy. After testicular cancer has been confirmed following orchiectomy, a computed tomography (CT) scan of the abdomen and pelvis, chest x-ray, and liver function tests (LFTs) are the next step in evaluation.

19. How common is testis cancer?

Despite the fact that testicular cancer accounts for only 1% of all male malignancies, it is the most common solid malignancy affecting males between the ages of 15 and 35 years. Advances in surgery and chemotherapy over the last few decades have improved survival. In fact, testicular cancer has become one of the most curable of all solid neoplasm. In the late 1970s, testicular cancer death accounted for 11.4% of all cancer deaths in the 25–34-year age group, with an overall 5-year survival rate of 64%. The most recent 5-year survival rate for testicular cancer in the United States is over 90%.

20. Is testicular carcinoma curable?

Yes. Therapy is selected according to histology, volume, staging (degree of dissemination), status of tumor markers, and previous therapy. Seminoma is traditionally curable with small doses of radiotherapy; large-volume seminoma or extranodal disease often warrants chemotherapy. Nonseminomatous germ-cell carcinoma (embryonal carcinoma, teratocarcinoma, choriocarcinoma) requires platinum-based chemotherapy, with retroperitoneal lymph node dissection selected according to persisting nodal masses.

21. What is the significance of acute pain and testicular enlargement after scrotal trauma?

Acutely painful posttraumatic testicular enlargement reflects rupture of the testicular capsule (tunica albuginea) with parenchymal extrusion and hematoma formation (hematocele). Pain may be extreme, with pallor, sweating, and nausea. Diagnosis may be confirmed in equivocal circumstances by scrotal ultrasound scanning. Patients managed conservatively usually recover spontaneously after an extended symptomatic convalescence, whereas scrotal exploration, evacuation of hematoma and infarcted tissue, and surgical repair of the testicular capsule contribute to a rapid benign recovery.

22. How is testicular carcinoma classified?

Testicular carcinoma is classified into germ cell and non-germ cell tumors. Germ cell tumors are subclassified into **seminoma** and **nonseminomatous** germ cell tumors (NSGCTs). NSGCTs include embryonal carcinoma, teratocarcinoma, teratoma, yolk sac tumor, and choriocarcinoma.

23. What is the most common type of testicular tumor?

Trick question. Seminoma is the most common type of testicular tumor (of all individual tumors), but NSGCT as a group is more common. Testicular cancer may be classified as follows:
- Seminomas—30–40% of all testicular tumors.
- NSGCT
- Embryonal carcinoma—20% of all testicular tumors that occur in 20–30-year-old men and is highly malignant. It grows rapidly and spreads to the lungs and liver.
- Teratocarcinoma—20%
- Teratoma—7% of adult cancers, 40% in young boys

- Choriocarcinoma
- Yolk sac tumor
- Stromal cell tumors—these tumors are made of Leydig cells, Sertoli cells, and granulose cells. They account for 3–4% of all testicular tumors. These tumors may secrete a hormone, estradiol, that can cause gynecomastia (excessive development of male breast tissue), one of the symptoms of testicular cancer.

24. Does age play a role in the type of testicular carcinoma seen?

Yes. In children, yolk sac tumors are more common (60%) followed by teratomas (up to 40%). Stromal cell tumors are nearly 20% of all childhood testicular tumors.

25. What are the risk factors for testicular carcinoma?

Although an exact cause of testicular cancer has not been identified, several predisposing factors may place some men at higher risk, including a past medical history of undescended testis, abnormal testicular development, Klinefelter syndrome, and previous testicular cancer. Other factors that are under investigation as a possible cause are exposure to certain chemicals and infection with the human immunodeficiency virus (HIV). A family history of testicular cancer may increase the risk. Vasectomy does not predispose individuals to testicular cancer.

BIBLIOGRAPHY

1. Berman JM, Beidle TR, Kunberger LE, Letourneau JG: Sonographic evaluation of acute intrascrotal pathology. AJR Am J Roentgenol 166:857–861, 1996.
2. Chinegwundoh FL: The post-traumatic painful testis. Postgrad Med J 72:251–252, 1996.
3. Doherty AP, Bower M, Christmas TJ: The role of tumor markers in the diagnosis and treatment of testicular germ cell cancers. Br J Urol 79:247–252, 1997.
4. Donohue JP, Foster RS, Little JS Jr, et al: Biology of metastases and its clinical implications: Testicular germ-cell tumors. W J Urol 14:197–203, 1996.
5. Flores LG II, Shiba T, Hoshi H, et al: Scintigraphic evaluation of testicular torsion and acute epididymitis. Ann Nucl Med 10:89–92, 1996.
6. Greenlee RT, Murray T, Bolden S, Wingo PA: Cancer statistics, 2000. CA Cancer J Clin 50:7–33, 2000.
7. Hendrikx AJ, Dang CL, Vroegindeweij D, Korte JH: B-mode and colour-flow duplex ultrasonography: A useful adjunct in diagnosing scrotal diseases? Br J Urol 79:58–65, 1997.
8. Herbener TE: Ultrasound in the assessment of the acute scrotum. J Clin Ultrasound Med 24:405–421, 1996.
9. Herr HW, Sheinfeld J, Puc HS, et al: Surgery for a post-chemotherapy residual mass in seminoma. J Urol 157:860–862, 1997.
10. Lewis AG, Bukowski TP, Jarvis PD, et al: Evaluation of acute scrotum in the emergency department. J Pediatr Surg 30:277–281, 1995.
11. Meares EM, Stamey TA: Bacteriologic localization patterns in bacterial prostatitis and urethritis. Invest Urol 5:492, 1968.
12. Moul JW, Heidenreich A: Prognostic factors in low-stage nonseminomatous testicular cancer. Oncology 10:1359–1368, 1996.
13. Mostofi FK: Testicular tumors: Epidemiologic, etiologic and pathologic features. Cancer 32:1186, 1973.
14. Oliver RT: Testicular cancer. Curr Opin Oncol 8:252–258, 1996.
15. Parkinson MC, Swerdlow AJ, Pike MC: Carcinoma in situ in boys with cryptorchidism: When can it be detected? Br J Urol 73:431–435, 1994.
16. Pels RJ, Bor DH, Woolhandler S, et al: Dipstick urinalysis screening of asymptomatic adults for urinary tract disorders. II. Bacteriuria. JAMA 262:1221–1224, 1989.
17. Peterson NE, Schwab R: Acute scrotal pain requires quick thinking and plan of action. Emerg Med Rep 13:11–18, 1992.
18. Rabinowitz R, Hulbert WC Jr: Acute scrotal swelling. Urol Clin North Am 22:101–105, 1995.
19. Schwaibold H, Fobbe F, Klan R, Dieckmann KP: Evaluation of acute scrotal pain by color-coded duplex sonography. Urol Int 56:96–99, 1996.

52. ERECTILE DYSFUNCTION

Iván Colón, M.D.

1. What is erectile dysfunction (ED)?

ED or impotence is the inability of a man to obtain or maintain a penile erection sufficient for intercourse and achieve his sexual needs or the needs of his partner. ED is distinct from infertility and also must be distinguished from unrealized ambitions of sexual potency. Erectile dysfunction can cause emotional and relationship problems and often leads to diminished self-esteem. It has many causes, most of which are treatable.

2. How common is erectile dysfunction in the United States?

An estimated 30 million men in the United States (10% of the male population) experience chronic erectile dysfunction, although as few as 5% seek treatment. Erectile dysfunction often may go undiagnosed because of embarrassment and reluctance to acknowledge symptoms and to pursue remedies. Annual estimates include more than 525,000 office visits and 30,000 hospital admissions for this disorder. It may affect 50% of men between ages 40 and 70 years. Transient lost or inadequate erection affects men of all ages.

3. What are the potential causes of ED?

Causes of ED are physiologic and psychological. Reduced blood flow to the penis and nerve damage are the most common causes. Erectile dysfunction may be categorized into organic and nonorganic causes:

Organic causes
- Trauma
- Inflammatory disorder: prostatitis
- Neurogenic disorders: spinal cord injury, multiple sclerosis, temporal lobe epilepsy, cerebrovascular accident, autonomic neuropathy, peripheral neuropathy
- Vasogenic disorders: arterial or venous
- Endocrine (hormonal): hypogonadism, decreased testosterone, hyperprolactinemia
- Systemic disorders: diabetes, hypertension, hypercholesterolemia, hyperthyroidism
- Pharmacologic impotence
- Miscellaneous factors: cigarettes, priapism, Peyronie's disease, dialysis, alcoholism, zinc deficiency, angina, arthritis, chronic obstructive pulmonary disease, postoperative dysfunction (abdominoperineal resection, prostatectomy, renal transplantation)

Nonorganic causes: All causes not qualifying as organic and involving basically psychogenic factors

4. What traumatic injuries may result in ED?

Excluding trauma-induced emasculation, injuries involving the spinal cord below the L1-L2 level and pelvic fracture with cicatrix-related or direct injury to the pudendal and genital arterial supply are most likely.

5. What are clues to psychogenic ED?

Clues to psychogenic impotence include descriptions of periodic erections or coitus, spontaneous nocturnal or early morning erections, or satisfactory potency in selected circumstances such as illicit romance or during drug or alcohol use. Psychogenic impotence typically involves patients in younger age groups and an absence of other potential pathologic influences. Psychogenic ED is equally deserving of every modality of care.

6. Can psychogenic ED be treated?

Psychological factors cause 10–20% of cases of impotence. These factors include stress, anxiety, guilt, depression, low self-esteem, and fear of sexual failure. Such factors are broadly associated with more than 80% of cases of impotence, usually as secondary reactions to underlying physical causes. Therapeutic remedies for psychogenic ED include psychiatric counseling, which may be prolonged and of variable benefit, and initiation of therapy to induce erection artificially. Successful therapy is often associated with progressive independence from such methods.

7. What are the differences between psychogenic and organic ED?

CHARACTERISTIC	ORGANIC	PSYCHOGENIC
Onset	Gradual	Acute
Circumstances	Global	Situational
Course	Constant	Varying
Noncoital erection	Poor	Rigid
Psychosexual problem	Secondary	Long history
Partner problem	Secondary	At onset
Anxiety and fear	Secondary	Primary

8. List the indications for psychiatric counseling.

Sex therapy
Ambiguous impotence
Psychiatric fitness for prosthesis
Preexisting functional impotence
Ethanol or drug abuse

Personality disorder
Hypochondriasis
History of psychiatric disorder
Situation impotence

9. Are objective means available for identifying or verifying nocturnal erections?

Erectile response to intracavernous injection of erection-inducing agents is satisfactory evidence of intact erectile physiology. Thus, referral to a urologist for this test may eliminate greater expense and help to direct therapy. Specific monitoring for nocturnal penile tumescence is largely abandoned as unimportant to the diagnosis.

10. What commonly used drugs or medications may deleteriously influence penile erection?

Diuretics
  Hydrochlorothiazide
  Spironolactone
Tranquilizers
  Phenothiazines
Antiandrogen
  Flutamide
Addictive and abused substances
  Alcohol
  Opiates
  Barbiturates
  Nicotine
  Cannabis
Alpha-adrenergic blocker
  Terazosin
Beta-adrenergic blockers
Anticholinergic agents
  Atropine
Antidepressants
  Tricyclics
  Monoamine oxidase (MAO) inhibitors

Antianxiety agents
  Benzodiazepines
Antihypertensive agents
  Hydralazine
  Clonidine
Antiparkinsonian agents
Antihistamines
Muscle relaxants
  Cyclobenzaprine
  Orphenadrine
Miscellaneous drugs
  Cimetidine
  Clofibrate
  Digoxin
  Estrogens
  Indomethacin
  Lithium carbonate
  Methysergide
  Metoclopramide
  Metronidazole
  Phenytoin

When it is suspected that an agent may be responsible for ED, discontinuation of the drug and rechallenge, if necessary, should be undertaken. The patient may also relate onset or exaggeration of ED with initiation of drug therapy.

11. What is the most frequent systemic disorder are associated with ED?

Diabetes may be the single most frequent cause of ED. Impotence occurs in 35–75% of diabetic men. Whereas many studies claim no correlation between impotence and duration and severity of diabetes, other reports assert that impotence affects 50% of male diabetics after 10 years. Impotence is often associated with peripheral or autonomic diabetic neuropathy. Patients with ED and poorly controlled hyperglycemia occasionally improve with careful medical management, but improvement is uncommon and limited. Artificial remedies are advised rather than a futile wait for spontaneous recovery.

12. Which laboratory tests are important in evaluating patients with ED?

Basic screening laboratory studies are essential in the evaluation of patients with ED. A screening total serum testosterone level is helpful in all patients. Normal serum testosterone values obviate the need for additional endocrine testing or exogenous testosterone therapy. The rare patient with hypogonadism characteristically presents with a serum testosterone level of ≤ 200 mg/dL, a small prostate; and small, soft testes (< 3.5 cm). Although changes in libido may suggest a decrease in testosterone, these changes are not always easily identified. A low libido may also be a sign of subclinical depression. If the total testosterone level is low, a free testosterone, luteinizing hormone (LH), and prolactin level should be the next tests to order. Impotence occasionally results from hyperprolactinemia (> 15–20 mg/dL), which is typically associated with subnormal testosterone and diminished libido. Because ED may be caused by diabetes and hypercholesterolemia, a serum glucose and lipid profile should also be ordered as screening tests.

13. What treatments are offered for erectile dysfunction?

Sex therapy	**Surgical treatment**
Medical treatment	Surgical penile implants
Oral medication	Semirigid prosthesis
Transurethral	Inflatable prosthesis
Intracavernous	Vascular reconstructive surgery
Hormonal therapy	Revascularization
Intramuscular	Venous ligation
Dermal patches	
Treatment of other endocrine disorders	
Vacuum devices	

14. What medical therapy is available for ED?

Medical Therapy for Impotence

AGENTS	DOSAGE
Oral agents	
Sildenafil (Viagra)	50–100 mg PO QD PRN
Verdenafil (Levitra)	5–20 mg/day PRN
Tadalafil (Cialis)	10–20 mg/day PRN
Yohimbine	6 mg three times/day
Dermal agents	
Testoderm	4–6 mg patch QD
Androderm	5 mg patch QD
Intramuscular agents (esterified testosterone)	
Propionate	50 mg three times a week
Cypionate (depo-testosterone)	200 mg every 2–3 weeks
Enanthate (Delatestryl)	200 mg every 2–3 weeks

Table continues on following page.

Medical Therapy for Impotence (Continued)

AGENTS	DOSAGE
Intracavernous	
Papaverine HCl	30–90 mg
Phentolamine	5 mg
Prostaglandin E$_1$	5–25 ng
Combination papaverine-phentolamine-prostaglandin	

Four oral medications are used to treat ED in men:

1. **Sildenafil (Viagra)** improves partial erections by inhibiting the enzyme that facilitates penile detumescence. It increases levels of cyclic guanosine monophosphate (cGMP), which causes the smooth muscles of the penis to relax, enabling blood to flow into the corpora cavernosa. Sildenafil is absorbed and processed rapidly by the body and is usually taken 30 minutes to 1 hour before intercourse. Patients with a cardiac history should be evaluated by a cardiologist. This medication is contraindicated with the concomitant use of nitrates.

2. **Verdenafil (Levitra)** is approved by the FDA for the treatment ED in men. It should be taken only as needed and no more than once a day. It is effective within 25–120 minutes, and the effect is delayed by fatty meal. It improved rates of penetration, intercourse success, and hardness with sexual experience in a broad population of men with ED and has been clinically shown to improve erectile function even in men who had other health factors, such as diabetes or prostate surgery. Side effects are similar to those of sildenafil. This medication should be taken concomitantly with nitrates and alpha-blockers used for the treatment of BPH or high blood pressure.

3. **Tadalafil (Cialis)** is effective within 16–30 minutes and should be taken 30 minutes to 12 hours before sexual activity. Its effect is *not* delayed by food. It often works within 30 minutes and stays effective for up to 36 hours, which is longer than both Viagra and Levitra. FDA approval is still pending as of this writing.

4. **Yohimbine** is expensive and of no objective benefit, although some patients claim improvement; placebo effect may explain the claim.

Transurethral therapy is another effective treatment for ED. The medications are delivered via the urethra and absorbed via the mucosa and act locally. Referral to a urologist is appropriate for additional therapy.

15. What is a vacuum erection device?

The vacuum erection device is a plastic tube that fits over the penis. Air is ejected from the tube by an attached hand pump, resulting in attraction of blood into the cavernosal tissues by negative pressure. An elastic constriction applied to the penile base maintains an erection satisfactory for coitus. Such devices are effective for many patients and have a low incidence of side effects. Cost ranges between $250 and $400 and may be partially covered by insurance. Battery-energized pump devices are available as affordable options. This device is indicated for the following conditions: ED; veno-occlusive dysfunction; and ED after radical prostatectomy, penile vascular surgery, removal of prosthesis, and venous grafting.

16. What role does penile or pelvic vascular surgery play in therapy for ED?

Penile vascular surgery is indicated for a small subset of patients with arteriogenic ED. This group consists mostly of young patients with discrete arterial lesions that are secondary to pelvic or perineal injuries. Surgery has a high failure rate; many early successes deteriorate later.

17. What are penile prostheses?

Penile prostheses are intracavernosal implants available to patients who fail or refuse other forms of treatment. Several models are available, including semirigid devices with malleability features for convenience and inflatable-deflatable hydraulic models. Semirigid devices are reliable and have a low failure rate. Improvements in materials and bioengineering have reduced the mechanical dysfunction of inflatable models, although cost remains significant.

18. Is there an effective treatment for premature ejaculation?

This variant of ED dominates clinical complaints of sexual inadequacy and deserves every therapeutic resource. Care traditionally has been reduced to reassurance and psychotherapy with disappointing results. Contemporary management favors methods developed for erectile failure, including intracavernous and intraurethral drugs and vacuum erectile devices. Benefit also has been described with low doses of selective serotonin uptake inhibitors, including fluoxetine (Prozac), 7.5–30 mg/day; sertraline (Zoloft), 50 mg/day; and clomipramine (Inapramil), 25–50 mg/day. Paradoxically, larger doses may increase sexual complaints.

BIBLIOGRAPHY

1. Brock G, Lue TF: Impotence. Monogr Urol 13:99–110, 1992.
2. Broderick GA, Schwartz S: Erectile dysfunction in diabetes. Hosp Pract 26:139–142, 147–155, 1991.
3. Carson CC: Erectile dysfunction in the 21st century: Whom we can treat, whom we cannot treat and patient education. Int J Impot Res 14(suppl 1):S29-S34, 2002.
4. Dorey G: Is smoking a cause of erectile dysfunction? A literature review. Br J Nurs 25:455–465, 2001.
5. Fallon B, Grahem H: Sexual performance and satisfaction with penile prosthesis in impotence of various etiologies. Int J Impotence Res 2:35–42, 1990.
6. Gilbert HW, Gingell JC: Vacuum constriction devices: Second-line conservative treatment for impotence. Br J Urol 70:81–83, 1992.
7. Gupta R, Kirschen S, Barrow R, et al: Predictors of success and risk factors for attrition in the use of intracorporal injection therapy. J Urol 157:1681–1686, 1997.
8. Lewis RW: Long-term results of penile prostheses implants. Urol Clin North Am 22:847–856, 1995.
9. Linet OL, Ogrinc FG: Efficacy and safety of intracavernosal alprostadil in men with erectile dysfunction: The Alprostadil Study Group. N Engl J Med 334:873–877, 1996.
10. McLean RH, Barrett DM: Patient and partner satisfaction with the AMS 700 penile prosthesis. J Urol 147:62–65, 1992.
11. Montorsi F, Guazzoni G, Barbieri L: Recovery of spontaneous erectile function after nerve sparing radical prostatectomy with and without early intracavernous injections of prostaglandin E-1: Results of a prospective, randomized trial [abstract]. J Urol 155(suppl):468A, 1996.
12. Montorsi F, Salonia A, Deho F, et al: The aging male and erectile dysfunction. World J Urol 20:28–35, 2002.
13. Moreland RB, Traish A, Mc Millin MA: PGE$_1$ suppresses the synthesis by transforming growth factor beta$_1$ in human corpus cavernosum smooth muscle. J Urol 153:826–834, 1995.
14. Mulcahy JJ, Eid F, Fair WF, et al: Treatment options for erectile dysfunction in the post-prostatectomy patient. Contemp Urol 9(suppl):3–22, 1997.
15. Newey J: Causes and treatment of erectile dysfunction. Nurs Stand 12:39–40, 1998.
16. Padma-Nathan H: Corporal pharmacotherapy for erectile dysfunction and priapism. Monogr Urol 17:51–64, 1997.
17. Padma-Nathan H, Auerbach SM, Barada JH: Multicenter, double-blind, placebo-controlled trial of transurethral alprostadil in men with chronic erectile dysfunction [abstract]. J Urol 155(suppl):496A, 1996.
18. Padma-Nathan H, Hellstrom WJG, Kaiser FE: Treatment of men with erectile dysfunction with transurethral alprostadil. N Engl J Med 336:1–7, 1997.
19. Porst H: The rationale for prostaglandin E$_1$ in erectile failure: A survey of worldwide experience. J Urol 155:802–815, 1996.
20. Sharlip ID: Evaluation and nonsurgical management of erectile dysfunction. Urol Clin North Am 25:647–659, 1998.
21. Spollett GR: Assessment and management of erectile dysfunction in men with diabetes. Diabetes Educ 25:65–73, 1999.

VIII. Common Disorders of the Renal and Urinary System

53. URINARY TRACT INFECTIONS

Randall R. Reves, M.D., M.Sc., and David W. Lehman, M.D., Ph.D.

1. Are urinalysis and urine culture always necessary to confirm the diagnosis of a urinary tract infection (UTI)?

No. By age 65 years, up to one third of women experience one or more episodes of cystitis, the great majority of which are uncomplicated. The risk of UTI increases with frequency of sexual intercourse. Other factors that increase the risk of UTI include recent use of a diaphragm with spermicide and a history of prior UTI. Such infections, which are usually caused by *Escherichia coli* (80%) or *Staphylococcus saprophyticus* (5–15%), follow predictable susceptibility patterns and respond to a short course of antimicrobial agents. Thus, a young woman with typical symptoms and signs of uncomplicated cystitis and with pyuria documented with a positive urine dipstick test for leukocyte esterase may be treated without urine microscopy or culture. If the leukocyte esterase test result is negative in such patients, microscopic examination of urine or a urine culture should be done.

2. How can one be certain that genitourinary symptoms in young women are caused by cystitis?

Dysuria may be caused by cystitis, urethritis, vulvovaginitis with or without urethritis, or noninfectious inflammatory processes such as chemical irritation. UTI is the cause of dysuria in about 50% of female patients. Among young women, cystitis is characterized by the abrupt onset of rather severe symptoms of urgency, dysuria, and urinary frequency, often with suprapubic or low back pain. Women with urethritis or vaginitis are more likely to report gradual onset of symptoms, vaginal discharge, and a recent new sexual contact; examination often reveals cervicitis or vulvovaginitis. Significant pyuria is strongly associated with UTI.

3. Define *significant pyuria.*

Most recent studies indicate that 8–10 leukocytes/mm^3 (as determined by cytometer) correlate with UTI. This level is probably similar to 10 cells per high power field on examinations of centrifuged urinary sediment.

4. What is the role of single-dose treatment of UTIs?

Uncomplicated cystitis in young women may be treated with a single dose of trimethoprim, trimethoprim-sulfamethoxazole (TMP-SMX), or a fluoroquinolone (which is far more expensive), but treatment failures are slightly higher than with 3-day courses of therapy. Beta-lactam drugs are less effective. In the United States, there is geographic variation in resistance of *E. coli* to TMP-SMX. The Infectious Diseases Society of America (IDSA) guidelines recommend using a fluoroquinolone for empirical therapy in areas where resistance to TMP-SMX is > 20% of *E. coli* isolates. Treatment for 7 days should be considered for women who are diabetic, are older than 50 years, are pregnant, have recently experienced a UTI or have had symptoms for over 1 week before treatment, or who use a diaphragm for contraception.

5. Should young women with repeated episodes of cystitis be evaluated differently?

Repeated episodes of cystitis usually are caused by recurrent episodes of infection rather than relapses of chronic infection. At least one culture should be done for confirmation, but cultures during recurrent infections are not necessary. Frequent recurrences can be managed by daily or thrice-weekly prophylaxis or postcoital prophylaxis. Self-diagnosis with prompt single-dose or 3-day treatment is an effective alternative and may minimize use of antibiotics.

6. Can recurrent cystitis in women be prevented without antibiotics?

High fluid intake, postcoital voiding, drinking cranberry juice, and other practices have been widely recommended to decrease the frequency of cystitis in young women. Pathophysiologically, frequent irrigation of the urethra and drainage of the bladder, including postcoital voiding, seem to complement immune mechanisms in aborting an early infection, but data to support these recommendations are limited. A retrospective case-control study showed a lower relative risk for UTI in young women who reported postcoital voiding. In the same study, tampon use, oral contraceptive use, voiding before sexual intercourse, and direction of wiping after a bowel movement did not correlate with UTI. A randomized, double-blind, placebo-controlled trial showed that daily consumption of 300 mL of cranberry juice decreased bacteriuria in elderly women. The previously proposed mechanism of urinary acidification was not supported by this study; the cranberry juice group had a higher median urinary pH (6.0) than control subjects (5.5). The beneficial effects of cranberry juice may be caused by compounds that inhibit bacterial adhesion to mucosal surfaces.

7. Why is a colony count > 10^5/mL of urine no longer the single standard for defining UTI?

Colony counts > 10^5/mL of a single species of bacteria are found in about 80% of patients with pyelonephritis; this concentration also reliably distinguishes between true (significant) asymptomatic bacteriuria and low-level contamination that occurs during specimen collection (frequently with several species). The value of > 10^5 is not useful in defining significant bacteriuria among several other populations (see table). Only 50% of young women with documented cystitis are correctly identified with such a definition.

Colony-forming Units (CFU)/mL of Urine Used to Define
Significant Bacteriuria among Different Populations

POPULATION	CFU/mL	COMMENTS
Patients with pyelonephritis	> 10^5	80% have > 10^5; most > 10^6
Asymptomatic patients	> 10^5	Repeat to confirm
Young women with cystitis	> 10^2	Pyuria/dysuria syndrome
Men with UTI	> 10^3	Contamination uncommon
Recently catheterized inpatients	> 10^2	CFUs usually increase; symptoms develop

8. How important is it to discriminate between upper and lower UTIs before considering a 3-day course of therapy?

Up to one third of women with symptoms of cystitis have been shown to have occult pyelonephritis. Nonetheless, single-dose antibiotic therapy is 85–95% effective, and 3-day treatment is even less likely to fail. When symptoms and signs of upper tract involvement are present, however, urine culture should be obtained and treatment for pyelonephritis should be given.

9. Should all patients with symptoms of pyelonephritis be admitted to the hospital?

Young women who have relatively mild symptoms without nausea and emesis that preclude oral therapy and for whom follow-up can be ensured may be treated as outpatients. Pyelonephritis during pregnancy should be treated in the hospital. Resistance to amoxicillin and first-generation cephalosporins is noted in 20–30% of bacteria that cause community-acquired pyelonephritis. Treatment may be initiated with TMP-SMX; if trimethoprim resistance is common in the community, a fluoroquinolone should be used. Two weeks of therapy appears adequate in most cases. Amoxicillin is less effective than TMP-SMX, even for susceptible strains.

Blood cultures should be obtained from patients requiring hospitalization; ≤ 20% are positive for bacteria. Options for initial empirical intravenous therapy include a third-generation cephalosporin such as ceftriaxone (1 g/day), a fluoroquinolone, or gentamicin for the usual gram-negative organisms. Ampicillin is often given initially in combination with ceftriaxone or gentamicin for the possibility of enterococci. After several days of intravenous therapy, treatment often can be completed with an oral agent.

10. What is the value of a Gram stain of uncentrifuged urine?

The detection of one or more bacteria per oil-immersion field correlates with a colony count $>10^5$/mL and identifies the organism in about 80% of cases of pyelonephritis. In addition, the detection of gram-positive cocci provides rapid indication of the possibility of enterococcus as the cause.

11. Should imaging procedures or urologic evaluations be used in all cases of pyelonephritis?

When fever and other symptoms fail to resolve after 72 hours of appropriate therapy, ultrasonography or computed tomography (CT) should be considered to look for obstruction, urologic abnormalities, or complications such as perinephric abscess.

12. When should a complicated UTI be suspected?

Complicated UTIs are defined as those caused by organisms resistant to antibiotics or occurring among patients with urinary tract abnormalities. The diagnosis of complicated infections should be considered in patients who recently received antibiotics or acquired infection nosocomially or after urinary tract instrumentation during urinary tract catheterization. UTIs are more likely to be complicated in men, diabetics, pregnant women, and immunosuppressed individuals.

13. What is the recommended therapy for complicated UTIs?

Recommendations vary, depending on the severity of the illness and the known or anticipated drug-susceptibility patterns of the infecting organism. A greater frequency of *Proteus* species, enterococci, and nosocomial pathogens such as *Pseudomonas aeruginosa* can be anticipated. Empiric therapy of seriously ill patients should include coverage for *P. aeruginosa* and *Enterococcus* species, pending culture results.

14. Should all men with a single UTI receive a urologic evaluation?

UTIs in men were previously considered to be complicated by definition, but later studies demonstrated that young men (age 18–50 years) occasionally experience uncomplicated cystitis. Sexual partners of women with vaginal colonization with *E. coli* or homosexual men engaging in insertive anal intercourse appear to be at greater risk. A 7-day course of therapy with pre- and posttreatment cultures is recommended. If the infection responds promptly, urologic evaluation may be deferred. Recurrent infections, pyelonephritis, and other complicating factors warrant urologic evaluation. Male infants and boys should be evaluated for structural abnormalities with an intravenous pyelogram (IVP). Men older than 50 years should be assessed for clinical symptoms suggestive of urinary tract obstruction, usually caused by benign prostatic hypertrophy (urgency, nocturia, and decreased flow rates). Men with symptoms of obstruction or recurrent infections should be evaluated with measurements of serum creatinine level and postvoid residual volume. IVP and cystoscopy are often required for further evaluation. Invasive procedures should be delayed until the acute infection has been treated.

15. What are the indications for repeat cultures after treatment of a UTI?

Routine posttreatment cultures of asymptomatic patients are not recommended except for patients with pyelonephritis, complicated UTIs, UTI associated with pregnancy, and infections in men. Follow-up cultures are usually obtained 2 weeks after treatment.

16. Who should be screened and treated for bacteriuria?

Only two patient groups are known to benefit from treatment of asymptomatic bacteriuria and to warrant screening with two separate urine cultures. Bacteriuria during pregnancy should be treated to prevent pyelonephritis and the risks of premature delivery. Patients with bacteriuria before urologic surgery should be treated to prevent infectious complications of surgery.

17. When should one consider treatment of a UTI for longer than 2 weeks?

Women with positive posttreatment culture results after having pyelonephritis may have subclinical pyelonephritis and may require 4–6 weeks of antibiotics for a cure. Men with positive posttreatment culture results may have either an upper urinary tract or prostatic source of infection and benefit from a 4–6-week course of therapy.

18. Should one treat patients with indwelling urinary catheters and positive urine cultures?

Bacteriuria in patients with chronic, indwelling urinary catheters should not be treated unless patients become symptomatic. Removal or replacement of catheters that have been in place for more than 2 weeks may be helpful. Bacteriuria in recently catheterized patients in the hospital frequently leads to clinically important UTI. Defining asymptomatic bacteriuria in patients in the intensive care unit is often difficult.

19. What is the significance of staphylococcal isolates from urine cultures?

S. saprophyticus is a recognized cause of cystitis in young women. *S. aureus* is an unusual cause of community-acquired UTI, and the diagnosis of staphylococcal bacteremia with or without a renal cortical abscess should be considered. Diabetes mellitus, hemodialysis, and intravenous drug use are predisposing factors for staphylococcal sepsis. Complications of pyelonephritis may lead to a perinephric abscess, usually caused by infection with *E. coli* or other enteric bacilli. Ultrasonography or CT is usually required to diagnose either type of renal abscess.

20. What factors may alter the vaginal flora and increase the risk of UTI?

The use of spermicides with or without a diaphragm for contraception increases the frequency of both vaginal colonization with uropathogens and UTIs. Estrogen deficiency in postmenopausal women leads to a decrease in the frequency of vaginal colonization with *Lactobacillus* species, a higher vaginal pH, and increased frequency of colonization with *E. coli*. Topical application of estriol has been shown to decrease the frequency of recurrent UTIs in postmenopausal women.

21. Describe the special considerations associated with UTIs in the elderly.

Factors that increase the rate of UTIs in the elderly include incomplete bladder emptying, incontinence, cystocele, decreased immune response, and the consequences of chronic disease, such as institutional living and more frequent hospital admissions. Bladder instrumentation is frequent, making the urinary tract the most common (40%) site of nosocomial infections. The presentation of UTI in elderly individuals may be atypical, lacking some or all of the classic symptoms and signs. Fever is not invariably present in elderly patients. The evaluation of elderly patients presenting with acute onset of confusion, lethargy, abdominal pain, and decline in functional status should include UTI in the differential diagnosis. Septic shock, a frequent complication of urosepsis in the elderly, causes a significant rate of mortality.

BIBLIOGRAPHY

1. Abrutyn E, Mossey J, Berlin JA, et al: Does asymptomatic bacteriuria predict mortality and does antimicrobial treatment reduce mortality in elderly ambulatory women? Ann Intern Med 120:827–833, 1994.
2. Fihn SD, Boyko EJ, Chen C-L, et al: Use of spermicide-coated condoms and other risk factors for urinary tract infection caused by staphylococcus saprophyticus. Arch Intern Med 158:281–287, 1998.
3. Foxman B, Gillespie B, Koopman J, et al: Risk factors for second urinary tract infection among college women. Am J Epidemiol 151:1194–1205, 2000.
4. Gratacos E, Torres P-J, Vila J, et al: Screening and treatment of asymptomatic bacteriuria in pregnancy prevent pyelonephritis. J Infect Dis 169:1390–1392, 1994.

5. Gupta K, Hooten TM, Roberts PL, et al: Patient-initiated treatment of uncomplicated recurrent urinary tract infections in young women. Ann Intern Med 135:9–26, 2001.
6. Gupta K, Sahm DF, Mayfield D, et al: Antimicrobial resistance among uropathogens that cause community-acquired urinary tract infections in women: A nationwide analysis. Clin Infect Dis 33:89–94, 2001.
7. Johnson CC: Definitions, classification, and clinical presentation of urinary tract infections. Med Clin North Am 75:241–252, 1991.
8. Kontiokari T, Sundqvist K, Nuutinen M, et al: Randomised trial of cranberry-lingonberry juice and *Lactobacillus* GG drink for the prevention of urinary tract infections in women. Br Med J 322:1571–1573, 2001.
9. Kunin CM: Urinary tract infections in females. Clin Infect Dis 18:1–12, 1994.
10. Lipsky BA: Urinary tract infections in men. Ann Intern Med 110:138–150, 1989.
11. Raz R, Stamm WE: A controlled trial of intravaginal estriol in postmenopausal women with recurrent urinary tract infections. N Engl J Med 329:753–756, 1993.
12. Strom BL, et al: Sexual activity, contraceptive use, and other risk factors for symptomatic and asymptomatic bacteriuria. Ann Intern Med 107:816–823, 1987.
13. Warren JW, Abrutyn E, Hebel JR, et al: Guidelines for antimicrobial treatment of uncomplicated acute bacterial cystitis and acute pyelonephritis in women. Clin Infect Dis 29:745–758, 1999.

54. SEXUALLY TRANSMITTED DISEASES

Simona Bratu, M.D., Michael Augenbraun, M.D., and Mary Ann De Groote, M.D.

1. Why should women be especially targeted for control of gonorrhea?

It is estimated that 600,000 new cases of infection caused by *Neisseria gonorrhoeae* develop each year in the United States. Although screening and treatment of all patients with gonorrhea is important, most men with new infection display symptoms and seek care. On the other hand, many women are asymptomatic until complications such as pelvic inflammatory disease (PID), tubal scarring, or ectopic pregnancy occur. Undiagnosed chronic pelvic infections are considered the major cause of infertility.

2. What are complications of gonorrhea other than urethritis, cervicitis, and PID?

1. **Pharyngeal infection** may be asymptomatic. A pharyngeal culture should be obtained in patients with a history of orogenital contact. Occasionally, overt pharyngitis and tonsillitis, with fever or cervical lymphadenitis may occur.

2. **Anorectal infection** occurs in women and men who have sex with men.

3. **Disseminated gonococcal infection** (DGI) occurs in up to 0.5–3 % of patients. Patients present with fever, tenosynovitis, petechial or pustular skin lesions, and occasionally septic arthritis.

4. **Perihepatitis,** also known as Fitz-Hugh–Curtis syndrome, is most often caused by *Chlamydia trachomatis* but also may be a rare complication of gonococcal infection.

5. **Tubo-ovarian abscess and pelvic peritonitis** are serious complications of *N. gonorrhoeae* infection that require hospitalization.

6. **Long-term complications** of gonorrhea include tubal scarring, which leads to ectopic pregnancy; infertility; and chronic pelvic pain.

7. **Gonococcal conjunctivitis** can present as acute, mucopurulent conjunctivitis.

3. What anatomic sites may be involved in women with *C. trachomatis* infection of the genital tract?

1. The **endocervix** is the most frequent site of infection. Patients may present with a vaginal discharge. On examination of the cervix, a yellow or green mucus is visible. Although not specific for *Chlamydia,* a swab obtained of the discharge reveals polymorphonuclear cells (PMNs) without gram-negative intracellular diplococci.

2. The **urethra** is also a common site of infection. In up to 65% of women with dysuria or urgency and a negative urine culture result for bacteria, *C. trachomatis* is the etiologic agent.

3. Numerous studies have shown that chlamydial infection of the **endometrium** may be the most common cause of endometritis and PID.

4. Damage to the **fallopian tube**s leading to obstructive infertility and ectopic pregnancy has been linked to *C. trachomatis*.

4. How is chlamydial infection diagnosed in women?

The diagnosis begins with a careful history. Chlamydial infection is most common in younger women (≤ 24 years old), women with a new sexual partner, and women who do not use barrier contraceptives. The patient may present with no symptoms, abdominal or pelvic pain, or vaginal or urethral symptoms. In most women, the cervix is the initial site of infection. Vaginal discharge, vaginal bleeding, and postcoital spotting may occur. On examination, the cervical discharge may be clear or mucopurulent, and cervical bleeding after using a culture swab is common. Culture for *C. trachomatis,* the gold standard, is not always available. Culture is performed using a Dacron swab (after mucus has been removed from the endocervix); specimens should be inoculated on special media and must be sent on ice within 24 hours. Other diagnostic modalities include direct fluorescent antibody, enzyme-linked immunosorbent assay, DNA probe, and nucleic acid amplification techniques such as polymerase chain reaction (PCR) and transcription-mediated amplification (TMA).

These techniques are more widely used than culture because of their ease of collection, transport, and performance. They carry a sensitivity rate of 75–90% and a specificity rate of 95%. Empirical therapy while the patient is still in the clinic is often begun before the results are confirmed. The treatment of choice is doxycycline or azithromycin. If the patient is pregnant, erythromycin or azithromycin may be used.

5. Why is therapy recommended for both gonococcal and chlamydial infections?

Persons infected with *N. gonorrhoeae* are often also infected with *C. trachomatis*. In fact, chlamydial infection accompanies 20–40% of gonococcal infections. Chlamydial treatment is safe and inexpensive.

Treatment for **gonococcal infections** involves one of the following:

- Cefixime, 400 mg orally in a single dose
- Ceftriaxone, 125 mg intramuscularly as a single dose
- Ciprofloxacin, 500 mg as a single dose
- Ofloxacin, 400 mg as a single oral dose
- Levofloxacin, 250 mg orally in a single dose

There are sporadic reports of fluoroquinolone-resistant gonococci from around the world. Fluoroquinolone resistance among gonococcal isolates is common in Asia and the Pacific, and increasing resistance rates are reported in western United States.

For **chlamydial infections,** the following are effective:

- Doxycycline, 100 mg twice daily for 7 days
- Azithromycin, 1 g orally as a single dose

6. Which organisms are thought to cause PID?

PID represents a spectrum of diseases of the upper genital tract in women and includes infection and inflammation of the endometrial tissue, tubes, and ovaries. It also may cause pelvic peritonitis. Symptoms include lower abdominal tenderness, adnexal tenderness, and cervical motion tenderness. PID may be caused by one or more organisms. The most common is *C. trachomatis,* but *N. gonorrhoeae* is also important. Polymicrobic infection, including facultative aerobic and anaerobic bacteria, also occurs. Laparoscopic cultures of fallopian tubes and culdocentesis from patients with PID often reveal a combination of aerobic and anaerobic organisms, such as *Bacteroides* species, *H. influenzae, Escherichia coli,* group B streptococci, *Gardnerella vaginalis,* and other anaerobic cocci. In addition, *Mycoplasma hominis* and *Ureaplasma urealyticum* may be etiologic agents of PID. These organisms are frequently isolated in the presence of *N. gonorrhoeae* or *C. trachomatis* from endocervical cultures.

7. Discuss the evaluation of a man who presents with urethritis.

Although some men may be asymptomatic, a history of urethral discharge, dysuria, itching, or recent diagnosis of a sexually transmitted disease (STD) in a partner should be ascertained. A Gram stain of the urethral discharge typically reveals increased PMN cells. Nucleic acid amplification tests on the urethral specimen are used for the detection of *N. gonorrhoeae* and *C. trachomatis*. A first-void urine sediment also may be used for diagnosis using new nucleic acid amplification tests for *N. gonorrhoeae* and *C. trachomatis*. The presence of intracellular gram-negative diplococci is diagnostic of gonorrhea. Because the Gram stain may miss some cases, a urethral swab for *N. gonorrhoeae* culture or DNA amplification tests should also be done. When PMNs are detected on a routine smear but no organisms are seen, the diagnosis of nongonococcal urethritis (NGU) is made. NGU is most frequently caused by *C. trachomatis*, but *U. urealyticum, Trichomonas vaginalis,* and other organisms also may be responsible.

Treatment of NGU consists of doxycycline or azithromycin. Because the coisolation of *N. gonorrhoeae* and *C. trachomatis* is common, patients with evidence of gonorrhea should be treated for both infections.

8. Name the three most common causes of genital ulcers.

1. **Herpes simplex virus (HSV).** In the U.S., HSV is the most common cause of genital ulcers and appears to be increasing.

2. **Syphilis.** The classic syphilitic ulcer is a painless, indurated chancre. Syphilis is a frequent cause of genital ulceration both in the United States and in developing nations.

3. **Chancroid.** This is a common cause of genital ulcers in the developing world; in the U.S., it occurs rarely. *Haemophilus ducreyi,* the etiologic agent, needs to be cultured on special media.

More than one pathogen may exist in a small number of lesions (3–10%). Less common causes are lymphogranuloma venereum and donovanosis (granuloma inguinale). The presence of a genital ulcer is a risk factor for transmission of the human immunodeficiency virus (HIV). All patients should be evaluated with syphilis serology. Other miscellaneous noninfectious causes include trauma, allergic reactions, Behçet's syndrome, malignancy, and Stevens-Johnson syndrome. Serologic tests for HIV should be done in patients with chancroid and syphilis and considered for patients with herpes simplex ulcers.

9. Describe the clinical stages and the consequences of untreated syphilis.

Syphilis is a systemic disease caused by the spirochete *Treponema pallidum.* Primary syphilis is manifested by a chancre that begins as a macule or single painless papule at the site of inoculation (usually on the genitals) and then becomes an indurated ulcer. Secondary syphilis, which usually appears 3–6 weeks after the initial chancre, includes a wide variety of signs and symptoms that reflect the systemic nature of the infection. The skin rash is a hallmark and characteristically appears on the palms and soles but may be highly variable. Lymphadenopathy, mucous membrane lesions, arthritis, hepatitis, nephrotic syndrome, meningitis, and cranial abnormalities may be seen with secondary syphilis. Syphilis is called the "great masquerader" because of the plethora of findings; most patients, however, display only one or a few of these findings.

If untreated, syphilis progresses to a latent stage with no evidence of disease, although serologic test results are positive. Early latent infection refers to a duration of < 1 year. Patients who have been infected > 1 year or for an unknown duration are considered to have late latent infection. In the preantibiotic era, approximately 25% of untreated patients with latent syphilis progressed to the tertiary stage, which includes gummas, granulomas of bones and soft tissues, cardiovascular symptoms, and neurosyphilis. Currently, rates of complications of unrecognized latent syphilis are probably lower because of the likelihood of receiving antibiotics with antisyphilitic activity for unrelated reasons.

10. How can laboratories assist clinicians in making the diagnosis of syphilis?

The definitive diagnosis of syphilis is made by demonstrating the presence of characteristic spirochetes on a darkfield examination or direct fluorescent antibody tests of infected tissue. However, two types of serologic tests assist in diagnosis: nontreponemal and treponemal. The first includes the rapid plasma reagin (RPR) and Venereal Disease Research Laboratory (VDRL) tests. The two specific treponemal tests are the fluorescent treponemal antibody-absorbed assay (FTA-ABS) and *T. pallidum* particle agglutination (TP-PA). The nontreponemal serologic tests may be quantitated and followed to assess response to therapy and to diagnose reinfection. The RPR and VDRL are associated with occasional false-positive results and must be confirmed with a specific treponemal test. Both abnormally high and low syphilis titers have been described in patients infected with HIV, but serologic tests remain reliable for the vast majority of patients. The diagnosis of neurosyphilis relies on serology of the cerebrospinal fluid (CSF) as well as abnormalities of CSF cell counts and protein levels.

11. Does the treatment of syphilis depend on the stage of infection?

Yes. Although the drug of choice for all stages is penicillin, late latent, tertiary, and neurosyphilis require a longer duration of therapy than primary, secondary, or early latent syphilis. Careful follow-up includes a medical history, physical examination, and serologic tests. Patients should be reexamined clinically and serologically at 6 and 12 months. Failure of nontreponemal test titers to decline fourfold by 6 months after therapy for primary or secondary syphilis may suggest the need to retreat. All patients should be tested for HIV. HIV-infected patients should be reevaluated at 3 months.

STAGE	THERAPY*
Primary	Benzathine PCN G, 2.4 million units IM once
Secondary	Benzathine PCN G, 2.4 million units IM once
Latent (early)	Benzathine PCN G, 2.4 million units IM once
Latent (late or unknown)	Benzathine PCN G, 2.4 million units IM weekly for 3 weeks
Neurosyphilis	18–24 million units aqueous crystalline PCNG daily for 10–14 days or 2.4 million units procaine PCN IM daily + probenecid, 500 mg 4 times/day for 10–14 days

*For HIV infection, PCN allergy, and treatment of pregnant patients, see Centers for Disease Control and Prevention: Sexually transmitted diseases treatment guidelines 2002. MMWR 51(RR-6):1–78, 2002.
PCN G = penicillin G; IM = intramuscularly.

12. Genital warts are caused by the human papilloma virus (HPV). Which malignant lesions are also linked to the virus?

HPV has been linked to cervical and vulvar cancer in women and squamous cell cancer of the penis and anus in men. Genital warts are commonly caused by HPV types 6 or 11. Other types, including 16, 18, 31, 33, and 35, have been associated with cervical dysplasia and cancer. External warts can be removed in a number of ways, including cryotherapy with liquid nitrogen or cryoprobe, podophyllin, and trichloroacetic acid or bichloroacetic acid, but recurrences are common. As alternatives to these provider-applied treatments, patients can be instructed to apply podofilox gel or imiquimod. Laser treatment and surgery are reserved for extensive warts. Intralesional interferon is an alternative treatment and has an efficacy comparable to the other treatment modalities; however, it is associated with significant side effects that limit its utility. Patients should be counseled about recurrences, use of condoms, and the importance of annual Papanicolaou smears (for women).

13. Which STD is caused by a protozoan?

Trichomoniasis is caused by the protozoan *Trichomonas vaginalis*. Signs and symptoms include vaginal inflammation and malodorous discharge. Some women and most men are asymptomatic. Occasionally, men have mild urethritis. Organisms can be demonstrated in 30–40% of sexual partners. Diagnosis can be made in the office by performing a microscopic evaluation of vaginal secretions and demonstrating typical motile organisms. Metronidazole is the only oral medication available in the United States for treatment of trichomoniasis. Sexual partners should be treated.

14. Differentiate between the clinical manifestations of primary and recurrent genital herpes infections.

Most cases of genital herpes are caused by HSV-2, but a small percentage are caused by HSV-1. Although the course may vary, primary disease is usually more severe. The patient lacks specific antibodies at the time of the lesions. Mucosal lesions may be multiple. Urethritis, cervicitis, lymphadenopathy, fevers, headaches, and occasionally aseptic meningitis or sacral nerve symptoms (urinary retention or laxness of the anal sphincter) may complicate primary genital herpes infection. Primary disease is often treated with acyclovir, famciclovir, or valacyclovir to reduce the duration of symptoms, although therapy does not cure or prevent latent infection.

Recurrent outbreaks tend to be milder. The small clusters of lesions usually crust over in a few days. Some patients have a prodromal tingling sensation, numbness, or paresthesias before the development of vesicles. Early treatment (i.e., on or before day one of lesions) can lessen the duration of lesions. In addition, daily therapy can suppress recurrences and is indicated if patients have frequent (e.g., > 6/year) recurrences. Options for suppression of recurrences or episodic treatment include acyclovir, famciclovir, and valacyclovir. The cost of treatment may be an important consideration. Patients with HIV may have prolonged or extensive disease.

15. Why are the diagnosis and treatment of genital herpes important? Describe both.

In addition to the morbidity associated with genital ulcers, HSV transmission to the newborn infant may occur at the time of delivery. The greatest risk occurs when the mother acquires a primary infection near the time of delivery. However, routine viral cultures do not predict viral shedding at the time of delivery; therefore, they are not recommended for pregnant women with recurrent genital herpes. Many specialists recommend cesarean section for women that present with recurrent genital herpes at the time of delivery.

In nonpregnant patients with HSV, clinicians should perform a careful examination with culture of suspicious lesions. Sexual transmission of virus is most efficient in the presence of overt lesions. However, virus can be shed in the absence of obvious lesions, and many cases are thought to be transmitted during asymptomatic periods. Patients should be advised to refrain from sexual activity in the presence of overt lesions. Condoms are not foolproof but should be encouraged during all sexual exposures. Sexual partners benefit from evaluation and counseling, even if they are asymptomatic. Serologic tests that can distinguish antibody to HSV-1 from HSV-2 are now available, but their utility in the clinical setting remains to be established.

16. Do STDs pose special risks to travelers?

All general guidelines apply to STDs during travel, but a few points deserve special mention:

1. Frequently, the incidence of STDs is much higher in developing countries than in most areas of the U.S. In addition to gonorrhea, chlamydia, and syphilis, two other important STDs—hepatitis B and HIV—are often more common. Hepatitis B antibody prevalence is well over 50% in some countries of Africa and Asia, and carriage of the surface antigen (HBsAg) may be as high as 25%. Unprotected sex in the developing world increases the risk of acquiring STDs that are uncommon in Western countries, such as chancroid, lymphogranuloma venereum, and granuloma inguinale.

2. HIV-1 and HIV-2 seroprevalence rates are high in certain areas of the world. The major route of transmission is heterosexual intercourse. Solid evidence suggests that the presence of an STD increases the risk of transmission of HIV.

3. Avoidance of high-risk sexual behavior is clearly the best course, but barrier contraception is also effective at decreasing the transmission of STDs. HBV vaccination is recommended for travelers who anticipate sexual contact with residents of areas with intermediate to high levels of HBV transmission.

BIBLIOGRAPHY

1. Ault KA, Faro S: Pelvic inflammatory disease: Current diagnostic criteria and treatment guidelines. Postgrad Med 93:85–91, 1993.

2. Centers for Disease Control and Prevention: Sexually transmitted diseases treatment guidelines 2002. MMWR 51(R-6):1–78, 2002.
3. Centers for Disease Control and Prevention: The Yellow Book: Health Information for International Travel. Atlanta, CDC, 2001–2002.
4. Freund KM: Chlamydial disease in women. Hosp Pract 27:175–186, 1992.
5. Hansfield HH: Recent developments in STDs. I: Bacterial diseases. Hosp Pract 26:47–56, 1991.
6. Hansfield HH: Recent developments in STDs. II: Viral and other syndromes. Hosp Pract 27:175–200, 1991.
7. Hansfield HH: Sex, science and society: A look at sexually transmitted diseases. Postgrad Med 101:268–278, 1997.
8. Holmes KK, Mardh PA, Sparling PF, et al (eds): Sexually Transmitted Diseases, 3rd ed. New York, Mc-Graw-Hill, 1999.
9. Jong EC, McMullen R (eds): The Travel and Tropical Medicine Manual, 2nd ed. Philadelphia, W.B. Saunders, 1995.
10. Mandell GL, Bennett JE, Dolin R (eds): Principles and Practice of Infectious Diseases, 5th ed. New York, Churchill Livingstone, 2000.
11. Mogabgab WJ: Recent developments in the treatment of sexually transmitted diseases. Am J Med 91(suppl 6A):140S–143S, 1991.
12. Parenti DM: Sexually transmitted diseases and travelers. Med Clin North Am 76:1449–1461, 1992.
13. Vinson RP, Epperly TD: Counseling patients on proper use of condoms. Am Fam Physician 43:2081–2085, 1991.
14. Woodridge WE: Syphilis: A new visit from an old enemy. Postgrad Med 89:193–202, 1991.

55. PROTEINURIA AND HEMATURIA

Moro O. Salifu, M.D.

1. What are the different methods of urine specimen collection?

Urine specimens should be collected with minimal contamination for urinalysis and culture. A freshly voided midstream urine specimen in the morning is preferred because it is noninvasive and gives the most concentrated and acidic urine, which preserves formed elements. It is ideal for urinalysis, culture, and determination of protein-to-creatinine ratio (a good estimate of 24-hour protein excretion). Because the collection is midstream, a moderately full bladder is required. At least 200 mL of urine should be voided before the specimen is collected. Contamination is avoided by foreskin retraction in men and good labial separation in women. Proper preparation includes gentle cleansing with cotton wool swabs moistened with saline. Even midstream urine collections in the majority of women demonstrate contamination unless cleaning instructions are clear. If it is impossible to obtain a good midstream urine specimen, as in patients with physical handicaps or children, a single catheterization or suprapubic aspiration may be required. For patients with indwelling Foley or condom catheters, urine specimens should be taken from above a clamp placed on the drainage tube. Specimens should never be taken from the bag itself because stasis will change the composition of formed elements.

Random urine specimens are not good for white blood cell (WBC) count or culture because they are often contaminated, but they may identify proteinuria or hematuria.

A 24-hour urine collection beginning at 8 A.M. and ending at 8 A.M. the next day is sometimes needed to quantify protein, creatinine, and electrolyte excretion. Urine specimens should be refrigerated immediately until examined, or the specimen should be reviewed while fresh to avoid changes in cellular and chemical composition.

2. What are the main components of urinalysis?

1. **Visual inspection.** The color and consistency of the urine should be assessed visually before centrifugation. Gross hematuria, marked pyuria, heavy crystalluria, and, occasionally, fun-

guria can be detected by visual inspection. A layer of foam at the top of the specimen is indicative of heavy proteinuria.

2. **Dipstick or chemical analysis.** Commercially available dipsticks measure a number of different components, including pH, glucose, ketones, hemoglobin, protein, leukocyte esterase, and bilirubin. Dipsticks screen most accurately for the presence of proteinuria, whereas microscopic analysis is a more informative method for the evaluation of hematuria. Dipstick evaluation of protein involves a pad that contains tetrabromophenol, which changes from yellow to green to blue as increasing amounts of protein are available for binding. Dipstick evaluation of hematuria involves hemoglobin or myoglobin to catalyse a reaction between hydrogen peroxide and the chromogen O-toluidine. When hemoglobin or myoglobin is present in the urine, the test pad turns blue.

3. **Microscopic analysis.** Fresh urine samples are aliquoted into a 10-mL test tube and centrifuged at 2500–3000 rpm for 5 minutes. The supernatant is poured off, and after resuspension, the sediment is poured onto a slide and placed under a coverslip. A bright-field microscope is commonly used for analysis of urinary sediment, although phase-contrast microscopy provides better vision of all elements. Microscopic analysis is commonly viewed without staining. This approach allows rapid preparation. Two magnifications are required, with the lower ($\times100$) for a general overview and the higher ($\times400$) for details and cell evaluation. The complete slide should be evaluated, which can take 10–15 minutes; most formed elements, however, adhere to the edges of the coverslip. Casts are reported as number per low power field and cells as number per high power field.

3. How should a patient be instructed to collect 24-hour urine?

The patient is instructed to void completely and discard the urine at 8 A.M. After that, all urine is collected for 24 hours, including the sample at 8 A.M. the next day, into a container, which must be refrigerated at all times. For protein and creatinine measurement, refrigeration alone is sufficient. For other chemical analyses, a container with a preservative supplied by the local laboratory should be used.

4. What is considered normal protein excretion?

Under physiologic conditions, urinary excretion of protein does not exceed 150 mg/day or 10 mg/dL. The main proteins normally excreted are albumin, immunoglobulins, immunoglobulin light chains, and Tamm-Horsfall protein. In some conditions, excessive proteinuria is benign, including functional proteinuria in patients with fever or after exercise; idiopathic transient proteinuria, as in patients with congestive heart failure; and orthostatic proteinuria.

5. What is considered abnormal protein excretion (proteinuria)?

A reading of 1+ protein on dipstick corresponds to 30 mg/dL (minimum 300 mg/day, assuming 1 L of urine is passed), 2+ corresponds to 100 mg/dL, 3+ to 300 mg/dL, and 4+ to > 500 mg/dL. Microalbuminuria, measured by special sensitive assays or in a 24-hour collection, defines albumin excretion between 30 and 300 mg/day. At this level, dipstick results are generally negative or only trace. Non-nephrotic proteinuria defines protein excretion of 300–3500 mg/day whereas nephrotic range proteinuria defines protein excretion in excess of 3500 mg/day. Nephrotic range proteinuria is the hallmark of the nephrotic syndrome, which predisposes to hypoalbuminemia, edema and hypercholesterolemia, infections with encapsulated organisms caused by loss of immunoglobulins, and thrombotic events caused by loss of antithrombin III and other anticoagulants in the urine.

6. What conditions produce false-negative and false-positive results for proteinuria on dipstick?

False-negative results for proteinuria occur when urine is extremely dilute or when Bence Jones protein (immunoglobulin light chains) is the predominant source of protein. Dipsticks are more sensitive to albumin. Sulfosalicylic acid should be added to determine whether immunoglobulin light chains are present.

False-positive results occur when urine is highly concentrated, when urine pH is > 8, when the dipstick has been immersed too long (> 30 seconds), and in the setting of gross hematuria when plasma proteins accompany blood.

7. What are the mechanisms of proteinuria?

The three types of proteinuria are glomerular, tubular, and overproduction proteinuria. Proteinuria is most commonly of glomerular origin, and albumin is the major component of protein that leaks through an abnormal glomerular basement membrane. Tubular proteinuria is caused by decreased tubular reabsorption of proteins contained in the glomerular filtrate, as in tubulointerstitial disorders. Overload proteinuria is secondary to increased production of immunoglobulin light chains, as in monoclonal gammopathies, or lysozyme, as in some forms of leukemia.

8. How does one evaluate a patient with proteinuria?

The first approach is to quantify the amount of protein in the urine by collecting a 24-hour urine specimen and determining rates of creatinine and protein excretion. Creatinine excretion rates are determined to assess the accuracy (total time) of urine collection. Men should excrete 15–25 mg/kg/day and women 12–20 mg/kg/day of urinary creatinine. Nephrotic range proteinuria is > 3.5 g/day. Protein-to-creatinine ratios have been found to be extremely useful in patients with established creatinine excretion rates, noncompliant patients, and patients for whom rapid diagnoses are sought. Ratios > 3.5 in a single voided sample represent > 3.5 g of proteinuria in 24 hours, and ratios < 0.2 represent < 0.2 g of proteinuria in 24 hours.

After quantitation, urine protein electrophoresis (UPEP) identifies if proteinuria is mainly in a glomerular pattern (albuminuria), tubular pattern (nonspecific), or overproduction (globulins). If UPEP is predominantly globulins, immunoelectrophoresis should be performed to identify the monoclonal component. Except for diabetes in which retinopathy is used as a marker of diabetic kidney disease, a kidney biopsy is often required to establish the cause of proteinuria.

9. What is the clinical significance of proteinuria?

Proteinuria is a sign of renal injury caused by intrinsic renal and a variety of diseases (see table), most of which progress to renal failure, resulting in death or need for dialysis or transplantation to sustain life. Microalbuminuria, especially in diabetics, indicates early renal damage as well as a marker of overall cardiovascular morbidity. It can be reversed by normalizing blood pressure (BP), using converting enzyme inhibitors or angiotensin II receptor blockers (ARBs). After the diagnosis of proteinuria is established, the goal of therapy is to induce remission (< 300 mg/day) with immunosuppression, normalizing BP, use of angiotensin-converting enzyme (ACE) inhibitors or angiotensin II receptor blockers. Strict BP control, with and without use of ACE inhibitors, has been shown to retard progression of chronic proteinuric kidney diseases.

Differential Diagnosis of Proteinuria and Hematuria

PROTEINURIA	HEMATURIA
Nephrotic range proteinuria	**Glomerular**
Focal segmental glomerulosclerosis	All forms of glomerulonephritis
Minimal change disease	Familial glomerular diseases
Membranous nephropathy	Alport's syndrome
Diabetes	Thin basement membrane disease
Amyloidosis	**Nonglomerular renal diseases**
Lupus nephritis class IV and V	Cystic kidney diseases
HIV nephropathy	Nephrolithiasis
NSAIDs, heavy metals	Renovascular disease
Non-nephrotic proteinuria	Interstitial nephritis
Postinfectious glomerulonephritis	Neoplastic diseases of the kidney
Membranoproliferative glomerulonephritis	Trauma
Rapidly progressive glomerulonephritis	**Extrarenal (ureter, bladder, prostate, urethra)**
IgA nephropathy	Calculi and infections
Lupus nephritis class I–III	Neoplasms
Vasculitis	Trauma, foreign body
Massive hematuria	Drugs (e.g., cyclophosphamide)

10. What is hematuria?

Hematuria is defined as the presence of > 4 red blood cells (RBCs) per high-powered field (HPF) of urine sediment. This usually corresponds to a trace or positive urine dipstick for blood. Healthy people may excrete transiently ≤ 1–3 RBC/HPF of urine sediment; however, if this is found on repeat urinalysis, further investigation should be performed. The term *microscopic hematuria* refers to that visible with the use of a microscope, and *macroscopic (gross) hematuria* refers to pink, red, brown, or cola-colored discoloration of the urine that must be confirmed by microscopy.

11. Are the characteristics of hematuria clinically useful?

Yes. Increased excretion of erythrocytes is a nonspecific finding and may be associated with bleeding at any site in the urinary tract. Patterns of hematuria usually are determined by four parameters:

1. Color and appearance of urine (gross or macroscopic vs. covert or microscopic hematuria)
2. Timing of the hematuria (persistent or constant, intermittent or recurrent)
3. Presence or absence of symptoms
4. Isolated hematuria or evidence of proteinuria, pyuria, or bacteriuria

12. What may cause false-positive hematuria?

A color of red or dark brown may be seen in conjunction with dyes in foods, including beets, paprika, and senna. Drugs such as rifampin, phenothiazines, and phenytoin (Dilantin) also may have this effect. Myoglobin also gives a red-brown color to the urine. After intravascular hemolysis, free hemoglobin may be excreted, giving a distinct red color to the urine. Hemoglobinuria or myoglobinuria is suspected when the dipstick is strongly positive for blood but microscopy shows only few or no RBCs. In women, menstrual blood occasionally finds it way into an improperly collected urine specimen. Such patients need to return when they are not having menstrual bleeding. Microscopically, yeast, calcium oxalate crystals, starch granules, and air bubbles have been mistaken for hematuria.

13. What are the causes of isolated hematuria?

Isolated hematuria is almost always caused by an extrarenal source. The major causes of both gross and microscopic hematuria include acute and chronic prostatitis or urethritis; hemorrhagic cystitis; renal stones; and tumors of the kidney, renal pelvis, ureter, bladder, prostate, and urethra.

14. How does one approach a patient with isolated hematuria?

Patients need repeat urinalyses to demonstrate persistent hematuria. Examination of the prostate and external urethra in conjunction with a urine culture is the basic first step in evaluation. A three-glass urine test is helpful in diagnosing lower urinary tract hematuria. The patient voids into three different containers. Hematuria only in the initial void suggests urethral bleeding, whereas hematuria in the terminal void suggests a prostatic or bladder origin. Intravenous pyelography and renal ultrasonography are the next tests to be performed if more information is needed. Renal stones, cysts, or urinary tract tumors can be identified in this fashion. Cystoscopy or retrograde pyelography may be needed to identify the source of bleeding. If these studies are uninformative, renal biopsy should be considered.

15. What suggests that hematuria may be renal in origin?

Associated proteinuria almost always suggests a renal origin of hematuria. However, in renal diseases in which proteinuria alone predominates (e.g., diabetes mellitus), evaluation for extrarenal sources of hematuria should be done, such as cystoscopy to screen for transitional cell carcinoma of the bladder.

Glomerular hematuria is suspected when there are dysmorphic erythrocytes (abnormalities in size, shape, and membrane appearance) or when there are RBC casts (RBCs enmeshed in Tamm-Horsfall protein) in the sediment. Glomerular hematuria is the hallmark of the nephritic syndrome, characterized by acute glomerulonephritis, hypertension, and edema. Phase-contrast microscopy is necessary to identify dysmorphic erythrocytes. RBCs from a nonglomerular source have normal and regular morphology (isomorphic erythrocytes). More recently, automated blood cell volume analyzers have been proposed to distinguish glomerular from nonglomerular hematuria. Decreased cell volumes are more commonly found in glomerular bleeding.

16. What is the most common cause of hematuria?

Extrarenal sites are the most common source of isolated hematuria. Of a consecutive series of 1000 patients with gross hematuria, 67% demonstrated a lesion in the bladder or lower urinary tract. The most common causes of gross hematuria originating in the kidney are nephropathy and polycystic kidney disease (see table in question 9). In 10–15% of patients, no cause for hematuria can be found.

17. Should hematuria in a patient taking anticoagulant therapy be worked up?

A normal urinary tract should not bleed spontaneously when a patient is taking anticoagulants. Up to 82% of such patients have a lesion somewhere in the urinary tract. Examples include renal cell carcinoma, vesicoureteral reflux, urethral strictures, cancer of the prostate or bladder, urinary tract infection, and stone disease.

BIBLIOGRAPHY

 1. Abuelo JC: Proteinuria: Diagnostic principles and procedures. Ann Intern Med 98:186–191, 1983.
 2. Anderson S: Proteinuria. In National Kidney Foundation: Primer on Kidney Diseases, 2nd ed. San Diego, Academic Press, 1998, pp 36–41.
 3. Antolak SJ, Mellinger GT: Urologic evaluation of hematuria occurring during anticoagulant therapy. J Urol 101:111–113, 1969.
 4. Ginsberg JM, Chung BS, Materese RA, Garella S: Use of single voided urine samples to estimate quantitative proteinuria. N Engl J Med 309:1543–1546, 1983.
 5. Glassock RJ: Hematuria and pigmenturia. In Massry S, Glassock R (eds): Textbook of Nephrology, vol. 1. Baltimore, Williams &Wilkins, 1989, pp 4.14–4.22.
 6. Haas M, Meehan SM, Karrison TG, Spargo BH: Changing etiologies of unexplained adult nephrotic syndrome. A comparison of renal biopsy findings from 1976–1979 and 1995–1997. Am J Kidney Dis 30:621–631, 1997.
 7. Kashtan CE: Hematuria. In National Kidney Foundation: Primer on Kidney Diseases, 2nd ed. San Diego, Academic Press, 1998, pp 36–41.
 8. Kubota M, Yamabe H, Ozawa K, et al: Mechanisms of urinary erythrocyte deformity in patients with glomerular disease. Nephrology 48:338–339, 1988.
 9. Larson TS: Evaluation of proteinuria. Mayo Clin Proc 69:1154–1158, 1994.
10. Raman VG, Peud L, Leu HA, Haskell R: A double-blind, controlled trial of phase-contrast microscopy by two observers for evaluating the source of hematuria. Nephrology 44:304–308, 1986.
11. Sutton JM: Evaluation of hematuria in adults. JAMA 263:2475–2480, 1990.

56. KIDNEY STONES

Jeffrey Pickard, M.D.

1. What is the likelihood that a person will develop kidney stones during his or her lifetime?

About 5–15% of people develop kidney stones during their lifetime.

2. Will a person who has had one kidney stone later develop another one?

Formerly, it was believed that first-time stone formers usually would not develop another stone, but the opposite is, in fact, true. In stone clinics, up to 80% of patients who have one episode of nephrolithiasis have another. However, population-based studies suggest that the recurrence rate is only 30–40% over 25 years.

3. List the five types of kidney stones.

Types of Kidney Stones

COMPOSITION OF STONE	CAUSES
1. Calcium oxalate	Primary hyperparathyroidism
	Idiopathic hypercalciuria
	Low urine citrate level
	Hyperoxaluria
	Hyperuricosuria
2. Calcium phosphate	Renal tubular acidosis
3. Uric acid	Low urine pH
	Hyperuricosuria
4. Struvite	Infection with bacteria that express urease
5. Cystine	Cystinuria

Adapted from Coe FL, Parks JH, Asplin JR: The pathogenesis and treatment of kidney stones. N Engl J Med 327:1141–1152, 1992.

4. What is the most common type of kidney stone?

Three fourths of all kidney stones are made of calcium oxalate. In fact, in normal urine calcium oxalate is concentrated to 4 times its solubility (i.e., the urine is supersaturated). However, nucleation (the nidus for crystal formation) usually occurs only when the concentration reaches 7 times solubility because of inhibitors of stone formation in normal urine, such as citrate (inorganic) and nephrocalcin (organic) About 10–20% of kidney stones are struvite (magnesium ammonium phosphate); 5% are uric acid; 5% have mostly hydroxyapatite or brushite (calcium monohydrogen phosphate); and < 1% are cystine.

5. How does hypocitraturia contribute to the formation of calcium stones?

Citrate forms soluble complexes with calcium oxalate in the urine to keep the crystals from coalescing to form stones. Women have higher urinary citrate levels than men, which may explain why women are less likely to develop stones.

6. What causes calcium oxalate stones?

The most common cause of calcium oxalate stones is idiopathic hypercalciuria, which is responsible for > 50% of all calcium oxalate stones. The two major types of idiopathic hypercalciuria are **absorptive,** in which calcium absorption is increased in the gut, and **renal,** in which a kidney defect leads to calcium wasting in the urine. In both types, serum calcium levels are usually normal. Differentiating between the two is usually unnecessary because the treatment is the same for both. Other causes include primary hyperparathyroidism, low urinary citrate level, hyperoxaluria, and hyperuricosuria.

7. What are the causes of hyperoxaluria?

The normal 24-hour urinary excretion of oxalate is ≤ 45 mg. Increase in dietary intake of foods that are rich in oxalate (spinach, rhubarb, beets, peppers, cocoa, chocolate, wheat germ, peanuts, pecans, okra, lime peel) may increase the concentration of oxalate in the urine to 60 mg/day. Urinary excretion of oxalate > 60 mg/day generally indicates an intestinal cause. Small bowel malabsorption, as in regional enteritis, increases intestinal absorption of oxalate. Primary hyperoxaluria is a rare disorder, which is inherited in an autosomal recessive pattern. Kidney stones start forming in childhood, and analysis of the urine reveals a marked increase in the concentration of oxalate (135–270 mg/24 hr).

8. What laboratory evaluation should be done in a person who develops a kidney stone?

A spot urine should be collected for culture and pH testing. A 24-hour urine and corresponding blood sample should be collected. Calcium, magnesium, phosphorus, uric acid, and creatinine should be measured in both. In addition, it is important to measure serum sodium and potassium and to analyze the urine for oxalate, citrate, volume, and cystine.

9. How do you prevent recurring stones in a patient with idiopathic hypercalciuria?

The answer depends on the specific cause based on stone analysis. All patients with stones probably benefit from increasing fluid intake, which increases urine volume and decreases concentrations. Dietary manipulation may be helpful for patients with hyperoxaluria (decrease dietary intake) or hypocitraturia (supplement with citrate), but calcium restriction is not helpful, as discussed below. Patients with calcium stones benefit from thiazides, which decrease urinary calcium by increasing fractional reabsorption of calcium from the distal tubule. It appears that reabsorbed calcium is shunted directly into bone. However, thiazides must be used for 2 years before a beneficial effect on stone recurrence is seen.

10. What is the value of dietary calcium restriction in patients with calcium stones?

Dietary calcium restriction is not helpful for preventing the recurrence of calcium stones and, in fact, may be harmful. In patients with idiopathic hypercalciuria, bone mineral is unusually labile. Those who restrict dietary calcium appear to compensate by increasing calcium resorption from bone, although this effect may not be universal. Some patients given a low calcium diet manifest a reciprocal hyperoxaluria, which can maintain calcium oxalate stone-forming potential even in the face of decreased urinary calcium. A recent randomized, controlled trial studied 120 men with idiopathic hypercalciuria and a history of stones. A diet low in calcium was compared with a normal calcium diet with reduced animal protein and salt. There was a $> 50\%$ relative risk reduction for recurrent stones in men who were given the reduced fat/sodium diet compared with men on a reduced calcium diet.

11. What analgesics are best for acute renal colic?

Narcotics have typically been first-line analgesics for controlling the pain of renal colic in both outpatient and inpatient settings. However, prospective trials using nonsteroidal anti-inflammatory drugs (NSAIDs) have shown them to be roughly equivalent in the ability to control pain, although the onset of pain relief from narcotics may be slightly faster. It appears that much of the pain is caused by the release of renal prostaglandins (primarily PGE_2) and localized inflammation, both of which may be counteracted by NSAIDs. It may be that combining narcotics (which act centrally) and NSAIDs (which act peripherally) may work better than either drug alone, but no studies have addressed this possibility.

12. What treatment should you recommend for an impacted stone?

Stones < 5 mm in diameter generally pass on their own, whereas stones > 7 mm generally do not. Stones in the distal ureter (i.e., below the pelvic brim) may be removed either ureteroscopically or by extracorporeal shock wave lithotripsy (ESWL). Although ESWL is less invasive than ureteroscopy, it is less effective in removing distal stones. Proximal stones ≤ 1 cm in diameter are best removed by ESWL. Stones ≥ 1 cm in the upper ureter may be treated by either of the above techniques or by percutaneous nephrolithotomy. Open surgery is done only if other modalities have failed or if the stones are unusually large or complex.

13. What beverages are best and worst for preventing recurrent stones?

This question was examined prospectively as part of the Health Professionals Follow-up Study, which included a cohort of 45,289 men 40–75 years of age with no history of kidney stones. Follow-up was for 6 years (242,100 person years). In addition, 81,093 women in the Nurses' Health Study were followed for 533,081 person years. After simultaneously adjusting for a variety of factors, the risk of stone formation was decreased for each 8-oz serving consumed daily of coffee, decaffeinated coffee, tea, beer, and wine. The risk was increased by apple juice and grapefruit juice. In contrast to a previously published report, these studies found no statistically significant effect for carbonated soft drinks.

14. How are struvite stones formed?

Struvite stones are caused by urine infected with urease-producing bacteria. Remember the two Ps, one K, and one E: *Proteus* species, *Pseudomonas* species, *Klebsiella* species, and *Enterococcus* species. *Escherichia coli* does not produce struvite stones.

BIBLIOGRAPHY

1. Bihl G, Meyers A: Recurrent renal stone disease: Advances in pathogenesis and clinical management. Lancet 358:651–656, 2001.
2. Borghi L, Schianchi T, Meschi T, et al: Comparison of two diets for the prevention of recurrent stones in idiopathic hypercalciuria. N Engl J Med 346:77–84, 2002.
3. Bushinsky D: Recurrent hypercalciuric nephrolithiasis: Does diet help? N Engl J Med 346:124–125, 2002.
4. Bushinsky DA: Kidney stones. Adv Intern Med 47:219–239, 2001.
5. Curhan CG, Willet WC, Rimm EB, et al: Prospective study of beverage use and the risk of kidney stones. Am J Epidemiol 143:240–247, 1996.
6. Curhan CG, Willet WC, Speizer FE, Stampfler MJ: Beverage use and risk for kidney stones in women. Ann Intern Med 128:534–540, 1998.
7. Gault MH, Longerich LL, Crane G, et al: Bacteriology of urinary tract stones. J Urol 153:1164–1170, 1995.
8. Labrecque M, Dostaler LP, Rousselle R, et al: Efficacy of nonsteroidal anti-inflammatory drugs in the treatment of acute renal colic: A meta-analysis. Arch Intern Med 154:1381–1387, 1994.
9. Lerolle N, Lantz B, Paillard F, et al: Risk factors for nephrolithiasis in patients with familial idiopathic hypercalciuria. Am J Med 113:99–103, 2002.
10. Morton AR, Iliescu EA, Wilson JWL: Nephrology: 1. Investigation and treatment of recurrent kidney stones. Can Med Assoc J 166:213–218, 2002.
11. Pearle MS: Prevention of nephrolithiasis. Curr Opin Nephrol Hypertens 10:203–209, 2001.
12. Porttis AJ, Sundaram CP: Diagnosis and initial management of kidney stones. Am Fam Physician 63:1329–1338, 2001.
13. Shokeir A: Renal colic: New concepts related to pathophysiology, diagnosis and treatment. Curr Opin Urol 12:263–269, 2002.
14. Wrenn K: Emergency intravenous pyelography in the setting of possible renal colic: Is it indicated? Ann Emerg Med 26:304–307, 1995.

57. URINARY INCONTINENCE

Edmund Bourke, M.D.

1. How common is urinary incontinence?

In elderly individuals, it is common. It is often not reported by community-dwelling elders, who attribute it to age and fail to mention it. In individuals who are 65 to 74 years old, estimates of 5–7% are reported; in those older than age 75 years, the incidence may approach 30%. A female-to-male ratio of 2:1 disappears after age 80 years. In nursing home patients, ≥ 50% have some urinary incontinence.

2. What are the consequences of urinary incontinence?

The morbidity of urinary incontinence falls into three categories:

1. **Physical consequences** include an increased incidence of urinary infections, pressure ulcers, perineal infections, sleep deprivation, and falls.

2. **Psychosocial consequences** include a loss of self-esteem, sexual dysfunction, decreased emotional well-being, social withdrawal, and impaired quality of life.

3. **Increased caregiver burden** may give way to a temptation for the inappropriate use of catheters for convenience, and it is a factor that contributes to the desire to institutionalize.

3. When it occurs, is incontinence usually permanent?

On the contrary, it is more often transient, and a transient, treatable cause should always be initially sought. The mnemonic DIAPPERS has stood the test of time as a useful memory aid.

D Delirium frequently causes incontinence. Moreover, incontinence may be the signal that alerts the clinician to the possible onset of delirium.

I Infection of the urinary tract may have incontinence as its sole clinical manifestation.

A Atrophic vaginitis or urethritis in postmenopausal women can present with incontinence, which resolves with topical estrogen.

P Pharmacologic agents can affect cognition, mobility, diuresis, bladder contractility, or sphincter tone.

P Psychological causes include depression and psychosis.

E Excessive urine output may be caused by caffeinated or other beverages at bedtime, potent diuretics, hyperglycemia, or hypercalcemia.

R Restricted mobility may be solved by, for example, giving the patient a urinal or bedside commode.

S Stool impaction may cause overflow or urge incontinence and pseudodiarrhea.

4. After these remediable factors are excluded, how is established urinary incontinence classified?

Generally, urinary incontinence is classified into one of three categories, but overlap with multifactorial components also occurs. These categories are **urge incontinence,** which is the most common in both genders; **stress incontinence,** which is the second most common cause in women; and **overflow incontinence,** which is the second most common cause in men.

5. Define the characteristics of urge incontinence.

It is characterized by an abrupt urge to empty the bladder that, more often than not, precludes getting to a toilet in time for normal voiding. It is caused by detrusor muscle instability or over-activity. The consequence is uninhibited bladder contractions sufficient to overcome urethral resistance, resulting in urinary leakage. It can result from:

- Lesions of the inhibitory pathways in the central nervous system (CNS), including advanced Alzheimer's disease, cerebrovascular accidents (CVAs), normal pressure hydrocephalus, and cervical stenosis
- Bladder lesions causing local detrusor instability, including infections, interstitial cystitis, neoplasms, and calculi

6. Is the nonpharmacologic approach to management of urge incontinence effective?

Yes, when a motivated patient and an encouraging clinician cooperate for success. A course of bladder retraining with timed voiding coupled with simple behavioral techniques to suppress precipitant urges can be very effective. Based on a bladder diary recording each void and leak, the patient initiates a wake-time and voiding schedule that is initially designed to minimize leaks. The time interval is gradually increased (e.g., by 30 minutes per week) as control improves. It may take about 2 months of rigorously staying the course to achieve a successful outcome. Meanwhile, various relaxation techniques are used to control urges that come on between voiding times. It is helpful to have the patient concentrate on getting through the urge by sitting or standing still and taking deep inspirations with slow expirations while conceptualizing the urge as a wave motion that passes after it peaks. When the urge is under control, the patient moves slowly to the nearest bathroom to void.

7. What can be done if the nonpharmacologic approach is unsuccessful?

Bladder-suppressant medication can be added. Because detrusor activity (bladder contraction) is cholinergically mediated, the judicious use of anticholinergics has proven useful. Oxybutynin (2.5 mg three times daily, titrating up as needed and changing to the extended release form, 5–20 mg once daily) is frequently effective in mitigating incontinence. The main side effects are constipation and dry mouth (a possible cause of polydipsia with return of incontinence). Urethral resistance to bladder contractions can be increased by alpha agonists as an alternative approach.

8. How important is urodynamic testing of urinary incontinence?

It is not usually needed as a routine. Its main role is when surgical treatment is being contemplated for bladder outlet obstruction or stress incontinence. Especially in the elderly population, in which the incidence of multifactorial components to the incontinence is increased, urodynamic studies are undertaken to assess the potential contributing factors that could reduce or nullify the benefit of a specific corrective surgery. Otherwise, studies such as cystometrics, fluoroscopic monitoring, and pressure-flow studies have not been shown to have clear benefits over good history taking and physical examination.

9. Define stress incontinence.

It is the result of failure of the bladder sphincter mechanism. Normal micturition results from the coordinated action of bladder contraction and urethral sphincter relaxation, reducing resistance to outflow. When urethral resistance is overcome in the absence of bladder contraction by increased intra-abdominal pressure, stress incontinence results. Impaired pelvic muscle support is the usual cause of reduced urethral resistance in women, particularly aging multiparous women in whom it is often aggravated by uterine or bladder prolapse. Less often, intrinsic sphincter damage may occur as, for instance, after radical prostatectomy in men. Coughing, laughing, the passage of flatus, and other causes of increased intra-abdominal pressure are the usual precipitants for leakage.

10. What treatments are available for stress incontinence?

Three treatments are available, each of which can be curative in appropriate patients.

1. Kegel's **pelvic muscle exercises** (see table) strengthen the muscular components of the urethral support system. Success can be impressive, but it depends crucially on the patient understanding of how to avoid contracting the wrong muscles (e.g., abdominal, buttock, and thigh muscles) and to isolate and appropriately contract the pelvic muscles. Motivation, perseverance, and encouragement are also essential because many weeks may be required to achieve the desired outcome.

Pelvic Muscle (Kegel's) Exercises

Pelvic muscles, like other muscles, can become weak or damaged. Pelvic muscle exercises strengthen weak muscles around the bladder.

- Start by doing your pelvic muscle exercises 3–4 times each week. Usually, it takes about 10 minutes to do the exercises. Your clinician will give you exact instructions about how many times you should perform the exercises and the number of times a day.
- Practice anywhere and anytime. It is usually best to begin practicing the exercises while lying on your bed. After you have mastered the exercises lying down, practice them sitting in a chair. Then advance to practicing them standing. Soon you will be able to do them anywhere.
- Never use your stomach, thigh, or buttock muscles. To find out whether you are also contracting your stomach muscles, place your hand on your abdomen while you squeeze your pelvic muscles. If you feel your abdomen move, then you are also using these muscles.
- Avoid holding your breath. Inhale and exhale slowly while counting. In time, you will learn to practice effortlessly.
- If you forget to do your exercises for several days, do not be discouraged. When you have realized that you have forgotten, begin your program again as instructed. Do not try to make up for lost days by doing more exercises, or you will have sore muscles.

After 4–6 weeks of following your prescribed exercise routine, you will begin to notice that you are having fewer urinary accidents. After 3 months, you will see an even bigger difference. It may help to keep a diary of the times you practice your exercises and the times that you leak urine. This will give you a picture of the progress you are making. If you are having problems, your clinician may suggest biofeedback, weighted vaginal cones, or electrostimulation to help you with pelvic muscle exercises.

Adapted from Busby-Whitehead J, Kinkade J, Granville L: Urinary Incontinence: Management in Primary Practice. Tool Kit 2, Practicing Physician Education Project, Robinson BE, ed. New York, The John A. Hartford Foundation and The American Geriatrics Society, 2000.

2. **Estrogen creams or vaginal tablets** may reduce stress (and urge) incontinence in some patients with atrophic urethritis and vaginitis, although evidence-based information is currently scant.

3. **Surgical correction** has an 85% cure rate in appropriately selected patients. Bladder neck suspensions that correct deficits in urethral support are effective. Concomitant corrections of significant cystoceles, rectoceles, or uterine prolapse are performed as indicated. When avoidance of surgery is advisable or preferred, pessaries may provide relief.

11. Explain what is meant by overflow incontinence.

Overflow incontinence is the result of bladder outlet obstruction, underactivity of the detrusor muscle, or both. The demonstration of an increased postvoid residual volume is axiomatic to diagnosis. Although this can be satisfactorily monitored sonographically, it should be initially established quantitatively by catheterization. A postvoid residual volume of > 60 mL is abnormal and suggests retention. Volumes 20-fold higher can be encountered. Benign prostatic hypertrophy (BPH), prostatic cancer, and urethral stricture are the most common causes of outlet obstruction, hence its much greater frequency in men. Outlet obstruction initially causes a weakened stream, terminal dribbling, hesitancy, and nocturia. Incontinence is not generally seen until the later stages. Detrusor underactivity, on the other hand, can result from neurologic defects, including neurogenic bladder from diabetes, Parkinson's disease, alcohol abuse, vitamin B_{12} deficiency, and spinal stenosis. It can also result from pressure atrophy consequent on chronic outlet obstruction.

12. How is overflow incontinence treated?

It depends on which of the two causes. Outlet obstruction has medical options if it is caused by BPH. They include alpha-blockers; finasteride; and, as has now been shown in a controlled trial, the complementary medicinal herbal extract saw palmetto. The need for surgical correction has decreased but still has an important role when medical treatment is inadequate. Less satisfactory is the management of detrusor underactivity. When possible, avoidance of anticholinergics or other drugs that decrease detrusor contractility is the first step. Double voiding and the use of suprapubic pressure are helpful in some situations. Pharmacotherapy has been disappointing, although bethanechol, when administered subcutaneously rather than orally, has been helpful in some patients. Otherwise, intermittent clean catheterization, including self-catheterization in patients with the motivation and required dexterity, has proven effective and safe compared with the use of indwelling catheters.

13. Let's get back to that multifactorial word used in question 3. What exactly is meant?

It means that more than one cause of incontinence may coexist. This is particularly common in elderly individuals. An example of double mechanism was mentioned in question 11: chronic outflow obstruction causes secondary fibrosis of the detrusor, with both contributing to overflow incontinence. Another such example is detrusor instability from local bladder irritation combined with detrusor overactivity caused by central nervous system lesions in which it may be very difficult to elucidate the predominant contributing factor. But, paradoxically, detrusor hyperactivity may also coexist with impaired detrusor contractility (detrusor hyperactivity with impaired contractility [DHIC]). The result is an elevated postvoid residual in the absence of outlet obstruction in combination with intermittent urge incontinence. This may be the most common cause of incontinence in frail elderly individuals and, in these patients, oxybutynin, so useful in pure urge incontinence, may precipitate acute retention from the resultant bladder relaxation. Finally, in women with stress incontinence, precipitating stressors may also trigger detrusor overactivity with concomitant urge incontinence occurring several seconds later.

14. When is an indwelling Foley catheter indicated in the management of chronic incontinence?

When other methods, already discussed, prove ineffective and timed diaper changes, intermittent clean catheterization, and condom catheters have failed or are deemed impractical to prevent skin breakdown with infected pressure ulcers.

15. What is the best way to manage an indwelling Foley?

Assume the universality of polymicrobial bacteriuria after the first month. Treat the bacteriuria only when it is symptomatic in order to avoid antibiotic overuse with the emergence of resistant strains. In turn, this obviates the need for routine urine cultures. Nonetheless, symptomatic infections do occur and require attention because the resultant morbidity can be serious, ranging from epididymitis to pyelonephritis to septicemia. Catheter blockage, which is common in alkaline urines, patients with infection-related bladder calculi, and women, requires early recognition and catheter change. Urinary leakage implies an ill-fitting catheter or Foley balloon, poor positioning, infection, or fecal impaction and should result in catheter replacement. If no such complications arise, there is no need to change catheters more frequently than every 4–6 weekly.

BIBLIOGRAPHY

1. Burgio KL, Locher JL, Goode PS: Combined behavioral and drug therapy for urge incontinence in older women. J Am Geriatric Soc 48:370–374, 2000.
2. Adapted from Busby-Whitehead J, Kinkade J, Granville L: Urinary Incontinence: Management in Primary Practice. Tool Kit 2, Practicing Physician Education Project, Robinson BE, ed. New York, The John A. Hartford Foundation and The American Geriatrics Society, 2000.
3. Fantl SA, Newman DK, Colling J, et al: Urinary Incontinence in Adults: Acute and Chronic Management. Clinical Practice Guideline No. 2, 1996 Update. Rockville, MD, US Department of Health and Human Services, Public Health Service, Agency for Health Care Policy and Research, 1996, AHCPR publication 96–0682.
4. Ouslander JG, Johnson TM: Urinary incontinence. In Hazzard WR, Blass JP, Ettinger WH, et al (eds): Principals of Geriatric Medicine and Gerontology, 4th ed. New York, McGraw-Hill, 1999, pp 1595–1614.
5. Poma PA: Nonsurgical management of genital prolapse: A review and recommendations for clinical practice. J Reprod Med 45:789–797, 2000.
6. Rackley RR, Appell RA: Evaluation and medical management of female urinary incontinence. Cleve Clin J Med 64:83–92, 1997.
7. Rhodes PR, Krogh RH, Bruskewitz RC: Impact of drug therapy on benign prostatic hyperplasia—specific quality of life. Urology 56:1090–1098, 1999.
8. Roberts RO, Jacobsen SJ, Rhodes T, et al: Urinary incontinence in a community-based cohort: Prevalence and healthcare seeking. J Am Geriatric Soc 46:467–472, 1998.
9. Scientific Committee of the First International Consultation on Incontinence: Assessment and treatment of urinary incontinence. Lancet 355:2153–2158, 2000.
10. Smoger SH, Felice TL, Kloecker GH: Urinary incontinence among male veterans receiving care in primary care clinics. Ann Intern Med 132:547–551, 2000.
11. Thom DH, Brown JS: Reproductive and hormonal risk factors for urinary incontinence in later life: A review of the clinical and epidemiological literature. J Am Geriatric Soc 46:1411–1417, 1998.

58. CHRONIC KIDNEY DISEASE

Moro O. Salifu, M.D.

1. What is chronic kidney disease (CKD)?

CKD (previously termed *chronic renal failure* or *chronic renal insufficiency*) is defined as any structural or functional kidney damage or a glomerular filtration rate (GFR) of < 60 mL/min lasting longer than 3 months. *Kidney damage* is defined as pathologic abnormalities or markers of damage such as elevations in blood urea nitrogen (BUN), serum creatinine, or abnormalities of the urine or imaging studies. The rationale for this definition is to allow for classification of various stages of CKD based on **GFR estimation** regardless of the underlying cause and to allow better understanding of the association of different stages with kidney and cardiovascular complications. The terms chronic renal failure or insufficiency, which were primarily based on etiology without standardization of function, are becoming obsolete.

2. What are the various ways to estimate GFR?

Accurate determinations of GFR require the use of inulin or iohexol clearance or a radio-labeled compound, such as iothalamate; however these methods are expensive and not widely available. Surrogate measures used to estimate GFR include creatinine clearance (CrCl) using the Cockcroft and Gault formula and 24-hour urine collection. More recently, the Modification of Diet in Renal Disease (MDRD; Levey) formula has been used, which is by far the best correlate of GFR. It is more complicated than the other methods but is widely available for use on pocket computers or at www.hdcn.com.

3. Why is the serum creatinine an insensitive measure of renal damage?

Both serum creatinine and CrCl are not sensitive measures of renal damage for two reasons. First, substantial renal damage can take place before any decrease in GFR occurs. Secondly, a substantial decline in GFR may lead to only slight elevation in serum creatinine, as shown in the figure. An elevation in serum creatinine is apparent only when the CrCl falls below 70 mL/min. Because creatinine is normally filtered as well as secreted into the renal tubules, the CrCl may substantially overestimate GFR (10–15%), especially as CKD progresses because of maximal tubular excretion.

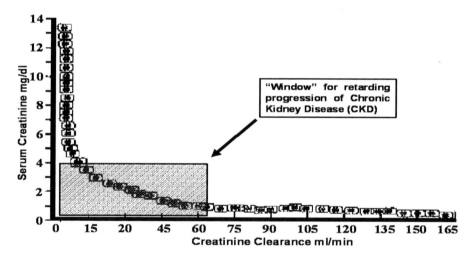

Creatinine clearance curve. Note that by the time serum creatinine begins to rise, creatinine clearance has fallen well below 70 mL/min.

4. How is the CrCl estimated?

The 24-hour urine CrCl is calculated by obtaining a 24-hour urine collection for creatinine and volume and then using the following formula:

$$CrCl \ (mL/min) = U/P \times V$$

where U is the 24-hour urine creatinine in mg/dl, P is the serum creatinine in mg/dl, and V is the 24-hour urine volume/1440 (number of minutes in 24 hours). Using the 24-hour urine creatinine in grams and the serum creatinine in milligrams,

$$CrCl \ (mL/min) = (creatinine \ [g/day]/serum \ creatinine \ [mg/dL]) \times 70$$

An adequate collection of 24-hour urine usually reflects a creatinine generation of 15–20 mg/kg in women and 20–25 mg/kg in men.

The relatively easy bedside formula (Cockcroft and Gault) may overestimate GFR by as much as 20% and should be used with caution. Using the patient's serum creatinine, age, and lean weight in kilograms:

CrCl (mL/min) = (140 − age) × weight (kg) / (72 × serum creatinine) in mg/dL (× 0.85 for women)

5. How is CKD classified?

Irrespective of the cause, CKD is classified into five stages as shown in the table. In **stage 1,** GFR is greater than 90 mL/min, and over 64% of the population fall into this category. In this category, diagnosis and treatment of comorbidities (e.g., hypertension, diabetes, and cardiovascular disease) are critical.

In **stage 2,** GFR is between 60–89 m/L/min and about 31% of the population fall into this category.

In **stage 3,** GFR is 30–59 mL/min with a prevalence of 4.3%. In addition to accurate assessment of renal injury and aggressive treatment of comorbidities, one must identify, evaluate and treat complications such as hyperparathyroidism, hypocalcemia, anemia, acidosis, malnutrition, uncontrolled hypertension, and volume overload.

Progression to **stage 4** is imminent in some patients despite all efforts. At this stage, patients are prepared for kidney replacement therapy by timely placement of vascular or peritoneal dialysis catheters. Patients with GFR < 20 mL/min can be listed to accrue time for cadaver renal transplantation. Renal replacement therapy is indicated when the GFR is < 15 mL/min with symptoms.

Classification of Chronic Kidney Disease

STAGE	GFR STATUS	GFR (mL/min/1.73m^2)	PREVALENCE % CKD IN 177 MILLION OF US POPULATION	ACTION
1	Kidney disease with normal or increased GFR	> 90	64.3	Diagnosis and treatment, treatment of comorbid conditions, slowing progression, cardiovascular risk reduction
2	Mildly impaired GFR	60–89	31.2	Estimating progression
3	Moderately impaired GFR	30–59	4.3	Evaluating and treating complications
4	Severely impaired GFR	15–29	0.2	Preparation for kidney replacement therapy
5	Kidney failure	< 15 (or dialysis)	0.1	Replacement (if symptomatic uremia)

Stages 1–4 are based on NHANES data 1998–1994 in persons older than age 20; stage 5 is based on USRDS data 2002.

6. Why does CKD progress overtime?

Reduction in nephron mass from the initial injury reduces the GFR. This reduction leads to hypertrophy and hyperfiltration of the remaining nephrons as well as to initiation of intraglomerular hypertension. These changes occur in order to increase the GFR of the remaining nephrons, thus minimizing the functional consequences of nephron loss. The changes, however, are ultimately detrimental because they lead to glomerulosclerosis and further nephron loss. In addition to the primary disease, proteinuria may exacerbate renal injury. Evidence suggests that protein resorption droplets in the proximal tubular epithelial cell stimulates a wide variety of cytokines that ultimately lead to tubular atrophy and interstitial fibrosis.

7. What are the symptoms of CKD?

Patients with stages 1–3 CKD may remain relatively asymptomatic. Patients with stages 4 and 5 have decreased production of erythropoietin, thus causing anemia; decreased production of vitamin D_3 resulting in hypocalcemia, secondary hyperparathyroidism, hyperphosphatemia, and renal osteodystrophy; reduction in acid, potassium, salt, and water excretion, resulting in acidosis, hyperkalemia, hypertension, and volume overload; and platelet dysfunction, leading to increased bleeding tendencies.

8. Describe the uremic syndrome.

Accumulation of toxic waste products (uremic toxins) with the signs and symptoms listed above is known as uremia. Classic uremic symptoms include pruritus, nausea, early morning vomiting, loss of appetite, weight loss, and change in sleep pattern and taste sensation. Uremia occurs at a GFR < 15 mL/min. Some uremic toxins (e.g., BUN, creatinine, phenols, guanidines) have been identified, but none can explain all the symptoms. Treatment of metabolic acidosis (with sodium bicarbonate) is recommended when serum bicarbonate levels reach 15 mg/dL, which may improve some symptoms. Untreated metabolic acidosis can lead to more protein catabolism and malnutrition.

9. What is the most common cause of CKD?

The most common cause of CKD is diabetes, accounting for 44% of all patients with CKD. The finding of diabetic retinopathy is highly predictive of diabetic kidney disease. Any level of proteinuria (including microalbuminuria) in a patient with diabetes is presumed to be diabetic kidney disease. A biopsy is not necessary to confirm the diagnosis in diabetes.

10. What other groups of patients are at risk for CKD?

- Patients with sonographic evidence of cystic kidney disease
- Those with history of tubulointerstitial disease, previous nephrotoxic injury
- Patients with known renovascular or other vascular disease
- Renal transplant recipients
- Patients with frequent urinary tract infections
- Patients with a family history of acute or chronic renal failure
- Individuals of black, Hispanic, or Native American origin
- Geriatric patients

Controversy exists concerning the role of hypertension in CKD, although it is clear that hypertension worsens any form of CKD.

11. Is there any link between CKD and cardiovascular disease?

Yes. Recent evidence suggests that microalbuminuria and CKD are independent predictors of cardiovascular disease, including coronary artery disease (CAD) and stroke.

12. How may the acute, usually reversible, causes of kidney diseases be classified?

Acute kidney disease can be easily classified into prerenal, intrarenal, and postrenal causes. A careful history, physical examination, especially to evaluate volume status (presence or absence of edema, orthostasis, neck veins, lung edema), and a review of the laboratory data are essential in determining the type of acute kidney disease. Distinguishing characteristics that can be used as an aid are listed in the table. The most common causes are as follows:

- Prerenal: decreased renal perfusion from cardiac failure or volume loss as a consequence of diarrhea, blood loss, poor intake, or renal vasculitis
- Renal: acute tubular necrosis, acute interstitial nephritis (i.e., drugs), acute glomerulonephritides
- Postrenal: complete or partial urinary obstruction

Diagnostic Indices in Prerenal, Intrarenal, and Postrenal Acute Renal Failure

TEST	PRERENAL	INTRARENAL	POSTRENAL
BUN (mg/dL)	↑↑	↑	↑
Serum creatinine (mg/dL)	↑	↑	↑
Serum BUN/creatinine ratio	> 20	< 20	< 20
Urine osmolality (mOsm/L)	< 500	< 400	< 400
Urine/serum creatinine ratio	> 49	< 20	< 20
FENa*	< 1	> 2	> 2
RFI†	< 1	> 1	> 1
Urine sediment	Normal	Cellular debris, casts	Cellular debris
Serum calcium (mg/dL)	↑	N/↓ ‡	N/↑ (pelvic malignancy)
Serum total protein (g/dL)	↑	N/↓	N/↓
Serum albumin (g/dL)	↑	N/↓	N/↓
Serum bicarbonate (mEq/L)	↑	↓	↓
Serum uric acid (mg/dL)	↑	N/↓ ‡	N/↓
Hematocrit (%)	↑	N/↓	N/↓

*Fractional excretion of sodium (FENa) = urine Na / serum Na × plasma Cr / urine Cr × 100.
†Renal failure index (RFI) = urine Na / urine Cr × serum Cr.
‡May be elevated if azotemia is a result of renal damage from hypercalcemia or hyperuricemia.

13. What findings suggest CKD rather than acute kidney failure?

Anemia, hypocalcemia and hyperphosphatemia, and small echogenic kidneys on ultrasound indicate CKD as opposed to simple acute kidney disease.

14. Which diagnoses resulting in CKD are suggested by large or normal size kidneys on ultrasound?

The classic diagnoses include polycystic kidneys, amyloid kidney, HIV nephropathy, hydronephrosis, and diabetic nephropathy.

15. What general strategies should you use to minimize the progression of CKD?

- Avoid and treat any acute reversible causes.
- Aggressively treat hypertension, maintaining a target blood pressure of 130/85 (125/75 in patients with > 1 g of proteinuria/day).
- Retard intrinsic renal disease progression by the use of drugs that inhibit the renin-angiotensin system. Angiotensin-converting enzyme inhibitors (ACEIs) are renoprotective in addition to their effects on hypertension, in any form of CKD. Angiotensin II receptor blockers (ARBs), which are more expensive, have also been shown to be effective.
- In diabetics, glycosylated hemoglobin should be maintained at < 7%.
- Correct lipid abnormalities and aggressively treat any comorbid conditions.

16. What is the leading cause of death in patients with CKD?

Cardiovascular disease is the leading cause of death in patients with CKD. Thus, primary and secondary cardiovascular disease prevention is critical in preventing morbidity and mortality.

17. When and why should anemia be treated in patients with CKD?

Anemia is an independent risk factor for mortality in CKD. Additionally, correction of anemia results in improved quality of life, prevention and reversal of left ventricular hypertrophy (LVH), and decreased mortality. After careful correction of underlying reversible factors that cause anemia (blood loss, folate or B_{12} deficiency), erythropoietin and iron should be provided to patients whose hemoglobin has fallen below the normal range as a consequence of loss of renal function. This is likely to occur when the creatinine clearance reaches 30 mL/minute.

18. What are the strategies to minimize progression of CKD?

1. **Distinguish between acute reversible from chronic kidney disease.** A good history, review of medical records, examination including orthostatic changes, and diagnostic indices illustrated in the table in question 12 will differentiate the various forms of acute kidney failure from CKD. Most of these acute diseases have specific treatments. Anemia, hypocalcemia, hyperphosphatemia, GFR estimation (by MDRD) < 60 mL/min/1.73 m^2 for over 3 months, and small echogenic kidneys on ultrasonography are indicative of CKD. Some CKD with normal to large kidneys include diabetic nephropathy, polycystic kidneys, hydronephrosis, HIV nephropathy, and amyloid kidney.

2. **Slow the rate of decline of GFR.** Ample evidence suggests that strict blood pressure control for both diabetic and nondiabetic CKD will slow progression of CKD. Target blood pressure should be < 130/85 or 125/75 if proteinuria > 1 g/day. Blood pressure control may require multiple agents. Drugs that inhibit the renin-angiotensin system (ACEIs and ARBs) have been shown to retard disease progression (renoprotective effect) when compared with conventional therapy and have additional cardiovascular benefits beyond blood pressure control alone. Both ACEIs and ARBs have been studied extensively and have been found to be renoprotective in any form of CKD. Blood sugar should be controlled in diabetics, with a target glycosylated hemoglobin (HbA$_{1c}$) of less than 7%. A low-protein diet (0.8–1.0 g/kg/day) in patients who do not show any evidence of malnutrition and correction of lipid abnormalities should be part of the strategic plan to slow disease progression. By these methods, progression of CKD has been remarkably and impressively reduced to that of aging (GFR loss of 0.1 mL/min/1.73 m^2/year) in some studies.

3. **Treat comorbid conditions aggressively and obtain appropriate early referrals to prevent other end organ damage.** The leading cause of death in patients with CKD is cardiovascular disease. Thus, cardiovascular surveillance should be a priority. Eye, foot disease, smoking, anemia management (with iron or recombinant erythropoietin), and bone disease management (with phosphate binders, vitamin D) should be addressed.

19. How should patients on ACEIs and ARBs be followed?

ACEIs and, less so, ARBs may be associated with an increase in serum potassium and creatinine levels in some patients because of inhibition of aldosterone synthesis and vasodilation of the efferent arteriole. An increase of more than 30% from baseline of serum creatinine or potassium should prompt dose reduction or withdrawal. The majority of patients, however, tolerate these drugs, and the drugs should be pushed to maximum doses to control blood pressure. Patients newly started on ACEIs or ARBs should have serum potassium and creatinine checked in about a week. Potassium-sparing diuretics, such as triamterene, spironolactone, and amiloride, should not be used in CKD unless in combination with a loop diuretic.

20. What are the six indications for acute dialysis in patients with acute or chronic kidney disease?

1. Life-threatening hyperkalemia
2. Profound metabolic acidosis
3. Pulmonary edema with hypoxemia
4. Toxic ingestions (lithium, theophylline, salicylates, methanol, or glycols)
5. Uremic pericarditis
6. Encephalopathy

21. Describe the acute management of the common CKD medical emergencies.

Pulmonary edema is best managed by emergent dialysis. Initial management with oxygen (or mechanical ventilation if severely hypoxemic), intravenous nitrates, morphine, or furosemide will decrease preload and buy time for dialysis. Initial treatment of hyperkalemia depends on the presence or absence of electrocardiographic (ECG) findings (widened PR interval, widened QRS complex, peaked T waves or sine waves in severe cases). When ECG findings are present, intravenous calcium gluconate or chloride (10% vials, repeated as needed until dialysis is available) is the initial drug of choice to stabilize the cardiac membrane. Cellular shift of potassium can then be enhanced by administration of intravenous sodium bicarbonate (50-mL vials), $D_{50}W$ (50-mL vials), and insulin (10 U). Blood sugar should be monitored to avoid hypoglycemia. Beta$_2$ agonists given as nebulization and repeated as needed may also shift potassium into cells.

Dialysis should be instituted emergently because these therapies are transient and do not remove the total body potassium excess. When ECG changes are absent and potassium elevation is modest ($<$ 6.5 mEq/L), orally administered sodium polystyrene sulfonate (Kayexalate in sorbitol, 1 g binds 0.5–1.0 mEq of potassium in the gut), 60 g, will reduce serum potassium by 0.8–1.0 mEq/L. The dose can be repeated every 4 hours until the estimated Kayexalate dose is given. Dialysis should still be considered for patients with severe hyperkalemia even in the absence of ECG changes because acidosis, which is normally present, will eventually exacerbate the hyperkalemia.

Uremic platelet dysfunction may increase the risk of gastrointestinal bleeding, which should be stopped endoscopically or surgically. However, packed red cell transfusion, early dialysis, administration of 1-deamino-8-D-arginine vasopressin (DDAVP) at 0.3 μg/kg as needed, and conjugated estrogens, 0.6 mg/kg intravenously daily for 5 days, may improve hemostasis. The duration of action of DDAVP is 4–6 hours, and it acts by increasing von Willebrand's factor from vascular endothelium. The mechanism of action of estrogens is not well understood, but its action may last up to 2 weeks. Coagulation factors are transfused only if indicated.

22. When is the best time to refer a patient to a nephrologist?

As soon as CKD is detected, patients should be referred for appropriate work up, estimation of GFR, and strategic planning to slow disease progression. Most patients can be followed by both nephrologists and primary care physicians. Poor patient outcomes (infections, vascular access problems, and death) are increased in untimely late referrals, in which uremia is imminent.

23. What is the most important aspect of patient preparation for renal replacement therapy?

Patient education is the most important element. Patients should be educated to understand and recognize symptoms of uremia to make informed choices on the available modalities such as hemodialysis, peritoneal dialysis, renal transplantation, or abstinence. Evidence suggests that transplantation offers the best rehabilitation in suitable candidates. The superiority of peritoneal dialysis over hemodialysis in the first 4 years of dialysis is still being debated; nonetheless, patient education on the benefits and risks of each modality will lead to an informed choice. After informed choice of therapy is made, the patient is referred for transplantation or dialysis access placement. The preferred dialysis access is a native arteriovenous fistula, but polytetrafluoroethylene grafts are also used in patients with poor peripheral veins. Temporary catheters should be avoided as much as possible because of their association with increase morbidity and mortality.

BIBLIOGRAPHY

1. Brenner BM, Cooper ME, de Zeeuw D, et al: Effects of losartan on renal and cardiovascular outcomes in patients with type 2 diabetes and nephropathy. RENAAL Study Investigators. N Engl J Med 345:861–869, 2001.
2. Campbell R, Sangalli F, Perticucci E, et al: Effects of combined ACE inhibitor and angiotensin II antagonist treatment in human chronic nephropathies. Kidney Int 63:1094–1103, 2003.
3. Gerstein HC, Mann JF, Yi Q, et al: Albuminuria and risk of cardiovascular events, death, and heart failure in diabetic and nondiabetic individuals. HOPE Study Investigators. JAMA 286:421–426, 2001.
4. Lewis EJ, Hunsicker LG, Clarke WR, et al: Renoprotective effect of the angiotensin-receptor antagonist irbesartan in patients with nephropathy due to type 2 diabetes. Collaborative Study Group. N Engl J Med 345:851–860, 2001.
5. Mann JF, Gerstein HC, Dulau-Florea I, Lonn E: Cardiovascular risk in patients with mild renal insufficiency. Kidney Int Suppl 84:192–196, 2003.
6. National Kidney Foundation Kidney and Dialysis Outcome Quality Initiative: http://www.kidney.org/professionals/doqi/kdoqi/tables.htm.
7. Parving HH: Hypertension and diabetes. The scope of the problem. Blood Press Suppl 2:25–31, 2001.

8. Pennell JP: Optimizing medical management of the patient with pre end stage renal disease. Am J Med 111:559–568, 2001.
9. Pereira BJ: Overcoming barriers to the early detection and treatment of chronic kidney disease and improving outcomes for end-stage renal disease. Am J Manag Care 8(4 suppl):S122-S135; quiz S136-S139, 2002.
10. Remuzzi G, Bertani T: Pathophysiology of progressive nephropathies. N Engl J Med 339:1448–1456, 1998.
11. Ruggenenti P, Perna A, Gherardi G, et al: Chronic proteinuric nephropathies: Outcomes and response to treatment in a prospective cohort of 352 patients with different patterns of renal injury. Am J Kidney Dis 35:1155–1165, 2000.
12. Ruggenenti P, Schieppati A, Remuzzi G: Progression, remission, regression of chronic renal diseases. Lancet 357(9268):1601–1608, 2001.
13. Salifu MO: Azotemia. Available online at http://www.emedicine.com/med/topic194.htm.
14. Stack AG: Impact of timing of nephrology referral and pre-ESRD care on mortality risk among new ESRD patients in the United States. Am J Kidney Dis 41:310–318, 2003.
15. UK Prospective Diabetes Study Group: Intensive blood-glucose control with sulphonylureas or insulin compared with conventional treatment and risk of complications in patients with type 2 diabetes (UKPDS 33). Lancet 352(9131):837–853, 1998.
16. US Renal Data System: USRDS 2002 Annual Data Report. Bethesda, MD, The National Institute of Health, National Institute of Diabetes and Digestive and Kidney Diseases, 2000.

IX. Common Problems of the Blood and Lymph System

59. ASYMPTOMATIC FINDINGS ON THE HEMOGRAM

Jeanette Mladenovic, M.D.

1. What value on the complete blood count (CBC) is helpful when the mean corpuscular volume (MCV) is disproportionately low in comparison with the mildly low hemoglobin (Hb)?

The major consideration is whether the low MCV results from iron deficiency or an abnormality of globin chain synthesis (i.e., thalassemia). Clues that suggest thalassemia trait rather than iron deficiency may be provided by the following: (1) a red cell count higher than expected for the hemoglobin *and* a near-normal mean corpuscular hemoglobin count (MCHC) or (2) a red cell distribution width (RDW) within the normal range. Microcytosis, when caused by to iron deficiency, is usually accompanied by a low red cell count, low MCHC, and high RDW. Because there are many instances in which the RDW may also be elevated in thalassemia trait, the finding of a low MCV and normal RDW has good specificity but poor sensitivity for thalassemia. The following table is an example of findings that strongly suggest these conditions.

	HEMOGLOBIN (G/DL)	MCV	RDW
Iron deficiency	8	74	> 15.3%
Chronic disease	10	86	Variable
Thalassemia syndromes	12	68	< 14%

2. When is the MCHC helpful?

An elevated MCHC with a mild or no anemia suggests the presence of hereditary spherocytosis, the most common hemolytic anemia that is related to a defect of the red cell membrane. Although anemia may or may not be present, an elevated reticulocytosis is hidden in the usually unremarkable MCV (making it higher than it otherwise should be). However, an elevated MCHC is characteristic. In fact, in children, an MCHC > 35 g/dL and an RDW > 14% were reported to have a sensitivity of 63% and a specificity of 100%. Therefore, this combination is useful as a screening tool for this hereditary disease.

3. What causes an elevated platelet count?

Thrombocytosis may result from primary or secondary causes. In primary thrombocytosis, an intrinsic defect in the stem cell leads to abnormally increased platelets, often irregular in size with variable granularity. Diseases such as polycythemia vera, chronic myelogenous leukemia, and essential thrombocythemia fall into this category. Secondary thrombocytosis is seen in patients with chronic inflammatory states, hemolysis, iron deficiency, gastrointestinal bleeding, and postsplenectomy syndrome. Chronic inflammatory states include malignancies and conditions that result in a cellular immune response (e.g., chronic infections and autoimmune disease). Patients with primary thrombocytosis may be at risk from bleeding or clotting with platelet counts higher than 1 million, whereas patients with secondary thrombocytosis rarely develop such high counts.

4. Besides infection, what causes leukocytosis?

Leukocytosis may be secondary or caused by primary bone marrow abnormalities. Secondary leukocytosis may be caused by demargination, accelerated release of cells from the marrow, increased production of white blood cells (WBCs), or even decreased removal of white cells from the circulation. Demargination may be seen with sepsis or any stress-mediated response, such as hypotension or hypoxia. Increased marrow release and production is seen with infection, inflammation (e.g., blood in a closed space), or even tumors that produce stimulatory factors (lung carcinoma). Primary leukocytosis occurs with leukemia. If the differential WBC count shows young WBCs (blasts or cells of earlier differentiation than metamyelocytes in the circulation), a primary marrow disorder (leukemia) is more likely.

5. Define lymphocytosis. With what disorders is it associated?

Lymphocytosis is defined as an absolute lymphocyte count $> 3.5 \times 10^9$/L. Lymphocytosis or a lymphoid leukemoid reaction may be seen in patients with viral infections, such as infectious mononucleosis, cytomegalovirus (CMV), measles, and pertussis (in children). Lymphocytes may be atypical in appearance, variable in size, and reactive. In an adult without evidence of infection, a persistent lymphocytosis $> 5 \times 10^9$/L suggests the diagnosis of chronic lymphocytic leukemia. Blood typing to determine that all lymphocytes are B lymphocytes confirms the diagnosis.

6. What is significant leukopenia?

Leukopenia is defined as a WBC count $< 4 \times 10^9$/L. Usually, as the count decreases, cells of the neutrophil series are most affected. The percentage of the WBC count of granulocytic lineage (bands and mature cells) determines the absolute neutrophil cell count and the risk of life-threatening infection. Patients with granulocyte counts $< 1 \times 10^9$/L are at risk of sepsis. Body temperature $> 38.3°C$ should be evaluated aggressively to determine the cause and treated empirically with broad-spectrum antibiotics that cover gram-negative (including *Pseudomonas* sp.) and gram-positive (including staphylococci) organisms. As the absolute count decreases, the association of fever with bacteremia increases.

7. What test should be ordered first to determine the cause of a prolonged prothrombin time (PT) or partial thromboplastin time (PTT)?

The first test that should be requested is a 1:1 mix, in which normal plasma is mixed with the patient's plasma and both PT and PTT are repeated. Complete correction suggests that prolongation is caused by factor deficiency. Failure to correct suggests the presence of inhibitors in the patient's plasma. Patients with liver disease often have two defects; thus, correction is incomplete. Alternatively, a prolonged PTT with evidence of inhibition is consistent with a lupus inhibitor.

8. What is the appropriate response when the hematocrit level is elevated above normal?

An increased hematocrit level may be caused by decreased plasma volume (relative erythrocytosis) or a true increase in the red cell mass (primary polycythemia vera or secondary erythrocytosis). At a hematocrit of 55%, the odds of a true increase are only 50/50, whereas at a hematocrit of 60%, the red cell mass almost certainly is increased. Thus, at levels in the 52–58% range, further testing is required to determined whether there is a true increase in the red cell mass. Because the measurement of red cell mass is not necessarily available, consultation with a hematologist may be required for further evaluation of a persistently elevated hematocrit level. Patients with elevated hematocrit levels should not undergo surgery or dye loads without evaluation because of the risk of thrombosis.

9. With automated counters, which abnormalities may cause a false change in CBC values?
Erythrocytosis: lipemia, very high WBC count
Pseudoanemia: cold agglutinins
Pseudothrombocytosis: red cell fragments or microcytic red cells
Pseudothrombocytopenia: clumped platelets
Pseudoleukocytosis: giant platelets
Pseudoleukopenia: leukoagglutination
Thus, unexpected values should be evaluated visually and usually are flagged for further laboratory analysis.

10. What is the significance of polychromatophilia and nucleated red blood cells (RBCs) on the peripheral blood smear?
Such findings suggest early release of cells from the marrow in response to erythropoietin or secondary to displacement of the marrow with other elements (myelophthisis). A reticulocyte count is required to determine which process caused the increase in early circulating RBCs..

11. What considerations should be used in interpreting the automated WBC differential?
Automated WBC counting is highly reliable ($> 90\%$ sensitivity) when the cell population of interest is large (i.e., $> 5\%$). However, at smaller numbers of cells, these instruments become less reliable. The instrumentation is designed to use a series of flags that will alert the clinician to the possibility that there may be an abnormal population or that the machine may be unreliable. Thus, blasts, atypical lymphoid cells, immature (shifted) neutrophils, and leukopenia all may result in flags whose accuracy and sensitivity should be further evaluated.

12. Define significant eosinophilia and significant basophilia.
Mild eosinophilia ($0.2–1.5 \times 10^9$ cells/L) may be seen in patients with mild skin disease, atopy, and allergic reactions. Marked eosinophilia is occasionally seen in patients with asthma (especially in the presence of *Aspergillus* spp.) or angioneurotic edema. Extremely high or progressively increasing numbers of eosinophils may also suggest tissue helminthic infection or eosinophilic syndromes related to any organ of the body or secondary to malignancies. Prolonged, marked elevation of eosinophils may lead to tissue damage caused by the eosinophils themselves. Eosinophilic leukemia is exceedingly rare.
Basophilia ($> 0.1 \times 10^9$) is seen in myeloproliferative diseases of all types. In the presence of leukocytosis or thrombocytosis, basophilia of any degree supports a diagnosis of primary myeloproliferative disease. Mild, transient basophilia also is seen with ulcerative colitis and allergic systemic or skin diseases.

BIBLIOGRAPHY

1. Gulati GL, Hyan BH: The automated CBC: A current perspective. Hematol Oncol Clin North Am 8:593, 1994.
2. Michaels LA, Cohen AR, Zhao H, et al: Screening for hereditary spherocytosis by use of automated erythrocyte indexes. J Pediatr 130:957, 1997.
3. Morris MW, Williams WJ, Nelson DA: Automated blood cell counting. In Beutler E, Lichtman M, Coller B, et al (eds): Williams Hematology, 6th ed. New York, McGraw-Hill, 2001.

60. ANEMIA

Jeanette Mladenovic, M.D.

1. Define anemia.

Normal hemoglobin levels are influenced by age, gender, ethnic group, altitude, and exposure to smoke. Normal values were calculated to a 95% reference range for a large population, thus providing the laboratory reference. Values for men are higher than for women, a finding attributed to testosterone. For children, the lower hemoglobin level at age 2 years (10.7 g/dL) increases gradually until normal limits are reached by age 15 and 18 years for girls and boys, respectively. Values for African Americans are approximately 0.5–0.6 g lower than for white Americans. It is important to compare the patient's hemoglobin values over time, thus determining when deviation from the norm occurs. Mild anemia may be important primarily as a barometer of a patient's overall health and as an early clue to disease.

2. Is anemia a normal concomitant of aging?

No. Early studies suggested that a decrease in hemoglobin with aging was of no clinical significance. However, more recently an increased mortality has consistently been seen in elderly men who have a hemoglobin < 13 g/dL (12 g/dL for women). The increased relative risk of mortality (up to two times) was seen, regardless of whether a cause for the anemia was readily detected or not. Therefore, these findings suggest that anemia in elder individuals is not a normal reflection of aging, but instead a marker for underlying disease.

3. What are the most common causes of anemia?

Iron deficiency	25%
Blood loss	25%
Anemia of chronic disease	25%
Megaloblastic anemias	10%
Hemolysis	10%
Other bone marrow failure	5%

4. Can anemia be diagnosed by a physical examination?

Physical examination is often diagnostic only indirectly when anemia is severe, by resting tachycardia, wide pulse pressure, hyperdynamic precordium, or evidence of high-output heart failure. Pallor is highly subjective and influenced by vascular tone and intrinsic skin hue. Even the absence of palmar creases in severe anemia is currently in question. When a patient appears pale in the face, conjunctiva, and mucous membranes, the physician is likely to order a complete blood count (CBC) to evaluate systemic illness. In most other instances, anemia is diagnosed asymptomatically or during the evaluation of other complaints.

5. What is pagophagia?

Pagophagia is an excessive appetite for ice. This feature of the history is considered to be quite specific for iron deficiency, even in the absence of anemia. It disappears with iron repletion.

6. When is a reticulocyte count helpful?

The reticulocyte count is the only available measure of daily marrow production. As such, it is the most important test for determining whether anemia is caused by increased red blood cell (RBC) destruction or inadequate marrow production. Normal production of RBCs is 1–2% per day. Thus, any number less than 2% in the patient with anemia is considered inadequate production, which may be caused by hematinic deficiencies (iron, vitamin B_{12}, folate); chronic inflammatory, endocrine, or renal disease; or infiltrating marrow diseases (e.g., tumor or primary stem cell failure).

However, when the reticulocyte count is > 2%, further analysis is required to determine whether chronic stimulated marrow production caused by increased destruction of RBCs is truly present. Because the reticulocyte count is expressed as a percentage of RBCs, measurement of daily production of RBCs requires correction of this percentage when the absolute RBC count is decreased (as in anemia). The following equation may be used to estimate the correction:

Corrected reticulocyte = observed hematocrit/45 × measured reticulocyte count. Alternatively, an absolute reticulocyte count > 90×10^9 is considered increased. When the absolute reticulocyte count is increased, a further correction is required for the increased length of time the reticulocyte spends in circulation; this is estimated by dividing the absolute count or the percentage in half.

Correction of the reticulocytes is a helpful reminder of underlying pathophysiology in the following circumstances: mild reticulocytosis with intramedullary hemolysis in B_{12} or folate deficiency when the underlying problem is hypoproliferative; after a single episode of acute hemorrhage with an appropriate marrow response; and in the instance of hemolytic disease, when it is necessary to determine whether the marrow is adequately responding (i.e., if the amount of iron or folate is sufficient to maintain the marrow production needed for the increased destruction or if the patient is entering an aplastic crisis).

7. How does the mean corpuscular volume (MCV) help in the differential diagnosis of anemia?

Classification of anemia has traditionally relied on the size of RBCs, as determined by the RBC volume. The normal MCV is 80–95 fl; values above and below this range define macrocytic and microcytic anemias, respectively. However, because the value represents the arithmetic mean of all RBCs, a mixed population of cells may contribute to the overall value. Furthermore, in several instances, a single deficiency may be masked by a combined deficiency. Thus, low or high values of the MCV are useful in directing the diagnosis, but a normal MCV does not exclude any of the causes that may contribute to the cause of anemia. The table below outlines the classification of anemia based on the MCV in conjunction with the reticulocyte count.

Practical Evaluation of Anemia

RETICULOCYTE	HALLMARK ON SMEAR	LABORATORY TESTS
< 2%, or < 25–50,000/μL		
MCV low	*Microcytosis*	
Iron deficiency	—	Low ferritin; low serum Fe/high TIBC, sat < 16%
Chronic disease	—	Ferritin low or may be < 100 μg/L Low serum Fe or low TIBC, Sat 20–30%
Thalassemia (αα-, β-minor, or HbE)	—	Hemoglobin electrophoresis
MCV high	*Macrocytosis*	
Vitamin B_{12} deficiency	Multilobed neutrophils	Low B_{12} level
Folate deficiency	Multilobed neutrophils	Low serum or RBC folate
Myelodysplasia or other stem cell defect	—	Diagnostic bone marrow aspiration and biopsy
MCV normal		
Early iron deficiency or chronic disease	Normal	As above
Renal or endocrine disease	Normal	As indicated
Marrow replacement or stem-cell diseases	Abnormal cells from the marrow; teardrops or nucleated red cells	Bone marrow biopsy
Mixed defects	Large and small cells, or normal	As needed from clinical suspicion

Table continues on following page.

Practical Evaluation of Anemia (Continued)

RETICULOCYTE	HALLMARK ON SMEAR	LABORATORY TESTS
Corrected > 2% or > 90,000/μL		
Extravascular hemolysis	Spherocytes	Direct and indirect Coombs' test result
Intravascular hemolysis	Abnormal RBC shapes and sizes	Tests for free hemoglobin, DIC evaluation
Intrinsic RBC defects	Clues: shapes, Heinz bodies	Evaluation for defect in RBC membrane, hemoglobinopathy, enzyme defects

MCV = mean corpuscular volume; TIBC = total iron-binding capacity; Sat = saturation; HbE = hemoglobin E; RBC = red blood cell; DIC = disseminated intravascular coagulation.

8. When may the red cell distribution width (RDW) be useful?

The RDW reflects the degree of homogeneity or heterogeneity in size among the RBCs. This measurement is meant to detect the degree of anisocytosis on a peripheral blood smear. It is a nonspecific measurement that needs to be considered in the context of the remainder of the hemogram and the patient. Oftentimes, an elevated value occurs in conditions in which marrow precursors see widely varying levels of nutrients (e.g., B_{12}, folate, iron). A wide RDW may be the first clue to iron deficiency, a manifestation of dual populations of cells, or a sign of anisocytosis caused by RBC fragments. A normal value, signifying a uniform cell population, may be helpful in distinguishing thalassemia minor from iron deficiency as a cause of microcytosis.

9. When should the clinician evaluate the peripheral blood smear?

Ideally, the smear should be evaluated in all patients with anemia or even leukocytosis, but this often becomes practically unfeasible and does not change the primary care provider's approach. Thus, it is important to determine when the smear should be further evaluated—a heretical but realistic approach. Often the smear needs to be viewed to confirm abnormalities detected by automated procedures before further work-up is pursued. Automated values require review of the smear in the following circumstances:

- Abnormal types of circulating cells (e.g., blasts or lymphocytes)
- Confirmation and evaluation of extremely high or low values of blood counts (especially platelets and neutrophils)
- RBC fragments of any type (e.g., teardrops, schistocytes, sickle cells)
- Perplexing hypoproliferative anemia, to look for clues of rouleaux (paraprotein) or mixed populations of cells (large and small)
- Anemia with reticulocytosis to search for spherocytes or other clues, such as shape abnormalities in hereditary membrane disease

10. What are the indications for a bone marrow aspirate or biopsy?

The provider should obtain consultation for the purpose of a bone marrow analysis under the following circumstances:

- Pancytopenia or bicytopenias
- A peripheral blood smear that shows abnormal early cells (i.e., blast, myelocytes) or evidence of myelophthisis (teardrops)
- For rare causes of anemia, such as sideroblastic anemia and pure RBC aplasia, which must be suspected because of unique clinical situations or in patients in whom the anemia is unexplained
- Severe thrombocytopenias
- Severe leukopenia
- Monoclonal serum protein
- Culture for granulomatous diseases in unique situations

A biopsy is not always indicated; however, when evaluation of cellularity or a search for tumor cells or other infiltrating disease is required, a biopsy is necessary along with the aspirate.

Although bone marrow examination has traditionally been advocated for the evaluation of iron stores, the diagnosis of iron deficiency is *usually* made by other means.

11. Which serum test should you order to diagnose iron deficiency?

Two laboratory tests are in common use to detect iron deficiency: the ferritin level, a measure of iron stores, and the serum iron saturation (serum iron/total iron-binding capacity = iron saturation). Both tests are unnecessary in the initial evaluation; on occasion, however, both may prove helpful.

In otherwise healthy individuals or in pregnant women in whom the total iron-binding capacity (TIBC) may be elevated, the ferritin level is a very reliable measure of iron stores. However, although values < 12 μg/mL are highly specific for iron deficiency, they are relative insensitive. A higher cutoff of 30 to 40 ng/mL improves the sensitivity upward to 98%, with < 30 ng/mL being a very reliable indicator of iron deficiency in pregnancy. Additionally, a normal ferritin value does not exclude iron deficiency, but a value > 100 ng/L is inconsistent with iron deficiency in otherwise healthy individuals.

The FE/TIBC, or iron saturation, with an elevated TIBC and a decreased serum iron may also diagnose iron deficiency when the value is < 16%. The presence of a low serum iron and a low or normal TIBC level is helpful in diagnosing the anemia of chronic disease.

12. When is the ferritin level likely to be falsely elevated?

Ferritin reflects true iron overload at values > 1000 μg/mL (hemochromatosis; hemosiderosis from blood cell dyscrasias). However, inflammation, infection, and liver disease with destruction of hepatocytes increase ferritin to values ranging from 100 to > 1000 μg/mL. A useful guide is to divide the ferritin level by three in the presence of inflammation in order to estimate the true ferritin level.

13. How common is iron deficiency in adolescents?

Approximately 10% of adolescent girls are iron deficient, although a much smaller percentage have anemia. Only 1% of adolescent boys and men are iron deficient. Several studies have suggested that iron deficiency may result in cognitive defects and decreased endurance in this age group. For these reasons, the American Academy of Pediatrics recommends checking the hemoglobin level at least once during adolescence. Additionally, evaluation of iron stores should be considered in adolescents at increased risk, including female athletes, vegans, those with heavy menstrual loss, and those who are underweight.

14. What is the significance of anemia in athletes (sports anemia)?

Anemia in endurance athletes, including long-distance runners and swimmers, appears to be multifactorial. Iron deficiency has been attributed to low-grade gastrointestinal loss, hematuria, and intravascular hemolysis. Likewise, a dilutional effect of plasma volume expansion may be seen. However, the diagnosis remains one of exclusion in populations at risk.

15. What are the hallmarks of the anemia of chronic disease (ACD)?

1. Nonprogressive anemia of 10–11 g% in most cases—but as low as 8 g% (Hct 25%)—is consistent with the diagnosis. The anemia parallels the severity of the underlying inflammatory disease. In this instance, inflammation is a broad term that includes systemic diseases accompanied by a major cellular inflammatory response. An elevated sedimentation rate often correlates with the presence of chronic disease. More recently, ACD has also been thought to occur in patients with diabetes or cardiovascular disease or more acutely after trauma. These situations, however, always required additional evaluation to be certain no other cause is present.

2. An MCV that is not increased and usually is mildly decreased

3. A low reticulocyte count (< 2% or 25,000/μL)

4. A low serum iron level

The pathophysiologic problem appears to be tissue avidity for iron and failure to release iron to the serum; a lower than normal erythropoietin level along with decreased erythropoietin responsivness; and shortened RBC survival, all apparently related to release of interleukin-1 and tumor necrosis factor. The ferritin level is often normal or even increased, but a low serum iron, often with a low TIBC, results in low iron saturation that characterizes the anemia of chronic disease in many, but not all, patients.

16. Are there other tests that might help in the diagnosis of iron deficient erythropoiesis?

Yes. Several other tests have been evaluated to aid in the diagnosis of anemia that is limited by iron availability. Among these is the zinc protoprophyrrin level, in which zinc substitutes for iron when it is unavailable in the last step of heme synthesis. However, zinc protoporphyrrin is then elevated in both the anemia of chronic disease and iron deficiency, making it far less sensitive than the ferritin test. The serum transferrin receptor, which is directly proportional to the rate of erythropoiesis and inversely proportional to tissue iron has been evaluated; however, clinical use of this test is actually no better than the serum ferritin test. Most recently, the reticulocyte hemoglobin content has been evaluated in patients with iron deficiency. The rationale is that the reticulocyte is the nearest relation to the erythrid precursor and demonstrates most readily if iron were to limit hematopoiesis. This test is promising, especially if the MCV is normal, even in the presence of chronic disease.

17. What further evaluation is required for the diagnosis of iron deficiency?

The cause of the iron deficiency must be evaluated. A chronic loss of 3–4 cc of blood per day (1–2 mg of iron) leads to iron deficiency. Although gastrointestinal (GI) blood loss may occur with common entities, including use of nonsteroidal anti-inflammatory drugs, aspirin, and anticoagulants; hemorrhoids; and various acid peptic entities (ulcers, esophagitis), they should not be assumed to be the cause. Chronic loss of iron from the lower GI tract as an initial manifestation of malignancy must always be considered. Additionally, consideration of celiac sprue as a cause of occult blood loss resulting in iron deficiency should also be considered if no other cause is found and the clinical setting is appropriate.

Another common cause of iron deficiency is menses. The history may provide clues to excessive menstrual loss such as menses > 7 days in duration, passage of clots greater than 2 cm in size, and inability to control flow with tampons. Even given these symptoms, excessive menstrual flow is poorly assessed by the medical history.

Urinary blood loss is not a cause of iron deficiency, unless excessive gross hematuria is chronically present or unless intravascular hemolysis is persistent (as in the presence of a cardiac valve that causes hemolysis or in rare blood disorders, such as paroxysmal nocturnal hemoglobinemia).

The above observations have led to the practical clinical recommendations that men with GI blood loss and women older than age 35–40 years require evaluation of iron deficiency anemia to exclude sources of occult GI blood loss caused by malignant, premalignant, or other treatable lesions.

18. Can a patient have both iron deficiency and chronic disease?

Yes. Iron deficiency is particularly common in patients with rheumatoid arthritis, although it may also be seen in other conditions. Clues to iron deficiency include a decrease in the usually low hematocrit of chronic disease, ferritin level < 100 μg/L, and a very low (5–10%) iron saturation. Oral iron supplementation may be given on a trial basis, with an anticipated increase in the hematocrit or hemoglobin level to low plateau levels consistent with the inflammatory state.

Iron deficiency may also occur with a defect in folate or vitamin B_{12} and initially high iron studies. Thus, normal iron study results in the presence of or at the initiation of treatment for folate or B_{12} deficiencies are not helpful in excluding iron deficiency. A more accurate reflection of iron stores is obtained when normal marrow maturation has resumed after replacement of B_{12} or folate.

19. How should patients with iron deficiency be treated?

Multiple preparations are available to treat iron deficiency, with variable amounts of iron available for absorption. Overall, GI side effects are related to the amount of iron, so that lower amounts of iron are better tolerated. Thus, ferrous gluconate or feosol may be better tolerated than traditional ferrous sulfate, 300 mg three times/day. However, the required rate of correction determines the choice of preparation. In any case, iron supplementation must be continued beyond correction of the anemia to replace iron stores ($\geq$ 3 months).

Failure to correct iron deficiency is caused by poor compliance, inadequate absorption, continued blood loss that exceeds supplementation, or incorrect diagnosis. Absorption may be enhanced by making certain the patient is taking iron between meals, by changing preparations or mode of administration, and by adding ascorbic acid. Systemic iron should be reserved for patients at extreme risk of malabsorption (e.g., inflammatory bowel disease).

20. When is parenteral iron therapy indicated?

Rarely. The ease of oral iron replacement, despite the issue of compliance, and the risk associated with parenteral therapy should lead to the use of parenteral iron only after careful consideration and clear indications. The most serious risk is anaphylaxis, which requires a test dose; other less serious adverse effects occur in as many as 10% of patients treated with iron dextran. A newer preparation, ferric gluconate, has a lower incidence of allergic reasions. Thus, prudence suggests that parenteral iron therapy should be given only after clear failure of iron absorption or when iron needs cannot be met by oral doses because of continued loss of iron through the GI tract or intravascular hemolysis. Intolerance to oral iron therapy should be considered an indication only in rare circumstances, if at all.

21. When is evaluation of the folate level useful?

Evaluation of folate level is rarely useful in the usual patients at risk, such as nutritionally deficient patients who consume alcohol or nutritionally replete patients who consume alcohol but have mildly elevated MCVs. Even a low serum folate level is easily and rapidly corrected by alcohol cessation or food intake. It is much more important to eliminate cobalamin as the cause of macrocytosis so as not to miss the potential for future neurologic defects caused by such a deficiency. If the cobalamin level is normal, folate deficiency may be treated with folate supplements. If the B_{12} level is low or borderline normal, further evaluation is necessary. Although folate, B_{12}, RBC folate, and iron levels are frequently ordered in the shotgun evaluation of anemia, the cost effectiveness of this approach is suspect. As a marker of malabsorption in high-risk patients or in the evaluation of a difficult-to-diagnose anemia with megaloblastosis, evaluation of levels of serum or erythrocyte folate levels is clearly useful.

22. In addition to the evaluation of a macrocytic anemia, when should vitamin B_{12} be measured?

In addition to the evaluation of macrocytic anemia caused by pernicious anemia, certain additional conditions are predictably associated with vitamin B_{12} deficiency, even in the absence of hematologic defects:

1. Gastrectomy, ileal resection, or malabsorption, because stores of vitamin B_{12} are large, deficiency is not suspected until years later; the average time to deficiency after gastrectomy is 5 years (2–12 years)

2. Neurologic complaints, especially with a peripheral neuropathy manifested by numbness and tingling, dementia, or evidence of posterior column disease, should prompt a search for cobalamin deficiency

3. Associated immune disease, including the following:

- Patients, usually young, who have combined variable immune deficiency or selective IgA deficiency
- Patients with autoimmune endocrinopathies, including Hashimoto's thyroiditis, Addison's disease, Graves' disease, and non–insulin-dependent diabetes
- Patients with other autoimmune disease, including vitiligo, myasthenia gravis, and primary ovarian failure

23. When should a patient's serum methylmalonate level be obtained?

It is possible for patients with near normal B_{12} levels to be B_{12} deficient. Additionally, cobalamin levels decrease during pregnancy, yet the patient is not truly B_{12} deficient. Methylmalonate, as a precursor of vitamin B_{12}, is elevated in true vitamin B_{12} deficiency. Thus, in patients with borderline B_{12} levels (usually 200–300 pg/mL), the finding of an elevated methylmalonate level is consistent with a deficient state.

24. How are patients with pernicious anemia treated?

The treatment of patients with pernicious anemia requires 1000 μg of cobalamin administered intramuscular daily for 1 week, with a maximal reticulocytosis seen by the end of the week. Therapy is then given weekly for the first month and then monthly for life. However, less painful therapy is currently available and efficacious. High-dose oral therapy (1–2 mg/day) has been effective; cobalamin is also available for sublingual use or as a nasal spray, with much more erratic absorption. Often, these therapies may be most effective after the initial course of parenteral therapy. Total correction of the hemoglobin should be expected in 2 months.

25. When is measurement of the erythropoietin level helpful?

Because the red cell mass is maintained within well-defined limits through a feedback mechanism regulated by the horomone erythropoietin, levels of the hormone should be appropriate for the level of hematocrit. Low levels of hormone are useful in diagnosing polycythemia vera, in which a high level is consistent with secondary serythrocytosis, and in determining the adequacy of the erythropoietic response to anemia, such as the blunted response in anemia of chronic disease. In the presence of very high levels, such as might be found in marrow failure states or HIV, additional hormone therapy is unlikely to be useful.

26. Which patients are candidates for therapy with erythropoietin?

1. Patients with chronic renal failure who are undergoing dialysis or predialysis
2. Patients with anemia during HIV infection when the erythropoietin level is < 500 IU/mL
3. Patients with malignancy or undergoing treatment for cancer, in whom anemia is severe enough to result in transfusions and is likely to respond to erythropoietin; treatment with erythropoietin may improve the anemia without exposing patients to the potential immunomodulating effect of transfusions
4. Patients who are anemic preoperatively, are scheduled for surgery in which blood conservation is likely to be inadequate, and who resist transfusions on religious grounds
5. Patients enrolled in a preoperative autologous donation program who are anemic at first donation and who are scheduled to undergo surgery (e.g., hip replacement) in which blood loss is expected to be between 1000 and 3000 mL

27. When may anemia be attributable to chronic renal failure?

The anemia of chronic renal failure, which is caused by deficient production of erythropoietin, is not likely to become manifest clinically until the creatinine clearance is < 40 mL/min. There is a rough correlation between creatinine and anemia, although this correlation cannot be extrapolated to the individual patient. With polycystic kidney disease, the erythropoietin level appears to be maintained; patients become anemic much later (if at all) in the natural course of the disease. With progressive renal failure, additional causes of anemia must be considered, especially iron deficiency and volume expansion.

28. What laboratory tests support the diagnosis of hemolysis or increased RBC destruction?

Measures of cellular breakdown of RBCs:

- **Bilirubin:** A slightly elevated bilirubin level may be a clue to underlying RBC destruction in the absence of a hepatic explanation. However, the liver can compensate tremendously for increased bilirubin production. Thus, values > 4 mg/dL are likely to reflect liver disease as well as excessive RBC breakdown.
- **Lactate dehydrogenase (LDH):** Although nonspecific for red cells or hemolysis, the presence of an elevated LDH level is consistent with the diagnosis of hemolysis.

Evidence of free hemoglobin:

- **Low haptoglobin:** This protein, one of the measurable carriers of free hemoglobin, decreases to undetectable levels as it is catabolized when it is bound to free hemoglobin. Thus haptoglobin may not be low in patients who have decreased RBC survival that is localized to the spleen (extravascular). Because haptoglobin may be elevated in inflammatory disease, the absolute value is not helpful clinically. However, an undetectable or very low level is consistent with hemolysis.
- **Free serum hemoglobin:** When overwhelming hemolysis is present, as in a mismatched transfusion reaction, free hemoglobin results in pink serum. Otherwise, hemoglobin is cleared and degraded quite rapidly.
- **Urine hemoglobin:** When haptoglobin is saturated, free hemoglobin dissociates into molecules that pass freely through the glomerulus and thus are detected in the urine when the tubular reabsorption threshold is exceeded. Therefore, urine hemoglobin is also a measure of hemolysis due to excessive RBC breakdown, if other mechanisms cannot clear serum hemoglobin.
- **Urine hemosiderin:** With excessive free serum hemoglobin, free heme pigment may precipitate in the distal tubular cells. Hemoglobin iron in the renal epithelial cell is rapidly stored as hemosiderin or ferritin. As the tubular cell sloughs, hemosiderin and iron can be measured in the urine. Thus, urine hemosiderin is a good measure of chronic intravascular hemolysis. After a single episode of hemolysis, measurement of urine hemosiderin may not show positive results for 2–3 days, but it may then persist for up to 14 days. Thus, it is a useful clue for an earlier event.

29. What classic disease results in extravascular hemolysis?

Autoimmune hemolytic anemia results in shortened RBC survival because of complement or antibody detection on the RBC membrane by the splenic macrophage. Hallmarks of the disease are the spherocyte and the direct Coombs'-positive antibody test in the presence of reticulocytosis. A spleen tip is palpable in 50% of patients. The majority of all other types of hemolytic anemia are is attributable to intravascular causes (including RBC mechanical or fibrinous breakdown in the vascular space) or intrinsic RBC defects.

30. What considerations should be given to optimizing hemoglobin concentration in patients with chronic anemia?

Although patients with chronic anemia appear to tolerate low hemoglobin better than patients with acute anemia, consideration should be given to optimizing oxygen-carrying capacity (by transfusion or erythropoietin) in certain circumstances:

- Patients with underlying symptomatic coronary artery disease
- Patients with poor exercise tolerance who wish to be more physically active (including patients with cancer or chronic inflammatory disease)
- Elderly patients who require surgery and are at risk for poor systemic perfusion that may result in stroke or myocardial infarction, for poor wound healing, and for infection postoperatively. Some evidence suggests that poor surgical outcomes are associated with anemia.

BIBLIOGRAPHY

1. Annibale B, Capurso G, Chistolini A, D'Ambra G: Gastrointestinal causes of refractory iron deficiency anemia in patients without gastrointestinal symptoms. Am J Med 111:439–445, 2001.
2. Beutler E, Lichtman M, Coller B, et al (eds): Williams Hematology, 6th ed. New York, McGraw-Hill, 2001.
3. Bruner AB, Joffe A, Duggan AK, et al: Randomized study of cognitive effects of iron supplementation in non-anemia iron-deficient adolescent girls. Lancet 384:992–996, 1996.
4. Cook JD: Clinical evaluation of iron deficiency. Semin Hematol 19:6–18, 1982.
5. Goodnough LT, Brecher ME, Kanter MH, Aubuchon JP: Transfusion medicine: Part I, II. N Engl J Med 340:438–447, 525–533, 1999.
6. Goodnough LT, Monk TG, Andriole GL: Erythropoietin therapy. N Engl J Med 336:933–938, 1997.

7. Goodnough LT, Skikne B, Brugnara C: Erythropoietin, iron and erythropoiesis. Blood 96:823–833, 2000.
8. Gulati GL, Hyun BH: Blood smear evaluation. Hematol Oncol Clin North Am 8:631–650, 1994.
9. Guyatt GH, Oxman AD, Willan M, et al: Laboratory diagnosis of iron deficiency anemia: An overview. J Gen Intern Med 7:145–153, 1992.
10. Izaks GJ, Westendorp RGJ, Knook DL: The definition of anemia in older persons. JAMA 281:1714–1717, 1999.
11. Jandl JH: Blood: Textbook of Hematology, 2nd ed. Boston, Little, Brown, 1996.
12. Kuzminski AM, Del Giacco EJ, Allen RH, et al: Effective treatment of cobalamin deficiency with oral cobalamin. Blood 92:1191–1198, 1998.
13. Mast AE, Blinder MA, Lu Q, et al: Clinical utility of the reticulocyte hemoglobin content in the diagnosis of iron deficiency. Blood 99:1489–1491, 2002.
14. Mast AE, Binder MA, Gronowski AM, et al: Clinical utility of the soluble transferring receptor and comparison with serum ferritin in several populations. Clin Chem 44:45–51, 1998.
15. Mladenovic J, Roodman D: Normocytic anemia. In Spivak J (ed): Textbook of Hematology. Baltimore, Johns Hopkins Press, 1993, pp 91–100.
16. National Kidney Foundation: K/DOQI clinical practice guidelines for chronic kidney disease: Evaluation, classification, and stratification. Am J Kidney Dis 39(suppl 1): S1–S266, 2002.
17. Osterborg A, Bradberg Y, Molostova V, et al: Randomized, double-blind placebo controlled trial of recombinant erythropoietin, epoietin beta, in hematologic malignancies. J Clin Oncol 20:2486–2494, 2002.
18. Rizzo JD, Lichtin AE, Woolf SH, et al: Use of epoetin in patients with cancer: Evidence-based clinical practice guidelines of the American Society of Clinical Oncology and the American Society of Hematology. Blood 100:2303–2320, 2002.
19. Robinson AR, Mladenovic J: Lack of clinical utility of folate levels in the evaluation of macrocytosis or anemia. Am J Med 110:88–90, 2001.
20. Swain RA, Kaplan B, Montgomery E: Iron deficiency anemia: when is parenteral therapy warranted? Postgrad Med 100:181–193, 1996.
21. Toh BH, Van Driel IR, Gleeson PA: Pernicious anemia. N Engl J Med 227:1441–1448, 1997.
22. Waters JS, O'Brien ME, Ashley S: Management of anemia in patients receiving chemotherapy. J Clin Oncol 20:601–603, 2002.

61. LYMPHADENOPATHY AND SPLENOMEGALY

Jeanette Mladenovic, M.D.

1. Why is it important to know the common drainage patterns of lymph nodes amenable to palpation?

Recognizing common drainage patterns of lymph nodes facilitates assessment of the anatomic location of infectious causes and potential serious pathology.

- Cervical nodes: Head, ears, eyes, nose, and throat (HEENT) area
- Submental and submandibular area: Salivary glands and mouth
- Pre- and postauricular area: Eyes, scalp, ears
- Supraclavicular nodes: Intrathoracic and intra-abdominal areas, ears, nose, and throat
- Axillary nodes: Breast and thorax
- Epitrochlear nodes: Hand and forearm
- Inguinal and femoral nodes: Pelvic area, external genitalia, and lower extremities

2. Which palpable lymph nodes suggest a malignancy?

- Supraclavicular nodes are generally not palpable. When they are enlarged, they suggest thoracic malignancy on the right and thoracic or upper gastrointestinal (GI) malignancy on the left (called a Virchow's node).
- Epitrochlear nodes are always abnormal, either because of infection or lymphoma.

- Enlarged femoral nodes complicating usually shotty inguinal adenopathy should raise suspicion.
- Enlarged periumbilical nodes (Sister Mary Joseph nodes) signify advanced GI malignancy.

3. Which palpable lymph nodes are probably benign?

1. Palpable nodes (1–2 cm) in the anterior cervical area are common under age 12 years and persist with diminishing frequency to age 30 years. In addition, almost all children have palpable axillary and inguinal adenopathy.

2. Mild insignificant bilateral inguinal adenopathy is common throughout life.

3. Isolated posterior cervical lymphadenopathy is usually benign.

4. What is the likely cause of a rapidly progressive fluctuant lymph node in a child?

This presentation is most consistent with an infection caused by staphylococci or streptococci that may occur without an obvious focus. Treatment consists of drainage and administration of appropriate antibiotics.

5. List the most common causes of generalized diffuse lymphadenopathy in the United States.

Infectious, inflammatory, and malignant diseases account for the majority of lymphadenopathy in clinical practice. Rare storage or lymph node diseases and, occasionally, hyperthyroidism also may present as generalized lymphadenopathy. If a patient has recently traveled to or is from an area with endemic parasitic infections, other causes must be considered.

CAUSES OF LYMPHADENOPATHY

Infectious diseases	Infectious mononucleosis, CMV, hepatitis A
	HIV, syphilis, toxoplasmosis
	Coccidiomycosis, histoplasmosis
Inflammatory diseases	Sarcoidosis
	Rheumatoid arthritis, SLE, dermatomyositis
	Serum sickness
	Drug reaction (phenytoin)
Malignant diseases	Non-Hodgkin's lymphoma
	Acute or chronic lymphoid or myeloid leukemias
Nonhematologic malignancies	Germ cell tumors, melanoma, breast cancer

6. What is the classic difference between the presentation of Hodgkin's disease and non-Hodgkin's lymphoma?

Non-Hodgkin's lymphoma spreads and often presents with diffuse lymphadenopathy. Classic Hodgkin's disease has a predictable pattern of spread in contiguous groups; thus, isolated lymphadenopathy in contiguously draining areas is more characteristic of Hodgkin's disease.

7. What finding on peripheral blood smear almost always accompanies the diagnosis of infectious mononucleosis?

Mononucleosis is the most common infectious cause of lymphadenopathy in young people. It is often accompanied by pharyngitis and constitutional symptoms. In > 95% of patients, the peripheral blood smear shows atypical lymphocytes. Atypical lymphocytes or lymphocytosis also may be seen in other conditions, such as cytomegalovirus, hepatitis, lymphoid malignancy (especially chronic lymphocytic leukemia), toxoplasmosis, serum sickness, and phenytoin lymphadenopathy.

8. Which complications of infectious mononucleosis should corticosteroid therapy be considered?

After a confirmed diagnosis of infectious mononucleosis (monospot or Epstein-Barr virus testing), corticosteroids may be indicated for obstructing tonsillar enlargement, autoimmune thrombocytopenia, severe granulocytopenia, or hemolytic anemia. Patients with splenomegaly should limit sports involvement to avoid rupture.

9. Name five common drugs that cause lymphadenophathy.

Phenytoin, allopurinol, carbamazepine, cephalosporins, and atenolol. Additionally, several other less common drugs can cause generalized lymphadenopathy.

10. How frequently is an enlarged lymph node malignant?

In primary care practices, lymphadenopathy is common; however, only approximately 1% of these lymph nodes are malignant.

11. When should a lymph node be biopsied?

Biopsy of a lymph node, in most instances, is a minor outpatient procedure. The timing of biopsy depends on the clinical presentation, age of the patient, and suspicion of the diagnosis. Certainly, systemic symptoms suggesting malignancy should prompt earlier diagnosis. Careful follow-up is essential because infectious lymphadenopathy usually improves or recedes in 14 days. Thus, sampling of the lymph node should be performed:

- When the node is very large (> 2 cm) or has associated skin changes with matting
- When the lymph node has increased in size in an area associated with a high incidence of malignancy
- When an isolated lymph node with no clear site of local infection has not receded in 3–4 weeks or when diffuse lymphadenopathy with no clear cause has not improved in 3–4 weeks

12. When is lymph node fine-needle aspiration (FNA) for cytology most useful?

FNA is helpful to confirm a suspected diagnosis of infection or metastatic malignancy. It is also useful in patients with HIV to determine other causes of adenopathy. However, it does not provide adequate tissue to distinguish architecture or type of lymphoma or to perform cellular or molecular studies that differentiate tumor origin. In lymphoma, biopsy is the procedure of choice in order to optimize diagnosis and time to treatment.

13. What is the significance of a nondiagnostic lymph node biopsy?

Lymph node biopsy provides a diagnosis in more than 50% of adults. Up to 25% of patients with nondiagnostic biopsies develop lymphoma in the following year. Thus, careful follow-up of a patient with a nondiagnostic biopsy is mandatory.

14. Does bilateral hilar lymphadenopathy always require a tissue diagnosis?

Isolated bilateral hilar adenopathy in a patient with characteristics and systemic manifestations of sarcoidosis may be followed. The classic patient is an African-American woman with erythema nodosum. However, asymmetry and additional symptoms should prompt aggressive diagnosis because the differential diagnosis includes lymphoma, lung carcinoma, tuberculosis, and histoplasmosis.

15. How are retroperitoneal lymph nodes evaluated?

Computed tomography (CT) or magnetic resonance imaging delineates the size of retroperitoneal nodes, including paraaortic nodal areas. The lymphangiogram is now rarely used. After lymph nodes are found on a CT scan, CT-directed lymph node biopsy may be undertaken. Another alternative, depending on the available expertise, is sonographically guided percutaneous biopsy of small lymph nodes in the abdomen, retroperitoneum, and pelvis. In one study, 86% (30 of 35 specimens) of lymph nodes of 2.0–2.5 cm were successfully biopsied.

16. What is the significance of massive splenomegaly?

Massive splenomegaly is most consistent with diseases of hematologic origin:

Myeloproliferative diseases
  Myelofibrosis
  Chronic myelogneous leukemia
  End-stage polycythemia vera or essential thrombocythemia
Neoplastic diseases
  Hairy cell leukemia
  Hodgkin's or non-Hodgkin's lymphoma
  Chronic lymphocytic leukemia
  Malignant reticuloendotheliosis

Other less common diseases are usually apparent from other symptoms and signs. Rarely, infiltrative disease (Gaucher's disease), infectious causes (malaria), or inflammatory diseases (sarcoidosis, Felty's syndrome) may present as isolated massive splenomegaly. Massive splenomegaly is seen with thalassemia major, but the majority of other hemoglobinopathies result in lesser splenomegaly.

17. What is the significance of a palpable spleen tip?

A palpable spleen tip usually suggests mild to moderate splenic enlargement (except in children) and may be caused by any of the diseases that cause diffuse lymphadenopathy because the spleen is yet another organ of the lymph system. Thus, systemic acute or chronic infection is the most common cause of palpable splenomegaly. Systemic inflammatory diseases that cause lymphadenopathy also may cause splenomegaly, with or without lymph node enlargement (e.g., rheumatoid arthritis, systemic lupus erythematosus). However, two other categories of diseases should be considered when a spleen tip is palpable:

Congestive diseases: Vascular congestion may be caused by portal vein hypertension, hepatic vein thrombosis, or portal or splenic vein thrombosis.

Hematologic diseases: Hemolytic disease caused by immune, enzyme, or membrane etiologies. Sickle cell disease of the SS variety is not accompanied by splenomegaly.

18. How can one evaluate the size and function of the spleen?

Besides physical examination, splenic size and consistency (cysts, tumors) may be evaluated by technetium scan, CT, or ultrasound, depending on the level of suspicion. Splenic function may be evaluated by viewing the peripheral blood smear. The finding of Howell-Jolly bodies suggests a nonfunctional spleen. A splenic scan with labeled red blood cells also may determine size and function.

19. Which patients manifest hypersplenism?

Hypersplenism consists of mild to moderate pancytopenia; various cell types are affected to varying detectable degrees. Cells are sequestered in the spleen as an exaggeration of the spleen's normal function. Thus, anemia with short survival, thrombocytopenia, and leukopenia constitutes hypersplenism, which usually complicates diseases that cause splenomegaly by congestion or hypertrophy of the phagocytic elements. There is no direct relationship between the level of blood counts and the size of the spleen. Infiltrative diseases (lymphoma, chronic lymphocytic leukemia) usually do not manifest hypersplenism.

20. What is a sentinel node?

A sentinel node is the first node that drains a tumor. For example, in patients with cutaneous melanoma, injection of a radioactive tracer at the site of the primary tumor (before wide excision) delineates the tumor's first draining node. This sentinel node is then removed and examined for metastatic tumor and helps to determine further lymph node dissection, therapy or both.

BIBLIOGRAPHY

1. Brady BS, Coit DG: Sentinel lymph node evaluation in melanoma. Arch Dermatol 133:1014–1020, 1997.
2. Crosby JH: The role of fine-needle aspiration biopsy in the diagnosis and management of palpable masses. J Med Assoc Ga 85:33–36, 1996.

3. Ferrer R: Lymphadenopathy: differential diagnosis and evaluation. Am Fam Physician 58:1313–1320, 1998.
4. Fijten G, Blijham GH: Unexplained lymphadenopathy in family practice: An evaluation of the probability of malignant causes and the effectiveness of the physician's work-up. J Fam Pract 27:373–376, 1988.
5. Fisher AJ, Paulson EK, Sheafor DH, et al: Small lymph nodes of the abdomen, pelvis, and retroperitoneum: Usefulness of sonographically guided biopsy. Radiology 205:185–190, 1996
6. Habermann TM, Steensma DP: Lymphadenopathy. Mayo Clin Proc 75:723–732, 2000.
7. Kelly CS, Kelly RE Jr: Lymphadenopathy in children. Pediatr Clin North Am 45:875–888, 1998.
8. Libman H: Generalized adenopathy: Clinical reviews. J Gen Intern Med 2:48–58, 1987.
9. Pierson FG: Staging of the mediastinum: Role of mediastinoscopy and computed tomography. Chest 103(suppl 4):3465–3485, 1993.
10. Vassilakopoulos TP, Pangalis GA: Application of a prediction rule to select which patients presenting with lymphadenopahy should undergo a lymph node biopsy. Medicine 79:338–347, 2000.

62. BLEEDING AND THROMBOCYTOPENIA

Jeanette Mladenovic, M.D.

1. What history is important in diagnosing a congenital bleeding disorder?

Careful inquiry into prolonged bleeding with minor common surgeries or insignificant trauma is the most helpful element of the history. Specifically, unusual or prolonged bleeding with circumcision, tonsillectomy, or tooth extraction provides strong clues. A history of hemarthrosis also is suggestive. The common congenital bleeding abnormalities of varying severity that present early or late in life include hemophilia A and B, von Willebrand's disease, and congenital platelet disorders. Of equal importance is the family history in patients who may be suspected of having a congenital abnormality. Even mild symptoms may be compatible with inherited disorders.

2. What are the major components of the hemostatic system?

The major components of the hemostatic system are platelets, blood coagulation proteins, and structural support of the vasculature. All components should be investigated in a bleeding patient or a patient with evidence of even a mild bleeding abnormality on physical examination. In acute bleeding, a structural lesion (e.g., postoperative bleeding) is likely when platelets and coagulation parameters are corrected. In a patient complaining of recurrent bruisability, failure to consider problems in vascular support may lead to a missed diagnosis (e.g., amyloidosis, vasculitis).

3. What abnormalities on physical examination suggest a bleeding disorder?

Major findings include petechiae, purpura (confluent petechiae), and ecchymoses. Isolated thrombocytopenia usually results in petechiae. However, petechiae are seen at lower levels of thrombocytopenia when the platelets are young and highly functional than when the defect is caused by poor production or dysfunctional platelets, as in myeloproliferative diseases. Ecchymoses, especially in areas not usually subjected to trauma, suggest abnormalities of the coagulation proteins, platelet dysfunction, or vascular fragility. The presence of mucosal bleeding from gingiva, spontaneous oozing, and fundic hemorrhages must also be determined, because they may have important clinical implications and consequences.

4. Characterize the differences in bleeding patterns when bleeding is caused by thrombocytopenia as opposed to the coagulation or fibrinolytic system.

- Bleeding with thrombocytopenia occurs immediately after trauma, but it is characteristically delayed in the presence of coagulation abnormalities.

- Bleeding with thrombocytopenia tends to be more superficial and profuse after vascular injury, but bleeding caused by coagulation abnormalities is more likely to be deep seated into muscles and joints.

5. What is the significance of "wet purpura"?

Wet purpura is confluent petechiae seen on mucosal surfaces, such as in the oral cavity. This finding, as opposed to petechiae and purpura found elsewhere, should raise the concern that the patient is at risk for life-threatening bleeding. The most serious of these, central nervous system (CNS) bleeding, is the most common cause of death attributable to thrombocytopenia.

6. What tests measure function of the coagulation system?

The prothrombin time (PT) and the activated partial thromboplastin time (aPTT) measure separate components of the coagulation system *in vitro*. A normal PT suggests that factor VII and other vitamin K–dependent factors contributing to the common pathway are functionally adequate. A normal aPTT suggests adequate function of factors VIII, IX, and XI. Prolongation of the PT or aPTT may be caused by inadequate levels of factors or to specific or nonspecific inhibitors.

7. In what circumstances are PT and PTT useful in the initial evaluation of a patient?

PT and PTT are useful in evaluating patients who have the following diseases or history:

Hematologic malignancies	History of bleeding
Hepatobiliary disease	Anticoagulant use
Malnutrition or malabsorption	Systemic lupus erythematosus

8. Are abnormalities of the coagulation system possible in patients with normal PT and PTT?

PT and PTT may be normal in rare patients with mild acquired von Willebrand's disease or abnormalities in factor XIII, alpha-2 plasmin inhibitor, or platelet procoagulant. If a strong history of bleeding (recurrent mucosal bleeding, large muscle hematoma with minimal trauma) is suspected, such disorders are still possible; referral to a hematologist is helpful.

9. List the critical levels of platelets that should direct assessment of bleeding risk.

20,000/mm³: Spontaneous bleeding in the absence of trauma is unusual until platelet counts fall below this level. Spontaneous bleeding is routinely seen with platelets counts of $< 5000/mm^3$.

50,000/mm³: This level is recommended to prevent bleeding after surgery and to maintain hemostasis postoperatively or with trauma.

100,000/mm³: This level, which is compatible with a normal bleeding time, may be required for patients who must undergo major surgery in which hemostasis is paramount (e.g., neurosurgery, cardiac surgery) or who have severe defects in the coagulation system or endogenous platelets before surgery.

10. What is pseudothrombocytopenia?

This is a reported low platelet count caused by platelet agglutination in the test tube that contains the anticoagulant ethylenediamine tetraacetic acid (EDTA). It is fairly common (0.1% of all normal individuals), and is caused by a naturally occuring autoantibody that reacts with the platelets when EDTA uncovers an epitope. Because the platelets are clumped, the white blood cell count is also spuriously elevated. The true count can be determined from the smear and by repeating the platelet count using another anticoagulant (e.g., heparin or citrate). This finding should be recorded in the patient's record.

11. How are platelets evaluated?

Platelets are evaluated by number and function. A low number should be confirmed by viewing the peripheral blood smear and estimating a count of 15,000/mm³ per single platelet viewed on high-power field. The presence of large platelets may help to diagnose immune destruction. Function is evaluated by bleeding time, which also is related to platelet number (100,000 platelets/mm^3 are needed for a normal bleeding time). Evaluation of bleeding time, however, is subject to variability in performance and in correlation with bleeding diathesis (especially preoperative or preprocedure evaluation). It may be most helpful in the positive diagnosis of a platelet defect, such as in von Willebrand's disease, or a myeloproliferative disease with thrombocytosis. In addition, the diagnosis of immune thrombocytopenia is corroborated by a short bleeding time with thrombocytopenia.

12. Should patients be screened preoperatively by a bleeding time?

The bleeding time has not proved to be useful in the routine evaluation of patients who are undergoing major surgery as a predictor of intraoperative or postoperative bleeding. A normal bleeding times does not exclude major hemorrhage, nor does it identify patients who have recently ingested aspirin. The best screening tools remain the medical history and physical examination. In the presence of a bleeding history, evaluation before surgery should include the bleeding time in addition to other tests of coagulation (platelet count, PT, and aPTT initially).

13. List the causes of bleeding in liver disease.

Abnormalities that lead to bleeding in liver disease may be attributable to structural, hemostatic, or therapeutic causes.

Structural causes
> Portal hypertension with varices
> Increased incidence of peptic ulceration and gastritis

Hemostatic causes
> Decreased hepatic synthesis of procoagulant proteins (fibrinogen; prothrombin; factors V, VII, IX, X, and XI)
> Decreased absorption and metabolism of vitamin K
> Decreased clearance of activated coagulation proteins

Therapeutic causes
> Dilution of proteins and platelets from massive transfusions
> Increase in bleeding with therapeutic endoscopy

14. Why are patients with renal failure at risk for increased bleeding?

Chronic uremia is associated with abnormalities in platelet function, which may be improved with dialysis (although the bleeding time does not correct). The bleeding diathesis may be corrected by desmopressin, cryoprecipitate, estrogen, or erythropoietin therapy, depending on which is most appropriate for the patient's clinical needs.

15. What contributes to thrombocytopenia in patients who chronically abuse alcohol?

Direct toxicity of alcohol: After alcohol is discontinued, the platelet count should increase and return to normal within 1 week in most patients.

Hypersplenism caused by portal hypertension: Hypersplenism alone should not lead to a platelet count significantly lower than 50,000–60,000/mm^3.

Folate deficiency: Folate is required for hematopoiesis; thus, folate deficiency may contribute to thrombocytopenia, usually when megaloblastosis and leukopenia are also evident.

16. Do patients with thrombocytopenia attributable to hypersplenism bleed?

Approximately one third or more of the platelet mass is sequestered in an enlarged spleen. Thus, the platelet pool is essentially normal, and is "clinically" available to the patient, if needed. Therefore, in patients with hypersplenism caused by portal hypertension, clinical bleeding is rarely seen in the absence of a structural lesion.

17. What diagnosis is likely in a young child with petechiae?

If the complete blood count demonstrates isolated thrombocytopenia, the likely diagnosis is immune thrombocytopenic purpura. This syndrome follows a viral exanthem or upper respiratory illness, and the majority of patients recover spontaneously, usually in 4–6 weeks. Diagnosis is made by the medical history; by evaluation of the peripheral blood smear, which shows isolated decreased numbers of large platelets; and by bone marrow aspiration, which eliminates an atypical presentation of a more severe hematologic disease as the cause. Transfused platelets are short lived and sensitize the patient; therefore, transfusion should be reserved for patients with severe bleeding. An increased incidence of CNS bleeding is seen with severe thrombocytopenia (< 5000–10,000 platelets/mm^3). If needed, prednisone is the drug of choice for initial therapy.

18. What drugs are the most common offenders in drug-induced thrombocytopenia?

Besides alcohol, the best-documented drugs in common practice that cause thrombocytopenia include thiazide diuretics, heparin, quinidine, and quinine (from tonic water), sulfathiazole, estrogens, and myelosuppressive chemotherapy. Many other drugs are suspect; the exact cause is documented in only 10% of patients with thrombocytopenia. Thus, the best confirmation of drug-induced thrombocytopenia is a prompt increase in platelet count after removal of the drug (in most patients, within 7–10 days). This reaction to a drug should be clearly documented in the patient's chart so that rechallenge does not occur.

19. Which viral infections are associated with thrombocytopenia?

Epstein-Barr virus (EBV), cytomegalovirus, HIV, varicella, mumps, rubella, parvovirus, and post-measle vaccination. In many instances, thrombocytopenia is transient; however, in others (i.e., EBV, HIV) it may be systained, and even life threatening.

20. How is disseminated intravascular coagulation (DIC) diagnosed?

Clinical setting: DIC should be considered in obstetric catastrophes or in severely ill patients with sepsis, hypoperfusion, nonviable tissue, massive cell breakdown, or malignancy.

Laboratory confirmation: Ongoing activation of the clotting system is evidenced by consumption of coagulation factors, platelets, and secondary fibrinolysis (as demonstrated by circulating dimers, a specific manifestation of plasmin cleavage). Thus, thrombocytopenia or prolongation of the PT and aPTT in the presence of a low fibrinogen level confirms DIC in the appropriate setting. Clinical bleeding correlates best with the fibrinogen level; patients with levels < 100 µg/mL are likely to require therapy. The presence of nonspecific fibrin degradation products and schistocytes on peripheral blood smear is confirmatory, but their absence does not rule out the diagnosis. However, marked elevation of D dimers, antigenic fragments released only during plasmin-induced lysis of crosslinked fibrinogen, is a specific marker of DIC. This test provides a reliable laboratory diagnosis of DIC.

21. What is gestational thrombocytopenia?

As a result of automatic platelet counts, asymptomatic thrombocytopenia has been recognized more frequently during normal gestation. The platelet count, normal before pregnancy, decreases in 8% of women during normal gestation. This thrombocytopenia may reach levels as low as 80,000/mm^3 at delivery but is not accompanied by bleeding or obstetric or fetal complications. The platelet count returns to normal after delivery. Gestational thrombocytopenia is *not* accompanied by hypertension, proteinuria, elevated liver enzymes, or progression to lower platelet counts; thus, it should not be confused with preeclampsia or the HELLP syndrome (*h*emolysis, *e*levated *l*iver enzymes, and *l*ow *p*latelet count).

22. What are the complications of platelet transfusions?

Platelet transfusions carry all of the risks of red blood cell (RBC) transfusions, with some additions. Febrile, nonhemolytic reactions are more common with platelets (especially with random donor platelets) than with RBCs. Although the risk of known viral pathogens has been minimized, platelet transfusions carry a higher risk of bacterial infections, frequently with skin saprophytes.

The effectiveness of platelet transfusions is easily decreased in the patient with fever, infection, hypersplenism, DIC, or treatment with amphotericin. Alloimmunization to platelet-specific antigens and human leukocyte antigen (HLA) may occur with regular transfusions. This problem should be suspected when a platelet increment 1 hour after infusion is less than approximately 7500/U (adjusted for body surface area of the patient).

23. When are patients who have used aspirin no longer at risk for bleeding?

Patients who discontinue aspirin for 3 days are likely to have enough newly produced, unaffected platelets to prevent bleeding. The platelets of such patients also may be used in a donor pool. Total replacement of the platelet pool does not occur until 8–16 days.

24. What is the hallmark of the thrombotic-thrombocytopenia purpura (TTP)?

TTP is a spectrum of disease that includes hemolytic uremic syndrome. In the past, the pentad of neurologic abnormalities, renal failure, fever, hemolytic anemia, and thrombocytopenia was thought to describe the clinical entity of TTP. In recent years, it has become clear that this spectrum is broader than previously thought, and it includes variants that range from very mild disease to life-threatening disease. Thus, in a patient with thrombocytopenia, the physician should carefully search for other signs and symptoms that could raise the suspicion of TTP; these include microangiopathic anemia and renal or neurologic complaints or abnormalities of varying severity. Even if mild initially, the patient may present with much more severe disease in future occurrences. This high index of suspicion is important because platelet transfusions may be detrimental and because appropriate therapy has radically changed the mortality rate of patients with this disease.

BIBLIOGRAPHY

1. Bell WR, Kickler TS: Thrombocytopenia in pregnancy. Rheum Dis Clin North Am 23:183–194, 1997.
2. Beutler E, Lichtman M, Coller B, et al (eds): Williams Hematology, 6th ed. New York, McGraw-Hill, 2001.
3. Cines DB, Blanchette VS: Immune thrombocytopenia purpura. N Engl J Med 346:995–1008, 2002.
4. Ebert ME, Berkowitz LR: Hemostasis in renal diseases: Pathophysiology and management. Am J Med 96:168–179, 1994.
5. George JN: Continuous update on drug-induced thrombocytopenia. Available at http://moon.ouhsc.edu/jgeorge.
6. George JN, Raskob GE, Shah SR, et al: Drug-induced thrombocytopenia: A systematic review of published case reports. Ann Intern Med 129:886–890, 1998.
7. Hassouna HI: Laboratory evaluation of hemostatic abnormalities. Hematol Oncol Clin North Am 7:1161–1249, 1993.
8. Hussein MA, Hoeltge GA: Platelet transfusion therapy for medical and surgical patients. Cleve Clin J Med 63:245–250, 1996.
9. Jandl JH: Blood: Textbook of Hematology, 2nd ed. Boston, Little, Brown, 1996.
10. Kitchens CS: Approach to the bleeding patient. Hematol Oncol Clin North Am 6:983–989, 1992.
11. Mammen EF: Coagulated defects in liver disease. Med Clin North Am 78:545–554, 1994.
12. Moake JL: Thrombotic microangiopathies. N Engl J Med 347:589–600, 2002.
13. Parker RI: Etiology and treatment of acquired coagulopathies in the critically ill adult and child. Crit Care Clin 13:591–609, 1997.
14. Peterson P, Hayes TE, Arkin CF, et al: The preoperative bleeding time test lacks clinical benefit. College of American Pathologists and American Society of Clinical Pathologists. Arch Surg 133:134–139, 1998.
15. Rutherford CJ, Frenkel EP: Thrombocytopenia: Issues in diagnosis and therapy. Med Clin North Am 78:555–575, 1994.

63. THROMBOSIS AND ANTICOAGULATION

Jeanette Mladenovic, M.D.

1. What are acceptable indications for chronic anticoagulation therapy?

Chronic anticoagulation may be indicated on a short-term (3–6 months) or long-term (lifelong) basis.

Short-term use
Pulmonary emboli
Proximal deep venous thrombosis (DVT)
New bioprosthetic mitral valves with sinus rhythm
Anterior wall transmural infarction with congestive heart failure

Long-term use (1 year or lifelong)
Cardiac disease
    Prosthetic mechanical valves
    Recurrent (not lone) or persistent atrial fibrillation
    Cardiomyopathy with left ventricular (LV) thrombus or emboli
    Rheumatic valve disease with embolism, atrial fibrillation, or atrium > 5.5 cm
    Recurrent emboli from noninfectious endocarditis or atrial myxoma
Acquired antiphospholipid antibody syndrome with recurrent emboli
Malignancy with recurrent emboli
Inherited disorders of hypercoagulability with recurrent emboli
Systemic emboli from unknown source

2. In what clinical conditions should heparin rather than warfarin be given?

Heparin should be administered in the acute management of thrombosis; for the prevention of thrombosis, especially in operative or hospitalized patients; and in patients in whom sodium warfarin is contraindicated.

Acute management
Venous thrombosis or thromboembolism
Acute thromboembolism
Unstable angina (3–5 days)

Prevention of thromboembolism
Preparation for cardioversion
General abdominal surgery
Orthopedic surgery of the lower extremity
Pregnant patients with history of thrombosis
Patients with known inherited hypercoagulopathy before surgery, pregnancy, and other
    situations at high risk for thrombosis

Warfarin contraindicated
Maintenance of anticoagulation during invasive surgical procedures
Pregnancy, as prevention or treatment for thromboembolism
History of warfarin skin necrosis
Warfarin failure in malignancy

3. What are the advantages of low–molecular-weight heparin (LMWH) compared with unfractionated heparin?

Because of its lower molecular weight and thus modified pharmacology, LMWH offers several advantages compared with unfractionated heparin:

- Longer circulating half-life
- Greater and more predictable bioavailability (less protein and cell binding)

- Less inhibitory effect on platelets and thrombin
- Lower incidence of thrombocytopenia
- Lower incidence of osteoporosis during prolonged administration

These differences translate into less need to monitor therapy and lower costs of care because patients may be managed on an outpatient basis and because they require fewer laboratory tests. Theoretically, heparin-associated bleeding is expected to be lower; however, this advantage has yet to be consistently demonstrated in clinical trials.

4. Can the effect of LMWH be measured?

Yes. A test of anti-Xa activity is required; the effect cannot be measured by the activated partial thromboplastin time (aPTT). However, before initiating therapy with LMWH, the platelet count, prothrombin time (PT), and PTT should be measured initially to determine the patient's underlying coagulation status. More importantly, anti-Xa activity should be assessed in patients with unexpected bleeding complications and in patients with renal failure; in addition, anti-Xa activity perhaps should be evaluated in patients weighing < 50 kg or > 80 kg. Although recommendations for the use of LMWH in pregnancy are evolving, if LMWH is used, anti-Xa activity should be monitored during the late stages of pregnancy.

5. Why must heparin be continued during initiation of warfarin therapy?

A time lag exists between the peak level of warfarin, the PT, and the therapeutic functional anticoagulation. This lag is caused by the time required for normal anticoagulation factors to disappear from plasma after their synthesis has ceased. Thus, the PT is maximally prolonged at 72 hours after warfarin administration, when levels of factor VII and protein C decrease, but the antithrombotic action does not peak until 7 days, when factors IX and X are significantly depressed. For this reason, heparin administration must continue for 3–5 days while warfarin is instituted. Large loading doses of warfarin are not indicated because they cannot hasten the initial action.

6. What is the international normalized ratio (INR)?

Warfarin impairs the synthesis of vitamin K–dependent coagulation factors in the liver. Because the PT reflects three of the four vitamin K–dependent coagulation factors, this test has historically been used to monitor the anticoagulant effect of warfarin. However, standardizing optimal therapeutic regimens has been difficult because the laboratory reagent used in the test (the thromboplastin) varies widely and, thus, produces significant variation in results. The INR compares the patient's PT with a population control adjusted for thromboplastin. Thus, the INR allows physicians to follow published recommendations for anticoagulation. Most indications require an INR of 2–3; the exceptions are patients with mechanical valves, arterial emboli, or recurrent emboli, in whom the INR should be maintained at 3.0–4.5.

7. When should fibrinolytic agents be considered?

Fibrinolytic agents activate plasminogen and are directed at the site of fibrin thrombi to cause dissolution. Currently, streptokinase (in some instances, the more expensive tissue plasminogen activator [TPA]) is indicated in following circumstances: acute coronary occlusion, acute peripheral artery occlusion, and massive pulmonary embolus resulting in hemodynamic compromise. Streptokinase also should be considered in the therapy of axillary vein thromboses and massive iliofemoral vein thromboses. Likewise, thrombolysis with fibrinolytic agents is used locally in thrombosed arteriovenous shunts and arterial or venous cannulas.

8. When is anticoagulation contraindicated?

In general:	Active bleeding
	Recent cerebrovascular hemorrhage
	Severe congenital or acquired defects in hemostasis
	Recent major surgery, especially of the central nervous system or eye
	Malignant hypertension

Heparin:	Thrombocytopenia with thrombosis
Warfarin:	Skin necrosis
	Pregnancy
Fibrinolytic agents:	Immediately after external cardiac massage
	Patients with a predisposition to intracranial bleeding, including those with untreated hypertension, head trauma or intracranial neoplasms
Relative contra-indications:	Severe hepatic or renal disease
	History of falling or unstable gait
	History of gastrointestinal (GI), genitourinary, or intracranial hemorrhage
	Requirement of high-dose salicylate or nonsteroidal therapy
	Poor compliance

9. How do other drugs affect the PT?

Numerous drugs affect warfarin therapy by various mechanisms. Recall of all specific drugs effects is impractical; thus, the *Physicians' Desk Reference* (PDR) or electronic drug reference should be consulted. In addition, the results of drug interactions in individual patients require regular monitoring (every 4–6 weeks when stabilized). However, some general classes of drugs and their effects should be commonly recognized as complicating warfarin therapy.

EFFECT ON WARFARIN THERAPY	DRUGS
Increased PT or INR through enhanced potency	
Reduced warfarin clearance or binding	Disulfiram
	Metronidazole
	Trimethoprim-sulfamethoxazole
	Phenylbutazone
Increased vitamin K turnover	Clofibrate
Decreased PT or INR through decreased potency	
Increased hepatic metabolism	Barbiturates
	Rifampin
Reduced drug absorption	Cholestyramine

10. Which clinical situations are likely to yield increased sensitivity to warfarin or bleeding while a patient is taking warfarin?

Systemic diseases
    Liver disease
    Renal disease
    Hyperthyroidism
Additive to other anticoagulant states
    Vitamin K deficiency
    Thrombocytopenia
    Therapy with heparin
    Therapy with aspirin

11. What is the risk of bleeding with use of warfarin?

Up to 10% of patients taking warfarin for 1 year have bleeding complications that require medical intervention. Fatal complications occur as frequently as 1 in 100 patient years of therapy, despite careful medical management. The highest risk for bleeding is at the initiation of therapy, when patients should be seen frequently. Factors that increase the risk for bleeding are underlying GI, urologic, or neurologic lesions and hypertension. Bleeding usually can be controlled by administration of vitamin K and infusion of fresh frozen plasma.

12. Who is at risk of bleeding from heparin?

Bleeding has not been prevented by frequent monitoring and does not correlate with any clinical assay. Bleeding after surgery or trauma may be severe. Certain patients are at particular risk:

- Patients taking drugs that inhibit platelet function
- Patients with renal failure
- Patients with thrombocytopenia
- Postmenopausal women
- Patients with underlying anatomic lesions

Bleeding usually can be managed by discontinuing heparin therapy. However, if necessary, rapid reversal can be accomplished by the slow administration of protamine sulfate, a specific antidote. Although reversal of LMWH by protamine sulfate may not be as complete when measured by persisting anti-Xa activity, clinical cessation of bleeding suggests its efficacy.

13. Should guaiac positivity and hematuria be attributed to vascular mucosal leak from anticoagulant therapy?

No, not until a structural lesion has been ruled out. Several studies have demonstrated the high incidence of demonstrable anatomic lesions in patients who bleed even while taking therapeutic doses of anticoagulant agents. Thus, the source of bleeding should be carefully evaluated.

14. How should patients with heparin-induced thrombocytopenia (HIT) be managed?

HIT is heralded by a decrease in platelet count to 50% of the original count over 5–15 days after initiation of heparin therapy. Because this is an immunologic reaction in patients who have been previously exposed to heparin, a precipitous decrease in platelet count may be seen earlier. Management consists of immediately discontinuing heparin. If the patient has an underlying thrombotic disorder, potential treatments include hirudin; vena cava interruption; or danaparoid, an LMWH that has proven effective in one randomized clinical trial. However, this or another LMWH should be tested against the patient's serum for the absence of crossreactivity. The immediate administration of warfarin is not recommended because it may exacerbate the HIT procoagulant state. If the patient develops HIT during prophylaxis against DVT, the standard of practice has been to discontinue heparin; however, some data suggest that such patients are also at risk for thrombotic episodes because of the HIT procoagulant state.

15. List 10 critical elements of education for all patients taking warfarin.

1. Take warfarin at the same time each day; never take extra doses to compensate for missed doses.

2. Report excessive bleeding or ecchymoses immediately.

3. Regularly check for blood in your stool and urine.

4. Notify your provider of all changes in medication.

5. Take aspirin or aspirin-containing drugs judiciously, only as recommended by your physician; use acetaminophen with care.

6. Avoid circumstances that lead to injury in normal daily activities.

7. Limit alcohol to a single beer or 1–2 oz of liquor daily.

8. Minimize dietary changes and erratic eating.

9. Women of child-bearing age should notify the provider of any delay in menses (3–4 days) when pregnancy may be possible.

10. Prevent epistaxis and learn techniques for its control.

16. List the indications for antiplatelet treatment.

Cardiovascular disease

Unstable angina
Primary and secondary prevention of myocardial infarction
Postoperatively for coronary bypass grafting or insertion of certain prosthetic valves

Cerebrovascular disease
    Transient ischemic attacks
    Secondary prevention of stroke
Renal disease
    Prevention of clotting in arteriovenous fistulas

17. Which systemic diseases are associated with an increased incidence of thrombosis?
- Chronic congestive heart failure
- Carcinoma, especially mucin-producing types
- Hyperviscosity from plasma proteins, red blood cells, or white blood cells
- Nephrotic syndrome
- Hematologic diseases (myeloproliferative diseases, paroxysmal nocturnal hemoglobinuria, hemoglobinopathies such as sickle cell disease)
- Homocystinuria
- Systemic lupus erythematosus (SLE) with lupus anticoagulant

18. Which physiologic, environmental, or iatrogenic conditions contribute to a hypercoagulable state?

Physiologic conditions	Environmental conditions
Stasis	Smoking
Pregnancy	**Iatrogenic conditions**
Postpartum status	Surgery
Increasing age	Oral contraceptive drugs

19. Who should be screened for an inherited or acquired disorder of hypercoagulability?
The most common inherited disorders that predispose to hypercoagulability are deficiencies of antithrombin III, protein C, and protein S. Proteins C and S are readily assessed either functionally or immunologically. Of patients with recurrent thromboses and a family history of thromboses, about 35% have an identifiable inherited defect in coagulation that appears causative. No known test predicts patients who will thrombose, but the following clinical clues should trigger screening for hypercoagulable states, either inherited or acquired:
- Thromboses at age < 40 years
- Thromboses in unusual sites
- Recurrent thromboses
- Recurrent spontaneous abortions
- Thromboses during pregnancy
- Warfarin necrosis (protein C)
- Resistance to heparin therapy (antithrombin III)

20. Why is the term *lupus anticoagulant* a misnomer?
The term is a misnomer because it refers to a group of antiphospholipid antibodies that prolong the aPTT but lead to thromboses in up to 30% of patients. Thus, it is a true hypercoagulable state associated with SLE but also found in other setttings, such as increased age, drug use (phenothiazines), and postinfection states. In women, it may present as recurrent spontaneous abortions. However, it also may be found in men, in whom the specificity of the antiphospholipid antibody may differ. Asymptomatic individuals do not routinely require treatment. If thrombosis occurs, heparin therapy and monitoring by heparin assay are indicated.

21. Name the known inherited thrombotic disorders. Which is most common?
It is currently estimated that ≤ 50% of patients with recurrent thromboses and 1 in 5 patients who present with initial venous thromboembolism may have an inherited hypercoagulable state. These include the following inherited abnormalities:

Abnormalities of activated coagulation factors
Activated protein C (APC) resistance (factor V Leiden mutation)
Protein S deficiency
Protein C deficiency
Antithrombin III deficiency
Heparin cofactor deficiency
Impaired clot lysis
Dysfibrinogenemia
Plasminogen deficiency
Metabolic defect
Homocysteinemia; homozygous and heterozygous disease
The most common of these to date is factor V Leiden mutation, which has an estimated prevalence of 4–6% in the general population; it is estimated to result in a five- to sixfold increase in thrombotic complications. However, to date, no evidence suggests that screening for this defect before surgery, pregnancy, or use of birth control pills is beneficial.

22. When should testing for APC resistance, protein S or C deficiency, and antithrombin III deficiency be done?
Acute thromboses and therapy with heparin or warfarin may alter levels of proteins C and S. Testing for APC resistance is also sensitive to anticoagulants, liver disease, and antiphospholipid antibodies. Optimally, levels should be measured when the patient is off therapy and asymptomatic. If the patient is on therapy, only a tentative diagnosis may be established if the level is decreased. In addition, because all defects are inherited autosomal dominant traits, confirmation of deficient levels in family members should be pursued. Testing for these deficiencies is best done in the reference laboratory; the results, which may be difficult to interpret, should be reviewed by a hematologist.

23. Should patients with hypercoagulable states be treated with lifelong anticoagulation after the first thrombosis?
No. Common practice is to place patients on chronic warfarin therapy after a second documented episode of thromboses. Patients with low levels of functional proteins and no episodes of thromboses require no treatment.

BIBLIOGRAPHY

1. Antiplatelet Trialists' Collaboration: Collaborative overview of randomized trials of antiplatelet therapy. I: Prevention of death, myocardial infarction, and stroke by prolonged antiplatelet therapy in various categories of patients. Br Med J 308:81–106, 1994.
2. Cook DJ, Guyatt GH, Laupacis A, Sackett DL: Rules of evidence and clinical recommendations on the use of antithrombotic agents. Chest 102(suppl):305–311, 1992.
3. Fihn S, McDonnell M, Martin D, et al, for the Warfarin Optimized Outpatient Follow-up Study Group: Risk factors for complications of chronic anticoagulation. Ann Intern Med 118:511–520, 1993.
4. Harris JM, Abramson N: Evaluation of recurrent thrombosis and hypercoagulability. Am Fam Physician 56:1590–1596, 1997.
5. Hirsh J, Poller L: The international normalized ratio: A guide to understanding and correcting its problems. Arch Intern Med 154:282–288, 1994.
6. Jandl JH: Blood: Textbook of Hematology, 2nd ed. Boston, Little, Brown, 1996.
7. Kelton JH, Warkentin TE: Heparin-induced thrombocytopenia. Postgrad Med 103:169–178, 1998.
8. Koniaris LS, Goldhaber SZ: Anticoagulation in dilated cardiomyopathy. J Am Coll Cardiol 31:745–748, 1998.
9. Meyer BJ, Chesebro JH: Treatment of arterial thromboembolic disease. Curr Opin Hematol 1:336–340, 1994.
10. Orsinelli DA: Current recommendations for the anticoagulation of patients with atrial fibrillation. Prog Cardiovasc Dis 39:1–20, 1996.

11. Petri M: Pathogenesis and treatment of the antiphospholipid antibody syndrome. Med Clin North Am 81:151–177, 1997.
12. Price DT, Ridker PM: Factor V Leiden mutation and the risks for thromboembolic disease: A clinical perspective. Ann Intern Med 127:895–903, 1997.
13. Raschke RA, Reilly BM, Guidry JR, et al: The weight-based heparin dosing nomogram compared with a "standard care" nomogram: A randomized controlled trial. Ann Intern Med 119:874–881, 1993.
14. Raskob GE, Durcia SS: Treatment of venous thromboembolism. Curr Opin Hematol 1:329–335, 1994.
15. Spandorfer JM, Merli GJ: Outpatient anticoagulation issues for the primary care physician. Med Clin North Am 80:475–491, 1996.
16. Thomas DP, Robert HR: Hypercoagulability in venous and arterial thrombosis. Ann Intern Med 126:638–644, 1997.
17. Weitz JI: Low molecular weight heparins. N Engl J Med 337:682–688, 1997.
18. Welch GN, Loscalzo J: Homocysteine and atherothrombosis. N Engl J Med 338:1042–1050, 1998.

64. SICKLE CELL DISEASE AND OTHER HEMOGLOBINOPATHIES

Jeanette Mladenovic, M.D.

1. How do globin abnormalities result in clinical hemoglobinopathies?

Hemoglobin, the major component of red cells, is a tetramer of four globin chains covalently linked to heme and arranged in two polypeptide chains. Each globin subunit is determined by inherited genes: two alpha genes on chromosome 16 and one nonalpha gene (normally beta) on chromosome 11. Thus, the hemoglobin in each cell may be composed of various globin types, depending on quantitative or qualitative defects in genes inherited from each parent. Remembering the genetic possibilities facilitates an understanding of the common clinical diseases. Alpha globin is inherited on four genes (two from each parent on chromosome 11), and the severity of quantitative defects (alpha thalassemias) increases with each missing gene. Because chromosome 16 contains a single gene not only for beta hemoglobin but also for other normal hemoglobins that are present in varying amounts during fetal and adult life, quantitative and qualitative defects commonly involve the beta gene. In addition, combined abnormalities may arise from quantitative or qualitative defects of genes on both chromosomes. The common abnormalities are as follows:

Qualitative defects in the beta gene are structural:

Hemoglobin S, C, E (usually caused by specific mutations)

Quantitative defects in both alpha and beta genes are seen with progressive defects in hemoglobin formation as demonstrated by microcytosis and varying clinical severity:

Alpha thalassemias: usually deletions of one or more genes

Beta thalassemias: quantitative defects in the beta gene

Hemoglobin Production

	ADULT RED CELLS	NEWBORN RED CELLS
Hemoglobin A: $\alpha_2\beta_2$	97%	20%
Hemoglobin A$_2$: $\alpha_2\delta_2$	2.5%	0.5%
Hemoglobin F: α_2, γ_2	< 1.0%	> 80%

2. Which groups in the United States are at risk for carrying a gene related to one of the common hemoglobinopathies?

GENE	ETHNICITY
S gene	1 in 12 African Americans
	Combined with beta thalassemia in people from the Mediterranean countries and Africa
C gene	1 in 50 African Americans
E gene	Southeast Asians, especially from Laos, Thailand, and Cambodia (almost 20% of Laotian and Cambodian refugee children in the United States.)
Beta thalassemia	Americans of African, Italian, and Greek descent
Alpha thalassemia	Americans of African (1 in 9 are affected), Southeast Asian, Chinese, Italian, and Greek descent

3. Why is it important to recognize the populations with high gene frequencies, even though the diseases may be clinically insignificant in patients who are heterozygous carriers?

Affected people may require genetic counseling. Because the genes follow Mendelian inheritance patterns, prevention or early knowledge of the homozygous state (especially sickle cell disease and beta thalassemia major) are possible with prenatal screening.

4. Which defects are lethal *in utero* or early in life?

Three major defects are severe and require serious genetic counseling or early recognition: **Alpha thalassemia** with four deleted genes leads to hydrops fetalis.

Beta thalassemia major (Cooley's anemia), a homozygous variant, leads to severe hemolysis, growth retardation, iron overload, and shortened survival.

Heterozygotes of beta thalassemia and hemoglobin E disease are similar to beta thalassemia major.

5. What abnormality causes sickle hemoglobin?

Because of a structural abnormality in the beta gene, a single amino acid substitution (i.e., valine for glutamic acid) creates an unstable hemoglobin instead of the normal beta hemoglobin. When the unstable hemoglobin deoxygenates, the normal biconcave red blood cell (RBC) becomes sickled, stiff, and sticky.

6. How does the primary care provider screen for hemoglobin?

The usual screen is a solubility test (deoxyhemoglobin S is poorly soluble). If the result is positive, a confirmatory test of hemoglobin electrophoresis should be performed. Sickle cell trait or disease is detected by the amounts of hemoglobin S, A, and F. The usual percentage of hemoglobin F and S should be known for patients with homozygous sickle cell disease because it may be helpful in therapy.

7. Who should be considered for screening and counseling for sickle cell hemoglobin?

All people who are not of Northern European origin should be considered for screening and appropriate counseling before general anesthesia or conception, at diagnosis of pregnancy, and neonatally. Appropriate counseling and screening of partners or family members should be offered if screening results are positive.

8. Should persons with heterozygous sickle cell disease be considered at high risk for insurance or employment purposes?

No. Affected people have normal life expectancy and no clinical illness related to hemoglobin. However, they may be unable to concentrate their urine and occasionally (at low oxygen tension) have asymptomatic splenic or renal infarcts; the latter may result in painless hematuria. They are not required to restrict athletic activity.

9. Describe the four major manifestations of sickle cell disease.

1. **Anemia.** Because of markedly shortened RBC survival, each patient has a characteristically low hematocrit level (usually between 18% and 30%) with a compensatory reticulocytosis. If the reticulocytosis is depressed by infection or folate deficiency, aplastic crises or critical anemia may develop emergently.

2. **Constitutional symptoms.** Growth and development are delayed because the illness presents in early childhood. In addition, patients soon become functionally asplenic; thus, overwhelming sepsis from encapsulated organisms poses a life-threatening risk.

3. **Acute pain crises.** Vasoocclusive phenomena lead to recurrent and unpredictable pain, which presents most frequently in the abdomen, joints, back, and chest. Patients usually are familiar with their own patterns of precipitating events and periodicity. A prior infection is known to precipitate crises. The chest syndrome is treated as both infection and infarction because the differentiation is not possible. Abdominal pain is particularly difficult to manage because it may mimic an acute abdomen. Joint crises may be accompanied by noninflammatory effusions.

4. **End-organ damage.** As patients with sickle cell disease reach adulthood, they experience end-organ damage in essentially all systems because of repeated microvascular occlusions. Most prominently affected are the lungs, heart, kidneys, bones, skin, and eyes. Macrovascular events are particularly apparent in the incidence of cerebral thromboses.

10. How should patients with painful crises be managed?

Patients with acute painful crises should be managed supportively with analgesia and hydration. Oxygen should be administered when low oxygen saturation is present. Infection should be ruled out or treated. Transfusion to decrease the percentage of hemoglobin S or to improve oxygen-carrying capacity should be reserved for severe illness or surgery; it usually is given with consultation of a hematologist.

11. Describe the presentation, pathophysiology, and treatment of acute chest syndrome.

Patients with SS, SC, or sickle-thal may present with this syndrome, which often is heralded by limb pain, minimal or extreme dyspnea, or both. Although a new pulmonary infiltrate may be present, many patients intially have no pulmonary findings on physical examination or chest radiograph, but they do have evidence of hypoxia on pulse oximetry. The disease course may be rapidly progressive, especially in patients older than age 20 years, requiring intubation. Treatment with antibiotics, (including a macrolide), matched transfusions, and even bronchodilators are important therapeutic modalities. The pathophysiology includes fat embolism and infection with any one of a number of community-acquired organisms (especially *Chlamydiae pneumoniae*). Mortality is as high as 9% in adults.

12. What preventive measures should primary care providers institute in the care of patients with sickle cell disease?

- Registration of patients into comprehensive sickle cell programs
- Immunizations: pneumococcal, *Haemophilus influenzae,* and hepatitis
- Prophylaxis: penicillin until puberty, malaria for travel to endemic areas
- Folate supplementation, especially before conception and during pregnancy
- Counseling of patients to avoid alcohol (dehydration) and tobacco (which may precipitate acute chest syndrome)
- Awareness of and monitoring for learning disabilities
- Regular ophthalmologic follow-up care
- Regular foot care and protective shoes
- Prompt treatment of all minor illnesses, especially those that may lead to dehydration
- Consideration of supply of analgesics for early prevention of painful crises

13. When should patients with sickle cell disease seek medical help?

Patients with sickle cell disease should be counseled to seek medical help in the following situations:

- Persistent fever ($> 101°F$)
- Chest pain, shortness of breath, or vomiting
- Prolonged new headache

14. When should primary care providers consider hospitalization for patients with the disease?

Primary care providers should hospitalize patients with sickle cell disease in the following situations:

- Tachypnea or signs of lung involvement
- Neurologic signs
- Abdominal pain with splenic or hepatic enlargement
- Swollen, painful joints
- Uncontrolled painful crises or loin pain
- Congestive heart failure or severe pallor

15. What therapies are available to diminish the effect of sickle hemoglobin on the clinical course of the disease?

Therapies are usually aimed at diminishing the percentage of hemoglobin S, often through monitored hypertransfusion programs for unique indications. Although hypertransfusion may appear to be an easy answer to decreasing the percentage of sickle hemoglobin, its routine use leads to iron overload and isoimmunization. In a national multicenter trial, hydroxyurea has been shown to reduce the frequency and severity of painful crises and the incidence of acute chest syndrome. In addition, bone marrow transplantation offers the potential for cure. Thus, therapy is available under the direction of specialized clinics or a hematologist.

16. Which patients should be considered for hydroxyurea therapy?

In the original randomized controlled trial, patients with sickle cell disease and three or more painful crises per year were given hydroxyurea therapy. This therapy was found to decrease the number of crises and to be cost-effective. In the long run, hydroxyurea could prove to be even more cost-effective if it decreases long-term complications for patients with SS disease.

17. Can sickle cell disease present late in life?

Yes. In some populations, disease severity varies considerably. Thus, hemolytic anemia should raise the possibility of sickle cell disease in a patient who belongs to a susceptible group and has not been screened previously.

18. What are the four major causes of death in patients with sickle cell disease?

Cardiopulmonary failure (including acute chest syndrome, which is now the most common cause of death in adults), renal failure, cerebrovascular events, and infection.

19. Is hemoglobin SS the only genotype associated with the phenotype of sickle cell disease?

No. Two additional disorders may mimic sickle cell disease. Sickle beta thalassemia (one gene for S and one for beta thalassemia) and sickle C (one S and one C gene on each of the two 16 chromosomes) present similarly to sickle cell disease. Sickle beta thalassemia may be seen in people of Mediterranean descent. If no beta chains are made, this condition may be difficult to distinguish from hemoglobin SS disease on electrophoresis. The life expectancy for patients with SC is approximately 2 decades longer (seventh decade) than the life expectancy for patients with homozygous SS disease.

20. What inherited hemoglobin abnormalities commonly result in microcytosis?

Prominent microcytosis is seen in three settings, alpha thalassemia trait, beta thalassemia trait, and hemoglobin E (heterozygous or homozygous). All may demonstrate a low mean cell volume in routine complete blood counts with no detectable anemia. Alpha thalassemia trait, a common asymptomatic finding in African Americans, may have a normal electrophoresis. If so, no further evaluation is usually necessary. A silent carrier of alpha thalassemia with one alpha gene missing has no detectable abnormalities. Electrophoresis in patients with beta thalassemia trait usually shows an increase in A_2 hemoglobin. Patients with hemoglobin E, both homo- and heterozygotes, may have microcytosis without anemia or only mild anemia. This condition may be diagnosed by electrophoresis.

21. What happens to patients with alpha thalassemia in whom three genes are missing?

This defect produces a compensated hemolytic disease, with anemia, reticulocytosis, many target cells, and precipitated beta chains in RBCs (called Heinz bodies).

22. What other hemoglobin abnormalities may cause a congenital hemolytic anemia?

The major defects in children or young adults who present with a relatively compensated hemolytic anemia are of three types: RBC enzyme defects (G6PD deficiency), RBC membrane defects, and other mutant hemoglobins. Many mutants of the beta genes lead to hemolytic anemia and often demonstrate precipitated hemoglobin as Heinz bodies. Whereas these mutants may result in a relatively compensated hemolytic anemia, their structural abnormalities may give rise to hemoglobins that have varying oxygen affinities or that are susceptible to precipitation with oxidant stress by drugs.

23. You are seeing a 34-year-old man with right upper quadrant pain and gallstones. Physical examination reveals, a palpable spleen tip. Additionally, his bilirubin level is elevated to 2.1 mg/dL. What test should help you make a diagnosis?

This patient may very well have hereditary spherocytosis, which it is a fairly common inherited disease (as high as 1 in 5000 individuals). This disease is heterogenous in its expression, with more severe disease presenting in childhood and milder disease remaining fairly assymptomatic. An elevated mean corpuscular hemoglobin concentration supports this diagnosis, which can be made by evaluation of the RBC membrane.

24. Which patients are at risk for gallstones?

All patients with congenital hemolytic anemias have an increased incidence of gallstones. In patients with sickle cell disease, the diagnosis is complicated by abdominal pain associated with sickle crisis and liver abnormalities that may result from repeated hepatic infarcts. Generally, cholecystectomy is recommended in symptomatic patients.

25. How may parvovirus affect patients with hemolytic anemia?

Parvovirus has a particular affinity for the developing RBCs, resulting in a cessation of mature RBC production. Thus, in patients who require high RBC production, as in all cases of hemolytic anemia, there is a precipitous decrease in hemoglobin concentration. Infection with parvovirus is the main cause of aplastic crises in patients with sickle cell anemia but also may cause precipitous anemia in other hemoglobinopathies. It represents a medical emergency in patients with hemolytic anemia. Red cell support and therapy with IgG should be initiated.

BIBLIOGRAPHY

1. Beutler E, Coller BS, Lichtman MA, et al (eds): Williams Hematology, 6th ed. New York, McGraw-Hill, 2000.
2. Bunn HF, Rosse W: Hemolytic anemias and acute blood loss. In Braunwald E, Fauci A, Hauser S, et al (eds): Harrison's Principles of Internal Medicine, 15th ed. New York, McGraw-Hill, 2002, pp 681–691.
3. Bunn HF: Pathogenesis and treatment of sickle cell disease. N Engl J Med 337:762–769, 1997.
4. Dabrow MB, Wilkins JC: Hematologic emergencies: Management of transfusion reactions and crises in sickle cell disease. Postgrad Med 93:183–190, 1993.

5. Davies SC, Oni L: Management of patients with sickle cell disease. Br Med J 315:656–660, 1997.
6. Jandl JH: Blood: Textbook of Hematology, 2nd ed. Boston, Little, Brown, 1996.
7. Kazazian HH: The thalassemia syndromes: Molecular basis and prenatal diagnosis. Semin Hematol 27:209–228, 1990.
8. Koshy M, Dorn L: Continuing care for adult patients with sickle cell disease. Hematol Oncol Clin North Am 10:1265–1273, 1996.
9. Moore RD, Charache S, Terrin ML, et al: Cost-effectiveness of hydroxyurea in sickle cell anemia. Am J Hemtol 64:26–31, 2000.
10. Steingart R: Management of patients with sickle cell disease. Med Clin North Am 76:669–682, 1992.
11. Vichinsky EP, Neumayr LD, Earles AN, et al: Causes and outcomes of the acute chest syndrome in sickle cell disease. National Acute Chest Syndrome Study Group. N Engl J Med 342:1855–1865, 2000.
12. Weatherall DJ: The hereditary anemias. Br Med J 314:492–496, 1997.
13. Weinberger M: Approach to the management of fever and infection in patients with primary bone marrow failure and hemoglobinopathies. Hematol Oncol Clin North Am 7:865–885, 1993.

X. Disorders of the Musculoskeletal System

65. PRINCIPLES OF MUSCULOSKELETAL INJURY AND SPORTS MEDICINE

Richard C. Fisher, M.D.

1. Describe the significant issues in acquiring a history from patients with musculoskeletal injury.

The time course of the injury is most important, particularly to separate acute injuries from chronic, recurrent, and repetitive use mechanisms. Knowing the mechanism of injury in severely traumatized patients often aids in identifying high-risk injury patterns. High-energy injuries, as in automobile or motorcycle accidents, have profound effects on multiple systems in addition to the musculoskeletal system. Low-energy injuries, such as simple falls, have different implications for patient survival and complications. Ask about previous treatment and response to the treatment in nonacute injuries.

2. During the initial evaluation of a severely traumatized patient, what are the priorities to consider?

As with all patients seen on an emergency basis, the ABCs (airway, breathing, and circulation) should take precedence over other examinations. The patient also should be evaluated for chest injuries, abdominal trauma, and head trauma before beginning definitive therapy for musculoskeletal injuries. The most important considerations in the musculoskeletal exam include pelvic fractures, spinal fractures, and long-bone injuries (e.g., femur and tibia). It is also necessary to determine whether any of the fractures are open. Pelvis and open long-bone injuries may entail significant blood loss and be accompanied by significant morbidity and mortality.

3. In evaluating a traumatized extremity, what are the principal tissue priorities to consider?

In order of importance, the six tissues to be considered are the vascular system, neurologic system, skin and underlying soft tissue, muscle–tendon units, joint and ligament complexes, and bone. The ultimate viability of the extremity depends on an intact vascular system, and avascular time is extremely important. Muscle ischemia longer than 6 hours often results in significant damage, which becomes irreversible at 8 hours. Changes in the skin often help to localize problems in an unconscious patient. If the patient has open wounds identify injury to underlying structures including bone, joints, or lacerations to muscle, tendon, vessels and nerves.

4. How may the vascular integrity of the extremity be evaluated?

Major arteries should be palpated, and the temperature and color of the extremity should be evaluated and compared with noninjured extremities, recognizing that extremities often feel cool in patients with shock. Capillary refill can be evaluated in the nail beds. If the pulses are difficult to palpate, the Doppler may be used. In cases of suspected major vascular injury, arteriography is indicated. High-risk injuries include (1) major injuries about the knee (e.g., knee dislocations, proximal tibia or distal femoral fractures), (2) injuries about the elbow (e.g., distal humeral fractures, which may involve the brachial artery), and (3) penetrating injuries in the vicinity of major vessels.

5. Briefly describe the pathophysiology and common causes of compartment syndromes.

The syndrome is caused by an increase in pressure within the muscle fascial compartments in either the upper or lower extremity. When intracompartmental pressure exceeds perfusion pressure, ischemic changes occur. Healthy muscle undergoes ischemic changes when the intracompartmental pressure is 10–20 mmHg below the diastolic pressure.

In trauma, the usual cause is direct damage to the muscle tissue, which causes swelling within the closed compartment. Other causes include arterial damage, burns, acute and chronic overuse syndromes, and drug overdose. Patients with bleeding disorders or those taking anticoagulant medications are at increased risk.

The clinical symptoms of pulselessness, pallor, paralysis, paresthesia, and pain may be obscured in unconscious or sedated patients. Keep a keen index of suspicion in these high-risk patients and use intracompartmental pressure monitoring. Treatment is by immediate surgical compartment release.

6. Describe the neurologic evaluation of an injured extremity.

The extremities should be checked for sensation and motor function with an attempt to cover all major peripheral nerves as well as dermatomes. Testing of the deep tendon reflexes also is helpful. Interruption of the tendon or muscle units may be mistaken at times for neurologic injury. Evaluate with serial exams to determine a change in status, which is an indicator of developing problems or improvement.

7. What are the stages of injury of a nonfunctioning peripheral nerve? Describe the prognosis for each.

1. **Contusion or neurapraxia** temporarily interrupts nerve conduction, but the nerve cell processes remain in continuity. Function usually returns within 6 weeks.

2. **Crush injury or axonotmesis** causes axon death below the injury. The axon must regrow distally from the point of injury before recovery occurs. Regrowth takes place at about 1 mm/day.

3. **Neurotmesis or complete division** of the nerve is associated with a laceration or injury from the sharp ends of a fractured bone. The nerve will not regain function without surgical repair.

8. Why does an open fracture require emergency management?

Exposure of the bone to outside contaminants has a high incidence of both soft tissue infection and osteomyelitis. The incidence of infection increases dramatically with the extent of the contamination of the wound, type of contamination (especially fecal material as in farm-related injuries), and delay in time to definitive debridement. Treat open fractures with tetanus prophylaxis and antibiotics. The patient should be transported to the operating room for thorough debridement and irrigation of the fracture to remove all possible contamination. In addition, the fracture should be properly stabilized. The goal is definitive debridement in < 6 hours from the time of injury.

9. What are the most commonly missed fractures in polytrauma patients?

The most commonly missed fractures involve the odontoid process, C7 vertebral body, scaphoid, radial head, pelvis, femoral neck, tibial plateau, and talus. The incidence of missed fractures is about 10%

10. Describe the initial treatment of a traumatized limb.

If a fracture, dislocation, or severe soft tissue injury is apparent or suspected, immobilize the limb in a temporary splint to prevent further damage and to help control discomfort. The splint should allow for extremity swelling and access for periodic neurologic and vascular examinations. U-shaped coaptation splints work well for most injuries.

11. Name some of the systemic conditions that are contraindications to participation in strenuous athletic activity.

Seizure within the past year; history of retinal detachment; active infection; cardiac conditions, such as cardiomegaly, aortic or mitral stenosis, and uncontrolled hypertension; uncontrolled asthma; and uncontrolled diabetes. Other conditions that should be considered carefully include spondylolisthesis with back pain, blood coagulation disorder, and possibly a solitary functioning kidney.

12. Describe the severity rating for muscle strains.

Muscle strains are graded into three stages, depending on the severity of the injury. **First-degree strains** consist of a mildly pulled muscle. The muscle–tendon unit remains intact. The muscle should be protected from use until painless function returns. **Second-degree strains** from a moderate pull to the muscle result in some tearing of muscle fibers, but continuity of the muscle–tendon unit is maintained. Signs and symptoms include impaired muscle function, moderate amounts of pain with muscle use or stretching, swelling, and ecchymosis. **Third-degree strains** are severely pulled muscles that disrupt the continuity of the muscle–tendon unit. Treatment depends on the site of the injury.

13. Any muscle–tendon unit may be injured by direct laceration. List the six most common sites of indirect third-degree muscle–tendon injuries.

1. Long head of the biceps tendon at the shoulder
2. Quadriceps tendon at its insertion into the patella
3. Patella tendon, which ruptures either from the surface of the patella or in midsubstance
4. Achilles tendon
5. Extensor tendon at the distal interphalangeal (DIP) finger joints
6. Flexor digitorum profundus tendon at the DIP joint

14. What are the stages of ligament injury?

Stage I injuries involve tearing of some of the ligament fibers without disruption of individual or collective fibers.

Stage II injuries involve tearing of multiple ligament fibers without disruption of individual or collective fibers. In both stage I and stage II injuries, the joint remains stable to testing. In more severe stage II injuries, however, tearing of the ligament fibers may involve partial disruption of the ligament complex. The joint may show mild instability but not complete laxity, and the exam is usually painful.

Stage III injuries involve complete disruption of the integrity of the ligament, usually with demonstrable instability. Treatment depends on the joint involved but generally is nonsurgical for stages I and II. Stage III injuries may require surgical repair or reconstruction.

15. Describe some of the basic principles for treating ligamentous injuries.

This area remains controversial, but it seems apparent that ligaments heal better and with greater strength with some type of controlled movement across the joint. Gross instability probably requires either surgical stabilization or brace stabilization during the healing process, but, when possible, early controlled motion gives a better long-term result than immobilization. Joint reinjury before completion of healing leads to prolonged disability and a less satisfactory outcome for the involved joint. Thus, early motion with protection against instability, with either surgery or orthoses, seems to give the best ultimate functional recovery.

16. Why does clipping in American football invoke a 15-yard penalty?

Clipping is a block from the posterolateral side at the level of the knee. The foot is usually planted on the ground, and a valgus force is produced across the knee. Clipping often results in a tear of the medial collateral ligament, anterior cruciate ligament, and medial meniscus. Treatment is surgical, and rehabilitation is often prolonged. Full functional recovery is not guaranteed.

17. Describe the signs and symptoms which make you suspicious of an anterior cruciate ligament tear.

The patient gives a history of a rotational or hyperextension injury to the knee followed by rapid swelling, pain, and, often, an unstable feeling with weight bearing. The physical exam demonstrates a painful, swollen knee with guarded motion. Lachman's test and the anterior drawer test may or may not demonstrate laxity in the acute setting but should become positive as the pain subsides. Radiographs are usually normal but may show a fracture of the rim of the lateral tibial plateau. Magnetic resonance imaging (MRI) examination is a reliable study for the cruciate ligaments and for associate meniscus tears. Women basketball and soccer players have a higher incidence of anterior cruciate tears than their male counterparts.

18. What principles should be followed in ordering radiographs for musculoskeletal injuries?

Generally, plain radiographs are indicated after examination of the patient and determination of the site to be examined; 90–90 radiographs are almost always indicated because deformities may be missed when only one view is taken. In addition, the joint above and the joint below the involved bone should always be included in the exam. Special studies, such as computed tomography (CT) or MRI, are indicated to evaluate certain fractures. Injuries most likely to require special imaging studies involve the calcaneus, tibia plateau region, pelvis, and spine. Occult fractures or stress fractures are often diagnosed earliest with MRI.

19. Under what special circumstances does musculoskeletal trauma lead to extreme blood loss that may be missed by the clinician?

Although blood loss needs to be monitored in all trauma patients, musculoskeletal injuries involving the femur, hip, and pelvis and all open fractures are especially prone to large amounts of blood loss. In closed fractures of the femur or pelvis, the loss may not be apparent, and many units of blood may be sequestered before external signs become obvious.

20. Occasionally, a patient presenting with a history of trauma may actually have a preexisting underlying condition responsible for the acute signs and symptoms. Name the more common conditions that may cause problems.

Underlying problems, such as infection and tumor, are often unmasked by simple and seemingly insignificant injury. Simple contusions may exacerbate symptoms or may cause a pathologic fracture. Acute symptoms from gout may be initiated by trauma and present at a site near or remote from the area of injury. Acute fractures and insufficiency fractures are often the first overt sign of severe osteoporosis. They may occur in older patients and in young patients with abnormalities of bone metabolism, such as estrogen deficiency and osteomalacia. Compartment syndromes follow minor trauma in patients with bleeding disorders.

21. Name the three most common delayed complications after musculoskeletal injury.

Compartment syndrome, fat embolism syndrome, and reflex sympathetic dystrophy (RSD). Compartment syndromes usually occur in the region of a long-bone fracture but may also occur in remote areas with muscle or crush injuries. Symptoms are usually present within the first few hours after injury. Fat embolism syndrome usually presents within 12–72 hours of multiple trauma, long-bone fractures, or burns. Symptoms include confusion, shortness of breath, tachycardia, and petechiae. The partial pressure of oxygen (PO_2) is low. RSD is usually seen late in the course of injury and presents as swelling, redness, and pain out of proportion to the underlying injury.

22. Describe the pathophysiology and presenting of a stress fracture.

Stress fractures are produced by overuse of the extremity with microdamage to the bone accumulating faster than it can be repaired. The symptoms are of gradual onset with a history of an increased activity about 3 weeks before the onset of pain. The symptoms are caused by repetition of the activity. This pattern of injury occurs commonly in runners when they quickly increase their distance or time. Some recent data suggest that patients prone to stress fractures have a decrease in bone density. In elite female athletes, decreased production of estrogen may lead to an increased incidence of stress injuries. Older patients with osteoporosis or osteomalacia may develop stress (insufficiency) fractures with no change in activity as their bone becomes less responsive to their normal stress level.

23. What are the common locations and treatment options for stress fractures?

The location depends on the activity producing the injury. The stress fracture was first described in the second metatarsal in association with prolonged walking. Fractures of the proximal tibia and mid- and proximal femur are common in runners. Fractures of the upper extremities are seen in gymnasts and others involved with prolonged upper extremity activities. Stress fractures associated with osteoporosis and osteomalacia also may be seen in the pelvis, scapula, and ribs. High-risk fractures associated with acute displacement or difficulty healing include tension side fractures in the femoral neck, anterior tibia, medial malleolus, and talus. These often require surgical stabilization. Others are treated with activity modification.

24. Describe the common signs and symptoms of spinal column injury.

The mechanism of injury is important in assessing the potential severity of spinal column and associated injuries. Falls from heights, diving injuries, and motor vehicle accidents are common mechanisms. Pain is usually reported at and below the level of injury, and a careful history should be taken with regard to neurologic symptoms, such as ascending numbness and loss of motor control. The physical exam should include evaluation of cutaneous reflexes, muscle power, muscle tone, deep tendon reflexes, sensation, and anal sphincter tone. Palpate the spine carefully for areas of tenderness and possible deformity. Treat a multiply injured patient as if a spinal column injury were present until history, physical exam, and radiographic studies prove otherwise.

25. What are the two most common areas of injury in the spinal column?

The two most common areas are the mobile parts of the column: the cervical spine and thoracolumbar junction.

26. What is the proper management of patients with suspected cervical spine injuries?

Patients should be immobilized initially in a rigid cervical collar, and anteroposterior and cross-table lateral radiographs should be taken. A careful neurologic examination should be performed and the presence or absence of cervical spine pain or tenderness determined. An unconscious patient should be assumed to have a cervical spine injury. In an awake patient with normal radiographs but spine pain and tenderness, the spine should be immobilized until the patient can perform adequate flexion and extension lateral radiographs. These radiographs evaluate soft tissue or ligamentous injury in the absence of acute fracture.

27. Which two injuries most commonly occur in combination with spinal column injuries?

Fractures of the calcaneus associated with lumbar spine fractures and head injuries associated with cervical spine injuries.

28. Discuss some of the diagnostic factors and treatment principles that apply to repetitive use disorder or cumulative trauma disorder.

This problem can be difficult to deal with in the clinical setting. Some of the important features include a chief complaint that is not clear and in which pain is a principal component. At times major psychosocial issues are involved, including depression and dramatization of symptoms. One should search for signs of stress in either the work or home environment and try to define the drug use history, disability, and duration of the symptoms. Treatment decisions should be made after a careful history, physical, and functional evaluation. Evaluation is often best undertaken by a team of people, including primary care physicians, physical therapists, psychologists, and others trained as case managers. Although it is tempting to think that surgical correction is curative, surgery should be approached with great care in patients with this symptom complex. Some of the musculoskeletal conditions that may seem to be part of this complex include carpal tunnel syndrome, cubital tunnel syndrome, thoracic outlet syndrome, and various types of tendinitis in both the upper and lower extremities.

BIBLIOGRAPHY

1. Beaty JH (ed): Orthopaedic Knowledge Update 6. Rosemont, IL, American Academy of Orthopaedic Surgeons, 1999.
2. Birrer RB (ed): Sports Medicine for the Primary Care Physician, 2nd ed. Boca Raton, FL, CRC Press, 1994.
3. Boden BP, Osbahr DC: High-risk stress fractures: Evaluation and treatment. J Am Acad Orthop Surg 8:344–353, 2000.
4. Fabian TC: Unraveling the fat embolism syndrome. N Engl J Med 329:961–963, 1993.
5. Greene WB (ed): Essentials of Musculoskeletal Care. Rosemont, IL, American Academy of Orthopaedic Surgeons, 2001.
6. Heckman JD, Bucholz RW (eds): Rockwood and Green's Fractures in Adults, 5th ed. Philadelphia, Lippincott Williams & Wilkins, 2001.
7. Millender LH, Conlon M: An approach to work-related disorders of the upper extremity. J Am Acad Orthop Surg 4:134–142, 1996.
8. Teitz CC, Hu SS, Arendt EA: The female athlete: Evaluation and treatment of sports-related problems. J Am Acad Orthop Surg 5:87–96,1997.
9. Whitesides TE Jr, Heckman MM: Acute compartment syndrome: Update on diagnosis and treatment. J Am Acad Orthop Surg 4:209–218, 1996.
10. Woo SLY, Vogrin TM, Abramowitch SD: Healing and repair of ligament injuries in the knee. J Am Acad Orthop Surg 8:364–372, 2000.

66. MONARTICULAR ARTHRITIS

David H. Collier, M.D.

1. List the most common diseases that present with an acutely warm, painful joint (monarticular inflammatory arthritis). Which of these diagnoses is the most critical?

- **Infections:** bacterial, mycobacterial, Lyme disease
- **Crystal-related diseases:** gout (monosodium urate [MSU], pseudogout (calcium pyrophosphate dihydrate [CPPD]), hydroxyapatite deposition disease (basic calcium phosphate [BCP])
- **Trauma:** hemarthrosis, internal derangement
- **Other:** osteoarthritis, avascular necrosis, foreign-body synovitis, coagulopathy, pigmented villonodular synovitis

Joint infection is one of the few rheumatologic emergencies. It must be diagnosed and treated quickly. If left untreated, bacterial infections can cause permanent damage to a joint in as early as 1 week. If treated promptly, they usually resolve without permanent damage. An infectious cause must be excluded in patients with acute monarthritis of uncertain cause.

2. What polyarticular diseases occasionally present with a monarticular arthritis?

Rheumatoid arthritis　　　　　　　Reiter's syndrome
Juvenile rheumatoid arthritis　　　　Psoriatic arthritis
Sarcoid arthritis　　　　　　　　　Enteropathic arthritis (associated with
Viral arthritis　　　　　　　　　　　ulcerative colitis or Crohn's disease)
Ankylosing spondylitis

3. Which conditions may mimic monarthritic conditions?

Inflammation around a joint, such as in a tendon, ligament, or bursa, may mimic a monarthritis. The typical patient with a truly inflamed joint guards the area from movement and will not allow any range of motion testing by the examiner. A patient with periarticular inflammation may allow careful movement of the joint and often localizes pain and tenderness to the area around the joint. Common areas of periarticular inflammation include the rotator cuff of the shoulder, olecranon bursa of the elbow, prepatella bursa of the knee, and greater trochanteric bursa of the hip. An effusion may be present in any of these cases.

4. What key information from the history can narrow the differential diagnosis for a monarthritis?

1. **Which joint is involved.** Gout commonly presents in the first metatarsophalangeal joint. Pseudogout and infections commonly present in the knee. Dactylitis is a common presentation of the spondyloarthropathies.

2. **Rapidity of onset.** Septic and crystal-induced arthritis tend to have a very rapid onset. Autoimmune or collagen vascular diseases tend to have less rapid onset.

3. **History of trauma, coagulopathy, or operations,** which may point to a traumatic cause or hemarthrosis.

4. **Previous attacks** may point to crystals or other inflammatory joint diseases.

5. **Age and sex.** In young patients, think of the spondyloarthropathies and rheumatoid arthritis; in older patients, consider gout and pseudogout. In men, consider gout, spondyloarthropathies, and hemochromatosis; in women, think of rheumatoid arthritis and systemic lupus erythematosus (SLE).

6. **History of intravenous (IV) drug use or recent corticosteroid use** may point to an infection or osteonecrosis of the bone.

5. What is the single most important test to determine the cause of an acute monarticular arthritis?

A sample of the synovial fluid aspirated from the inflamed joint.

6. Explain the helpful information that can be obtained from the evaluation of joint fluid.

Although several tests are available to analyze joint fluid, examination of the fluid for white and red blood cell counts with differentials, assessment of crystals, and microbiologic cultures for infectious organisms are the most useful. White blood cell counts > 2000 cells/mm^3 are consistent with inflammation; the highest counts are seen with septic joints, although crystals and pseudosepsis in rheumatoid arthritis or the spondyloarthropathies may give very high counts. A Gram stain, even in the presence of crystals, should be done; if the results are negative, however, a negative culture result is required to exclude suspected diagnosis of septic arthritis. A noninflammatory arthritis is suggested by the finding of < 2000 cells/mm^3.

Examination of the fluid for crystals requires a rose-quartz filter and a polarizing microscope. Gout is confirmed by the presence of negatively birefringent, needle-shaped crystals, which appear yellow with the slow wave of the polarizer parallel to the crystals. Pseudogout is suggested by small, rhomboid positively birefringent crystals, which appear blue with the slow wave of the polarizer parallel to the crystals.

7. Does an overlying cellulitis preclude aspiration through the apparently infected area?

No. A diagnosis of septic arthritis must be pursued, if suspected. However, before the aspiration, systemic antibiotics should be given for the cellulitis. Hemarthrosis caused by a coagulopathy, either congenital or acquired, is a relative contraindication to arthrocentesis. If a septic joint is suspected in this case, try to reverse the coagulopathy before arthrocentesis.

8. What radiographic findings are helpful in the differential diagnosis of arthritis?

Although frequently normal, radiographs may reveal a fracture or osteonecrosis of the bone. Soft-tissue swelling, periarticular osteopenia, and joint space loss followed by erosions at the site of the capsular insertion into the bone are characteristic of inflammatory arthritides. Crystal-induced arthritis may show dramatic erosions or calcified cartilage (pseudogout) with intact cartilage space. In contrast, osteoarthritis demonstrates cartilage loss in stress areas, with sclerosis along the joint line and osteophyte formation. The contralateral joint radiograph may serve as basis for comparison.

9. List other diagnostic studies that are useful in the initial evaluation of monarthritic conditions.

1. **Complete blood count.** Leukocytosis may be seen in bacterial infections of the joint.

2. **Cultures of blood, urine, or a suspected site of infection** are useful when a septic joint is considered because most joints become septic as a result of hematogenous spread.

3. **Serum prothrombin and partial thromboplastin times** when a coagulopathy or hemarthrosis is considered.

4. **Erythrocyte sedimentation rate** is nonspecific but usually elevated in inflammatory processes.

5. **Serum uric acid level** is sometimes helpful in gout. However, a normal serum uric acid level does not exclude gout, nor does a high uric acid level confirm a diagnosis of gout.

6. **Antinuclear antibodies and rheumatoid factor** are occasionally helpful if early SLE or rheumatoid arthritis is suspected. Antinuclear antibodies are frequently positive in the pauciarticular form of juvenile rheumatoid arthritis and indicate which patients should be followed for iritis. However, these test results can be positive in a variety of diseases, including chronic infections, liver disease, and malignancies and in elderly patients.

10. What are the most likely causes of an acute monarthritis in an elderly person hospitalized for a medical or surgical problem?

The most likely causes are gout, pseudogout, and infection.

11. List additional factors that may precipitate an attack of gout.

1. Drugs that cause a change in uric acid level. Common examples can be remembered by the mnemonic **CAN'T LEAP:**

Cyclosporine	**L**asix (furosemide)
Alcohol	**E**thambutol
Nicotinic acid (niacin)	**A**spirin (low dose)
Thiazides	**P**yrazinamide

2. Exercise, weight reduction, hyperalimentation, and fluid shifts
3. Trauma, hemorrhage, infection
4. Dietary excess of purines
5. Radiation therapy and chemotherapy for malignancies

12. Which joints are most commonly involved in gout?

The first metatarsophalangeal (MTP) joint is involved in > 50% of initial attacks and over time is involved in > 85% of patients (this condition is termed *podagra*). After the MTP, the joints most frequently involved are the joints of the foot, instep, ankles, and heel, followed by the knees, wrists, fingers, and elbows. Gout in elderly individuals frequently presents as polyarticular inflammation in the fingers and wrists.

13. Does crystal deposition only occur in joints?

No. Deposition of MSU, CPPD, and BCP in periarticular tissue may present as acute attacks of tendinitis or bursitis.

14. Should a fluid-filled bursa be aspirated?

A fluid-filled bursa, especially one that appears inflamed, should be approached in a manner similar to acute monarthritis. Infections, crystalline-induced arthritis, and traumatic causes need to be excluded. Thus, aspiration of fluid for Gram stain, culture, and crystal analysis is indicated in the first episode of bursitis. If infection is clinically suspected, intravenous antibiotics should be administered for 2–4 days, followed by 10–14 days of oral antibiotics covering *Staphylococcus aureus* or streptococci and daily aspiration of the bursa until little fluid is obtained or the white blood cell count is low. If sterility of the synovial fluid is assured, bursitis may be treated with aspiration, compression dressing and extensor pads, nonsteroidal anti-inflammatory drugs (NSAIDs), or steroid injection, which shortens the course of the disease.

15. How should gout be treated acutely?

Therapy of gout is effective if begun early in the attack. Gout responds well to NSAIDs. Indomethacin is commonly used but should be avoided in patients with congestive heart failure, cirrhosis, renal disease, or a history of gastrointestinal (GI) bleeding. The selective cyclooxygenase type II (COX-2) inhibitors, such as celecoxib, rofecoxib, valdecoxib, and in the future, etoricoxib, parecoxib, and lumiracoxib, cause fewer ulcers and stomach upset and are commonly used to treat acute attacks of gout. Colchicine, the traditional specific therapeutic intervention, is helpful when the diagnosis is uncertain; however, the frequency of GI side effects usually makes it a less popular alternative. Intravenous colchicine must be used carefully because it has a highly sclerosing effect on veins. Oral colchicine should not be given for 1 week after intravenous colchicine. Oral or intramuscular adrenocorticosteroids are used when NSAIDs and colchicine are contraindicated or in cases resistant to both therapies. If none of these drugs can be used, intraarticular steroids may be considered.

16. Why should the level of uric acid not be treated during an attack of gout? What is the treatment for symptomatic hyperuricemia?

An acute attack may be prolonged or precipitated when the level of uric acid is treated. Thus, it is wise to wait 4 weeks or more before instituting therapy to lower the level of uric acid. Treatment is begun after it is determined whether the patient is an overproducer or underexcretor of uric acid. Underexcretors are the most common type. Probenecid is a cost-effective drug to treat underexcretors (in the absence of renal disease or tophi); allopurinol treats both underexcretion and overproduction but may cause exfoliative dermatitis. Sulfinpyrazone is also used for underexcretors. New treatments for hyperuricemia, including uricase (which metabolizes uric acid), oxypurinol (a safer and effective metabolite of allopurinol), and other xanthine oxidase inhibitors, maybe available soon. Starting an agent that lowers uric acid levels may precipitate an attack of gout. It is wise to prevent these acute gouty attacks by using concomitant colchicine or NSAIDs for 6 months to 1 year.

17. What are the indications for chronic treatment of symptomatic hyperuricemia?

Therapy is usually lifelong. Indications for therapy with antihyperuricemic drugs include:
- Three or more attacks of gout within 2 years
- Renal stones (urate or calcium)
- Tophi
- Chronic gouty arthritis with bony erosions
- Asymptomatic hyperuricemia with serum uric acid > 12 mg/dL or 24-hour urinary excretion > 1100 mg

18. What is pseudogout? How does it present?

Pseudogout is an acute arthritis related to the release of CPPD crystals into the joint. It may mimic a gouty attack, although it tends to be less painful and takes longer to reach peak intensity than gout. It usually affects one joint but may be polyarticular. The most frequently involved joints are large joints, the knee being the most common (this condition is termed *gonagra*). If left untreated, the acute attack usually resolves within 1 month; the patient is asymptomatic between attacks.

19. What is the spectrum of CPPD deposition disease?

Acute synovitis caused by CPPD crystals is not the only presentation of CPPD deposition disease. This disorder may present in a polyarticular fashion, mimicking rheumatoid arthritis; it may complicate osteoarthritis or appear like an atypical osteoarthritis; or it may be noted as calcified hyaline and fibrocartilage on radiographs in asymptomatic patients. Rarely, it may behave as a pseudoneuropathic or pseudo-Charcot joint. These clinical presentations frequently overlap. CPPD deposition increases in incidence with age. Acute attacks are precipitated by the same physical factors that precipitate gouty attacks.

20. How is pseudogout treated?

Therapy for pseudogout is symptomatic and based on NSAIDs. Colchicine also leads to improvement and may be given prophylactically for frequent recurrence. Joint aspiration may provide symptomatic relief, and glucocorticoid injection is an option, although it should be used with care. There is no therapy to prevent crystalline deposition.

21. Which joints are most likely to become bacterially infected?

Usually bacteria are hematogenously spread from a remote focus. Organisms resist serum and reticuloendothelial defenses and colonize synovial tissue. This resistance accounts for the increased likelihood of infection in a damaged joint or impaired host and in joints with the greatest amount of synovium. Therefore, the most commonly affected joints are the knee, hip, shoulder, ankle, wrist, and elbow. The most common joints affected in intravenous drug abusers include the vertebral column, sacroiliac joint, sternoclavicular joint, knee, and ankle, often on the side used for drug injection. Such patients usually have staphylococcal infections, but atypical infections are noted in many case reports.

22. What organisms are commonly responsible for acute pyogenic arthritis in adults?

ORGANISM	INCIDENCE (%)
Neisseria gonorrhoeae	50
Staphylococcus aureus	35
Streptococcus pyogens	10
Gram-negative bacilli	5
Mycobacteria, fungi	< 1

Suspicion or diagnosis of septic arthritis requires intravenous antibiotic therapy.

23. How does the presentation of gonococcal arthritis differ from nongonococcal arthritis?

Gonococcal arthritis often begins as a migratory polyarticular disorder that progresses to a monarticular joint problem. It often is accompanied by two extra-articular manifestations:
- Tenosynovitis, usually in the dorsum of the hands, feet, wrists, and Achilles tendons
- A rash that can be tender vesicopustular lesions on a erythematous base or hemorrhagic papules

24. What is the definition of chronic monarticular arthritis?

The usual definition is persistence of symptoms in a single joint for longer than 6 weeks. The most likely diagnosis shifts from crystals and bacterial infection to more indolent diseases, such as spondyloarthropathies, mycobacterial or fungal septic arthritis, avascular necrosis, and internal derangement.

25. List the diseases most likely to cause chronic monarticular arthritis.

Inflammatory	Noninflammatory
Spondyloarthropathies	Osteoarthritis
Mycobacterial infection	Avascular necrosis of bone
Fungal arthritis	Internal derangement
Lyme arthritis	Synovial chondromatosis
Sarcoid arthritis	Pigmented villonodular synovitis
Unusual presentation of rheumatoid arthritis or SLE	Synovioma
Foreign-body synovitis	

26. What other tests should be considered for a chronic monarthritis?
- Mycobacterial and fungal cultures
- Radiograph of the sacroiliac joint to look for spondyloarthropathy
- Chest radiograph to look for evidence of sarcoid and possibly evidence of mycobacteria. However, < 50% of chest radiographs are abnormal in patients with mycobacterial arthritis.
- Tuberculin skin test to document exposure to mycobacteria
- Serologic tests for Lyme disease, rheumatoid factor, and antinuclear antibody

BIBLIOGRAPHY

1. Baker DG, Shumacher HR: Acute monoarthritis. N Engl J Med 329:1013–1020, 1992.
2. Calin A, Taurog JD (eds): The Spondylarthritides. New York, Oxford University Press, 1998.
3. Carias K, Panush RS: Acute arthritis. Bull Rheum Dis 43:1–4, 1994.
4. El-Gabalawy HS, Duray P, Goldbach-Mansky R: Evaluating patients with arthritis of recent onset. JAMA 284:2368–2373, 2000.
5. Espinoza L, Goldenberg DL, Arnett FC, Alarcon GS (eds): Infections in Rheumatic Diseases: A Comprehensive Review of Microbial Relations to Rheumatic Disorders. Orlando, FL, Grune & Stratton, 1988.
6. Goldenberg DL, Reed JI: Bacterial arthritis. N Engl J Med 312:764–771, 1985.
7. Ho G, DeNuccio M: Gout and pseudo-gout in hospitalized patients. Arch Intern Med 153:2787–2790, 1993.
8. Klippel JH, Dieppe PA (eds): Practical Rheumatology. London, Mosby-Wolfe, 1995.
9. Mankin HJ: Nontraumatic necrosis of the bone (osteonecrosis). N Engl J Med 326:1473–1479, 1992.
10. McCarty DJ: Crystals and arthritis. Dis Month 40:253–299, 1994.
11. Sack K: Monoarthritis: Differential diagnosis. Am J Med 102:30S-34S, 1997.
12. Schumacher HR: Crystal-induced arthritis: An overview. Am J Med 100(suppl 2A):46S-52S, 1996.
13. Shmerling RH: Synovial fluid analysis: A critical reappraisal. Rheum Dis Clin North Am 20:503–512, 1994.
14. Shoen RP, Moskowitz RW, Goldberg VM: Soft Tissue Rheumatic Pain: Recognition, Management, and Prevention, 3rd ed. Baltimore, Williams & Wilkins, 1996.

67. POLYARTICULAR ARTHRITIS

David H. Collier, M.D.

1. List the most common diseases that present with acute polyarthritis.

Inflammatory arthritis
Rheumatoid arthritis (RA)
Systemic lupus erythematosus (SLE)
Psoriatic arthritis
Reiter's syndrome
Sarcoid arthritis
Polyarticular gout
Juvenile rheumatoid arthritis (JRA)
Hypertrophic pulmonary osteoarthropathy

Infections
Neisseria gonorrhoeae
Bacterial endocarditis
Lyme disease
Meningococcal
Viral (e.g., hepatitis B and C, parvovirus, HIV, rubella)
Acute rheumatic fever

2. List the most common diseases that present as chronic (persisting > 6 weeks) polyarthritis.

Inflammatory
RA
SLE
Psoriatic arthritis
Reiter's syndrome
Polyarticular gout
Pseudogout
Enteropathic arthritis
Sarcoid arthritis
Polymyalgia rheumatica
Polymyositis
Mixed connective tissue disease (MCTD)

Noninflammatory
Osteoarthritis
Hypermobile joint syndrome
Hemochromatosis
Paget's disease
Polyarticular gout
Calcium pyrophosphate deposition disease

3. Describe how age, gender, and family history can be useful in the differential diagnosis of polyarticular disease.

Some types of arthritis are more common in certain age groups and gender.
• **Young:** RA, spondyloarthropathies, SLE
• **Old:** gout, pseudogout, polymyalgia rheumatica
• **Male:** gout, ankylosing spondylitis, Reiter's syndrome, hemochromatosis
• **Female:** RA, SLE
Types of arthritis that run in families include RA, SLE, spondyloarthropathies, gout, and osteoarthritis (hereditary generalized osteoarthritis and hereditary Heberden and Bouchard nodes).

4. How may the temporal pattern of joint involvement in polyarthritis be helpful in the differential diagnosis?

Polyarthritic diseases present in three types of temporal patterns. The characteristic arthritides associated with these patterns are as follows:

Migratory pattern. Symptoms and signs appear in joints and then remit and go to other joints. Examples are gonococcal arthritis, rheumatic fever, and early Lyme disease.

Additive pattern. Symptoms and signs appear in some joints and remain as other joints become involved. This pattern is seen in patients with RA, SLE, psoriatic arthritis, Reiter's syndrome, and MCTD.

Intermittent pattern. This pattern presents as an acute polyarticular attack with a complete remission, followed by a recurrent bout of a polyarticular attack. Examples of this pattern are gout, pseudogout, sarcoid arthritis, and sometimes RA, psoriatic arthritis, and Reiter's syndrome.

5. Name the two most common causes of chronic polyarthritis.
Osteoarthritis and RA.

6. How do the history and physical examination help to determine whether complaints of polyarticular arthritis are more likely caused by rheumatoid arthritis or osteoarthritis?

	RHEUMATOID ARTHRITIS	OSTEOARTHRITIS
History		
Morning stiffness	Usually > 1 hr	Usually < ½ hr
Movement	Improves stiffness	Increases pain
Systemic symptoms	Common	Uncommon
Physical examination		
Inflammation	Warm, occasionally red	Rare
Swelling	Invariable	Variable
Symmetry	Characteristic	Variable
Joints	Distal small joints	Variable
Hands and feet	PIP joint, MCP joint	DIP joint, first CMC joint, first MTP joint

7. Clinical osteoarthritis can be placed into six categories. Name them.
    1. **Primary generalized osteoarthritis.** Inheritance is autosomal dominant in women and recessive in men. Commonly affected joints are proximal interphalangeal, (PIP) distal interphalangeal (DIP), first carpometarcarpal (CMC), knees, and spine.
    2. **Inflammatory or erosive small-joint osteoarthritis.** Found primarily in postmenopausal women and in some cases familial; this category of disease involves the DIP and PIP joints. The patient usually has a negative rheumatoid factor, normal sedimentation rate, and no systemic symptoms.
    3. **Isolated nodule osteoarthritis** usually begins after age 45 years and is inherited. The patient has Heberden nodes over the DIPs and Bouchard nodes over the PIPs.
    4. **Unifocal large joint osteoarthritis** usually affects the hip or knee. Congenital hip problems are notable.
    5. **Multifocal large joint osteoarthritis** usually affects both hips or knees.
    6. **Unifocal small joint osteoarthritis** commonly affects the first CMC or first metacarpophalangeal (MTP) (bunion).

8. How is rheumatoid arthritis (RA) diagnosed?
    RA is diagnosed by a constellation of clinical and laboratory abnormalities, often appearing over a 1-year period. Criteria developed by the American College of Rheumatology have a high sensitivity (90–95%) and specificity (89%) in establishing the diagnosis but cannot be used to exclude early disease. These criteria were developed mainly for studies on patients with RA. Four of the seven following criteria should be observed by a physician for 6 weeks:
    1. Morning stiffness of more than 1 hour's duration
    2. Polyarticular arthritis (simultaneous involvement of three or more joint areas)
    3. Arthritis of the hands or wrist
    4. Simultaneous symmetric arthritis
    5. Rheumatoid nodules
    6. Positive rheumatoid factor
    7. Typical radiographic changes of rheumatoid arthritis in the hands adjacent to affected joints

9. Is RA a disease only of joints?

No. The spectrum of RA ranges from mild, seronegative disease to high titers of rheumatoid factor accompanied by vasculitis. Patients with RA may have rheumatoid nodules, small and medium vessel vasculitis involving the skin and peripheral nerves, pleuropericardial or pleuropulmonary disease, eye disease (episcleritis, scleritis), and Felty's syndrome. About one third of patients have associated secondary Sjögren's syndrome or sicca syndrome with dry eyes and dry mouth. Carpal tunnel syndrome is common.

10. What other diseases in addition to rheumatoid arthritis may include subcutaneous nodules?

SLE	Rheumatic fever
Tophaceous gout	Vasculitis
Erythema nodosum	Panniculitis
Scleroderma with calcinosis	Sarcoid
JRA	Type II hyperlipoproteinemia

11. What is the standard therapeutic approach to patients with RA?

1. Education by trained professionals.

2. Occupational and physical medicine to instruct patient about joint protection, assistive devices, range of motion (ROM) exercises, and use of heat and cold.

3. First-line pharmacologic therapy for control of pain and inflammation is usually nonsteroidal antiinflammatory drugs (NSAIDs), either traditional NSAIDs or the newer cyclooxygenase-2 (COX-2) inhibitors, prescribed at optimal doses as tolerated. In the past, if the disease was not adequately controlled, a second-line agent or disease-modifying antirheumatic drug (DMARD) was started. With the realization that 70% of RA patients have radiographic damage in their joints within 2 years, a more aggressive approach is used. A DMARD is started very early after the diagnosis of RA.

4. The main second-line agents initiated early are methotrexate, hydroxychloroquine, sulfasalazine (alone or in combination with each other), leflunomide, and azathioprine. Oral or injectable gold and penicillamine were standard treatments in the past but are rarely used today. Other nonbiologic agents used include cyclosporine, mycophenolate mofetil, cyclophosphamide, and minocycline. The dramatic change in therapy is the use of biologic agents. These include antibodies to tumor necrosis factor-alpha (TNF-alpha) (infliximab and adalimumab), receptors to TNF-alpha (etanercept), and a cloned natural inhibitor of interleukin-1 (anakinra). The new biologic agents can be used alone or in combination with other DMARDs. The biologic agents usually control symptoms rapidly and can stop joint space loss and erosions. They are increasingly being used in early disease as a way of preventing joint destruction. Low doses of prednisone are used as a bridge to control symptoms until the second-line agents take effect.

12. What is the characteristic difference between the arthritis in RA and SLE?

Both are a polyarticular symmetric inflammatory arthritis that most commonly affects the hands (PIPs, MCPs, wrists) and feet. SLE, however, is nonerosive and has reducible deformities. Alignment abnormalities, swelling, pain, and even subcutaneous nodules may be seen in both diseases.

13. What is the "gel" phenomenon?

The gel phenomenon refers to the complaint of stiffening with inactivity and is characteristic of systemic arthritides. Typically, it develops with prolonged sitting or is manifest as morning stiffness that requires loosening with a hot shower or activity. Quantitating the morning stiffness may be helpful in gauging the severity of the disease and its response to therapy.

14. Describe the four major characteristics of the spondyloarthropathies.

1. Seronegative arthritis (absence of rheumatoid factor and nodules)

2. Asymmetric involvement of peripheral joints (often in the lower extremity), usually accompanied by sacroiliitis (whether symptomatic or evident only on radiographs) and often by spondylitis involving the posterior intervertebral apophyseal joints

3. Involvement of synchondroses (cartilaginous junction between bones), specifically in the vertebral bodies and discs, pubic symphysis, and manubriosternal joints

4. Enthesopathies or inflammation at insertions of ligaments, tendons, and fibrous structures into the bone

15. How are the spondyloarthropathies characterized?

Spondyloarthropathies are characterized by the level of involvement of the sacroiliac joint:

Bilateral sacroiliitis	**Unilateral sacroiliitis**
Ankylosing spondylitis	Reiter's disease
Enteropathic arthropathies caused by ulcerative colitis or Crohn's disease	Psoriatic arthropathy

Other diseases, such as Whipple's disease and Behçet's syndrome, may present with sacroiliitis but are not spondyloarthropathies.

16. What five questions about back pain may distinguish an inflammatory cause, as seen with a spondyloarthropathy, from a mechanical one?

1. *Did the back pain begin before age 40 years?* Most mechanical back problems start after age 40, but most spondyloarthropathies are symptomatic before age 40 years.

2. *Was the onset of pain insidious?* The pain of ankylosing spondylitis typically has a slow, vague onset, whereas most mechanical back problems start suddenly.

3. *Has the pain persisted for over 3 months?* More than 80% of acute back injuries improve after 3 months, whereas pain of the spondyloarthropathies is slowly progressive.

4. *Is the pain worse in the morning and associated with morning stiffness?* A major complaint of most patients with inflammatory problems is severe back stiffness and pain in the morning, which lasts more than 1 hour. Mechanical back problems typically improve after a night's rest.

5. *Does the pain improve with exercise?* Moving the back exacerbates pain caused by a mechanical problem, whereas a patient with ankylosing spondylitis may exercise each morning to feel more comfortable and to carry out daily activities.

17. What physical maneuvers may point to a diagnosis of spondyloarthropathies?

1. **Measurement of spinal ROM.** Mark two points on the back, one at the base of the low back in the L5–S1 area and one 10 cm above this mark. The patient is asked to bend over in an attempt to touch the toes. A normal change between the two marks is 5 cm, or a total ROM of 15 cm. A smaller change suggests restricted ROM of the lower spine.

2. **Palpation of the sacroiliac joints:** Pressure on the pelvis while the patient lies on the side or back may elicit pain over the sacroiliac joint. Pain in the sacroiliac joint may be brought out by Gaenslen's maneuver, in which the patient lies on the side, flexes the ipsilateral hip (knee to chest), and then hyperextends the contralateral hip.

18. What five organ systems may be involved in patients with spondyloarthropathies?

1. **Eyes:** iritis, uveitis, or conjunctivitis
2. **Skin:** psoriasis, keratoderma blenorrhagicum (similar to psoriasis)
3. **Cardiovascular system:** aortitis, conduction defects
4. **Pulmonary system:** apical pulmonary fibrosis
5. **Gastrointestinal tract:** diarrhea, ulcerations of the small and large intestines

19. What constitutes Reiter's syndrome?

Reiter's syndrome is a type of reactive arthritis. Typically, it is an acute, asymmetric arthritis of the lower extremities, sometimes accompanied by dactylitis (sausage digit). It may be isolated to joints or include systemic illness characterized by fatigue, fever, and weight loss. Classic accompanying or intercurrent manifestations involve the following three systems:

1. **Urethritis or cervicitis** (including prostatitis and salpingitis)
2. **Ocular manifestations,** ranging from sporadic conjunctivitis to debilitating uveitis
3. **Mucocutaneous disease,** ranging from painless oral or genital ulceration to keratoderma blenorrhagicum, a psoriatic-like skin lesion typically on the palms and soles

20. What organisms have been associated with patients who develop reactive arthritis?

The following organisms have been cultured from stool or genitourinary discharge: *Chlamydia trachomatis, Neisseria gonorrhoeae, Shigella flexneri, Yersinia enterocolitica, Campylobacter jejuni, Borrelia burgdorferi,* and *Salmonella* species. *Salmonella, Borrelia* and *Neisseria* species may cause true septic arthritis as well as reactive arthritis. Other organisms have also been implicated.

21. Psoriatic arthritis can present in five different patterns of joint involvement. Name them.

1. Asymmetrical oligo- or polyarthritis of peripheral joints
2. Chronic symmetrical polyarthritis, with or without skin lesions
3. Rapidly destructive arthritis (arthritis mutilans)
4. Spondylitis, with or without peripheral arthritis
5. Isolated arthritis of the DIP joints

22. When should the human leukocyte antigen B27 (HLA-B27) be assessed in patients suspected of having a spondyloarthropathy?

Seronegative spondyloarthropathy probably arises from interactions of a susceptible genetic background and an environmental factor that induces the disease. HLA-B27 is strongly associated with the spondyloarthropathies, especially in white people ($> 80\%$ of white people with ankylosing spondylitis are HLA-B27 positive). However, in Japanese and Africans, HLA-B27 is associated with $< 50\%$ of cases. Of 100 people who are HLA-B27-positive, only two have a spondyloarthropathy. Thus, it is a poor screening test. HLA-B27 may be helpful in family counseling or in particularly enigmatic cases in which every piece of evidence may help to determine a probable diagnosis.

23. What is the treatment of the spondyloarthropathies?

Traditionally, patients with ankylosing spondylitis respond well to exercise, and daily exercise is encouraged. Good posture should be emphasized because if the patient fuses his or her back, the back should be straight and not bent over. Standard drug treatment includes traditional NSAIDs or COX-2 selective agents. Sulfasalazine and methotrexate are used if peripheral joints are involved. Patients with psoriatic arthritis in an RA pattern of joint involvement are treated as if they had RA. The anti–TNF-alpha biologic agents have a dramatic effect on the spondyloarthropathies and seem to control the symptoms and inflammation in both axial and peripheral joints. Bisphosphates are used in patients with osteoporosis secondary to their inflammatory disease.

24. What skin lesions may lead to the diagnosis of a patient presenting with polyarthritis?

- Psoriatic plaque—psoriatic arthritis
- Keratoderma blenorrhagicum—Reiter's syndrome
- Butterfly rash, discoid lupus, subacute cutaneous lupus, or photosensitive skin rash—SLE
- Erythema marginatum—acute rheumatic fever
- Erythema nodosum—sarcoid arthritis, enteropathic arthropathies
- Erythema chronicum migrans—Lyme arthritis
- Vesicopustular lesions or hemorrhagic papules—gonococcal arthritis
- Heliotrope rash on eyelids or erythema of the upper chest—dermatomyositis
- Gottron's papules overlying the extensor aspects of the MCP and PIP joints of the hands—dermatomyositis

- Gray/brown skin hyperpigmentation—hemochromatosis
- Thickened skin—systemic sclerosis

25. What rheumatic conditions are possible in a patient with Raynaud's phenomena and polyarticular complaints?

Systemic sclerosis (prevalence: > 90%)
Mixed connective tissue disease (prevalence: 80%)
SLE (prevalence: 10–40%)
Sjögren's syndrome (prevalence: 30%)
Polymyositis or dermatomyositis (prevalence: 20%)
Cryoglobulinemia (prevalence: 10%)

26. What tests may be helpful in evaluating a patient with polyarthritis?

Complete blood count	Urinalysis
Erythrocyte sedimentation rate	Synovial fluid analysis
Antinuclear antibodies (ANA)	Radiographs
Rheumatoid factor	Others to consider:
Liver enzymes	Thyroid-stimulating hormone
Serum creatinine	Calcium, phosphorus, albumin
Serum uric acid	Iron studies

CONTROVERSY

27. Are antibiotics of benefit in the therapy of reactive arthritis?

Treatment of reactive arthritis has classically centered on NSAIDs. Refractory cases are treated with sulfasalazine, corticosteroids, methotrexate, other immunosuppressive drugs, and now the new biologic agents. In the past, antibiotics were thought to play no role. However, chlamydia-induced disease was shown to respond to a 3-month course of long-acting tetracycline. The effectiveness of other antibiotics remains to be determined.

BIBLIOGRAPHY

1. American College of Rheumatology Ad Hoc Committee on Clinical Guidelines: Guidelines for the management of rheumatoid arthritis. Arthritis Rheum 39:713–722, 1996.
2. Bornalaski JS: Acute rheumatologic disorders in the elderly. Emerg Med Clin North Am 8:341–359, 1990.
3. Calin A, Elswood J, Rigg S, Skevington SM: Ankylosing spondylitis—an analytical review of 1500 patients: The changing pattern of disease. J Rheumatol 15:1234–1238, 1988.
4. Calin A, Porta J, Fries JF, Schurman DJ: Clinical history as a screening test for ankylosing spondylitis. JAMA 237:2613–2614, 1977.
5. Epstein JH, Zimmerman B, Ho G: Polyarticular septic arthritis. J Rheumatol 13:1105–1107, 1986.
6. Granfors K: Do bacterial antigens cause reactive arthritis? Rheum Dis Clin North Am 18:37–48, 1992.
7. Harris ED: Rheumatoid arthritis: Pathophysiology and implications for therapy. N Engl J Med 322:1277–1289, 1990.
8. Hochberg MC, Altman RD, Brandt KD, et al: Guidelines for the medical management of osteoarthritis: Part I. Osteoarthritis of the hip. Arthritis Rheum 38:1535–1540, 1995.
9. Hochberg MC, Altman RD, Brandt KD, et al: Guidelines for the medical management of osteoarthritis: Part II. Osteoarthritis of the knee. Arthritis Rheum 38:1541–1546, 1995.
10. Hughes RA, Keat AC: Reiter's syndrome and reactive arthritis: A current view. Semin Arthritis Rheum 24:190–210, 1994.
11. Klippel JH, Dieppe PA (eds): Practical Rheumatology. London, Mosby-Wolfe, 1995.
12. Lipsky PE, van der Heijde DM, St Clair EW, et al: Infliximab and methotrexate in the treatment of rheumatoid arthritis. N Engl J Med 343:1594–1602, 2000.
13. Pinals RS: Polyarthritis and fever. N Engl J Med 330:769–774, 1994.
14. Sergent JS: Polyarticular arthritis. In Ruddy S, Harris ED, Sledge CB (eds): Kelley's Textbook of Rheumatology, 6th ed. Philadelphia, W.B. Saunders, 2002, pp 379–385.

68. LOW BACK PAIN

Joseph C. Anderson, M.D.

1. Why should primary care providers develop expertise in the management of low back pain?

Low back pain is one of the most common presenting symptoms in a doctor's office. Approximately 75% of all adults experience back pain during their lives. A recent survey found that low back pain accounted for almost 15 million office visits, ranking it as the fifth most common complaint by patients. In addition, disability from chronic back pain is growing at an alarming rate. Practitioners should be prepared to help patients with low back pain maintain functional status. Although > 90% of all patients will have resolution of their symptoms, the practitioner should be vigilant about identifying diseases that may present as low back pain, such as aortic aneurysm.

2. Which structures in the body may be a source of low back pain?

Musculoskeletal structures	Visceral structures
Vertebral periosteum	Renal organs
Outer layers of the anulus fibrosus	Gastrointestinal organs
Nerve roots	Pelvic organs (e.g., prostate, ovary, uterus)
Apophyses	Aorta
Posterior longitudinal ligaments	Endocrine organs

3. Which potentially serious diagnoses should be considered in the evaluation of low back pain?

Osteomyelitis, malignancy, aortic aneurysm, and unstable spine fractures.

4. What are the relative frequencies of diseases that cause low back pain?

Unfortunately, a large percentage ($\leq 85\%$) of patients cannot be given a definite diagnosis. Fewer than 5% of all patients with low back pain present with sciatic complaints. Another small fraction ($< 5\%$) have malignancy, infection, fracture, or visceral disease as a cause of pain.

5. In addition to a careful history aimed at determining the organic cause of pain, what additional information should be elicited from patients with low back pain?

Practitioners should extract a thorough and careful history from patients because the differential diagnosis of low back pain encompasses many organ systems. However, it is also important to question patients about motor vehicle accidents, sports injuries, and previous back surgery. In addition, a full employment history as a date of eligibility for disability should be obtained. The practitioner also should ask about lifestyle behavior such as weight, exercise, and smoking.

6. What clues in the history may indicate that the patient may have a spondyloarthropathy?

In addition to the insidious onset and morning stiffness, most patients are men younger than age 40 years. A history of inflammatory arthritis of the hips or knees may also indicate the presence of a spondyloarthropathy.

7. Most mechanical back pain is relieved by bed rest. What diagnoses may be considered when low back pain persists despite bed rest?

Malignancy and spondyloarthropathy are two diagnoses in which pain may persist even after bed rest. Malignancy also may be suspected in the presence of weight loss or history of malignant disease. Spondyloarthropathies tend to present with an insidious onset of pain and morning stiffness.

8. What are good predictors of compression fractures?

Steroid use and age older than 70 years are good predictors for the presence of compression fractures. Although trauma may be a cause, most patients have no history of trauma.

9. What is sciatica? What does it indicate?

Sciatica is a sharp, burning pain radiating posteriorly or laterally down the leg past the knee, often in association with numbness. Such pain is usually increased with coughing and sneezing. The complaint of sciatica is a clue to nerve root irritation and may herald neurologic compromise. The presence of sciatica usually signifies disc herniation, which most commonly occurs at the level of L4–L5 or L5–S1; however, sciatica also may be seen in spinal stenosis.

10. What characteristic history suggests the diagnosis of spinal stenosis?

Spinal stenosis is a degenerative disease of the spine and thus usually begins after age 50 years. Neurologic symptoms are not localized and are often bilateral because the process involves multiple vertebrae. These problems are ameliorated by spinal flexion and are exacerbated by extension of the spine. Therefore, patients complain of pseudoclaudication or back pain accompanied by lower extremity pain with paresthesias or dysesthesias that worsen with standing but are not present in the sitting position.

11. What maneuvers should be performed during the physical examination of patients who present with low back pain?

1. **Inspection of the back,** including identifying leg length discrepancies and spinal curvature abnormalities.

2. **Palpation of the vertebral column and the sacroiliac joints.** Point tenderness may be found in malignancy or infection, whereas sacroiliac (SI) joint tenderness suggests spondyloarthropathies.

3. **Range of motion (ROM) of the spine.** Two lines are drawn (at L5–S1 and 10 cm above), and the distance between the two lines is measured during spinal flexion. A distance of < 15 cm during flexion suggests decreased ROM and may be one of the earliest manifestations of spondyloarthropathy. This test is called the Schober test.

4. **Straight leg raising.** With the patient supine, the examiner raises the affected leg in the extended position. Pain at < 60° signifies nerve root irritation.

5. **Motor exam.** See the table below for correlation of nerve with muscle innervation. Foot dorsiflexion testing is particularly useful.

6. **Sensory exam.** Careful attention must be paid to the dermatomal or lack of dermatomal distribution of numbness. The saddle area must be included.

7. **Reflexes,** especially the ankle reflexes, are diminished when the S1 nerve root is affected. Although ankle reflexes decrease with age, unilateral loss of ankle reflexes at any age should alert the practitioner.

NERVE	MOTOR	SENSORY	REFLEX
L1	Hip flexion	Back and groin	Cremasteric
L2	Hip adduction	Back	Cremasteric
	Hip flexion	Anterior thigh	
L3	Same as L2 and knee extension	Back	Patellar
		Upper buttock	
		Anterior thigh	
L4	Knee extension	Medial foot and calf	Patellar
L5	Toe extension	Lateral lower leg	Tibialis posterior
	Ankle dorsiflexion	Medial dorsum of foot	
S1	Ankle plantar flexion	Sole and heel	
	Knee flexion	Lateral foot	Achilles
S2	Ankle plantar flexion	Posterior upper and lower leg	None
	Toe flexion		
S3	No test	Medial buttocks	Bulbocavernosus
S4	No test	Perirectal	Bulbocavernosus
S5	No test	Perirectal	Anal

12. What is the utility of plain radiographs of the spine?
Plain radiographs, although inexpensive, are often not helpful or even misleading. Because by age 50 years, two thirds of adults have narrowing between vertebrae and 20% have osteophytes, radiographs are of greatest use after trauma or when systemic disease is suspected from the history or physical examination.

13. What routine laboratory studies may be helpful clues in the diagnosis of a patient with low back pain?
An elevated sedimentation rate (ESR) suggests malignancy and infection. A complete blood count, urinalysis, and assessment of calcium and alkaline phosphatase levels may be considered in patients who are older than 50 years, have failed conservative management, or have signs or symptoms suggestive of systemic disease.

14. When should an HLA-B27 test be ordered?
The HLA-B27 test should be considered only when the radiographs are normal but the clinical history, setting, and physical exam are perplexing and highly suggestive of a spondyloarthropathy.

15. When are other imaging tests indicated?
A bone scan may detect malignancy or infection before a radiograph. However, bone scans are not specific and do not detect lytic lesions. Computed tomography (CT) or magnetic resonance imaging (MRI) should be ordered when surgery is contemplated. Both are sensitive for disc pathology. However, a recent study found evidence of disc herniation in a significant percentage of asymptomatic patients.

16. What is the cauda equina syndrome?
The cauda equina syndrome is the constellation of bowel dysfunction with or without urinary retention, saddle anesthesia, and bilateral leg weakness or numbness. This syndrome constitutes a true surgical emergency.

17. When should back pain result in surgical referral?
- Cauda equina syndrome (emergency)
- Progressive or severe neurologic deficit at presentation (presence of fever should suggest epidural abscess as an emergency)
- Persistent neurologic deficit and sciatica after 4–6 weeks of conservative management
- Persistent pain or neurologic deficit associated with spinal stenosis or spondylolisthesis

18. How should patients with acute back pain be managed?
1. Education
   - Explanation of symptoms
   - Advise to return for worsening symptoms
   - Strong reassurance about the natural history (resolution expected)
   - Counseling: weight loss, smoking cessation (if applicable)
2. Activity
   - Limit activity only as desired (2–3 days) in patients with neurologic deficits
   - Bed rest should be prescribed for longer periods ($\leq$ 1 week) for patients with neurologic deficits
3. Pain control
   - Nonsteroidal anti-inflammatory drugs (NSAIDs) may control inflammation and pain but should be used with caution in elderly patients and patients with renal disease
   - Narcotics and muscle relaxants should be used only for short, well-defined periods (1 week)
   - Heat may be used as desired after the acute injury
4. Follow-up: 1 month–6 weeks if the patient does not improve

19. What is the role of exercise in the treatment of low back pain?

An exercise program, in the absence of neurologic deficit, should be encouraged. Stretching exercises for the lower back and extremities and general aerobic fitness may improve back mobility, increase energy levels, and decrease recurrent acute episodes of back pain. Such a program may begin within 2 weeks of the acute episode, assuming that it has resolved.

20. What are the indications for hospitalization?

The patient should be hospitalized only if surgery is contemplated. Traction has not been shown to be beneficial in the treatment of low back pain.

21. What methods may be used to determine whether a patient is a malingerer?

Waddell reported five ways to elicit nonorganic signs in a patient who amplifies symptoms:

1. **Spinal loading or rotation.** Lightly press down on the patient's head and rotate the patient's hips and pelvis. These maneuvers should not cause back pain.

2. **Nonorganic tenderness.** If lightly touching the paraspinal muscles causes pain, the patient may be amplifying the symptoms.

3. **Distraction straight-leg raising.** When the patient is seated, straighten the leg while asking about the knee. This maneuver should produce pain in the back, causing the patient to lean backward, especially if the straight leg-raising test is positive.

4. **Inappropriate sensory findings.** Check for reproducibility of sensory abnormalities as well as dermatomal distribution.

5. **Overreaction during examination**

Kummel recently reported that the finding of limitation of shoulder motion causing low back pain is more specific than Waddell's signs for a poor prognosis for return to work.

22. List five basic principles in treating patients with chronic back pain.

Only 10% of all patients with back pain develop chronic symptoms. Patients must understand that complete resolution of chronic pain is an unrealistic goal. The mnemonic **TREAT** summarizes the approach to preventing chronic back pain:

T = Transfer some responsibility to the patient. The patient must adhere to lifestyle changes such as weight loss and smoking cessation.

R = Reassurance. The patient should understand that the back pain is not life threatening and should not interfere with most activities of daily living.

E = Early mobilization. The patient should understand that activity will not be detrimental and may be beneficial.

A = Avoid drug dependency. It is unrealistic for the patient to expect total relief from medication.

T = Titrate medications upward only for short, preset periods during occasional flare-ups.

23. What therapeutic modalities have a role in chronic back pain?

Steroid injections have been shown to alleviate back pain for short periods (up to 4 months) in patients with sciatic complaints. A recent study of 158 patients confirmed the short-term benefit but failed to show any long-term effect of injection treatment. Patients with disc pain who fail conservative treatment may be candidates for this treatment.

24. What role does chiropractic medicine play in back pain?

Despite methodologic flaws in studies supporting spinal manipulation for low back pain, its use appears to have some efficacy in acute low back pain. A recent study found that the cost per episode of back pain was less for patients who saw a primary care practitioner than those who saw a chiropractor. However, there was a higher rate of satisfaction among patients who went to chiropractors than among patients who saw a primary care practitioner. Another study suggests that patients who receive osteopathic manipulation may require fewer medications including analgesics, anti-inflammatory drugs, or muscle relaxants. One trial comparing physical therapy and chiropractic manipulation to use of an educational booklet found that the interventions gave minimal benefit but at additional cost. Thus, chiropractors may have a role in acute back pain, especially if the added expense is not burdensome to the individual.

25. What measures have been shown to be effective in preventing back pain?
Increasing aerobic capacity and increasing back and leg strength through exercise have been shown to decrease the recurrence of low back pain. Unfortunately, education and lumbar supports have not been shown to be effective in preventing low back pain. Observational studies suggest that weight loss and smoking cessation may prevent the occurrence of low back pain.

CONTROVERSY

26. Should strict bed rest be prescribed for all patients with acute low back pain, even if sciatica is present?
Strict bed rest has been the cornerstone of conservative treatment. The rationale is to limit disc pressure so that the disc may resume its previous form. However, most low back pain does not originate with the disc. Furthermore, little evidence supports bed rest as a therapeutic modality. Deconditioning, loss of muscle, and demineralization of bone are among the deleterious effects of just a few days of bed rest. On the other hand, the back must be given sufficient recovery time to prevent chronic injury.

A recent randomized, controlled study found that patients who continued normal activities as tolerated had better recovery than patients who were prescribed bed rest. Statistically significant differences were noted in duration of pain, pain intensity, lumbar flexion, and ability to work.

Thus, it appears unwise to prescribe bed rest for patients without neurologic deficits or sciatic complaints. Individualized treatment plans should be the rule with an emphasis on early mobilization. Patients with a neurologic deficit should stand periodically to decrease the negative effect of bed rest. Standing causes only a slight increase in disc pressure over the supine position.

BIBLIOGRAPHY

 1. Andersson GB, Lucente T, Davis AM, et al: A comparison of osteopathic spinal manipulation with standard care for patients with low back pain. N Engl J Med 341:1426–1431, 1999.
 2. Assendelft W, Koes B, Knipschild P, Bouter L: The relationship between methodological quality and conclusions in reviews of spinal manipulation. JAMA 274:1942–1948, 1995.
 3. Borenstein D: Chronic low back pain. Rheum Dis Clin North Am 22:439–454, 1996.
 4. Borenstein D: Epidemiology, etiology, diagnostic evaluation and treatment of low back pain. Curr Opin Rheumatol 9:144–150, 1997.
 5. Borenstein D, Wiesel S: Low Back Pain: Medical Diagnosis and Comprehensive Management, 2nd ed. Philadelphia, W.B. Saunders, 1995.
 6. Carette S, Leclaire R, Marcoux S, et al: Epidural corticosteroid injections for sciatica due to herniated nucleus pulposus. N Engl J Med 336:1634–1640, 1997.
 7. Carey T, Garrett J, Jackman A, and the North Carolina Back Pain Project: The outcomes and costs of care for acute low back pain among patients seen by primary care practitioners, chiropractors, and orthopedic surgeons. N Engl J Med 333:913–917, 1995.
 8. Cherkin DC, Deyo RA, Battie M, et al: A comparison of physical therapy, chiropractic manipulation, and provision of an educational booklet for the treatment of patients with low back pain. N Engl J Med 339:1021–1029, 1998.
 9. Deyo R, Loeser J, Bigos S: Herniated lumbar intervertebral disk. Ann Intern Med 112:598–603, 1990.
10. Deyo R, Roinville J, Kent D: What can the history and physical exam tell us about low back pain? JAMA 268:760–765, 1992.
11. Deyo RA, Weinstein JN: Low back pain. N Engl J Med 344:363–370, 2001.
12. Hall S, Bartleson J, Onotrio B: Lumbarspinal stenosis. Ann Intern Med 103:271–275, 1985.
13. Hart L, Deyo R, Cherkin D: Physician office visits for low back pain: Frequency clinical evaluation, and treatment patterns from a U.S. national survey. Spine 20:11–19, 1995.
14. Jensen M, Brant-Zawadzki M, Obuchowski N, et al: Magnetic resonance imaging of the lumbar spine in people without back pain. N Engl J Med 331:69–73, 1994.
15. Kummel B: Nonorganic signs of significance in low back pain. Spine 21:1077–1081, 1996.

16. Malmivaara A, Hakkinen U, Aro T, et al: The treatment of acute low back pain—bed rest, exercises, or ordinary activity? N Engl J Med 332:351–355, 1995.
17. Spaccarelli K: Lumbar and caudal epidural corticosteroid injections. Mayo Clin Proc 71:169–178, 1996.
18. Waddell G, McCulloch JA, Kummel E, Vernner R: Nonorganic physical signs in low back pain. Spine 5:117–125, 1980.

69. HIP AND KNEE PAIN

Richard C. Fisher, M.D.

1. What information do you need to begin an investigation of the etiology of hip and knee pain?

1. **Localization of pain.** Pain originating in the lumber spine or posterior pelvis may be felt about the sacral iliac joints, gluteal muscles, and posterior thighs. Pain from bursae or tendons is sharply localized. Hip joint pain is often felt in the anterior groin area or medial thigh and knee in the distribution of the obturator nerve.

2. **Onset and duration of pain.** Onset is slow in inflammatory conditions but rapid with trauma or infections. If trauma is suspected, try to obtain a history the mechanism of injury. Try to determine if recent situational changes have occurred. Pain from degenerative arthritis usually increases gradually but may be accelerated by changes at work or in the family or other lifestyle changes.

3. **Relation of pain to activities.** It is important to know whether the pain occurs at rest, whether it has changed the lifestyle of the patient, and whether it requires the use of walking support such as a cane or walker. Pain referred from the lumbar spine often increases with sitting.

4. **Previous treatment.** Ask what treatment the patient has tried and if it provided any relief.

5. **Associated systemic symptoms.** Of specific importance are back pain, abdominal complaints, other joint involvement, and associated fever, chills, and malaise.

2. What is the first change in the physical examination of a patient with a disorder of the hip joint?

Loss of joint motion, usually internal rotation, is affected first. Measure hip motion with the patient supine and include flexion, extension, abduction, adduction, and internal-external rotation. Note any loss of motion that is associated with pain. Other findings include a limp and decreased circumference of the thigh caused by secondary disuse atrophy. At times, pain with deep palpation is noted over the anterior aspect of the hip joint.

3. List the most common causes of hip joint pain.

Degenerative, inflammatory, and occasionally infectious arthritides
Avascular necrosis of the femoral head
Villonodular synovitis
Stress (insufficiency) fractures
Paget's disease
Tumors, especially metastatic lesions

4. What is the differential diagnosis of traumatic hip pain in elderly patients?

The most obvious consequence of trauma to the hip region in elderly patients is a fracture of the proximal femur. Occasionally, the initial radiographs appear normal, but the patient continues to have varying degrees of pain with activity. In such situations, establishing the correct diagnosis is important. The most common abnormalities include simple contusion of the soft tissue, fractures of the greater trochanter, occult fractures of the pelvis, and occult fractures of the femoral neck or intertrochanteric region. The latter are the most significant because an initial occult fracture may become displaced without appropriate treatment. Focused routine radiographs may show a fracture line; if no fracture is seen, the diagnosis may be confirmed with a magnetic resonance imaging (MRI) scan. MRI is useful in assessing occult femoral neck fractures immediately after injury. Stress (insufficiency) fractures and metastatic disease cause hip pain in this age group and may or may not be associated with a history of trauma.

5. What common problems may masquerade as hip and thigh pain?
- Spine problems
- Atraumatic pelvis fractures (pelvic insufficiency fractures)
- Lower abdominal abnormalities, including tumors and infections
- Meralgia paresthetica (compression of the lateral femoral cutaneous nerves)
- Claudication of the internal iliac artery

6. Name the common causes of avascular necrosis of the femoral head.

Among the many causes of avascular necrosis, the most common are trauma (e.g., femoral neck fracture or hip dislocation), use of corticosteroid medication, alcohol overuse, rapid decompression (caisson disease), sickle cell disease; and radiation.

7. Describe the treatment options for avascular necrosis.

Initial treatment should include protective weight bearing and physical medicine modalities such as range of motion (ROM) and muscle strengthening. Antiinflammatory medication is of value for symptomatic pain relief. After structural changes occur in the femoral head, the surgical options should be considered. The value of surgical decompression of the femoral head remains controversial. Decompression in the stage before radiographic changes but after changes on MRI studies may improve the prognosis for revascularization without collapse, but this approach remains unproved. After the femoral head has begun to deform, decompression may not be helpful. Osteotomy or total joint replacement is indicated at this stage.

8. What are the manifestations of overuse syndromes in the region of the hip and knee?

1. **Stress fractures.** The most commonly seen overuse problem is stress fractures in the proximal or mid femur or proximal aspect of the tibia. Of greatest concern is a stress fracture of the femoral neck and intertrochanteric region, which often results in displaced fractures. Patients with this diagnosis should be removed from weight bearing immediately and considered for referral to an orthopedic surgeon for surgical stabilization.

2. **Soft tissue injury.** Soft-tissue injuries develop from repetitive motion of the fascia lata over the greater trochanter (greater trochanteric bursitis) and lateral femoral condyle (iliotibial friction syndrome) of the femur.

3. **Tendinitis.** Quadriceps and patella tendinitis are more frequent in young patients at the tendon insertion sites.

9. Briefly discuss the diagnosis approach and treatment options for patients presenting with a painful, snapping hip.

The "snapping hip syndrome" is not uncommon, although it is not always painful. The three major causes include (1) the popping of the iliotibial band over the greater trochanter of the femur, often associated with trochanteric bursitis; (2) a popping on the medial side of the hip associated with the iliopsoas tendon; and (3) various intra-articular lesions, including loose bodies, old fractures, labral tears, or hypertrophic synovium. Diagnosis is made largely by the clinical examination, although plain radiographs may show bony fragments within or about the hip joint. Iliopsoas bursography may be confirmatory for popping secondary to the iliopsoas tendon on the medial side of the hip. All conditions are best treated conservatively with rest or avoidance of symptom-producing activities. Anti-inflammatory medication and stretching exercises likewise should be part of the rehabilitation program. Steroid injections into the bursal area or iliopsoas tendon may be of value. Surgical treatment is rarely necessary.

10. Which bursae about the hip or knee are most commonly involved in clinical symptoms?

Greater trochanteric bursa, prepatellar bursa, infrapatellar bursa, and pes anserinus bursa seem to be the most commonly involved. Others include the iliopsoas bursa and occasionally the ischiogluteal bursa (with prolonged wheelchair use).

11. Describe the treatment for bursitis and tendinitis.

Initial treatment consists of rest from aggravating activities. Rest may be supplemented with application of ice and use of nonsteroidal anti-inflammatory agents (NSAIDs). Various physical therapy modalities are also effective, including ultrasound treatments. When conservative therapy is not effective, injections of corticosteroids into the bursa or tendon sheath may be indicated. The use of steroids about ligaments and tendons should be considered carefully because the alteration of collagen synthesis may lead to tendon or ligament rupture. The same is not necessarily true of bursitis. Surgical excision of the bursa or release of the tendon sheath is occasionally indicated for unremitting and disabling cases.

12. List the more common atraumatic causes of knee pain.

Because knee trauma is extremely common, it is important in evaluation of knee pain to elicit any history of injury. Atraumatic causes of knee pain, which may be associated with an effusion, include inflammatory or infectious arthritis, patella femoral arthritis, gout or other crystal-induced arthropathy, and synovial hypertrophy due to pigmented villi nodular synovitis. Other less common causes, which may not be associated with knee effusions, include avascular necrosis of the femoral or tibial condyles, sympathetic reflex dystrophy, and stress fractures. Intra-articular hip abnormalities often refer pain to the knee area via common obturator nerve innervation.

13. Explain the diagnostic features of meniscus injuries of the knee. Is age a factor?

Most meniscus injuries are associated with young athletic patients, but a second peak occurs in older patients because degenerative tears associated with early degenerative arthritis. Critical elements in the history of both groups include recurrent swelling, catching or locking that precludes full extension, buckling or giving way with weight bearing, and limitation of usual activities. Physical findings are medial or lateral joint line tenderness, a positive McMurray test result, effusion, and limited extension. In general, the clinical evaluation has a low accuracy rate for predicting meniscus injuries, and MRI may be helpful.

14. Enlargement about the knee may be associated with bursitis, knee effusion, or generalized swelling. How are the three differentiated?

Prepatellar bursitis causes fluid accumulation between the skin and the patella. A fluctuant area superficial to the bony patella is palpable.

A **knee effusion** elevates the patella, which is readily palpated beneath the skin with no intervening fluid. In addition, the suprapatellar pouch, which extends approximately 3 fingerbreadths above the superior pole of the patella, feels full superiorly, medially, and laterally.

Generalized swelling in the knee, as occurs from acute injuries, is not localizable to either the bony patella or the suprapatellar pouch. Swelling is diffuse, usually extends to the proximal tibia and distal femur, and is often circumferential in nature. It is frequently associated with ecchymosis.

15. What are the most common causes of knee effusions?

1. **Traumatic effusions** usually contain blood or a mixture of blood and synovial fluid. The fluid may contain fat droplets in the presence of an associated fracture.

2. **Post-traumatic effusions** occur after meniscal tears, ligamentous injuries, or other destabilizing injuries of the knee. Post-traumatic effusions show an increased amount of normal-appearing synovial fluid.

3. **Inflammation,** as seen in rheumatoid arthritis or gout, often causes an effusion with an abnormal synovial analysis.

4. **Purulent fluid** is seen in both acute and chronic infections.

16. What are the indications for joint aspiration?

The aspiration should be done for diagnostic purposes. After trauma, the knee occasionally swells to the extent that it becomes tense and painful. Removing a portion of the bloody joint fluid relieves the patient's pain temporarily. After aspiration, the fluid should be examined visually to determine whether it is purulent, translucent, or bloody and should be sent to a laboratory for culture, cell count, crystal exam, and other specific tests, as needed.

17. Describe the classic signs and symptoms associated with early degenerative arthritis of the knee.

The history usually includes pain with weight-bearing activities. Often patients report removal of a meniscus or a ligamentous injury some years before. A mild effusion may be present, and crepitus is felt with joint motion. The early radiographic changes include flattening of the femoral condyles, osteophyte formation beginning at the joint margins, and narrowing of the cartilage space. The latter is best evaluated with weight-bearing radiographs.

18. A 52-year-old man presents with early degenerative arthritis of both knees that limits his normal activities. He would like to know his treatment options. What would tell him?

1. **Maintain knee ROM and muscle strength** with an active rehabilitation program and avoid traumatic activities entailing running or jumping. Consider selective load transfer bracing when needed.

2. **Medications:** Acetaminophen may be taken for pain control, and NSAIDs help with both analgesia and inflammation. The chondroprotective supplements glucosamine and chondroitin sulfate possibly have a positive metabolic effect on the chondrocyte by slowing matrix degradation.

3. **Injections:** Intra-articular corticosteroids dramatically decrease symptoms but, over time and repeated injections, exert a deleterious effect on cartilage metabolism. Viscosupplementation therapy using a hyaluronic acid derivative has been shown to relieve symptoms and may a positive effect on cartilage repair.

4. **Cartilage substitution:** A variety of techniques are being tried to replace damaged or absent articular cartilage. Although some seem to be useful, they remain controversial and await appropriate studies.

19. Describe the history and physical findings associated with patellofemoral disease.

The major finding in the history is pain with walking up or down stairs or inclines, rising from a chair, and kneeling. The pain is felt directly beneath the patella and associated with crepitus or a rough feeling as the patella glides over the femoral condyle. On physical examination, the patella may track laterally as the knee reaches full extension. Patellar instability is evaluated by palpation with the quadriceps muscle rested and the knee extended. The patient becomes apprehensive as the patella is pushed to the lateral side. Hamstring tightness is a common associated finding.

20. What treatment is available for patella femoral joint pain?

The treatment depends to some extent on the cause of the pain. In general, treatment is symptomatic, as in other inflammatory conditions, and consists of rest, ice or heat, and NSAIDs. Protection of the patella femoral joint is sometimes possible with a patellar orthosis or a special type of taping to correct malalignment. Physical therapy consists primarily of short arc quadriceps-strengthening exercises and hamstring stretching. In patients with severe malalignment and recurrent subluxations or dislocations, surgical correction protects the underlying articular cartilage. The value of arthroscopic or open patella debridement and shaving remains controversial.

21. When are imaging techniques useful in the evaluation of knee problems?

Imaging techniques are useful for bony lesions such as osteochondritis dessicans, fractures, tumors, and early degenerative changes. Routine radiographs are indicated for the initial evaluation. MRI has become increasingly useful for diagnosing soft tissue problems such as meniscal and anterior and posterior cruciate injuries and for evaluating possible bony or soft tissue tumors about the knee. Arthrograms have been largely supplanted by MRI for the evaluation of meniscal injuries, although an arthrogram may still be of value in diagnosing the size and extent of popliteal cysts. Ultrasound is also useful for evaluating popliteal cysts and distinguishing fluid-filled from solid lesions. Computed or plain tomography is of value in evaluation of certain fractures, particularly in the proximal area of the tibia and distal femur.

22. When is total hip or total knee arthroplasty indicated?

Replacement arthroplasty is a serious undertaking and should be used only in patients with no other alternatives for treatment. Failure of arthroplasties may result in either a flail or a fused joint. Arthroplasty should be recommended only as an end-stage procedure when the joint is destroyed by an arthritic or traumatic process beyond the point at which conservative measures are effective. The failure rate in young patients is high, and surgery is usually discouraged before age 60 years. However, in young patients who have incapacitating joint destruction and are not candidates for either osteotomy or arthrodesis, arthroplasty may be an appropriate procedure.

23. What are the expected outcomes from total hip or total knee arthroplasty?

The expected outcome is return to a pain-free functional status. Rarely does the involved joint regain full ROM or become totally pain free. The goal is return of enough function to allow activities of daily living and low-impact recreational activities. The major short-term complications are infection (reported incidence of 0.5–4.0%) and mechanical failure (reported incidence of 5% at 2 years). Both complications usually require revision surgery. The major long-term complication is mechanical failure or loosening, which is reported in the range of 10–40% at 10-year follow-up.

24. Discuss the treatment options for pyogenic infections of the hip and knee joint.

The choice of open drainage, arthroscopic drainage, or needle drainage of pyogenic infections remains controversial, although experts agree that some type of drainage is needed. Antibiotics also are mandatory in the treatment of these potentially destructive infections. In general, the two most important considerations are the type of organism involved in the infection and ease of access to the joint. The most destructive organisms include the gram-negative bacilli and staphylococci; streptococci and gonococci are known to be relatively benign. Joint accessibility is important for adequacy of drainage and monitoring of the clinical response.

Pyogenic hip joint infections in children should be treated with open drainage. Treatment of other joints remains controversial. No clear evidence indicates an advantage of one treatment over another for adult hips and knees. If clinical response is not adequate within 3–4 days of aspiration, open or arthroscopic drainage is indicated. Failure of needle drainage is probably related to the virulence of the organism and inability to evacuate loculated areas within the joint. Acute infections that occur after total joint arthroplasty should be treated by open drainage.

BIBLIOGRAPHY

1. Allen WC, Cope R: Coxa saltans: The snapping hip revisited. J Am Acad Orthop Surg 3:303–308, 1995.
2. Beaty JH (ed): Orthopaedic Knowledge Update 6. Rosemont, IL, American Academy of Orthopaedic Surgeons, 1999.
3. Berman AT, Hermantin FU, Horwitz SM: Metastatic disease of the hip: Evaluation and treatment. J Am Acad Orthop Surg 5:79–86, 1997.
4. Cole BJ, Harner CD: Degenerative arthritis of the knee in active patients: Evaluation and management. J Am Acad Orthop Surg 7:389–402, 1999.
5. Fulkerson JP, Shea KP: Disorders of patellofemoral alignment. J Bone Joint Surg 72A:1424–1429, 1990.
6. Greene WB (ed): Essentials of Musculoskeletal Care. Rosemont, IL, American Academy of Orthopaedic Surgeons, 2001.
7. Jackson RW: The painful knee: Arthroscopy or MR imaging? J Am Acad Orthop Surg 4:93–99, 1996.
8. Jackson DW, Scheer MJ, Simon TM: Cartilage substitutes: Overview of basic science and treatment options. J Am Acad Orthop Surg 9:37–52, 2001.
9. Solomon DH, Simel DL, Bates DW, et al: Does this patient have a torn meniscus of ligament of the knee? JAMA 286:1610–1620, 2001.
10. Teitz CC, Garrett WE, Miniaci A, et al: Tendon Problems in Athletic Individuals. Instructional Course Lectures, vol. 46. Rosemont, IL, American Academy of Orthopaedic Surgeons, 1997.

70. SHOULDER AND ELBOW PAIN

Richard C. Fisher, M.D.

1. What questions are important in taking a history from a patient presenting with shoulder or elbow pain?

1. Time of onset and patient's perception of the cause of pain, such as a fall or other trauma, overuse, or systemic illnesses

2. Duration of the pain and its change over time

3. Anatomic location of maximal discomfort

4. Activities that increase or decrease the pain

5. Functional limitations caused by the pain, specifically decreased range of motion (ROM), inability to use the arm for certain activities of daily living (ADLs), and difficulty sleeping

6. Treatment modalities that have been tried and their effect

2. Outline the common anatomic areas where shoulder pain is experienced.

- Acromial clavicular joint: infection, separation, osteolysis (*A* in figure)
- Subacromial region: bursitis, impingement, degenerative arthritis, rotator cuff tears (*B* in figure)
- Mid-humerus: biceps tendon rupture (anterior), cervical radiculopathy (posterior) (*C* in figure)
- Mid-clavical region: clavical fracture, brachial plexus neuritis (*D* in figure)

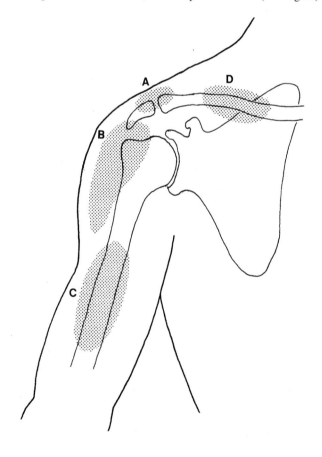

3. Describe the visible deformities that may suggest the cause of the patient's pain.

After trauma, deformity may be seen with acromioclavicular (AC) separations, shoulder or elbow dislocations, and fractures of the clavicle and humerus. AC separations show a prominence, swelling, or both at the AC joint and may be accompanied by an abrasion over the tip of the shoulder. Patients with anterior shoulder dislocations have a hollow area inferior to the acromion with a palpable humeral head more distally. The arm is held in abduction and cannot be adducted to the side. Patients with posterior dislocations are unable to rotate externally. Elbow dislocations show a prominence of the distal humerus or olecranon with loss of motion. Fractures of the clavicle are usually in the midportion and present with swelling, bony angulation, or both. Some fractures of the mid-humerus have visible angular deformity. Pain of neurogenic origin may be associated with muscle atrophy about the shoulder and arm region. The most common abnormality is atrophy of the deltoid muscle after axillary nerve injury or of the supraspinatus and infraspinatus muscles after compression injuries to the suprascapular nerve. Patients with spastic neuropathies often have an internal rotation contracture at the shoulder.

4. What common sites refer pain to the shoulder and upper arm region?
- Cervical spine
- Brachial plexus
- Thoracoabdominal region, including tumors of the lung, ischemic heart disease, subphrenic abscesses, and gastric and gallbladder disease

5. How are the causes of referred pain differentiated?

Referred pain caused by cervical spine and brachial plexus abnormalities usually is accompanied by local discomfort that is aggravated by motion of the neck and palpation over the brachial plexus. Neurologic deficits may be present. In patients with thoracic and abdominal problems, symptoms are referable to those areas and usually accompanied by physical findings or radiographic abnormalities.

6. Describe the differential diagnosis of a patient presenting with an acute swollen shoulder or elbow that is red, warm, and painful and not associated with recent trauma.

The most important condition to exclude is acute septic arthritis, which can be diagnosed by aspiration of the fluid and examination for cell count, crystals, Gram stain, and culture. Other conditions to consider include an inflammatory arthropathy, such as gout or rheumatoid arthritis, and a neuropathic or Charcot joint. The latter is often associated with syringomyelia. Other conditions include diabetes, syphilis, leprosy, Charcot-Marie-Tooth disease, and rarely, congenital-indifference-to-pain syndrome. The diagnosis is usually confirmed by radiographic changes showing osteolysis and osseous fragmentation of the periarticular structures.

7. Name the common locations of compression neuropathies of the shoulder, upper arm, and elbow region.

Suprascapular nerve entrapment occurs as the nerve transverses the suprascapular notch on the superior border of the scapula. The presenting complaint is weakness of shoulder abduction and external rotation as well as diffuse, nonspecific shoulder pain. Atrophy of the scapular fossa muscles is usually present. Suprascapular nerve entrapment is often seen in throwing athletes and patients performing other repetitive motions. **Thoracic outlet syndrome** is commonly associated with pain after using the upper extremity in the elevated or abducted position and with symptoms of ulnar nerve dysfunction. **Ulnar nerve compression** at the olecranon groove of the elbow is one of the most common compression neuropathies of the upper extremity. **Median nerve compression** by the pronator muscle in the proximal forearm is seen less frequently.

8. Describe the diagnostic features of thoracic outlet syndrome.

Usually the patient complains of pain in the shoulder region with radiation into the arm. If the arm is held in the abducted position, the palpable pulse at the wrist decreases, and a bruit may be audible over the subclavian artery. This test also may produce pain and dysesthesias in the upper extremity. The ulnar nerve is most commonly involved, but median and radial nerves also may be affected. The elevated arm stress test is conducted with the arms placed overhead and posterior. The patient open and closes his or her fists repeatedly for several minutes. A positive test result reproduces symptoms. Cervical spine radiographs show cervical ribs or abnormal transverse processes known to be associated with thoracic outlet stenosis. Additional imaging only helps to rule out other problems.

9. What are the diagnostic features and treatment options for ulnar nerve entrapment at the elbow?

Diagnostic signs include (1) a positive Tinel's sign (tingling sensation with percussion of the nerve) result at the olecranon groove on the medial aspect of the distal humerus and (2) motor and sensory changes in the ulnar nerve distribution distal to the elbow. Electromyography and nerve conduction tests are confirmatory in most cases if the diagnosis is unclear. Treatment initially consists of rest with a splint or sling and often a trial of anti-inflammatory medications. Corticosteroid injections are hazardous because of the tight compartment in which the nerve travels at the medial epicondyle. Surgical decompression is indicated for persistent symptoms or progressive neuropathy, especially muscle weakness.

10. Name the most common sites of bursitis in the shoulder and elbow region.

The **subacromial bursa** can be palpated directly distal to the tip of the acromion process on the lateral aspect of the shoulder. If inflamed, it is tender to palpation and painful with shoulder abduction approaching 90°. This is an integral part of the shoulder impingement syndrome. **Olecranon bursitis** produces swelling directly over the tip of the olecranon process, which is tender to palpation. In acute cases, the surrounding skin appears red and indurated. Olecranon bursitis is differentiated from an infected bursa by the lack of systemic signs of infection and by the results of aspiration.

11. Discuss the common lesions in the elbow region that are secondary to repetitive trauma.

The most common problem is **lateral epicondylitis** (tennis elbow), which is caused by repetitive use of the upper extremity for a variety of activities, such as tennis or gripping a hammer or saw. **Medial epicondylitis,** although less frequent, results from similar activities, including golf. In both conditions, the area directly over the epicondyle at the insertion of the extensor or flexor muscle mass is usually tender. On the lateral side, other causes of pain include **entrapment of the radial nerve** just distal to the elbow and **inflammation of the anular ligament** about the radial head.

12. Explain the initial treatment protocol for medial and lateral epicondylitis.

Initial treatment includes avoidance of aggravating activity, ice before and after use, and antiinflammatory medication. Physical therapy modalities and a graded biceps- and triceps-strengthening program are useful. A tennis elbow band, which fits just below the elbow, acts as a damper for the extensor muscle mass and may be beneficial during activity. If noninvasive therapy has not helped, an injection with corticosteroid may be tried. Surgical release and reimplantation of the extensor muscle mass into the lateral epicondyle may be indicated in resistant cases.

13. What are the clinical findings of acute impingement syndrome?

A history of pain with overhead activities felt in the subacromial area radiating to the deltoid muscle insertion (see question 2). There is often pain with sleeping on the involved side and a history suggesting overuse. Physical findings include tenderness in the subacromial region; pain with shoulder abduction, flexion, and external rotation; and a positive impingement test result (elevating the internally rotated arm against resistance).

14. List the pathologic stages of shoulder impingement syndrome.

The major stages include inflammation, fibrosis and scar formation, and overt tendon rupture. The inflammatory stage results from overuse in the region, which causes swelling about the bursa or adjacent tissues so that the greater trochanter impinges on the acromion with abduction and internal rotation of the arm. If treatment fails or repetitive activity continues, the tissues become fibrotic and scarred and lead to a decreased ROM of the shoulder joint. After the rotator cuff tendon, which includes the predominantly supraspinatus and infraspinatus muscles, ruptures, shoulder function is greatly altered and abduction is not possible. The late-stage impingement syndromes are sometimes associated with degenerative changes in the AC joint, which may lead to osteophyte formation and increased impingement in that region.

15. Describe the treatment for shoulder impingement syndrome.

The inflammatory stage is reversible and is treated with rest, physical therapy, nonsteroidal anti-inflammatory medications (NSAIDs), and steroid injection in selected patients. The stage of fibrosis and scarring is accompanied by a decreased ROM. This phase is also reversible initially but becomes less so with time and repetitive activities. Treatment should begin with the same modalities as in the inflammatory stage, but some patients may benefit from surgical decompression, either open or with the arthroscope. After the tendons of the supraspinatus or infraspinatus and teres major rupture, surgical reconstruction is usually needed to regain function. In some patients, pain can be relieved with nonsurgical modalities.

16. What are the diagnostic features of rotator cuff tear?

A history of decreasing function and increased pain about the shoulder is fairly typical. The pain is often worse at night or when the patient lies in the supine position. Degenerative tears occur over a long period after repetitive use. Traumatic tears usually are associated with an injury that the patient can identify as the onset of symptoms. The physical examination typically demonstrates the patient's inability to abduct the arm beyond 30–40°. If the arm is passively abducted above 90°, the patient can maintain the arm in this position. On lowering the arm, the patient loses control at about 90°, and the arm becomes painful as it falls. Often patients learn to maneuver the arm into abduction by circumducting the shoulder. Useful imaging techniques include computed tomographic (CT) arthrography and magnetic resonance imaging (MRI). Rupture of the long head of the biceps tendon is associated with rotator cuff pathology and may either precede of follow a rotator cuff tear.

17. Describe the common mechanisms of injury in the shoulder region.

Falls onto the outstretched arm and hand commonly result in injuries at many levels, including the radial head, supracondylar area of the humerus, humeral shaft, and midclavicle area. If the arm remains tucked close to the side in a position of adduction, a fracture of the proximal humerus is likely. Such a fall is typical among older people, who may slip while holding a grocery bag. Falls onto the tip of the shoulder, often accompanied by an abrasion, are the classic cause of AC separations. This mechanism is common with forward falls from bicycles and horses. Injuries with the arm abducted are associated with shoulder joint dislocations.

18. Explain the etiology of AC joint pain.

Acute injuries result in a range of joint stability from mild stretching of the AC ligaments with no instability (grade I) to complete tear of the AC and coracoclavicular ligaments (grade III). Degenerative arthritis occurs *de novo* or after trauma. It is diagnosed by radiographic changes of cartilage space narrowing and osteophyte formation. The inferior joint osteophytes contribute to the symptoms of shoulder joint impingement. Distal clavical osteolysis is an inflammatory condition associated with rheumatoid arthritis and from overuse common in weight lifters. Septic arthritis presents as an acute, red, painful, swollen joint best diagnosed by aspiration.

19. Why should an axillary radiographic view be obtained of all shoulder injuries?

Dislocations caused by trauma to the abducted arm usually result in an anterior dislocation of the shoulder; the humeral head is anterior and usually inferior to the glenoid cavity. The incidence of posterior dislocations caused by trauma is about 10%. Seizures, however, result in a much higher incidence of posterior dislocations. Care should be taken in diagnosis because the joint often appears normal in the anteroposterior radiograph. Thus, it is important to obtain an axillary view in all suspected cases of shoulder dislocation. Recurrent dislocations require much less trauma and sometimes occur with simple reaching activities.

20. A patient presents with shoulder pain and loss of motion over the past 6–8 months. What shoulder consider in attempting to reach a diagnosis?

Shoulder motion is lost after trauma and overuse (impingement) syndromes because of pain. It is important, but at times difficult, to determine the underlying abnormality. Treatment should begin with restoration of motion via physical therapy and anti-inflammatory medication. Preventing the loss of motion in the early stages in most important. The frozen shoulder syndrome is an idiopathic loss of motion without a prior abnormality. Pain accompanies the progressive loss of motion. Type I diabetes is the most common risk factor, but the syndrome is also associated with hypothyroidism, Parkinson's disease, and cerebral hemorrhage.

21. Describe the treatment for acute and recurrent dislocations of the shoulder.

The recurrence rate for a first-time shoulder dislocation depends on the age of the patient. Patients in the second and third decades of life at the time of the initial dislocation have a recurrence rate as high as 70%; the rate decreases with age. Although the efficacy of treatment is controversial, the initial step consists of immobilization with the arm in a position of adduction and internal rotation; limited ROM exercises should begin at 2–3 weeks. Abduction and external rotation of the shoulder should be limited for 6–8 weeks, and sporting and other high-risk activities should be avoided. The decision to perform surgical stabilization of the shoulder is based on the number and ease of recurrent dislocations and the inconvenience or risk to the patient caused by repeated dislocation.

22. List some of the common skeletal tumors about the shoulder area that may present with a predominant symptom of pain.

In young people, several benign lesions are common, including chondroblastoma, which usually occurs in the proximal humeral epiphysis; exostosis, which sometimes is associated with multiple familial osteochondromatosis; and unicameral cysts, which are more common in children than adults. Malignant tumors include osteosarcoma and chondrosarcoma. Chondrosarcomas seem to have a predilection for the pelvic and shoulder girdle areas. Metastatic disease is common in the humerus, as is multiple myeloma. Although such lesions are rare, the possibility that they underlie shoulder pain make it especially important to obtain radiographs before proceeding with steroid injections or other treatment for benign conditions.

23. Describe the pattern of involvement of the elbow and shoulder region with the various types of arthritis.

Rheumatoid arthritis and osteoarthritis frequently affect the elbow, shoulder, and AC joints. AC joint disease may follow discreet episodes of previous trauma. The humeral head is a common site of avascular necrosis with collapse and destruction of the humeral articular surface. Post-steroid avascular necrosis seems to be the most common cause. Other less common causes include sepsis, neuropathy (see question 7), Paget's disease, and gout.

24. Briefly describe the principles of treatment for arthritis of these joints.

If the arthritis is caused by a systemic condition, treatment of the underlying systemic disease is indicated. For degenerative or osteoarthritis, NSAIDs and gentle physical measures monitored by physical therapy are appropriate. Synovectomy is sometimes indicated for early rheumatoid arthritis in the elbow; resection arthroplasty of the AC joint is a satisfactory procedure that usually follows conservative care and a trial of steroid injections into the joint area. Total joint arthroplasty of the shoulder and elbow are indicated when other treatment has failed.

25. What are the expected results of total shoulder and elbow arthroplasties?

Total shoulder arthroplasty has shown results comparable to those of knee and hip procedures. A 90% relief of pain can be expected initially, but the long-term failure or revision rate is 10–20% at 10 years. The cause of the joint destruction makes some difference in the outcome. Patients with osteonecrosis or degenerative arthritis have better results than patients with rheumatoid arthritis. The worst results are seen in traumatic arthritis after fractures about the shoulder with scarring and interruption of the rotator cuff tendons. Total elbow arthroplasty is less reliable than arthroplasty of the shoulder, but with new techniques, it is becoming a more efficacious procedure. Its primary indication is joint destruction caused by inflammatory arthritis, but satisfactory results can be expected in patients with posttraumatic arthritis.

BIBLIOGRAPHY

1. Alpert SW, Koval KJ, Zuckerman JD: Neuropathic arthropathy: Review of current knowledge. J Am Acad Orthop Surg 4:100–108, 1996.
2. Beaty JH (ed): Orthopaedic Knowledge Update 6. Rosemont, IL, American Academy of Orthopaedic Surgery, 1999.
3. Dawson DM: Entrapment neuropathies of the upper extremities. N Engl J Med 329:2013–2018, 1993.
4. Greene WB (ed): Essentials of Musculoskeletal Care, 2nd ed. Rosemont, IL, American Academy of Orthopaedic Surgery, 2001.
5. Jobe FW, Ciccotti MG: Lateral and medial epicondylitis of the elbow. J Am Acad Orthop Surg 2:1–8, 1994.
6. Kasser JR (ed): Orthopaedic Knowledge Update 5 Home Study Syllabus. Rosemont, IL, American Academy of Orthopaedic Surgeons, 1996.
7. Leffert RD: Thoracic outlet syndrome. J Am Acad Orthop Surg 2:317–325, 1994.
8. Posner MA: Compressive ulnar neuropathies at the elbow: I Etiology and diagnosis. J Am Acad Orthop Surg 6:282–288, 1998.
9. Shaffer BS: Painful conditions of the acromioclavicular joint. J Am Acad Orthop Surg 7:176–188, 1999.
10. Warner JJ: Frozen shoulder: Diagnosis and management. J Am Acad Orthop Surg 5:130–140, 1997.

71. HAND PAIN

Richard C. Fisher, M.D.

1. What are the most common categories of atraumatic hand pain?

Referred pain from the shoulder or cervical spine
Overuse syndromes
Inflammatory conditions
Compression neuropathies
Arthritis

2. List the common compression neuropathies involving the forearm and hand.

1. Median nerve compression at the wrist (carpal tunnel syndrome)
2. Anterior interosseous syndrome (pain in the proximal forearm associated with weakness of thumb tip to index finger tip pinch)
3. Pronator syndrome (median nerve compression in the region of the pronator teres muscle)
4. Ulnar nerve compression at the wrist joint within Guyon's canal
5. Radial nerve compression at the wrist (Wartenberg's syndrome)

3. How is carpal tunnel syndrome diagnosed?

The classic history includes pain at night that is sufficient to wake the patient from sleep. Pain may be referred to the elbow and shoulder. In addition, the patient may have pain with repetitive hand use, a feeling of clumsiness, and numbness and tingling in the median nerve distribution on the radial side of the hand. Physical findings include decreased sensation in the thumb, index and long fingers, and half of the ring finger (with two-point discrimination > 5 mm); weakness of thumb opposition; dysesthesias with percussion of the median nerve at the wrist (Tinel's sign); reproduction of the carpal tunnel symptoms with acute flexion of the wrist (Phalen's sign); or direct median nerve compression at the wrist. Radiographs may show changes attributable to an old fracture or other lesion in the bone, but these are rare causes of carpal tunnel syndrome. Electrodiagnostic studies help to confirm the diagnosis by showing prolonged sensory and motor latency and decreased conduction velocity across the wrist.

4. List the general medical conditions that may be associated with carpal tunnel syndrome.

Hypothyroidism	Hemophilia
Rheumatoid arthritis	Pregnancy
Multiple myeloma and amyloidosis	Hemodialysis
Diabetes mellitus	

5. What is the best approach for treating carpal tunnel syndrome?

The primary treatment includes decrease in repetitive activities, workplace and workstyle modifications, night splints, and nonsteroidal anti-inflammatory drugs (NSAIDs). Injection of corticosteroids into the carpal canal is controversial but might be helpful if care is taken not to injure the median nerve. Surgical release of the transverse carpal ligament is necessary if neurologic deficit or pain persist after conservative treatment. Carpal tunnel syndrome associated with pregnancy usually resolves at term, so surgical treatment is not indicated.

6. What is reflex sympathetic dystrophy (RSD)?

RSD is characterized by pain, swelling, discoloration, and stiffness in the hand and distal forearm after trauma. The symptoms are usually out of proportion to those expected from the instigating trauma.

1. Pain may be of a cutting or searing nature, usually worsens with range of motion (ROM), and usually is felt with light touch.

2. Swelling usually is extensive in and about the hand and often spreads from the point of initiation to encompass the whole distal aspect of the extremity.

3. Discoloration often begins as redness accompanying the swelling, changes to a dusky color in secondary stages, and may become pale in the chronic stages.

4. Stiffness initially is caused by pain with attempted ROM, but as the fibrosis progresses, the joints become markedly limited in their ROM. The final stages may actually be painless despite marked limitations of function.

5. Osteoporosis is seen initially as spotty areas of demineralization and later progresses to involve the entire extremity.

7. Explain the relationship of the shoulder–hand syndrome to RSD.

The physical findings in both conditions are similar, but patients with shoulder–hand syndrome usually report a history of proximal trauma to the neck or shoulder region, chest injury, cervical spine disc disease, myocardial infarction, gastric ulcer, or Pancoast's tumor. The physical findings in shoulder–hand syndrome include tenderness and stiffness of the shoulder and elbow in addition to the hand symptoms in RSD.

8. What do de Quervain's syndrome and trigger fingers have in common?

Both hand abnormalities result from stenosing tenosynovitis. The two most commonly involved areas are the tendon sheaths of the abductor pollicis longus and extensor pollicis brevis (de Quervain's syndrome) and the flexor tendon sheaths in the palm (trigger finger syndrome).

De Quervain's syndrome is caused by a repetitive use of the hand, especially the thumb, and is characterized by mild swelling over the tendon sheath at the radial styloid as well as tenderness to palpation and pain with adduction of the thumb across the palm. Treatment consists of splinting, NSAIDs, injection of corticosteroids into the tendon sheath, or surgical release of the tendon sheath on the radial side of the wrist.

Trigger finger deformities involve a tendon nodule at the opening of the flexor sheath at about the level of the distal palmar crease. The nodule becomes entrapped either within or outside the tendon sheath and makes a snapping sensation accompanied by discomfort in the area of the nodule when the *involved finger* or thumb is flexed or extended. Treat initially with a splint and NSAIDs. Corticosteroid injection into the tendon sheath and surgical release of the sheath opening are indicated for persistent problems.

9. Describe the expected outcome after steroid injections for de Quervain's disease and trigger finger. What are the complications of such treatment?

Injection and immobilization of de Quervain's tenosynovitis show a success rate of about 60%. In trigger finger, the success rate is about 90%. The complications of steroid injection in this area include tendon ruptures, subcutaneous atrophy if injection is outside the sheaths and into the subcutaneous fat area, and loss of skin pigmentation if the steroid extravasates beneath the skin. Infection in the vicinity of the injection site is a contraindication to injection treatment.

10. Patterns of arthritic involvement of the joints of the hand are somewhat characteristic of the specific diagnosis. Name the regions commonly involved with osteoarthritis and rheumatoid arthritis.

Osteoarthritis involves the distal interphalangeal joints, predominantly with production of Heberden nodes or distal osteophytes. In addition, the first metacarpophalangeal (MCP) joint and the first carpometacarpal joint (Bennett's joint) of the thumb are common sites of degenerative change. Rheumatoid arthritis involves predominantly the proximal interphalangeal and metacarpophalangeal joints of the hand as well as the intracarpal joints at the wrist. Synovial hypertrophy is common at the wrist and digital joints, and late changes typically include swan-neck deformity and ulnar deviation at the MP joints.

11. What are the common causes of posttraumatic midwrist discomfort?

Several entities may follow minimal trauma to the wrist that may be overlooked initially but manifest at a later time. The most common is fracture of the scaphoid bone that has progressed to nonunion, often with avascular necrosis of the proximal fragments. If left untreated, it leads to late degenerative changes. Various syndromes of carpal instability that follow intercarpal ligament injury may cause diastasis of the carpal bones. The most common is scapholunate separation. Kienböck's disease (avascular necrosis of the lunate) follows trauma or a congenital discrepancy between the length of the radius and the ulna. Radiographic changes include irregular density of the lunate, often with collapse or change in shape of the bone. In addition, the most common location for ganglion cysts is the dorsal aspect of the wrist; these cysts can sometimes become painful because of impingement with the extensor tendons. A mass is usually palpable, and its size often changes in relation to activity.

12. Name the causes of ulnar wrist pain.

The most significant aspect of the ulnar side of the wrist involves the distal radial ulnar joint in association with the triangular fibrocartilage complex, which completes the articulation of the carpal bones at the wrist. Tears or abnormalities in this cartilaginous complex may lead to pain and a snapping sensation with use. Injuries may be traumatic, resulting in tears of either the ulnar or radial attachment or through the midsubstance of the cartilage plate. Degenerative tears of the cartilage result from adjacent carpal arthritis or instability. Begin treatment with rest, NSAIDs, and consultation with the occupational therapist. Carefully selected surgical treatment may be necessary. Other causes of pain include dislocation or arthritis of the distal radioulnar joint and tendinitis in an unstable extensor carpi ulnaris tendon.

13. A patient presents with swelling and pain about the index and long fingers after being bitten by a playful cat. How should the patient be treated? What are the likely organisms involved?

About 50% of cat bites become infected, and the most prevalent organism is *Pasteurella multocida,* although staphylococcus, streptococcus, and anaerobic organisms are also common. Lavage small or superficial wounds and begin antibiotics (oral amoxicillin, 500 mg twice a day for 5 days). If it is believed that the joint or tendon sheath has been perforated or the bone contaminated, surgical exploration and irrigation are indicated. Wounds should not be closed. Remember tetanus and rabies prophylaxis.

14. Describe the clinical presentation of common hand infections.

Infection usually follows some type of puncture injury and involves several characteristic locations. Perionychia often develops around the nail bed on the dorsal aspect of the digit. Volar infections may involve the closed space of the palmar side of the tip of the digit (felon), which becomes red, swollen, and exquisitely tender. Because of the many spaces in the hands, swelling of the palmar surface with tenderness is the first sign of a deep space infection. If the tendon sheath is involved, the finger is held in a moderately flexed position and becomes painful with attempted passive extension or active flexion. In addition, fullness and tenderness may be palpated in the distribution of the tendon sheath into the palm. Because of the lymph drainage pattern, the swelling secondary to infection eventually involves the dorsal aspect of the hand, although the primary focus of the infection is usually on the palmar surface. Prompt treatment is imperative and usually involves both antibiotics and surgical drainage.

15. Discuss the common tumors that involve the hand.

The common benign lesions include ganglion cysts, giant cell tumors of tendon sheaths, epidural inclusion cysts, and enchondromas. The first three are soft tissue lesions that are easily treatable with simple excision. Enchondromas occur most commonly within the bones of the phalanges, usually are not clinically symptomatic until the bone fractures through the cyst, and are most often diagnosed by incidental radiographs. Primary malignant musculoskeletal tumors or metastatic tumors of the hand, although not unknown, are extremely rare.

BIBLIOGRAPHY

1. Abrams RA, Botte MJ: Hand infections: Treatment recommendations for specific types. J Am Acad Orthop Surg 4:219–230, 1996.
2. Beaty JH (ed): Orthopaedic Knowledge Update 6. Rosemont, IL, American Academy of Orthopaedic Surgery, 1999.
3. Chidgey LK: The distal radioulnar joint: Problems and solutions. J Am Acad Orthop Surg 3:95–109, 1995.
4. Green WB (ed): Essentials of Musculoskeletal Care, 2nd ed. Rosemont, IL, American Academy of Orthopaedic Surgeons, 2001.
5. Idler RS (ed): The Hand: Examination and Diagnosis. New York, Churchill Livingstone, 1990.
6. Morgan WJ, Slowman LS: Acute Hand Injuries in Athletes: Evaluation and Management. J Am Acad Orthop Surg 9:389–400, 2001.
7. Szabo RM: Nerve entrapment syndromes in the wrist. J Am Acad Orthop Surg 2:115–123, 1994.

72. FOOT CARE

Stephen F. Albert, D.P.M., C.Ped.

1. What are the three most common foot problems in the United States?

Based on the 1990 National Health Interview Survey, ingrown nails and other toenail problems, foot infections, and corns and calluses are the three most common foot problems. Each of these problems troubles more than 11 million civilian, noninstitutionalized Americans.

Incidence of Foot Problems in the United States, 1990

PROBLEM	NUMBER IN MILLIONS
Ingrown nails or other toenail problems	11.3
Foot infection, including tinea and warts	11.3
Corns and calluses	11.2
Foot injury	5.6
Flat feet	4.6
Bunions	4.4
Arthritis of toes	3.9
Toes and joint problems	2.5
Bone spurs	0.95
Nerve damage to foot	0.23
Clubfoot	0.16
Others	2.7

2. What are the chances of success when an ingrown nail is treated by avulsion only?

At 1-year follow-up the success rate is poor. Ingrown toenails most commonly affect the great toes, but any digit may be involved. Although the condition may occur in either sex and at any age, it is seen most frequently in boys and young men. A prospective British study randomized 163 patients with ingrown nails into three groups: total nail avulsion, nail edge excision, and nail edge excision with chemical cautery (phenolization) of the germinal nail matrix. The recurrence rates at 1 year were 73%, 73%, and 9%, respectively. Phenolization of the germinal nail matrix can be performed by primary care practitioners, but the technique requires attention to procedural details. Underapplication of phenol may result in a greater than expected rate of recurrence, whereas overapplication may result in a persistent draining periungual wound that is prone to infection.

3. Why is foot care important to patients with diabetes mellitus?

Twenty-five percent of patients with diabetes develop related foot problems. Foot ulcers and amputation rank high among the many disabling complications of diabetes. Multiple foot problems may quickly progress to a critical point; without immediate and definite measures, amputation may soon follow. Of all nontraumatic amputations, 50–70% occur in patients with diabetes. Although the precise location and number of amputations are unknown, it is estimated that 56,000 per year involve the foot and leg.

4. Which factors contribute to amputations in diabetics?

Infection and gangrene are common causes of diabetic amputations. Contributing causes include minor trauma, cutaneous ulceration, and failure of wound healing. All of these factors are exacerbated by the nearly universal occurrence in diabetics of peripheral neuropathy (motor, sensory, and autonomic), peripheral arterial disease, and mechanical dysfunction in the lower extremities.

5. Plantar calluses and plantar warts are often confused. How do clinicians differentiate between the two?

Warts (verruca plantaris) result from viral infection, whereas a plantar callus (also called tyloma or plantar keratoma) is a dermal response to the vertical and shear forces of standing and walking on a foot with mechanical dysfunction, osseous plantar prominences, or a thinned plantar fat pad. Both are painful, visible skin lesions that are exacerbated by weight bearing.

Warts may be solitary with a clearly circumscribed border or mosaic with a patchy and irregular border. They have a rough surface with hypertrophic papillae and are tender with side-to-side squeezing. Individual papillae may become darkly colored from capillary hemorrhage secondary to standing and walking. Plantar warts are surrounded and covered by keratotic tissue. They may or may not be associated with an osseous plantar prominence. After paring, a "cauliflower" center is visible, the patient experiences pain, and pinpoint capillary hemorrhages readily appear.

Initial management of discrete plantar warts most commonly involves patient application of 40% salicylic acid plasters every 2–3 days after removal of overlying hyperkeratosis. Removal of macerated hyperkeratosis is best accomplished if the patient soaks the foot for 5 minutes in water and then uses an emory board or pumice stone only on the treated area, avoiding the surrounding skin. Salicylic acid paint (10%) with lactic acid (10%) in flexible collodion may be used for mosaic warts or warts that coalesce over larger areas. The paint is commonly applied once daily and, again, is most effective if the macerated hyperkeratotic tissue is removed. Caution is advised when using salicylic acid at this concentration in patients with neuropathy and peripheral vascular disease. Physicians should supervise closely the use of any caustic agents for verruca.

Plantar callus presents as a hyperkeratotic mass at a site of friction or pressure. The lesion consists of raised, often clear, compressed layers of stratum corneum without a definite border. The more severe lesions may be pared below the level of the surrounding skin without pain or pinpoint capillary hemorrhage. Calluses are commonly managed by periodic paring of the hyperkeratosis and use of cushioning innersoles or foot orthoses to alleviate mechanical dysfunction and to accommodate osseous plantar prominences and thinned plantar fat pads.

6. What advice about foot care should be given to vascularly impaired or diabetic patients?

1. Wash and inspect the feet daily.
2. Use foot creams or lubricating oils, except in toe webs.
3. Cut toenails straight; do not bevel the sides.
4. Do not attempt to cut corns or calluses.
5. Avoid self-medication and extreme temperatures.
6. Do not walk barefooted.
7. Wear appropriate shoes and inspect the insides daily.
8. Seek early medical care for all skin lesions.
9. Do not delay medical care for abrupt foot swelling.

7. What guidelines assist patients in attaining properly fitting shoes?

Properly fitting shoes are necessary to avoid aggravating or precipitating foot problems. A recent study of 356 women aged 20–60 years found that 88% wore improperly fitting shoes. Proper fit implies correct shape and size. The shape of the foot and shoe should match. Both feet should be measured. Size should be assessed while the patient stands in both shoes; there should be approximately 1 cm between the tip of the longest toe and the distal aspect of the shoe, the metatarsal heads should be in the widest part of the shoe (particularly the first metatarsal), and the heel should have a snug fit. In feet with high insteps (pes cavus), laces are preferred. For feet subject to edema, shoes should be purchased later in the day. It is important to be aware that shoe size tends to increase with age.

8. What medical diseases are commonly associated with foot deformity?
Diabetes mellitus, rheumatoid arthritis, and gout.

9. How often does rheumatoid arthritis affect the feet?
Rheumatoid arthritis involves the feet in > 50% of patients. Patients commonly present with hallux valgus, hallux varus, hallux rigidus, hammertoes, fibular deviation at the metatarsopha- langeal joints, or rheumatoid nodules (or a combination of these symptoms). The distribution is symmetric, particularly at the distal metatarsals, with warmth, tenderness, and edema. The metatarsal heads often become plantarly prominent as the nonfunctional joints develop mechan- ical adaptations, including dislocation of the digits and displacement of the plantar fat pad. Ra- diographs show demineralization at the ends of the metatarsals, with joint space narrowing, ar- ticular erosions, soft-tissue edema, joint malalignment, and eventually subluxation. Women are affected more commonly than men.

10. What condition should be suspected in a normal-appearing foot with lateral forefoot pain, a joint of maximal tenderness at the third intermetatarsal space, normal radiographs, and negative laboratory test results?
Intermetatarsal neuroma, also known as Morton's neuroma, is often a diagnostic challenge. Foot radiographs, ultrasound, nerve conduction velocity, magnetic resonance imaging, clinical laboratory tests, and visual appearance of the foot usually reveal nothing out of the ordinary. The diagnosis is made through history and examination of the foot. The patient commonly indicates a sharp, lancinating, radiating pain in the lateral forefoot that is relieved by removal of the shoe and massage. Palpation or squeezing of the affected intermetatarsal interspace and numbness or burning in the associated toes are common features.

A neuroma of the foot is an irritative process of the common digital nerve that supplies the plantar aspect of adjacent toes. The term *neuroma* is a misnomer because the entity does not demonstrate neoplastic growth of nerve tissue or fibers; instead, histopathology reveals degener- ative changes with perineural fibrosis. Repetitive microtrauma or constriction is the presumed un- derlying causes. Intermetatarsal neuroma occurs in all adult age groups and affects women nine times more frequently than men. The third intermetatarsal interspace is most often involved. Con- servative measures include steroid or local anesthetic injection, accommodative padding to sep- arate the metatarsal heads, physical therapy, or orthotics. Neurectomy of the affected area is the treatment of choice; the rate of patient satisfaction is reported to be 93%.

11. Which patients should be referred to podiatrists routinely and acutely?
Podiatrists treat the full spectrum of foot problems. They excel in treating the chronic recur- ring foot problems that tend to increase as people age, particularly when periodic care is required, when prior interventions by a primary care provider have not been successful, or when the diag- nosis is unclear. Of the acute presenting foot conditions, by far the most potentially devastating are infections in diabetic, immunocompromised, or vascularly compromised patients. Primary care providers should be aware that podiatrists' educational credentials, interests, and expertise vary. In general, hospital-affiliated, residency-trained, board-certified podiatrists are better pre- pared to deal adeptly with acute conditions.

12. What is the likelihood that osteomyelitis underlies a diabetic foot ulcer when the ulcer does not appear inflamed?
In one study, as many as two thirds of 12 patients had clinically unsuspected osteomyelitis. Many practitioners believe that the radionuclide spatial resolution among the numerous bones and joints of the foot is inadequate and that none of the imaging modalities are entirely specific for osteomyelitis. Many advances in imaging modalities since 1993 allow more accurate diagnosis of osteomyelitis. The use of TC-99 hexamethyl propyleneamine (HMPAO)–labeled leukocyte scan (Ceretec) and magnetic resonance imaging are superior to prior techniques. No matter what

imaging modality is used, it is quite difficult to differentiate foot osteomyelitis in diabetics from diabetic osteopathy or osteoarthropathy (Charcot foot).

13. Injections into the foot are often painful for patients. What methods can be used to decrease patient discomfort, excluding systemic medication?

The addition of 6.25% sodium bicarbonate to lidocaine in local anesthesia of the foot decreased pain by 50% in a double-blind study. Adjunctive use of skin refrigerant further decreases the pain involved in the initial needle stick.

14. What is the significance of a normal white blood cell (WBC) count in a suspected diabetic foot infection?

The diagnosis of diabetic foot infections are made primarily on the basis of clinical signs and symptoms. A study completed by Armstrong et al. found that in patients with active foot infections, 56% had WBC counts within normal limits. Therefore, a WBC count should be used as an adjunctive test in the diagnosis of diabetic foot infections.

15. What are the clinical manifestations of plantar fasciitis?

Sharp pain, aching, or stiffness at the plantar or plantar medial aspect of one or both heels. The pain is often at its worst upon arising in the morning or after sitting down for an extended period and then resuming activity, creating hobbling or limping for a few minutes before comfortable walking can be resumed. In periods of exacerbation during walking or standing, moderate or severe pain may persist. Palpation of a point of maximal tenderness at the medial plantar calcaneal tubercle is quite common. Dorsiflexion of the foot followed by dorsiflexion of the toes stretches the plantar fascia and usually elicits symptoms.

16. What is the role of night splints and shoe modifications in the treatment of plantar fasciitis?

Several investigators have stated that the use of night splints and shoe modifications is a viable alternative to foot orthotics in the therapy of plantar fasciitis. The use of night splints is often a complicated treatment modality. The night splint device is cumbersome in application and use. The theory that plantar fascial pain is the result of contractures and muscle tightening while sleeping is controversial. The concept behind the night splints is to prevent the plantar fascia from contracting. This theory does not explain the common presentation of increased pain upon activity and relief during rest. Studies show, however, that the use of a functional orthotic for ≤ 3 months relieved the symptoms of plantar fasciitis in 90–95% of patients.

17. Do older people with a history of multiple falls exhibit greater foot impairment than their peers who have fallen only once or not at all?

A cross-sectional, retrospective study from Sydney, Australia, seems to assert so. Investigators studied the relationship among foot problems, balance, and functional ability in community-dwelling older people to determine whether older people with a history of multiple falls exhibit greater foot impairment than those who have not fallen or who have fallen once only. A total of 135 community-dwelling men and women aged 75–93 years (mean age $\pm$ standard deviation, 79.8 $\pm$ 4.1) were studied. A foot problem score was determined from the following: postural sway; coordinated stability; stair ascent and descent; an alternate stepping test; timed 6-m walk; and tests of vision, sensation, strength, and reaction time. The results revealed that 87% of the sample had at least one foot problem. Women had a significantly higher foot problem score than did men. The foot problem score was significantly associated with performance on the coordinated stability test, stair ascent and descent, alternate stepping test, and timed 6-m walk. Multiple regression analyses revealed that the foot problem score was a significant independent predictor of performance in the coordinated stability test, stair ascent and descent, and alternate stepping test. Subjects with a history of multiple falls had a significantly higher foot problem score than did those who had not fallen or who had fallen once only, but the prevalence of individual foot conditions or the presence of foot pain did not differ between these groups. In conclusion, foot problems are common in older people and are associated with impaired balance and performance in functional tests. Furthermore, older people with a history of multiple falls have greater foot impairment than once-only or non-fallers. These findings provide further evidence that foot problems are a falls risk factor and suggest that the cumulative effect of multiple foot problems is more important in increasing falls risk than the presence or absence of individual foot conditions.

18. Which plays a greater role in plantar fascial heel pain, body mass index (BMI) or foot structure?

BMI appears to play a greater role in heel pain than does foot structure. A prospective, descriptive study was performed at Oakwood Healthcare medical clinics by Rano et al. to determine the BMI of patients with heel pain and of a control group of patients presenting for other reasons. A questionnaire was used to obtain information in each of the patient groups and to determine the characteristics of patients with plantar fascial heel pain. Standard weight-bearing lateral radiographs were taken to determine overall foot structure. Although height was comparable, patients with heel pain had a higher BMI (30.4 ± 0.7) than those without heel pain ($28.2 \pm 0.7, P = 0.04$). Control patients also reported a higher level of activity. Fifty-one percent exercised three or more times per week for more than 20 minutes each time, but $< 50\%$ that (25.4%) of heel pain patients did so. Whereas, 50% of the heel pain patients had been treated by other providers before visiting the clinic, $< 25\%$ of these patients had been instructed to lose weight by a physician. The authors believe that a BMI of 25 (the target for decreased cardiovascular risk) represents a reasonable goal for weight loss that may reduce heel pain.

19. What is the most effective topical agent that could be used as an alternative to oral antifungal therapy for onychomycosis?

Topical ciclopirox solution 8% (Penlac nail lacquer) has no known drug interactions, requires no laboratory monitoring, and is the first topical prescription approved by the Food and Drug Administration for treatment of onychomycosis. It is indicated for mild to moderate onychomycosis, and studies show it is not equally effective as the oral agents. The ability to apply the lacquer daily (it goes on like nail polish) and remove buildup are important aspects of prescribing this medication.

BIBLIOGRAPHY

1. American College of Foot Surgeons: Ingrown Toenail: Preferred Practice Guidelines. Park Ridge, IL, American College of Foot Surgeons, 1991.
2. Armstrong D, Perales T, Murff R, et al: Value of white blood cell count with differential in the acute diabetic foot infection. J Am Podiatr Med Assoc 86:224–227, 1996.
3. Awbrey BJ, Bernardone JJ, Connoly TJ: Prospective Evaluation of Invasive and Noninvasive Treatment Protocols for Plantar Fasciitis. Rehabilitation R & D Progress Report. Baltimore, Department of Veterans Affairs, 1989.
4. Bild DE, Selby JV, Sinnock P, et al: Lower extremity amputation in people with diabetes: Epidemiology and prevention. Diabetes Care 12:24–31, 1989.
5. Blume P, Dey H, Daley L: Diagnosis of pedal osteomyelitis with Tc-99M HMPAO labeled leukocytes. J Foot Ankle Surg 36:120–126, 1997.
6. Boulton AJM: The diabetic foot. Med Clin North Am 72:1513–1530, 1988.
7. Cicchinelli LD, Corey SV: Imaging of the infected foot: Fact or fancy? J Am Podiatr Med Assoc 83:10, 1993.
8. Frey C, Thompson F, Smith J, et al: American Orthopedic Foot and Ankle Society women's shoe survey. Foot Ankle 14:2, 1993.
9. Friedman H, Jules K, Springer K, Jennings M: Buffered lidocaine decreases the pain of digital anesthesia in the foot. J Am Podiatr Med Assoc 87:219–223, 1997.
10. Greenberg L, Davis H: Foot problems in the US: The 1990 National Health Interview Survey. J Am Podiatr Med Assoc 83:475–483, 1993.
11. Grieg JD, Anderson JH, Ireland AJ, Anderson JR: The surgical treatment of ingrowing toenails. J Bone Joint Surg 73B:121–133, 1991.

12. Janisse DJ: The art and science of fitting shoes. Foot Ankle 13:257–262, 1992.
13. Keh RA, Ballew KK, Higgins KR, et al: Long-term follow-up of Morton's neuroma. J Foot Surg 31:93–95, 1992.
14. Krupski WC: Growth factors and wound healing. Semin Vasc Surg 5:249, 1992.
15. Luskin R, Battista A: Peripheral neuropathies affecting the foot. In Jahss M (ed): Disorders of the Foot and Ankle, vol. 3, 2nd ed. Philadelphia, W.B. Saunders, 1991, p 2122.
16. Menz HB, Lord SR: The contribution of foot problems to mobility impairment and falls in community-dwelling older people. J Am Geriatr Soc 49:1651–1656, 2001.
17. Miller S: Morton's neuroma: A syndrome. In McGlamry D, Banks A, Downey M (eds): Comprehensive Textbook of Foot Surgery, vol. 1. Baltimore, Williams & Wilkins, 1992, pp 309–311.
18. Patton JP, Murdoch DP, Lindsey J, Young G: Rheumatoid arthritic foot: Two manifestations with case studies. J Am Podiatr Med Assoc 83:270–275, 1993.
19. Pecoraro RE, Reiber GE, Burgess EM: Pathways to diabetic limb amputation. Basis for prevention. Diabetes Care 13:513–521, 1990.
20. Rano JA, Fallat LM, Savoy-Moore RT: Correlation of heel pain with body mass index and other characteristics of heel pain. J Foot Ankle Surg 40:351–356, 2001.
21. Rogoff R, Tinkle J, Bartis D: Unusual presentation of calcaneal osteomyelitis. J Am Podiatr Med Assoc 87:125–130, 1997.
22. Schauwecker DS: The scintigraphic diagnosis of osteomyelitis. Am J Roentgenol 158:9–18, 1992.
23. Sussman KE, Reiber G, Albert SF: The diabetic foot problem—a failed system of health care? Diabetes Res Clin Pract 17:1–8, 1992.
24. Wapner K, Sharkey P: The use of night splints for treatment of recalcitrant plantar fasciitis. Foot Ankle 12:135–137, 1991.

73. FIBROMYALGIA AND RELATED SYNDROMES

Olga Dvorkina, M.D., and Danny C. Williams, M.D.

1. Define soft-tissue rheumatism.

The term *soft-tissue rheumatism* (i.e., nonarticular rheumatism) defines a heterogeneous group of common ailments that affect musculoskeletal structures other than the joints. Symptoms may arise from the muscles, tendons, ligaments and their bony insertion sites (entheses), or bursae. Pain and functional loss are usually attributed to inflammation but may occur in its absence. Soft-tissue disorders are categorized according to their distribution: focal (e.g., bursitis, tendinitis), regional (e.g., myofascial pain syndrome), or diffuse (e.g., fibromyalgia, chronic fatigue syndrome).

2. What is fibromyalgia?

Fibromyalgia is a chronic, generalized musculoskeletal pain syndrome of unknown etiology. Fibromyalgia is not a disease but a distinct, chronic pain syndrome characterized by multiple somatic symptoms and widespread muscle tenderness. The term *fibromyalgia* is preferred over *fibrositis,* the syndrome's previous designation, which erroneously implies an inflammatory disorder. In the clinical setting, fibromyalgia simply identifies a patient population that exhibits similar symptoms and signs.

3. Who develops fibromyalgia?

Fibromyalgia is predominantly a disorder of middle-aged women (80–90%). Although peak age of onset is 35–50 years, fibromyalgia may occur in anyone, including children (usually adolescents) and elderly people. The prevalence of fibromyalgia is estimated to be 2% in the general population. Familial aggregation has been reported, suggesting the possibility of genetic predisposition.

4. In what settings may fibromyalgia be seen?

Fibromyalgia may develop at any time, either spontaneously or in relation to a stressful life event, such as a flulike illness, whiplash injury, or divorce. Despite temporal association of precipitating events with fibromyalgia inception, no evidence of a causal relationship has been demonstrated. Fibromyalgia may also be seen in patients with established, chronic illnesses such as rheumatoid arthritis, alcoholism, and AIDS. Up to 25% of patients with rheumatoid arthritis, systemic lupus erythematosus (SLE), or ankylosing spondylitis meet American College of Rheumatology (ACR) criteria for fibromyalgia. In patients with chronic diseases (e.g., SLE), careful evaluation for fibromyalgia may prevent unwarranted therapeutic alterations (e.g., prescribing corticosteroids) for symptoms actually attributable to the chronic pain syndrome.

5. Describe the clinical features of fibromyalgia.

The essential features of fibromyalgia are diffuse subjective pain and physically demonstrable areas of muscle tenderness (i.e., tender points). Profound fatigue, nonrestorative sleep, and diffuse stiffness are also major manifestations. Other associated symptoms include headaches (tension or migraine), dizziness, sicca, atypical chest pain, irritable bowel syndrome, irritable bladder, arthralgias with subjective joint swelling, restless leg syndrome, nondermatomal paresthesias, cognitive dysfunction, and depression. Raynaud's phenomenon with cold intolerance and mitral valve prolapse is common. Symptoms may be exacerbated by factors such as physical and mental stress, weather changes, inactivity, repetitive exercise, and poor sleep.

6. What are tender points?

Aside from a nonspecific, alpha electroencephalogram (EEG) sleep anomaly, multiple tender points are the only physical finding in patients with fibromyalgia. Tender points are discrete areas (2–3 cm in diameter) of normal-appearing skin at which application of digital pressure elicits focal pain. Adequate pressure is the pressure required to blanche the thumbnail (4 kg/cm^2). Palpation of a tender point should generate pain and frequently causes a sudden withdrawal response, called the "jump sign." Control points (e.g., central forehead, anterior mid-thigh, and thumbnail) are used to differentiate fibromyalgia from somatoform disorders and malingering.

7. How does myofascial pain differ from fibromyalgia?

Myofascial pain differs from the diffuse pain of fibromyalgia by being localized to a specific region, usually a single muscle or closely related muscle group (e.g., temporomandibular joint syndrome). Trigger points, which are typical of myofascial pain syndromes, consist of palpable abnormalities (taut band or thickened nodule) usually found in the bellies of traumatized muscles. Palpation of a trigger point produces local tenderness and, unlike palpation of tender points, generates referred pain throughout the involved muscle or muscle group. In general, tender points should not be equated with trigger points, but they may coexist in the same patient.

8. How is fibromyalgia diagnosed?

The clinical diagnosis of fibromyalgia is based on the 1990 ACR classification criteria. A patient is classified as having fibromyalgia if both of the following criteria are present.

1. Widespread pain for ≥ 3 months affecting all four body quadrants and the axial skeleton
2. Palpable, subjective pain in 11 of the following 9 pairs of tender points (see figure):

Occipital	Lateral epicondyle (2 cm distally)
Low cervical (posterolateral C5–C7)	Gluteal (upper, lateral quadrant)
Trapezius (mid, upper fold)	Greater trochanter (2 cm posteriorly)
Supraspinatus (origin)	Knee (medial fat pad)
Second rib (costochondral junction)	

Note the following pearls:

- Palpate one tender point at a time.
- Palpate with sufficient pressure to blanch the nail bed.

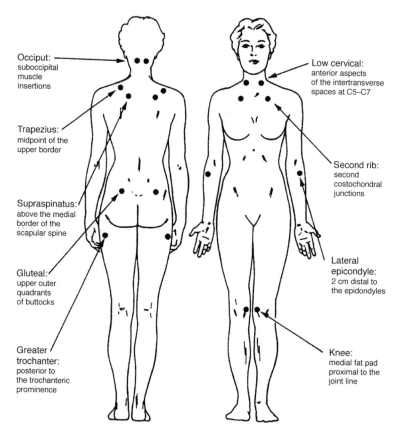

Occiput:
suboccipital
muscle
insertions

Low cervical:
anterior aspects
of the intertransverse
spaces at C5–C7

Trapezius:
midpoint of the
upper border

Supraspinatus:
above the medial
border of the
scapular spine

Second rib:
second
costochondral
junctions

Gluteal:
upper outer
quadrants
of buttocks

Lateral
epicondyle:
2 cm distal to
the epidondyles

Greater
trochanter:
posterior to
the trochanteric
prominence

Knee:
medial fat pad
proximal to the
joint line

The tender points of fibromyalgia. (From Freundlich B, Leventhal L: The fibromyalgia syndrome. In Schumacher HR Jr, Klippel JH, Koopman WJ (eds): Primer on the Rheumatic Diseases, 10th ed. Atlanta, Arthritis Foundation, 1993, pp 247–249; with permission.)

- Because most of the tender points appear at articulation sites, locate a tender point at the posterior midcalf to convince the patient that he or she has a muscle pain syndrome rather than arthritis.

9. In a setting of generalized chronic pain syndrome, what other treatable conditions need to be ruled out? What is the differential diagnosis of fibromyalgia?

Many systemic illnesses may present with the clinical features of fibromyalgia. Likewise, fibromyalgia may mimic many systemic diseases; however, as a clinical entity, fibromyalgia is not a systemic disorder. There are no consistent physical or laboratory abnormalities in patients with fibromyalgia. Therefore, evidence of inflammation or systemic disease suggests diagnoses other than fibromyalgia. The following select disorders may share features with fibromyalgia:

- Rheumatoid arthritis (early)
- Spondyloarthritis (early)
- SLE
- Sjögren's syndrome
- Polymyositis
- Polymyalgia rheumatica
- Giant cell arteritis
- Generalized osteoarthritis
- Drug-induced myopathy
- Chronic fatigue syndrome (CFS)
- Myofascial pain syndrome
- Paraneoplastic disorders
- Hyper- or hypothyroidism
- Hyper- or hypoparathyroidism
- Viral infections
- Metastatic cancer
- Somatoform disorders or depression

The most commonly occurring conditions are hypothyroidism, medication use (especially lipid-lowering drugs and antiviral agents), polymyalgia rheumatica, hepatitis C, sleep apnea, parvovirus infection, cervical stenosis or Chiari malformation, and somatoform disorders or depression. The less common conditions are autoimmune disorders (e.g., SLE; rheumatoid arthritis, especially early in the course of disease), endocrine disorders (e.g., Addison's disease, Cushing's syndrome, hyperparathyroidism), Lyme disease, eosinophilia-myalgia syndrome, tapering of corticosteroids, and malignancy.

Caution: Fibromyalgia is not a diagnosis of exclusion because it also may occur in patients with systemic disease.

10. What laboratory screening tests are useful in helping to rule out treatable conditions in the diagnosis of fibromyalgia?

In patients with fibromyalgia alone, laboratory investigations and imaging study results are typically normal. Thus, screening tests are performed to determine whether a systemic disease (see above) is generating fibromyalgia-like symptoms. The following investigations are useful in the diagnosis of fibromyalgia:

Essential	Optional (select patients)
Complete blood count and differential	C-reactive protein
Erythrocyte sedimentation rate	Rheumatoid factor
Serum electrolytes, creatinine	Antinuclear antibody
Serum calcium, phosphate, magnesium	Hepatitis profile
Liver function tests	Serum protein electrophoresis
Creatine phosphokinase	Radiographs
Urinalysis	Bone scan
Thyroid-stimulating hormone	

Note: Formal neuropsychological testing may be appropriate in select patients to exclude subtle organic brain dysfunction.

11. What is known about the pathophysiology of fibromyalgia? Is polysomnography useful in the diagnosis of fibromyalgia?

It is increasingly evident that the primary abnormality is caused by changes in the central nervous system, leading to exaggerated pain perception—the so-called central sensitization. Several studies have demonstrated elevated levels of substance P and nerve growth factor in the cerebrospinal fluid of fibromyalgia patients compared with control subjects. Sleep disturbance is common in fibromyalgia (75%), and some patients exhibit EEG alterations during polysomnography testing. A distinct pattern, the alpha EEG sleep anomaly, is observed and appears to be associated with nonrestorative sleep, pain, and fatigue. It represents intrusion of an arousal state pattern (alpha rhythm) onto the nonrapid eye movement (NREM) patterns of restorative sleep. The alpha EEG sleep anomaly is not a consistent or specific finding among patients with fibromyalgia; it has also been demonstrated in other disorders and in asymptomatic, normal people. Thus, polysomnography should not be used in the evaluation of fibromyalgia unless symptoms of sleep apnea or narcolepsy are reported. It also has been suggested that fibromyalgia patients have reduced hypothalamic-pituitary axis responsiveness as well as diminished levels of growth hormone. Many patients with fibromyalgia demonstrate abnormalities of autonomic function and low baseline sympathetic tone. No specific pathology in the muscles of fibromyalgia patients has been demonstrated thus far.

12. Describe the nonpharmacologic management of patients with fibromyalgia.

Reassurance is a major therapeutic tool for patients with fibromyalgia. Many patients suspect that their symptoms are the result of occult malignancy, crippling arthritis, or an emotional disturbance or aberrant psyche. The latter suspicion is usually reinforced by the patient's family, friends, or physician. Simply providing a diagnosis may be therapeutic. Local measures such as heat packs, gentle massage, gentle stretching exercises, and avoidance of cold may provide temporary relief. The best therapeutic intervention at present is the adoption of a graduated (progressing over 4–6 months) aerobic exercise program. The goal is to perform low-impact, aerobic activity so that patients exercise 3 times/week, 30 minutes each session, and at 70% of their maximal heart rate. Aquatic aerobics, stationary bicycle riding, and brisk walking seem to be most effective. Older patients or patients with cardiac risk factors may warrant an initial exercise treadmill test to determine exercise tolerance. Other potentially helpful modalities include fibromyalgia self-help groups, biofeedback, stress reduction exercises, vapocoolant spray and stretch techniques, and acupuncture.

Pearl: A useful analogy is the "pain thermostat." It is important to explain to the patient that during the development of fibromyalgia, the "pain thermostat" in the brain has been reset so that even mild, external stimuli are abnormally perceived as painful. A routine exercise program serves to reset the pain thermostat threshold to normal limits. The key to the fibromyalgia exercise program is that the patient must progress in minute increments with reasonable goals, akin to losing weight. Too aggressive a program causes postexercise flareups and subsequent avoidance of exercise.

13. Is pharmacologic management of patients with fibromyalgia effective?

The pharmacologic management of patients with fibromyalgia assumes a trial-and-error approach because there is no consistent underlying abnormality, symptoms are typically heterogeneous, and individual response is variable. Medical therapy should be tailored to the individual in an effort to relieve specific symptoms that may perpetuate the fibromyalgia condition. Examples include disturbed sleep, anxiety, depression, muscle spasms, restless leg syndrome, and stiffness. Pharmacologic management should be directed toward functional improvement rather than eradication of the chronic pain, which may be unrealistic. Functional improvement may foster participation and compliance with an exercise program (see above). The following medications may be effective in some patients with fibromyalgia:

Analgesics	Hypnotics	Antidepressants
Acetaminophen	Antihistamines	Tricyclics
Aspirin	Zolpidem	Serotonin reuptake inhibitors
NSAIDs	Melatonin	**Local therapy**
Tramadol	Antidepressants	Tender point injection
Muscle relaxants	Tranquilizers	
Anticonvulsants	Topical capsaicin	

Analgesics and muscle relaxants provide variable relief from the symptoms of fibromyalgia. Narcotics and benzodiazepine derivatives may exacerbate symptoms and are not recommended for patients who exhibit the potential for chronic pain. Systemic steroids have no role in the treatment of fibromyalgia. A trial of nonsteroidal anti-inflammatory drugs (NSAIDs) is warranted in most patients, but the response is variable and may result only in improved stiffness.

Pharmacologic therapy for fibromyalgia is directed primarily at improving the quality of restorative sleep with low doses of cyclobenzaprine (10–30 mg) or amitriptyline (10–50 mg) administered 2–3 hours before bedtime. If these agents are unsuccessful, other antidepressants may be used in successive trial-and-error fashion. A novel nonbenzodiazepine hypnotic, zolpidem (5–10 mg taken at bedtime), may improve sleep quality in some patients. For the restless leg syndrome, dopacarbidopa and new dopa agonists may be useful. In people with symptoms of autonomic dysfunction, low doses of beta-blockers may be helpful, as can increased fluid and sodium intake.

Tender point injection with local anesthetics with or without corticosteroids may be effective in select patients, especially if one or two tender points seem more painful than the rest. Knowing which tender points to inject is the usual dilemma.

Pearl: Fibromyalgia is not amenable to pharmacologic therapy alone. The ideal therapeutic program uses a multidisciplinary approach with education, cardiovascular fitness training, cognitive behavioral therapy, and pharmacologic treatment.

14. What is the relationship of fibromyalgia to pregnancy?

No controlled studies of fibromyalgia in pregnancy have been done so far. However, it is suggested that pregnancy may worsen the symptoms of fibromyalgia, especially in the third trimester. Pharmacologic treatment of symptoms related to fibromyalgia should be reviewed carefully for possible teratogenic effect. Women with fibromyalgia have a higher risk of postpartum depression.

15. What is the prognosis for patients with fibromyalgia?

The few long-term outcome studies suggest that prognosis in fibromyalgia depends on the population studied. For example, patients in community clinics fare better than patients at tertiary care centers. The prognosis for children (73% remission at 30 months) is better than for adults (24% remission at 24 months in community clinics). Overall, most adults continue to have chronic symptoms, regardless of treatment. Over a period of years, a patient's symptoms can shift considerably from musculoskeletal concerns to fatigue, headaches, or irritable bowel syndrome. Remissions are uncommon, but symptoms tend to improve with time. No evidence suggests that fibromyalgia evolves into systemic disease.

16. Are fibromyalgia and CFS the same disorder?

Considerable overlap exists between CFS and fibromyalgia if patient demographics and clinical features are compared. The greatest difference lies in their diagnostic criteria, not in the patients. The 1994 Centers for Disease Control and Prevention (CDC) case definition of CFS requires the presence of chronic fatigue ($\geq$ 6 months) and four of the following symptoms ($\geq$ 6 months): impaired memory or concentration, sore throat, tender cervical or axillary lymph nodes, muscle pain, multijoint pain, new headaches, unrefreshing sleep, and postexertion malaise. In contrast to the fibromyalgia classification criteria, there are no physical criteria for CFS in the CDC case definition. Nonetheless, 70% of patients with CFS have tender points. Likewise, 90% of patients with fibromyalgia have fatigue. Because of their clinical similarity, these syndromes are perhaps different manifestations of the same disorder.

Note: No data indicate that a persistent infection (e.g., Epstein-Barr virus) is responsible for CFS or fibromyalgia.

17. Is fibromyalgia a psychological disorder?

It is unlikely that fibromyalgia represents a pure psychological disorder. In tertiary care centers, only 30–35% of patients with fibromyalgia exhibit psychological problems such as increased mental stress, anxiety, or depression. Furthermore, some patients respond to subtherapeutic doses of antidepressants, whereas others have no improvement at all, despite full therapeutic doses. With little evidence for the biomedical model (true tissue pathology) to explain fibromyalgia, attention has been directed to the psychosocial model. This model attempts to relate altered pain perception, sleep disturbance, fatigue, psychological distress, and other symptoms to subtle changes in the neuroendocrine, immune, and psychological systems. The evolving paradigm categorizes fibromyalgia as one of several **affective spectrum disorders,** which share a common but unknown etiology. Examples include fibromyalgia, CFS, migraine headache, irritable bowel syndrome, and major depression.

18. Should patients with fibromyalgia receive disability compensation?

Disability compensation for fibromyalgia remains a controversial issue, even though initial consensus guidelines have been established. Most of the controversy stems from an inability to measure objectively the impact of a patient's self-reported symptoms. Another contested issue is whether trauma (i.e., motor vehicle accident) can *cause* fibromyalgia. To date, no studies demonstrate that fibromyalgia can be directly induced by trauma. Symptom severity may be best determined by a combination of health status instruments (e.g., Health Assessment Questionnaire), visual analog scales, psychological testing, and formal functional or work capacity assessments. Tender points, the only objective finding, do not correlate with symptom severity. It is estimated that 10–15% of patients with fibromyalgia have functional impairment severe enough to merit disability; however, the majority of patients are able to work productively despite their symptoms. Seeking disability compensation has been shown to affect outcome adversely.

BIBLIOGRAPHY

1. Bennet RM: Fibromyalgia and the facts: Sense or nonsense. Rheum Dis Clin North Am 19:45–59, 1993.
2. Bennet RM: The fibromyalgia syndrome. In Kelley WN, Harris ED Jr, Ruddy S, Sledge CB (eds): Textbook of Rheumatology, 5th ed. Philadelphia, W.B. Saunders, 1997, pp 511–519.
3. Bennet RM: The rational management of fibromyalgia patients. Rheum Dis Clin North Am 28:181–189, 2002.
4. Clauw DJ: Fibromyalgia and diffuse pain syndromes. In Primer on the Rheumatic Diseases, 12th ed. Atlanta, Arthritis Foundation, 2001, pp 188–193.
5. Fukuda K, Strauss SE, Hickie I, et al: The chronic fatigue syndrome: A comprehensive approach to its definition and study. Ann Intern Med 121:953–959, 1994.
6. Geel SE: The fibromyalgia syndrome: Musculoskeletal pathophysiology. Semin Arthritis Rheum 23:347–353, 1994.
7. Goldenberg DL (ed): Controversies in Fibromyalgia and Related Conditions. Rheumatic Disease Clinics of North America, vol. 22, no. 2. Philadelphia, W.B. Saunders, 1996.
8. Goldenberg DL: Fibromyalgia, chronic fatigue syndrome, and myofascial pain syndrome. Curr Opin Rheumatol 8:113–123, 1996.
9. Goldenberg DL: Fibromyalgia and related syndromes. In Klippel JH, Dieppe PA (eds): Rheumatology, 2nd ed. St. Louis, Mosby, 1998, pp 15.1–15.12.
10. Masi AT (ed): Fibromyalgia and myofascial pain syndromes. In Baillière's Clin Rheumatol 8:4, 1994.
11. Moldofsky H: Sleep and the fibrositis syndrome. Rheum Dis Clin North Am 15:91–103, 1989.
12. Sheon RP, Moskowitz RW, Goldberg VM (eds): Soft Tissue Rheumatic Pain, 3rd ed. Baltimore, Williams & Wilkins, 1996.
13. White KP, Manfred H, Teasell RW: Work disability evaluation and the fibromyalgia syndrome. Semin Arthritis Rheum 24:371–381, 1995.
14. Wolfe F: The fibromyalgia syndrome: A consensus report on fibromyalgia and disability. J Rheumatol 23:534–539, 1996.
15. Wolfe F, Smythe HA, Yunus MB, et al: The American College of Rheumatology 1990 criteria for the classification of fibromyalgia: Report of the Multicenter Criteria Committee. Arthritis Rheum 33:160, 1990.

XI. Common Disorders of the Nervous System

74. DEMENTIA

Edmund Bourke, M.D.

1. Define dementia.

Dementia is a decline in cognition manifested by:

- One essential feature is impairment of short-term memory that interferes with the ability to recall previously known information and to learn new information, and
- Impairment of at least one of the following: language (dysphasia); recognition or identification of objects despite intact sensory function (agnosia); performance of motor activities despite intact motor function (apraxia); or planning, organizing, sequencing or thinking abstractly (executive function).

There are two qualifiers: impairment should be severe enough to interfere with social or occupational functioning, and it must not occur exclusively during the course of delirium.

2. What conditions are most readily confused with dementia?

Four conditions need to be excluded before establishing the diagnosis: delirium, psychiatric disorders, mental retardation, and mild cognitive impairment (MCI).

3. How do you distinguish between delirium and dementia?

The cardinal distinguishing features are:

- Delirium is an acute confusional state that is usually more abrupt in onset. However, dementia may escape notice in the early stages until it is abruptly brought to the attention by a stressor such as a bereavement, family squabble, or change to an unfamiliar environment.
- Decreased attention span is highly characteristic of delirium and is only a late development in the course of dementia.
- Altered arousal, either decreased with lethargy or increased with agitation or hypervigilance, is frequent but not invariable in delirium. Again, it is only a late manifestation of delirium.
- Delirium is characterized by waxing and waning in the level of consciousness, often throughout the course of a single day. These features often compound attempts at mental status evaluation.
- Delirium is usually associated with a precipitating cause. Infectious and iatrogenic causes are the most common. However, in elderly individuals, numerous other conditions, ranging from acute cardiac events to fluid-electrolyte derangements, that ordinarily present differently in younger age groups may be manifested by delirium, and a reference source may need to be consulted to minimize overlooking potential causes.

4. Do delirium and dementia frequently coexist?

Yes. The frequency of delirium is significantly increased in dementia, because dementia lowers the threshold for delirium. For example, a temperature of 105°F would render most of the readers of this chapter delirious. On the other hand, a superimposed delirium could complicate much lesser degrees of fever in demented patients. Numerous days of solitary confinement may induce delirium in the sturdiest prisoner, as can the sensory deprivation that accompanies the onset of darkness in an unfamiliar environment in a patient with underlying and sometimes previously unrecognized dementia ("sundowning"). However, neither the diagnosis nor the quantitation (e.g., the Mini Mental Status Examination [MMSE]) of dementia is reliable if delirium is present.

5. Explain what is meant by *pseudodementia*.

Major depression can masquerade as dementia, especially dementia of the subcortical variety, in elderly individuals. The characteristic psychomotor retardation may hinder the motivation to recall or learn, thereby mimicking memory impairment. The ability to concentrate and make decisions may be ineffective, and a variety of tests of cognitive function may reveal inaccuracies. Any components of suicidality are, of course, a red alert for depression and should always be sought; early morning waking or deep feelings of guilt may be useful pointers. Conversely, coping adaptations characteristic of early dementia (e.g., the patient's making note of where he parked his car or placed his various medications on the mantelpiece) may be disregarded in pseudodementia. A history of depression or bipolarity helps in the diagnosis. Such patients, however, are not immune from developing true dementia. Moreover, secondary depression is a common complication of true dementia, and the judicious use of antidepressants in such instances can improve both function and the quality of life.

6. Are there other psychiatric illnesses that need exclusion before dementia is diagnosed?

Yes. Occasionally, schizophrenia has a late onset, more often in women. A stable elderly schizophrenic patient who has stopped taking her medication could mislead a physician unaware of the patient's history. Hypomania tends to be less florid in elderly patients but can also exacerbate on cessation of medications. Unlike pseudodementia, the distinction from true dementia is more readily apparent as soon as these conditions are given consideration.

7. Name the most common cause of dementia.

Alzheimer's disease remains the number one cause. It affects 4% of people aged 70–79 years and 11% of people older than age 80 years. It requires autopsy confirmation for definitive diagnosis; hence, some geriatricians prefer the term *dementia of the Alzheimer type* on clinical grounds.

8. What are the other common causes of dementia?

The second-place cause is currently in dispute. Until recently, vascular dementia (commonly called multi-infarct dementia) ranked second in frequency. However, recent studies open the possibility of a relatively new dementia syndrome, diffuse Lewy body (DLB) disease, an entity with suggestive clinical features but currently requiring retrospective autopsy confirmation. The dementia associated with Parkinson's disease may rank number four. Not infrequently, the label *multifactorial* is applied (e.g., Alzheimer's and cerebrovascular disease). Other causes include Pick's disease, trauma, anoxic encephalopathy, Wilson's disease, AIDS, Creutzfeldt-Jacob disease, and (most importantly) a number of uncommon but potentially reversible conditions (see question 10).

9. What is DLB disease?

In recent years, DLB disease has received increased attention. To make the diagnosis clinically requires dementia and at lease one of the following: detailed visual hallucinations, parkinsonian signs, and alterations of alertness or attention. Lewy bodies are also characteristic of autopsy findings in Parkinson's disease, but they tend to be localized to the extrapyramidal system rather than diffuse. Clinically, there may be overlap between DLB disease and either Alzheimer's or Parkinson's disease. At our present level of understanding, treatment is as for Alzheimer's.

10. What is the goal of evaluating patients who may have dementia?

There are several important goals. This is necessary to stress because of the tendency to focus on what has traditionally been, and indeed remains, its first goal to the exclusion of others.

The first goal is to look for a reversible cause or component. To find one is uncommon, but when done in a timely fashion—there are a few more important things one can do in medicine—one saves a human mind. As soon as the diagnosis of dementia is made, one searches for 10 causes that could at least be partially reversible. Alcohol dementia heads the list. In the early acute stage of Wernicke's encephalopathy, intravenous administration of thiamine constitutes a medical emergency. Progression to Korsakov's psychosis more often represents an irreversible stage, although thiamine should be tried.

Patients with vitamin B_{12} deficiency occasionally present with mental status change characterized by impaired cognition without anemia or subacute combined degeneration of the cord. A raised mean cellular volume (MCV) level may be the first clue. Folate deficiency remains on many lists, although definitive proof is not established. Thyroid function, however, must always be checked because hyperthyroidism and (more often) hypothyroidism may both present with features of dementia. Normal pressure is characteristically manifested by ataxia and urinary incontinence in addition to dementia. Other conditions in which intervention might mitigate the progression of dementia include subdural hematoma; other space-occupying intracranial lesions; cerebral vasculitis (e.g., systemic lupus erythematosus [SLE]); and infections of the central nervous system (CNS), including syphilis and, rarely, viral (e.g., herpes) encephalitis.

11. Are there additional goals of treating patients with dementia?

1. Early in the course of the disease is the time to pursue with family, and when possible, with the patient, advance directives, both medical and legal, while it is still possible to ascertain patient preferences.

2. Discussion of long-term care options should be initiated early to permit time to make arrangements and emotional adjustments. Most patients with dementia ultimately require placement.

3. Early initiation of nonpharmacologic therapies is aimed at delaying the progression of the disease, including adult day health care facilities that provide appropriate stimulation, recreational therapy, patient support groups, and other activities aimed at maximizing function; enhancing quality of life; and improving cognition, mood, and behavior.

4. Institution of pharmacotherapy is aimed at dementia and its complications. The most commonly used agents to delay progression of Alzheimer's disease are cholinesterase inhibitors such as donepezil (Aricept). Less established cognitive enhancers include selegiline, vitamin E, nonsteroidal anti-inflammatory drugs (NSAIDs), and the complementary medicinal ginkgo biloba. Aspirin is axiomatic in vascular dementia. The judicious use of a variety of pharmacologic agents to manage complications such as mood disorders (e.g., antidepressants) or behavioral disturbances not controlled by nonpharmacologic means requires consideration.

5. Provision of education and support systems for caregivers, including opportunities for respite care and other modifiers of caregiver burden and burnout in order to maximize the capacity and duration of managing patients in their home environments.

12. What is meant by the term MCI?

MCI is a term endorsed by the American Academy of Neurology for individuals who do not meet the clinical criteria of dementia outlined above but who are cognitively (usually memory) impaired. Although progression to dementia occurs in some, in whom represents a dementia prodrome, this is by no means invariable. It was estimated in one 4-year follow-up study that 12% of dementia patients per year convert to Alzheimer's disease.

13. Should patient's with dementia be prohibited from driving cars?

In the case of advanced dementia, the answer is, of course, yes. But in the case of early dementia, we encounter a bone of contention. Recommendations to stop driving should not be given lightly. The car may be the patient's sole source of transportation. Driving cessation can decrease activity and increase symptoms of depression and dependence. However, elderly impaired drivers are a potential hazard to themselves and to others. Some states (e.g., California) require reporting of Alzheimer's disease to the health department, which forwards the information to the Department of Motor Vehicles. A history of traffic accidents or evidence of significant spatial or executive dysfunction requires careful scrutiny of driving ability. In cases of doubt, referral for a formal driving education evaluation by a skilled occupational therapist may be helpful.

14. Are any quantitative assessments of dementia available?

Yes. Perhaps the best, because it has been most thoroughly validated, is the MMSE of Folstein (see figure). The top score is 30. It is influenced by educational level so that a highly educated individual may have a normal score despite being affected by dementia. By contrast, elderly patients with lower levels of educational achievement may have low MMSE scores with no decline in function. The usefulness of the test is mainly to provide a baseline from which to judge rates of decline and responses to therapeutic interventions.

MAXIMUM SCORE	SCORE	
5	( )	**ORIENTATION** What is the (year) (season) (date) (day) (month)? *One point for each correct response.*
5	( )	Where are we (state) (county) (town or city) (hospital) (floor)? *One point for each correct response.*
3	( )	**REGISTRATION** Name 3 common objects (e.g., "apple, table, penny"). *One point for each correct response.* **Count trials and record. Trials:**_____
5	( )	**ATTENTION AND CALCULATION** Serial 7's, backwards. *One point for each correct response.* Stop after 5 answers. Alternatively, spell "WORLD" backwards. *One point for each correct response.*
3	( )	**RECALL** Ask for the 3 objects repeated above. *One point for each correct response.*
2	( )	**LANGUAGE** Name a pencil and a watch
1	( )	Repeat the following: "No ifs, ands, or buts."
3	( )	Follow a 3-stage command: "Take a paper in your right hand, fold it in half, and put it on the floor." *One point for each correct response.*
1	( )	Read and obey the following: CLOSE YOUR EYES.
1	( )	Write a sentence.
1	( )	Copy the following design.
Maximum Total 30	**Total Score**	

The Mini Mental State Examination. Suggested guidelines for determining the severity of cognitive impairments: mild: MMSE $\geq$ 21; moderate: MMSE 10–20; severe: MMSE $\leq$ 9. (Adapted from Folstein MF, Folstein SE, McHugh PR: Mini-Mental State: A practical method for grading the cognitive state of patients for the clinician. J Psychiatry Res 12:189–198, 1975.)

15. Is there an indication for laboratory investigations or imaging in Alzheimer's patients?

A general **laboratory** evaluation, including a complete blood cell count (CBC); blood chemistries, including liver function tests, thyroid-stimulating hormone (TSH) and vitamin B_{12} levels; and syphilis serology, is recommended. The history and physical examination may suggest other tests (e.g., Kayser-Fleischer ring, Rx ceruloplasmin).

The role of **imaging** is more controversial. A noncontrast head computed tomography (CT) scan should suffice to rule out normal-pressure hydrocephalus or a space-occupying lesion as a cause of dementia. Neither magnetic resonance imagine (MRI) nor positron emission tomography (PET) scanning have a definitive role in the clinical evaluation of dementia at this stage.

Lumbar puncture is not generally indicated unless an index of suspicion points toward encephalitis, syphilis serology is positive, or other atypical features are present. Finally, cerebrospinal fluid examination for apoprotein E genotype has been useful in some forms of inherited Alzheimer's disease; it has been found to be of value in the management of individual patients.

16. Can primary care providers unwittingly contribute to making dementia worse?

Unfortunately, this is a common phenomenon. Aging per se can increase the sensitivity of the brain to pharmacologic agents. Polypharmacy, in which physicians so often play a contributory role, has a compounding effect. A vital first step in guarding against this is to have the patient or family member bring all medications, prescribed and otherwise, for the physician's review. Medicines that primarily effect the CNS are an obvious source and should be eliminated whenever possible. A large number of other agents may affect cognitive ability as a side effect; these include antihistamines, nonsteroidals, and a host of others. In case of any doubt, the *Physicians Desk Reference* should be consulted.

BIBLIOGRAPHY

1. American Psychiatric Association: Diagnostic and Statistical Manual of Mental Disorders, 4th ed. Washington, D.C., American Psychiatric Press, 1994.
2. Bourgeois MS, Schulz R, Burgio L: Interventions for caregivers of parents with Alzheimer's disease: A review and analysis of content, process and outcomes. Int J Aging Hum Dev 43:35–92, 1996.
3. Cummings J, Benson DF: Dementia: A Clinical Approach. Boston, Butterworth, 1992.
4. Elie M, Cole MG, Primean FJ, et al: Delirium risk factors in elderly hospitalized patients. J Gen Intern Med 13:204–212, 1998.
5. Froelich TE, Robinson JT, Inouye SK: Screening for dementia in the outpatient setting: The time and change test. J Am Geriatric Soc 46:1506–1511, 1998.
6. Hanlon JT, Shimp LA, Semla TP: Advances in geriatrics: Drug-related problems in the elderly. Ann Pharmacother 34:360–365, 2000.
7. Kokmen E, Whisnant JP, O'Fallon WM, et al: Dementia after ischemic stroke: A population-based study in Rochester, Minnesota (1960–1984). Neurology 46:154–159, 1996.
8. Lyketsos CG, Sheppard JM, Steele CD, et al: Randomized, placebo-controlled, double blind clinical trial of sertraline in the treatment of depression complicating Alzheimer's disease: Initial results for the depression in Alzheimer's disease study. Am J Psychiatry 157:1686–1689, 2000.
9. Peterson RC, Smith GE Waring SC, et al: Mild cognitive impairment: Clinical characteristics and outcomes. Arch Neurol 56:303–308, 1999.
10. Post SG, Whitehouse PJ: Fairhill guidelines on ethics of people with Alzheimer's disease: A clinical summary; Center of Biomedical Ethics Case Western Reserve University, and the Alzheimer's Association. J Am Geriatric Soc 45:1423–1429, 1995.
11. Rabins PV, Lykelsos CG, Steele CD: Practical Dementia Care. New York, Oxford University Press, 1999.
12. Roger S, Friedhoff L: The efficacy and safety of donepezil in patients with Alzheimer's disease. Dementia 7:293–303, 1996.
13. Sluck AE, Walthert JM, Nikolaus T, et al: Risk factors for functional status decline in community living elderly people: A systematic literature review. Soc Sci Med 48:445–469, 1999.
14. Small GW: Treatment of Alzheimer's disease: Current approaches and promising developments. Am J Med 104:325–385, 1998.
15. Small GW, Robins PV, Baerz PP, et al: Diagnosis and treatment of Alzheimer's disease and related disorders: Consensus statement of the American Association for Geriatric Psychiatry, the Alzheimer's Association, and the American Geriatrics Society. JAMA 278:1363–1371, 1997.

75. TREMOR

C. Alan Anderson, M.D., and Richard L. Hughes, M.D.

1. Define tremor.

Tremor is an involuntary, unwanted movement characterized by a rhythmic oscillation ranging in frequency between 1 and 12 or more Hz.

2. What four questions help to classify a tremor?

1. Where in the body does it occur? Is it restricted to the hands?
2. Is it unilateral or asymmetric?
3. Does it occur at rest or with movement?
4. Is it affected by sustained posture (postural or static tremor), movement (kinetic, action, or intention tremor), or a specific activity such as writing (task-specific tremor)?

3. What causes rest tremor?

Nearly all resting tremors are related to parkinsonian-like states. Possible diagnoses include Parkinson's disease, drug-induced parkinsonism, focal brain injury from stroke, other degenerative disorders, tumor, trauma, and infections.

The tremor of Parkinson's disease is typically 4–6 Hz, asymmetric, and "pill-rolling" in appearance. The diagnosis of Parkinson's disease is supported by the presence of bradykinesia, rigidity, stooped posture, loss of postural reflexes, and festinating gait. Treatment includes anticholinergic agents (trihexyphenidyl, benztropine), dopamine precursors (levodopa), dopamine agonists (bromocriptine, pergolide, ropinirole), monoamine oxidase inhibitors (selegiline), and catechol-o-methyltransferase inhibitors (entacapone).

4. Which drugs are most commonly responsible for drug-induced parkinsonism?

Drug-induced parkinsonism most commonly results from neuroleptic or antiemetic agents (e.g., metoclopramide). Occasionally, the antidepressant amoxapine is responsible. Treatment of drug-induced parkinsonism is removal of the offending drug.

5. What causes postural tremor?

The most common causes are familial tremor and essential tremor. Essential tremor, which occurs sporadically, and familiar tremor, which follows an autosomal dominant pattern of inheritance, have identical characteristics. The head and distal upper extremities are most often affected. The tremor may begin at any time from childhood to late in life and is slowly progressive. It rarely persists at rest but worsens with use of the limb. Many patients describe temporary improvement of essential or familial tremor with alcohol. This response is so specific that it is helpful diagnostically. Conventional therapy includes beta-blockers, primidone, or injections of botulinum toxin.

Parkinson's disease occasionally involves a postural tremor that coexists with a resting tremor. Patients with Wilson's disease may present with postural tremor. The tremor of Wilson's disease varies in amplitude and frequency and is more prominent proximally. Patients often have psychiatric problems, liver disease, and other abnormal movement.

6. Why do excitement and caffeine produce tremor?

All people experience a low-amplitude tremor with frequency of 6–12 Hz when they maintain a fixed posture. This normal physiologic tremor may be exaggerated with anxiety, excitement, fatigue, caffeine, thyrotoxicosis, hypoglycemia, alcohol withdrawal, hysteria, and drugs. The most commonly involved drugs are stimulants, lithium, beta-adrenergic agents, theophylline, and valproate. Exaggerated physiologic tremor may be suppressed by removing or minimizing the underlying cause; if necessary and tolerated, beta-blockers or anxiolytics may be used.

7. Characterize a kinetic tremor.

Kinetic (or action) tremors are usually irregular, jerky, severe, and ataxic; they are caused by diseases of the cerebellum or its outflow tracts. They may affect the trunk and limbs and interfere with all activities. Specific causes include chronic toxicity from alcohol, phenytoin, or other drugs and structural brain lesions such as from multiple sclerosis, tumors, infection, stroke, and trauma. Hysteria should be considered if no obvious cause is present.

8. What is a task-specific tremor?

A task-specific tremor occurs only with repetitive hand–arm activity, such as writing. It is similar to the focal dystonia known as writer's cramp. Psychological factors are common, but cause and effect remain uncertain. Treatment includes beta-blockers, anxiolytics, or anticholinergics, but the best results are achieved with injections of botulinum toxin.

9. What principles should be followed in treating patients with tremor?

Tremor alone is rarely a painful or life-threatening disease. The classification of the tremor should direct treatment, and the clinical response to therapy may help diagnostically. Treatment should be started slowly to minimize side effects, with the response measured over weeks to months.

10. What is the role of botulinum toxin injections?

Botulism is a potentially fatal disease caused by a neuromuscular junction toxin produced by the anaerobic bacterium *Clostridium botulinum*. The toxin can be purified and injected into muscles to reduce excessive contractions, including those that cause tremor. As experience grows, more tremors are treated with botulinum toxin, but results are mixed at best. Botulinum toxin is best for dystonias, chronic focal tremor, and spasms.

BIBLIOGRAPHY

1. Adams R, Victor M, Ropper A: Tremor, myoclonus, focal dystonias, and tics. In Victor M, Ropper A (eds): Principles of Neurology, 7th ed. New York, McGraw-Hill, 2001.
2. Calne D: Treatment of Parkinson's disease. N Engl J Med 329:1021–1027, 1993.
3. Hallett M: Classification and treatment of tremor. JAMA 266:1115–1117, 1991.
4. Jankovic J, Fahn S: Physiologic and pathologic tremor. Ann Intern Med 93:460–465, 1980.
5. Lou J, Jankovic J: Essential tremor. Neurology 41:234–238, 1991.

76. MUSCLE WEAKNESS

Michele A. Ferguson, M.D., and Richard L. Hughes, M.D.

1. Describe the three patterns of muscle weakness that aid in determining its cause.

1. The **upper motor neuron** or **elective pattern** of weakness involves the extensor muscles of the upper extremity and the flexor muscles of the lower extremity. This pattern is seen in cerebral hemisphere lesions, subdural hematomas, stroke, and tumor. The patient assumes a posture of arm flexion and adduction with wrist drop and leg extension that causes a spastic gait and circumduction of the affected leg.

2. **Proximal muscle weakness** involving the muscles of the shoulder and pelvic girdle usually occurs in patients with myopathy, which may be inherited (muscular dystrophy) or acquired (polymyositis, hypothyroidism).

3. A **distal pattern** of weakness involving primarily the hands and feet is seen in inherited conditions and in peripheral nerve disease associated with diabetes, trauma, and amyotrophic lateral sclerosis (ALS).

2. What physical maneuvers permit the best functional assessment of weakness?

Weakness may be evaluated both functionally and formally. Functional testing is carried out by the observation of simple everyday tasks such as walking on the heels and toes, rising from a chair without assistance or use of hands, stepping onto a stool or step, raising the arms above the head, buttoning a shirt or closing a zipper, or "burying" eyelashes. Such observation of everyday activities allows an assessment of functional impairment.

3. How is muscle strength graded?

Formal testing of muscle strength involves isolating individual muscles or muscle groups for evaluation. Strength is graded with a 6-point scale developed by the Medical Research Council:
    5 = Normal power
    4 = Active movement against gravity and resistance
    3 = Active movement against gravity only
    2 = Active movement with gravity removed
    1 = A trace or flicker of muscle contraction
    0 = No muscle contraction detectable
This scale has significant shortcomings because of the high degree of interobserver variability and subjectivity; 90% of patients tend to be evaluated at grade 4.

4. What is the most common motor neuron disease in adults?

ALS is the most common motor neuron disease in adults. It affects men more commonly than women, typically presents between 40 and 60 years of age, and is primarily a clinical diagnosis. Patients usually complain of weakness, atrophy, fasciculations, and muscle cramps. Some patients also have dysarthria and dysphagia. Diagnosis is based on a combination of diffuse upper and lower motor neuron findings and a rapidly progressive course.

Electromyography (EMG) proves most useful by demonstrating diffuse denervation; studies of the cerebrospinal fluid (CSF) are characteristically normal. After the diagnosis is confirmed, supportive measures such as physical therapy and symptomatic treatment for aspiration or depression are helpful.

5. In which patients should physicians consider the diagnosis of Guillain-Barré syndrome (GBS)?

The most frequent cause of acute muscle weakness from a peripheral neuropathy is GBS. The clinical picture is dominated by acute weakness (duration of hours to days), with only minor asymmetries, that usually begins in the legs and ascends but occasionally begins in the arms or face and descends. Maximal weakness may occur distally or proximally and may involve both bulbar and respiratory muscles, making intubation necessary. Reflexes range from diminished to absent; sensory aberrations and autonomic dysfunction are not uncommon. CSF protein levels may remain normal early in the course of the disease but usually increase after the first week and peak within 4–6 weeks. The protein peak often coincides with the maximal amount of weakness. The CSF may demonstrate a mild leukocytosis. EMG studies support the diagnosis by demonstrating delayed nerve conductions.

Because GBS has an immunopathogenic basis, plasmapheresis or intravenous immunoglobulins are used to limit the severity and duration of disease. Supportive care to maintain respiratory functions and to avoid infections has dramatically reduced the mortality of GBS. Mortality from GBS is nearly 0% in the era of ICU care and modern respiratory support.

6. Describe the course of botulism.

Botulism occurs 12–48 hours after the consumption of contaminated food. It progresses rapidly over a matter of hours, causing death if respiratory support is not available.

7. What are the first symptoms of botulism?

Symptoms of cranial nerve dysfunction appear first, including diplopia, ptosis, blurred vision, dysphagia, and dysarthria. Dilated, fixed pupils are a classic sign of botulism but often are not present. The five cardinal features of botulism, as outlined by the Centers for Disease Control and Prevention, are (1) absence of fever, (2) normal mental status, (3) normal or slow pulse, (4) no sensory dysfunction, and (5) symmetric neurologic dysfunction. Respiratory failure may precede the onset of significant limb weakness. Treatment strategies include the removal of unabsorbed toxin via cathartics and emetics, neutralization of circulating toxins with antitoxins, and compensation for neurologic deficits through vigorous support.

8. How is myasthenia gravis differentiated from botulism?

Myasthenia gravis rarely presents as fulminantly as botulism and typically begins with progressive fatigability accompanied by intermittent diplopia, ptosis, dysarthria, and dysphagia. Most patients report that symptoms worsen throughout the day and improve after periods of rest. Diagnostic tests for myasthenia gravis include the edrophonium chloride test, repetitive nerve stimulation, and measurement of serum antibodies to acetylcholine receptors.

Although both myasthenia gravis and botulism are disorders of neuromuscular transmission, the pathology is quite different. Whereas botulism results from impaired release of acetylcholine at peripheral synapses, myasthenia gravis involves impaired binding of acetylcholine to postsynaptic receptors, which are blocked by antibodies. Treatments for myasthenia gravis include immune modulation and thymectomy.

9. What is the difference between weakness and fatigue?

Patients often complain of "weakness" when they are actually fatigued. Fatigue is defined as a lessened capacity for work, whereas weakness is a state of reduced power. The diagnosis of weakness is often clarified by a history of decreased strength or decreased muscular contraction with normal force. Some patients have both weakness and fatigue.

Patients with fatigue often state that they are "tired all the time" or "exhausted." They often have decreased interest in otherwise routine exertion and decreased initiative. Fatigue is to be expected with sleeplessness, prolonged exertion, and excessive work. However, fatigue associated with a psychiatric disorder is often worse in the morning, increases with mild activity, and generally relates more specifically to some activities than to others. Fatigue is often the first symptom of psychosocial stress and interferes with mental activity.

10. Which medical disorders may present as fatigue?

Medical disorders that may produce fatigue include common viral infections, hepatitis, tuberculosis, Lyme disease, mononucleosis, metabolic or endocrine disorders (e.g., Addison's disease, hypothyroidism, diabetes, hyperparathyroidism, anemia), and occult malignancy. Nutritional deficiencies and other causes of poor health also may present as fatigue. Fatigue is a common problem for patients with multiple sclerosis.

11. What are myopathies?

The myopathies are a heterogeneous group of primary muscle disorders. They are characterized by clinical and laboratory evidence of muscle destruction with or without inflammation.

Inflammatory myopathies include polymyositis, dermatomyositis, inclusion body myositis, and infectious myopathies. They typically present as a chronic proximal muscle weakness accompanied by pain. EMG studies, elevated serum creatine phosphokinase (CPK) level, and muscle biopsy are helpful in making the diagnosis.

Noninflammatory myopathies include both inherited and endocrine myopathies. Common inherited myopathies include Duchenne's muscular dystrophy and the adult form, Becker's muscular dystrophy, which are both X-linked disorders that are accompanied by calf hypertrophy. Endocrine myopathies include hyperthyroid, hypothyroid, and steroid-induced myopathies.

12. Which myopathies are not accompanied by an elevated level of CPK?

Classically, the level of CPK is not elevated in steroid-induced myopathy. It may be elevated in hypothyroidism because of decreased renal clearance, and it is characteristically elevated in inflammatory myopathies. In common inherited myopathies, although the muscles are not painful, the CPK level may be markedly elevated.

13. When may steroid use cause myopathy?

Steroids can induce dramatic proximal weakness. Despite reports of onset within a few weeks or with low doses (e.g., 15 mg of prednisone), myopathy typically occurs in chronic users of high-dose steroids. Many steroids have a discrete dose threshold above which weakness predictably occurs. Similar weakness occurs with excessive endogenous production of glucocorticoids, as in Cushing's disease or ectopic production of adrenocorticotropic hormone (ACTH). Fortunately, such myopathies resolve with correction of the endocrine condition or withdrawal of the steroid.

BIBLIOGRAPHY

1. Campbell W, Swift T: Differential diagnosis of acute weakness. South Med J 74:1371–1375, 1981.
2. Dalakas MC: Polymyositis, dermatomyositis, and inclusion-body myositis. N Engl J Med 325:1487–1498, 1991.
3. Riggs JE: Adult-onset muscle weakness. Postgrad Med 78:217–226, 1985.
4. Rowland LP (ed): Merritt's Textbook of Neurology, 10th ed. Philadelphia, Lippincott Williams & Wilkins, 2000.
5. Victor M, Ropper A (eds): Principles of Neurology, 7th ed. New York, McGraw-Hill, 2001.

77. NUMBNESS AND TINGLING

Michele A. Ferguson, M.D., and Richard L. Hughes, M.D.

1. When should a complaint of numbness and tingling raise the concern of a primary care provider?

Numbness and tingling, also known as *paresthesias* (or, if painful, *dysesthesias*), can originate anywhere in the nervous system, either peripheral or central. If severe or clearly localized to a focal brain or spinal cord lesion, the complaint may herald a serious condition, especially if the symptoms are continuous and progressive.

Fortunately, paresthesias are usually of little significance, especially if fleeting. For example, everybody experiences a limb "falling asleep" from compression of the ulnar, sciatic, or peroneal nerves, and simple anxiety with hyperventilation commonly produces paresthesias of the face, hands, and legs.

2. Describe the pathway of sensory fibers.

Sensory information is first registered in various specialized nerve endings in the skin, subcutaneous tissue, and deep tissue. It is then conveyed via the peripheral nerves to the dorsal roots. Here the fibers enter the spinal cord and split into the dorsal columns (proprioception and vibratory sense) and the spinothalamic tracts (pain and temperature). These tracts ascend into the medulla, where the proprioception/vibration fibers synapse and cross over to form the medial lemniscus, whereas the pain/temperature fibers ascend laterally. All sensory information converges in the thalamus. From there the final step is through the deep white-matter tracts of the internal capsule to the sensory cortex, located in the parietal lobe of the brain. A lesion at any point in these pathways may produce sensory symptoms, including paresthesias, hypoesthesia (lack of sensation), or hyperesthesia (increased sensation).

3. What clues suggest that a lesion in the sensory cortex produced the paresthesias?

Lesions in the sensory cortex also produce objective signs. Examples include astereognosis, the inability to identify simple objects (e.g., paper clips, keys) placed in the hand by texture and shape, and graphesthesia, the inability to identify letters or numbers scratched on the palm. Many patients also have mild hemiparesis. Because many processes may affect this area of the brain, neurologic consultation is needed if more than subjective paresthesias are present on examination.

4. When may a cerebrovascular event cause isolated sensory loss?

Lacunar or small strokes result from small-vessel occlusions in the internal capsule, thalamus, or brainstem. The major symptoms of such purely sensory strokes is objective numbness to pain and temperature in the contralateral face, arm, and leg. Thalamic infarction may cause a long-lasting, painful "numbness" that is refractory to treatment.

An unusual but important situation is the lateral medullary infarction, also known as Wallenberg syndrome. Symptoms include numbness of the ipsilateral face but contralateral body. This split sensory loss occurs as the fibers responsible for facial sensation travel to the cervical spinal cord before crossing and synapsing in the thalamus. Other signs and symptoms of lateral medullary syndrome include hoarseness, ipsilateral Horner's syndrome, hiccoughs, vertigo, and ipsilateral ataxia.

5. What signs and symptoms suggest a lesion in the spinal cord?

Spinal cord lesions produce symptoms and signs at or below their cervical, thoracic, or lumbar level. The face is spared. Other clues include back pain, Lhermitte's sign (electric shocks or tingling sensations down the back with forward flexion of the neck), bladder dysfunction, and a discrete level at a sensory dermatome.

6. How common is paresthesia as a presentation of multiple sclerosis (MS)?

Patients with MS commonly experience unilateral or bilateral paresthesias from demyelinating plaques in the cerebral hemisphere or spinal cord. Paresthesias may be the first symptoms, but typically they are associated with other signs, such as upper motor neuron weakness, incontinence, ataxia, or optic neuritis (blurred vision in one eye).

7. Do herniated discs cause numbness and tingling?

Yes. In addition to pain, herniated discs may produce paresthesias radiating to the shoulder, arm, and hand (cervical) or the buttocks, thigh, and foot (lumbar). Less commonly, other serious lesions may produce sciatica, including epidural abscess, strategically placed tumors, and osteophytes impinging on the neural foramina. Serious causes are usually suspected by the presence of excruciating pain, fever, or tenderness.

8. Where do the most common causes of numbness and tingling originate?

The most common causes of numbness and tingling originate in the peripheral nerves. Both polyneuropathies and mononeuropathies have paresthesias as prominent symptoms. The causes of polyneuropathy are numerous, but the most common are diabetes, infection with the human immunodeficiency virus (HIV), alcohol abuse, nutritional deficiencies (including vitamin B_{12}), drugs (chemotherapeutic agents), and idiopathic factors. The most common cause of hand paresthesias is carpal tunnel syndrome.

9. Why do polyneuropathies typically follow a stocking-glove pattern?

The patient with polyneuropathy typically has paresthesias in a stocking distribution, because these branches of the nerves are farthest from the cell bodies in the dorsal root ganglion. As neuropathies progress, the patient may experience similar symptoms in a glove distribution in the hands.

10. Which classic polyneuropathy is life-threatening and treatable?

A life-threatening but treatable polyneuropathy is Guillain-Barré syndrome or acute idiopathic demyelinating polyneuropathy (AIDP). Patients experience mild-to-severe symmetric paresthesias in the feet, legs, or thigh in association with progressive paralysis and areflexia. The syndrome may progress to respiratory failure requiring mechanical ventilation. Effective treatments include plasmapheresis or intravenous immunoglobulin. The recurrent form of this process is called chronic idiopathic demyelinating polyneuropathy (CIDP).

11. How does a claw hand deformity develop?

Compressions of the ulnar nerve at the elbow or "funny bone" produce paresthesias in the ulnar aspect of the hand, the fourth and fifth fingers. If the condition is longstanding, atrophy may be seen in the first dorsal interosseous muscle on the dorsum of the hand in the web space between the thumb and the index finger. In a complete palsy, the claw hand deformity develops.

12. What causes a peroneal palsy?

Compression of the peroneal nerve at the fibular head occurs in bedridden patients, habitual leg crossers, and diabetics; it also may be associated with surgery, overly tight compression stockings, and trauma. In the days before soft luggage, peroneal palsy was called palsy of the "suitcase nerve," because hard valises often repetitively traumatized the lateral knee. Patients experience paresthesias and hypoesthesias down the lateral leg to the dorsum of the foot; footdrop may result from weakness of the tibialis anterior muscle.

13. What neural lesions do *not* produce numbness and tingling in the nervous system?

Amyotrophic lateral sclerosis (ALS, motor neuron disease) is a disease of the anterior horn cells and long motor tracts; sensory symptoms directly exclude ALS. **Neuromuscular junction disease** (e.g., myasthenia, botulism) and **myopathies** (polymyositis and muscular dystrophy) produce weakness without sensory symptoms or signs.

14. What clues suggest a psychiatric cause?

Be wary of the patient who complains of paresthesias in nonanatomic distributions. On repeated examination, the location of the symptoms often changes. Anxious patients often note decreased hearing, vision, smell, or taste. Many have typical functional complaints in other organ systems and historically have suffered from depression, anxiety, or stress-related disorders.

15. When should electromyographic (EMG) studies be ordered?

EMG and nerve conduction studies may be helpful in the diagnosis and prognosis of patients with nerve, plexus, and root lesions. EMG is not helpful in patients with diseases of the central nervous system except to exclude concomitant peripheral disease. Its usefulness depends on the clinical setting. Neurologic consultation is advisable before requesting EMG testing.

16. Any closing thoughts?

Remember—try to localize the lesion by the pattern of numbness and sensory loss and by associated findings. Most confusion is due to imprecise descriptions of sensory symptoms. Patients often use "numb" or "dead" for either sensory changes or weakness. With a clear description, good localization, and knowledge of the patient's medical history, the etiology of the numbness or tingling becomes apparent.

BIBLIOGRAPHY

1. Devor M: Neuropathic pain and injured nerve: Peripheral mechanisms. BMJ 47:619–630, 1991.
2. Greenberg DA, Aminoff MJ, Simon RP (eds): Clinical Neurology, 5th ed. New York, McGraw-Hill, 2002.
3. Kanchardani R, Howe JG: Lhermitte's sign in multiple sclerosis: A clinical survey and review of the literature. J Neurol Neurosurg Psychiatry 45:308–312, 1982.
4. Manusov EG: Late life migraines accompaniments: A case preventative and literature review. J Fam Pract 24:541–544, 1987.
5. Patten JP: Neurological Differential Diagnosis, 2nd ed. London, Springer-Verlag, 1996.
6. Schmahmann JD, Leifen D: Parietal pseudo-thalamic pain syndrome: Clinical features and anatomic correlates. Arch Neurol 49:1032–1037, 1992.
7. Victor M, Ropper AH (eds): Adams and Victor's Principles of Neurology, 7th ed. New York, McGraw-Hill, 2001.

78. CEREBROVASCULAR DISORDERS

C. Alan Anderson, M.D., and Richard L. Hughes, M.D.

1. What is the difference between a transient ischemic attack (TIA) and a cerebrovascular accident (CVA)?

The nomenclature for stroke is less than ideal. Both CVA and TIA refer to ischemia in the brain that results in neurologic deficits. If the clinical deficit resolves by 24 hours, the ischemia is termed TIA. If the deficit is persistent at 24 hours, even if it resolves over a few days, the ischemia is called CVA or stroke. The nomenclature becomes more complicated because 30–50% of patients with clinically defined TIA actually have permanent abnormality in the brain on computed tomography (CT) or magnetic resonance imaging (MRI) or at autopsy. Thus, TIAs and stroke represent a continuum of ischemic injury to the brain.

2. What is the value of the history and physical examination in patients with obvious stroke?

In most instances, the history and physical examination explain the pathophysiology of the event. For example, small-vessel thrombosis or lacunae are associated with a history of hypertension and risk factors for arteriosclerosis (advanced age, high cholesterol, smoking, diabetes). Patients often awaken with the deficit and commonly present with either pure motor or pure sensory findings with proportional involvement (equal impairment of the face, arm, and leg). Some patients with cerebral embolism have a history of cardiac arrhythmias, valvular disease, or myocardial infarction (MI). Artery-to-artery embolism is also common, as suggested by the finding of carotid bruits. The onset of an embolic deficit is immediate and is usually associated with activity or physical exertion. Because superficial vessels are usually affected, a combination of cortical problems (aphasia, neglect) with motor and sensory findings and nonproportional involvement (greater involvement of face and arm than leg) is common.

3. Can a migraine cause a stroke?

Yes. The rare migraine that causes a stroke, however, must be differentiated from the more common complicated migraine, which presents with a neurologic deficit that resolves within 20–30 minutes. Actual strokes cause persistent symptoms and objective deficit. A careful search for unusual causes of stroke, such as hypercoagulable states and inflammatory conditions, is indicated before stroke is attributed to migraine.

4. How frequently does a CVA or TIA present as a seizure?

A seizure is the first manifestation of ischemia in 5–10% of embolic strokes. A seizure rarely, if ever, complicates a small or lacunar stroke.

5. What other medical conditions can mimic a stroke?

Seizure or Todd's paralysis	Systemic infections	Demyelinating disease
Complicated migraine	Peripheral nerve disease	Toxic and metabolic disorders
Trauma	Transient global amnesia	Meningoencephalitis
Brain abscess	Psychiatric illness	Hypertensive encephalopathy

6. Why should patients with ischemic events be rapidly evaluated?

The risk of recurrent stroke is highest in the first few days and weeks after an initial stroke or TIA. Therefore, it is crucial that patients have an appropriate evaluation to prevent, if possible, a second ischemic event. Furthermore, about 20% of acute cerebral infarcts progressively worsen during the first 24 hours after onset. Rapid, thorough clinical evaluation and management can prevent progressive brain injury.

7. What mistakes during early management of patients with a CVA may worsen injury?

Overtreatment of hypertension   Failure to prevent aspiration

Failure to treat dehydration   Failure to treat concomitant cardiac disease

8. Is contrast CT necessary to evaluate patients with an acute CVA?

Generally, no. An acute imaging study, such as a CT scan, is useful mainly to exclude the presence of hemorrhage. If the patient has a history of malignancy that theoretically could metastasize to the brain, a CT scan with contrast or an MRI scan is worthwhile.

9. Is anticoagulation indicated in patients with acute stroke?

The use of anticoagulation for stroke is controversial. Anticoagulation is used to prevent recurrent embolization in either cardiogenic emboli (i.e., atrial fibrillation) or noncardiogenic emboli (i.e., artery-to-artery). It is not clear whether anticoagulation should begin immediately or after a few days. The duration of anticoagulation varies with the risk of recurrence. For example, atrial fibrillation and valvular diseases usually require anticoagulation for life. Transient conditions, such as MI and carotid artery injuries (e.g., dissection), may need only short-term anticoagulation.

10. When is thrombolytic therapy indicated in patients with an acute stroke?

Recombinant tissue plasminogen activator (r-TPA) was approved by the Food and Drug Administration for use in acute ischemic stroke in 1996. Recent studies with the thrombolytic agent streptokinase demonstrated no benefit and reported a higher mortality rate in patients who received the drug. Streptokinase is contraindicated in patients who have had strokes.

Approval of r-TPA therapy in acute stroke was based in large part on the results from the National Institute of Neurological Disease and Stroke (NINDS) r-TPA Study Group. The study looked at outcome in patients with acute ischemic stroke treated with intravenous r-TPA given within 3 hours form the onset of symptoms. Outcome at 3 months after stroke was significantly better in the r-TPA–treated group. The patients' age, race, or sex; stroke location; and stroke mechanism did not influence benefit from the drug. There was no significant difference between the r-TPA–treated and placebo groups in mortality, although r-TPA–treated patients fared slightly better, despite a significantly higher incidence of symptomatic hemorrhage during the first 24 hours after treatment. Based on these results, r-TPA is a recommended treatment if it can be given within 3 hours of onset of acute ischemic stroke. If the patient awakens from sleep with deficit, the last time they were known to be well is used to calculate the time from onset. The use of r-TPA requires careful patient selection. There is increasing evidence that using intra-arterial TPA is an acceptable alternative. One of the advantages of intra-arterial administration is that a diagnostic study is first performed to clearly delineate the vascular occlusion. A higher local concentration of TPA can be infused, with a dramatically lower systemic effect. This allows the use of intra-arterial therapy in many patients who have a contraindication to intravenous r-TPA. If a patient would qualify for either treatment, there is a trend, yet to be proven, suggesting that the more severe deficits may have better out comes with intra-arterial therapy, and the small- to moderate-sized infarctions may do better with intravenous (IV) r-TPA, largely because of the delays in getting intra-arterial therapy organized.

11. What factors are contraindications to the use of IV r-TPA in treatment of stroke?

- Onset > 3 hours before therapy
- Rapidly improving deficit
- Isolated, mild neurologic deficits
- Possible hemorrhage on CT
- Early changes of major infarction on CT
- Stroke in previous 3 months
- Head trauma in previous 3 months
- Major surgery within past 14 days
- Recent MI
- Gastrointestinal (GI) or urinary tract bleeding within prior 21 days
- Seizure at onset of stroke
- Prior intracranial hemorrhage
- Use of oral anticoagulants
- International normalized ratio (INR) > 1.7
- Use of heparin within past 48 hours
- Prolonged partial thromboplastin time (PTT)
- Blood glucose < 50 mg/dL or > 400 mg/dL
- Platelet count < 100,000/mL
- Pretreatment systolic blood pressure (BP) > 185 mmHg
- Pretreatment diastolic BP > 110 mmHg

12. Does every patient with a CVA or TIA need an echocardiogram?

No. However, the mechanism of the stroke should be defined in every patient. Cardiac ultrasound, either transthoracic or transesophageal, has demonstrated unsuspected cardiac sources for emboli in many patients, including common sources, such as atrial fibrillation, prosthetic valves, endocarditis, and mural thrombi, as well as paradoxical emboli through a patent foramen ovale (PFO). Young victims of stroke (< 45 years old) have a 2–3 times greater prevalence of PFO than age-matched control subjects, suggesting that PFO plays an important role in causing strokes.

13. How much aspirin is required to prevent stroke?

The initial recommendation was 4 aspirin/day, but recent evidence has demonstrated that 1 aspirin/day is as effective as higher doses. It may be possible to reduce the dose further; for example, 80 mg/day or 1 aspirin 3 days/week may eventually become the standard. Reducing the dose of aspirin reduces the risk of GI and perhaps cerebral hemorrhages. Ticlopidine, clopidogrel, and dipyridamole with aspirin (Aggrenox) are newer antiplatelet agents that may be more effective than aspirin in the first year after a stroke or TIA. They are good alternatives when therapy with aspirin or warfarin fails or is contraindicated.

A small number of patients with hyperaggregable platelets need higher doses of aspirin to block platelet aggregation effectively. Currently, no standard guidelines specify which patients need platelet aggregation testing. Such testing may be considered in patients in whom aspirin therapy has failed, young patients, migraineurs, or patients without typical risk factors for stroke.

14. Should hospitals have stroke centers?

In large hospitals that care for many patients with strokes, there is overwhelming data that a dedicated stroke unit improves patient outcomes. There is a movement in metropolitan areas, states, and nationally to set up a system of stroke centers similar to the coronary centers that were established for patients with acute MI. This process should result in the actual designation of institutions as stroke centers sometime around 2004.

With information from recent clinical trials, carotid endarterectomy has become a less controversial topic. Results from the North American Symptomatic Carotid Endarterectomy Trial (NASCET) and the Asymptomatic Carotid Atherosclerosis Study (ACAS) provide reasonable data for selecting patients for surgery. It has been established that after a successful endarterectomy, the risk of a stroke in the affected vascular distribution is reduced, probably for many years. Both studies demonstrated that the risks of surgery increase as the severity of carotid disease increases. Finally, it is clear that the angiographic and surgical morbidity and mortality rates vary greatly among individual patients, institutions, and surgeons.

Symptomatic patients who have had either a TIA or a stroke and have carotid stenosis of ≥ 70% benefit from an endarterectomy performed by an experienced surgeon. Because the benefit of the surgery is obvious after a few months, older patients, if robust, are reasonable candidates for the procedure. Asymptomatic patients with carotid stenosis of ≥ 60% also benefit from the surgery, but the criteria for patient selection are less clear. Relatively healthy ACAS patients reduced the risk of stroke by 50% over a 5-year period with endarterectomy and aggressive management of modifiable risk factors. The perioperative morbidity and mortality rates were < 3%. The overall risk of stroke, with or without surgery, is not great, making the option to use medical therapy alone reasonable, even if somewhat less effective. For patients who are fragile, aged, or in poor health, medical therapy is best. For younger, healthier patients, carotid endarterectomy is a reasonable option that should be fully discussed.

BIBLIOGRAPHY

1. Adams H, Adams R, Brott I, et al: Guidelines for the early management of patients with ischemic stroke: A scientific statement from the Stroke Council of the American Stroke Association. Stroke 34:1056–1083, 2003.
2. Adams RD, Victor M: Cerebrovascular disease. In Victor M, Ropper A (eds): Principles of Neurology, 7th ed. New York, McGraw-Hill, 2001.

3. European Carotid Surgery Trialists Collaborative Group: MRC European Carotid Surgery Trial: Interim results for symptomatic patients with severe (70–90%) or mild (0–29%) carotid stenosis. Lancet 337:1235–1243, 1993.
4. Executive Committee for the Asymptomatic Carotid Atherosclerosis Study: Endarterectomy for asymptomatic carotid artery stenosis. JAMA 273:1421–1428, 1995.
5. Gent M, Blakely JA, Easton JD, et al: The Canadian American Ticlopidine Study (CATS) in thromboembolic stroke. Lancet 1:1215–1220, 1989.
6. North American Symptomatic Carotid Endarterectomy Trial Collaborators: Beneficial effect of carotid endarterectomy in symptomatic patients with high grade carotid stenosis. N Engl J Med 325:445–453, 1991.
7. Sauer J, Starkman S: State of the art medical management of acute ischemic stroke. J Stroke Cerebrovasc Dis 6:189–194, 1997.
8. Special Writing Group of the Stroke Council AHA: Guidelines for thrombolytic therapy for acute stroke: A supplement to the guidelines for management of patients with acute ischemic stroke. Circulation 94:1167–1174, 1996.

79. HEADACHE

Catherine Amlie-Lefond, M.D.

1. How common are migraines?

Migraine affects 1.7% of 7-year-olds, 5.3% of 15-year-olds, 17% of women, and 6% of men.

2. Characterize the four migraine syndromes.

1. **Common migraine** occurs in 5–10% of the population and accounts for about 80% of all migraines. Symptoms include throbbing headache, nausea and vomiting, pallor, and sensitivity to light and noise. The headache usually lasts for hours and often is relieved by sleep.

2. **Classic migraine,** which occurs in about 1% of people, has features of a common migraine as well as preceding or associated neurologic symptoms, which often include visual phenomena, such as scotomata or fortification spectra (zigzag lines).

3. **Basilar artery migraine** is rare and usually occurs in young women. It is associated with symptoms referable to the territory of the vertebral and basilar arteries, such as vertigo, dysarthria, ataxia, and quadriplegia.

4. **Complicated migraine** is associated with focal neurologic symptoms and signs that outlast the headache and occasionally are permanent. In rare cases, migrainous neurologic symptoms may precede the headache or occur without headache.

3. How should migraine headaches be treated?

Therapy for migraine is divided into two stages: (1) treatment of acute migraine and (2) chronic therapy to prevent and reduce the severity of headaches. Standard therapy for a moderately severe headache consists of nonsteroidal anti-inflammatory drugs (NSAIDs; e.g., ibuprofen, 600 mg every 4 hours), vasoconstrictors (Midrin, Cafergot), or analgesics (Fiorinal, acetaminophen with codeine), often accompanied by a sedating antinausea drug (metoclopramide or hydroxyzine). More severe headaches are treated with dihydroergotamine (DHE-45; 0.5–1.0 mg intramuscularly), usually combined with sedating antinausea supplement. Sumatriptan (6 mg subcutaneously) is highly effective in the treatment of acute, severe migraine. It may be self-injected by the patient, thus avoiding emergency department visits. Oral and nasal sumatriptan are also available but may not be as efficacious as the subcutaneous form. Other selective 5-HT receptor agonists effective in migraine include zolmitriptan, naratriptan, and rizatriptan. Triptans can trigger vaso-occlusive ischemia and should be used cautiously in patients at risk for cardiovascular or cerebrovascular disease. Chronic therapy to prevent migraines includes tricyclic antidepressants, beta-blocking agents, valproic acid, serotonin antagonists, and calcium channel blockers. Most agents have not been irrefutably proved to be effective, however.

4. How does cluster headache differ from migraine?

Cluster and migraine headaches differ in their epidemiology, presentation, and treatment. Migraine is more common in young women; cluster headache is more common in middle-aged men. Cluster headache is defined by multiple episodes of unilateral orbital pain that last 0.5–1.5 hours/day over several weeks. The headache may be accompanied by unilateral conjunctival injection, lacrimation, sweating, or even Horner's syndrome.

5. How should cluster headache be treated?

Individual headaches are sometimes relieved by inhaled oxygen (6–8 L/min; 100% oxygen mask for 10–15 minutes), subcutaneous sumatriptan, or dihydroergotamine. Clusters of headaches may be abbreviated with prednisone (60 mg/day for 7 days, followed by a rapid taper) and verapamil. Verapamil should be continued until the patient has been headache-free for 2 weeks, and then the drug should be tapered. Chronic cluster headaches can be treated with verapamil, lithium, or valproic acid.

6. Define tension headaches. How are they treated?

The classic dichotomy of vascular (i.e., migraine and cluster) and tension (muscle contraction) headaches is useful but not fully accurate. The typical bandlike fronto-occipital tension headaches are presumably caused by increased contraction of scalp muscles attributable to life stress.

Treatment is usually with NSAIDs; more potent analgesics are rarely used. However, many patients have headaches with features of both vascular and tension types. Such headaches are best treated as common migraine.

7. What characteristics of a headache should raise the suspicion of intracranial disease?

No headache is pathognomonic for brain tumor, although the classic triad of headache, vomiting, and papilledema may be seen in those with brain tumors. Nonetheless, the physician must recognize headaches that are signs of intracranial disease. Such headaches may awaken patients from sound sleep and be more severe in the early morning. The pain usually progressively worsens over days or weeks and is increased by changing posture, cough, or Valsalva effort. Changes in mental status or focal neurologic signs also may be present. New-onset seizures in combination with headache often herald serious brain lesions.

8. When should benign intracranial hypertension (BIH) be considered as a cause of headache? Is it actually benign?

BIH, also called *pseudotumor cerebri,* is elevated intracranial pressure of unknown cause. It often is associated with obesity, pregnancy, and use of oral contraceptives, vitamin A, tetracycline, or steroids. It usually presents in young women as a headache that is worse upon waking. The headaches often respond poorly to treatment. Papilledema is present, often along with visual symptoms such as blurring, enlarged blind spot, constricted visual fields, or even blindness.

BIH is not benign. Without proper therapy (weight loss; discontinuance of inciting medications; and treatment with acetazolamide, corticosteroids, lumboperitoneal shunt, or optic nerve sheath fenestration), visual loss may be permanent.

9. What medical emergency is suggested by a unilateral headache in an elderly patient?

Temporal arteritis, or giant-cell arteritis, is a disease of the elderly that presents with headache centered over the temporal artery or around the eye. It also may be associated with fever, anorexia, myalgias, malaise, weight loss, or leukocytosis. On palpation, the temporal artery is prominent and tender. The diagnosis is suggested by a sedimentation rate > 50 mm/hour. Definitive diagnosis depends on temporal artery biopsy, which shows granulomatous inflammation. The diagnosis represents an emergency because the central artery of the retina, a branch of the ophthalmic artery, may become thrombosed, causing unilateral or bilateral blindness in > 25% of patients. Prednisone, 50–80 mg/day, may diminish headache and help to prevent blindness.

10. What should be done for a patient who complains of intense, sharp, stabbing pains through the eye?

Lancinating or "ice pick" pains are a common phenomenon. They are sudden, brief (< 10 sec), highly localized, piercing pains, often through or behind one eye, temple, occiput, or ear. They may first hit one spot, then another. They are common in migrainous and anxious patients but also occur in many other settings. They are always benign, do not require brain imaging, and are too brief to be treated. The best therapy is to reassure the patient.

11. What condition is suggested by a patient with daily or constant headache who takes daily NSAIDs, acetaminophen, vasoconstrictors, or analgesics?

The patient probably has drug withdrawal rebound headaches. He or she needs consultation and treatment by a specialist experienced in the management of severe headaches, chronic pain, and drug withdrawal. Hospitalization may be required.

12. What is the best way to prevent post–lumbar puncture headaches (PLPHAs)?

PLPHAs are positional headaches occurring in the upright position associated with low cerebrospinal fluid (CSF) pressure and presumably are caused by traction on dural attachments. PLPHAs are best avoided by using the smallest diameter needle possible for the lumbar puncture, inserting the bevel (if the needle is beveled) parallel with the dural fibers, and replacing the stylet before withdrawing the needle. The volume of CSF removed is not a risk factor for PLPHA. Prolonged recumbency after lumbar puncture and increased hydration have not been shown to prevent PLPHA, although some physicians advise these practices.

BIBLIOGRAPHY

1. Evans RW, Armon C, Frohman EM, Goodin DS: Assessment: Prevention of post–lumbar puncture headaches. Neurology 55:909–914, 2000.
2. Johnson RT, Griffin JW, McArthur JC (eds): Current Therapy in Neurologic Disease, 6th ed. St. Louis, Mosby, 2002.
3. Raskin NH: Headache. In Appel SH (ed): Current Neurology, vol. 10. Chicago, Year Book, 1990, pp 195–219.
4. Saper JR, Silberstein SD, Gordon CD, et al: Handbook of Headache Management: A Practical Guide to Diagnosis and Treatment of Head, Neck and Facial Pain, 2nd ed. Philadelphia, Lippincott Williams & Wilkins, 1999.
5. Silberstein SD: Intractable headache: Inpatient and outpatient treatment strategies. Neurology 42(suppl 2), 1992.
6. Silberstein SD, Goadsby PJ, Lipton RB: Management of migraine: An algorithmic approach. Neurology 55(suppl 2):S46–S52, 2000.
7. Touchon J, Bertin L, Pilgrim AJ, et al: A comparison of subcutaneous sumatriptan and dihydroergotamine nasal spray in the acute treatment of migraine. Neurology 47:361–365, 1996.

WEBSITE

Headache specialist David C. Haas, M.D.: http://www.hscsyr.edu/haasd/index.html.

80. DIZZINESS AND SYNCOPE

Richard L. Hughes, M.D., and B. Jane Distad, M.D.

1. What is the first thing to do when a patient complains of dizziness?

Because dizziness is a vague term, it is critical to understand the patient's definition. The first task is to distinguish dizziness from complaints referable to weakness, visual disturbances, or seizures. The second task is to distinguish between vestibular and nonvestibular types of dizziness. Vestibular dizziness or vertigo is accompanied by a sensation of movement, whereas nonvestibular dizziness is often described as a sensation of lightheadedness or imbalance.

2. What are the most common causes of dizziness?

The key role of the primary care physician is to identify the common causes of dizziness: postural hypotension, positional vertigo, hyperventilation, and multiple sensory deficits. Thus, unnecessary referrals and expensive testing are often avoided.

3. What historical data are important in suggesting the cause of dizziness?

Vestibular causes are suggested by episodic attacks that may be precipitated by positional changes and often are accompanied by nausea and vomiting, with or without hearing loss or tinnitus. Nonvestibular causes usually result in a prolonged sensation of lightheadedness brought on by stress, hyperventilation, or standing and perhaps accompanied by palpitations, perspiration, paresthesias, and pallor. Syncope may result. The patient should be questioned about a history of head injury, recent viral infections, diabetes, or psychiatric disturbance.

4. Which medications most notably cause dizziness?

Antibiotics (e.g., gentamicin, streptomycin), anticonvulsants, high-dose salicylates, antiparkinsonian agents, and antihypertensives may be responsible. Any sedative medication may cause fatigue and unsteadiness that some patients call "dizziness."

5. Describe the specific elements of the evaluation of a dizzy patient.

The cardiovascular examination pays special attention to pulse and blood pressure (standing and supine), murmurs, arrhythmia, and carotid bruits. The examination also should focus on evidence of impacted wax and ear infection as well as a brief assessment of hearing loss. Hyperventilation for 2–3 minutes may reproduce the symptoms and confirm the diagnosis of primary hyperventilation. A careful neurologic examination with special attention to cranial nerve and cerebellar function is critical to exclude signs of a focal process.

6. When are laboratory tests helpful in evaluating a patient with dizziness?

Laboratory tests are dictated by the history and examination. A complete blood count and electrolyte panel are needed when the patient equates dizziness with "feeling generally unwell." A routine electrocardiogram (EKG) should be performed to search for evidence of cardiac disease. An imaging study (computed tomography [CT] or magnetic resonance imaging [MRI]) is useful when focal brainstem abnormalities, such as acoustic neuromas or multiple sclerosis, are suspected. Audiometry is useful in patients with hearing loss and tinnitus. Other tests, such as electromyogram, electroencephalography (EEG), brainstem-evoked potentials, and cervical spine films, are usually not needed.

7. After a diagnosis of dizziness of vestibular origin is made, is the patient treatable?

Yes. Most dizziness or tinnitus of vestibular origin is self-limited. Symptomatic treatment with transdermal scopolamine, meclizine (Antivert), or dimenhydrate (Dramamine) is helpful for vertigo. Promethazine hydrochloride (Phenergan) or trimethobenzamide (Tigan) is usually effective for controlling associated nausea. Vestibular exercise therapy may be useful in benign positional or posttraumatic vertigo.

8. Which serious central nervous system diseases may cause new-onset vertigo?

1. **Posterior circulation cerebrovascular disease** typically is associated with brainstem or occipital lobe complaints.

2. **Acoustic neuroma,** when unilateral, typically is associated with hearing loss in the telephone range.

3. **Other posterior fossa tumors** are associated with slow onset and coordination difficulties.

4. **Multiple sclerosis** typically is associated with more than one neurologic abnormality as well as episodic symptoms.

9. Can seizures cause dizziness?

Yes. **Complex partial seizures** may present with an aura of dizziness, vertigo, or unsteadiness. Without clear evidence of epilepsy, the diagnosis may require EEG monitoring. Complex partial seizures are easily treated with appropriate anticonvulsants. **Basilar migraine,** an odd variant of complicated migraine, may be accompanied by lightheadedness, vertigo, or ataxia.

10. What systemic disorders may cause dizziness or even brief alterations of consciousness?

Hypoglycemia; allergic reactions; drug or alcohol blackouts; and orthostasis caused by loss blood, volume, or electrolytes (adrenal insufficiency).

11. Describe syncope.

Syncope is a brief loss of consciousness that occurs while standing and causes the patient to collapse to the floor. Syncope is usually preceded by a warm or "floating" feeling and sometimes by changes in vision. Such premonitory symptoms typically last a fraction of a second but may occasionally be prolonged. When patients experience premonitory symptoms and sit or lie down to prevent syncope, the condition is termed "presyncope."

After the patient hits the floor, unconsciousness lasts from a few seconds to 1 minute. During the period of unconsciousness, muscle twitches, called myoclonic jerks, may be observed. When prominent, they are mistaken for seizures. Only rarely, however, does syncope induce a truly generalized tonic-clonic seizure. When patients try to stand too quickly, syncope commonly recurs; the autonomic system may require a few minutes to recover sufficiently to allow maintenance of an erect posture. Typically, patients are not confused or disoriented.

12. Is it important to discover the cause of syncope?

Most causes of syncope in the United States are not serious. Episodes of simple fainting or vasovagal syncope account for approximately 50% of all events. For neurologists and cardiologists who sees a small subset of high-risk patients with syncope, a serious diagnosis is more common, accounting for another 20% of cases. This bias explains the variation in opinion on the seriousness of syncope, which depends on which group of patients is seen. Approximately 20% of patients have no known diagnosis after evaluation.

13. How do I know who is safe?

Perhaps the most important role of the primary care physician is to recognize and treat appropriately (or leave alone) simple vasovagal syncope or fainting. A good history includes the instigating event (if any), premonitory symptoms, and typical resolution of the syncopal episode. If the neurologic and cardiovascular examination results are normal, little more needs to be done.

Common triggering mechanisms include heat and dehydration combined with physical stress or startle. Examples include fainting at the sight of blood or instrumentation, micturition syncope, tussive syncope, Valsalva syncope (e.g., while diving, weightlifting, trumpet playing), and the notorious tendency of people to faint at church services or weddings. Military recruits often faint during routine immunizations. If the patient cannot recall a triggering event, a witness may help.

14. Which cardiovascular abnormalities are associated with syncope?

Cardiac syncope requires a 50% decrease in cardiac output and thus is a harbinger of serious cardiac disease. Mechanical, ischemic, and arrhythmic causes may lead to syncope. Mechanical lesions include aortic and pulmonary obstruction, including hypertension. Arrhythmias, including complete heart block, sick sinus syndrome, and brady- or tachycardias, may cause syncope. Ischemia caused by myocardial infarction or aortic dissection may also present with syncope. Thus, any syncopal patient older than age 50 years or with known cardiac abnormalities on EKG or physical examination requires further evaluation.

15. When should prolonged EKG monitoring be performed in the evaluation of syncope?

Certainly, patients with a history, physical examination, or routine EKG suggestive of cardiac disease should have prolonged EKG monitoring. However, prolonged EKG monitoring provides diagnostic information in only 20% of syncopal patients older than 50 years with no clues pointing to cardiovascular disease. Further study is needed to determine the cost–benefit ratio.

16. What is the value of invasive testing in the diagnosis of syncope?

A thorough history and examination, an EKG, and 24-hour cardiac monitor should be performed in older patients. If no abnormalities or clues are found, additional invasive testing, such as electrophysiology or coronary angiography, head CT, or EEG, seldom adds significant information.

17. How useful is the tilt table?

Unfortunately, a tilt table can make anyone faint, regardless of what symptoms they may have had in church last week. Perhaps the most useful information results from inducing a faint in the patient with an unexplained loss of consciousness, which confirms that the episode was indeed a faint rather than another type of spell (such as hysteria). Many investigators have remarked on the negative electrophysiologic studies of patients who have simple faints on the tilt table. However, the tilt table is not a good screening device to determine who may need a more involved evaluation.

18. Define "drop" attacks.

Drop spells are vaguely defined attacks that usually affect older patients, especially women. Patients experience a sudden "giving way" of the legs, fall, and may injure themselves but do not lose consciousness. The cause is not known. After a thorough history, physical, and EKG are performed, no additional evaluation is needed.

19. Can strokes or neurologic problems cause syncope?

Yes. Patients with basilar artery ischemia may lose consciousness but usually have vertigo, unsteadiness, dysesthesia, weakness, or blindness. Furthermore, basilar artery ischemia usually involves a longer period of unconsciousness than simple syncope. Epilepsy is always a concern in patients whose syncope was unwitnessed or who do not recall the event. Typical postictal clues, such as headache, confusion, fatigue, tongue biting, or incontinence, are found. Many neurologic disorders cause fainting by loss of normal blood pressure and pulse responses to standing. Both central degenerative disorders (e.g., Alzheimer's disease, Parkinson's disease, Shy-Drager syndrome) and peripheral nerve disorders induce autonomic impairment sufficient to cause syncope.

20. What is the natural history of syncope?

Because most syncope occurs in the older population, mortality may be high. For simple vasovagal syncope, the 1-year mortality rate is < 5%, but the 1-year mortality rate for cardiac syncope is 20–30%. Electrophysiologic testing has probably increased understanding of the disorder more than it has changed mortality rates.

BIBLIOGRAPHY

1. Brandt TH, Daroff RB: Physical therapy for benign paroxysmal vertigo. Arch Otolaryngol 42:290–293, 1980.
2. Hart GT: Evaluation of syncope. Am Fam Physician 51:1941–1952, 1995.
3. Kapoor WN: Workup and management of patients with syncope. Med Clin North Am 79:1153–1170, 1995.
4. Kapoor WN, Hammil SC, Gersch BJ: Diagnosis and natural history of syncope and role of invasive electrophysiologic testing. Medicine 69:160–175, 1990.
5. Kaufmann H: Neurally mediated syncope: Pathogenesis, diagnosis and treatment. Neurology 45:S12–S18, 1995.
6. Manolis AJ, Linzer M, Salem D, Estes NAM: Syncope: Current diagnostic evaluation and management. Ann Intern Med 112:850–863, 1990.
7. McGee SR: Dizzy patients: Diagnosis and treatment. West J Med 162:37–42, 1995.
8. Samuels MA: Manual of Neurology, 4th ed. Boston, Little, Brown, 1991.
9. Troost BT, Patton JM: Exercise therapy for positional vertigo. Neurology 42:1441–1444, 1992.
10. Victor M, Ropper AH (eds): Adams and Victor's Principles of Neurology, 7th ed. New York, McGraw-Hill, 2001.

81. SEIZURE DISORDERS

Archana Shrestha, M.D., and Richard L. Hughes, M.D.

1. Define epilepsy.

The International League of Epilepsy defines epilepsy as an ongoing propensity to have seizures in the absence of provoking circumstances. Thus, withdrawal seizures, childhood febrile seizures, and seizures during cardiorespiratory arrest do not constitute epilepsy.

2. When does the onset of epilepsy most frequently occur?

Although the onset of seizure disorders may occur at any age, the incidence of first seizure has been found to be highest in patients younger than age 20 years.

3. Describe the different forms of epilepsy.

Primary generalized epilepsies begin in a widespread fashion, involving the entire cortex (i.e., generalized rather than focal pathology). They often follow an autosomal dominant pattern of inheritance with incomplete penetrance. The onset is usually in childhood (for example, 5–7 years of age for absence seizures or puberty for juvenile myoclonic epilepsy). Patients typically have a normal neurologic examination and normal IQ. The possible types of seizure include absence (petit mal), generalized tonic-clonic (grand mal), atonic (often called "drop attacks"), and myoclonic (often described simply as "jerks").

Acquired epilepsies begin focally but often invade the entire brain (generalized), thus making the focal onset difficult to confirm. Genetic factors may create a predisposition, but the onset is highest under age 20 years and over age 60 years. Although some patients with acquired epilepsy have clear evidence of a focal brain lesion by history, examination, or neuroimaging, most are normal. Common seizure types include complex partial seizures (which affect mentation without loss of consciousness), simple partial seizures (which do not alter mentation), and secondarily generalized seizures (grand mal seizures immediately preceded by a brief complex partial or simple partial seizure).

4. When do traumatic seizures usually occur?

When the cause of trauma to the cortex is known, the onset of seizure disorder is most likely to occur within 1 year of injury, although it may occur several years later.

5. Should prophylactic anticonvulsants be given to patients with significant head trauma?

No. The prophylactic administration of currently available anticonvulsant medications after trauma or disease of the central nervous system (CNS) probably does not alter the risk of developing a seizure disorder.

6. When is CNS imaging warranted in the evaluation of new-onset seizure?

When the clinical manifestations of seizure disorder fit one of the syndromes of primary generalized epilepsy, with an appropriate family history, response to medications, and electroencephalographic (EEG) findings, imaging of the brain may be unnecessary, unless specific findings or elements of the history suggest coexisting focal neuropathology. In contrast, evaluation of acquired seizure disorders always includes an imaging study of the brain in an attempt to elucidate the cause of the presumed focal cortical injury. The differential diagnosis is voluminous and includes almost all illnesses and mechanisms known to cause injury to the cortex.

7. How is epilepsy treated?

The choice of medication depends on the form of epilepsy. This is why it is important to distinguish the acquired seizure disorders, such as those after head injury or stroke, from the primary generalized epilepsies, in which seizures began without any particular brain insult.

The acquired epilepsies by far the most common seizure type seen in adults. In general, carbamazepine (Tegretol) or phenytoin (Dilantin) are the first-line agents. Because of the cosmetic side effects of phenytoin (facial coarsening, hirsutism), women are often started on carbamazepine, and men on phenytoin. For those who fail these medications because of efficacy or side effects, any of the other agents can be tried. These include divalproex sodium (Depakote), lamotrigine (Lamictal), felbamate (Felbatol), topiramate (Topamax), tiagabine (Gabitril), gabapentin (Neurontin), zonisamide (Zonegran), and the newest addition, levetiracetam (Keppra).

Patients with absence seizures as the only manifestation of their primary generalized epilepsy can be treated with ethosuximide (Zarontin). In general, divalproex sodium (Depakote) is the first-line agent for all of the primary generalized epilepsies. Alternatives include lamotrigine, topamax, and zonisamide.

On occasion, the barbiturates (phenobarbital, primidone, mephobarbital) can be helpful in refractory cases. Most patients find these agents quite sedating, so they have gone out of favor. Nonetheless, for patients who do not seem to tolerate the newer agents, some find great success with use of the barbiturates.

8. Are two drugs better than one in the treatment of seizures?

No. In general, polypharmaceutical treatment of seizures is not necessary and may be disadvantageous. Although the beneficial effects of most of the antiepileptic medicines may be additive, the side effects are synergistic and typically accumulate faster than the benefits. Most patients have the best profile of benefit/side effects with the use of a single, appropriately chosen, optimally titrated medication.

9. Can generic drugs be used to treat seizures?

The answer to this used to be a resounding no. However, the changes in the coverage for medications has led to more epileptics using generic medications. Because of the narrow therapeutic windows that most epileptics must maintain, differences in manufacturers and bioavailability can cause breakthrough seizures or excess drug toxicity, especially for patients who are diverted from one generic manufacturer to another. Secondary costs such as extra blood levels and emergency department visits often make the change to generic agents a cost-negative proposal.

That said, for patients who are able to find a consistent manufacturer for a generic medication or for patients who are easily controlled with a wide therapeutic window, generic medications can be cost saving.

10. What are possible causes for an increase in seizure frequency?
Possibilities include medication; noncompliance; changes in antiepileptic medication (including generic substitution); addition of another medication that may interact with the antiepileptic medication; and physical, psychological, or emotional stress (e.g., infections, sleep deprivation).

11. What are common causes of nonepileptic seizures?
This broad list includes almost all illnesses and mechanisms known to cause acute injury to the cortex. Common causes include electrolyte and other metabolic disturbances, CNS infections, trauma, tumors, stroke, drug effects, and alcohol.

12. Can some patients eventually discontinue their seizure medications?
Yes. However, patients with a primary generalized seizure disorder generally have to be on lifelong medication. Patients with an acquired seizure disorder who have a normal neurologic examination, a normal imaging study, and a repeat EEG (before stopping medication) that has no epileptiform activity and who have remained seizure-free for approximately 2 years may attempt slow titration off anticonvulsant medication.

13. How frequently should laboratory tests be used to monitor patients on therapy?
In general, a complete blood count, assessment of electrolytes, and liver function tests should be obtained before initiating therapy with antiepileptic medications and repeated 1–2 months later. The value of routine repetition of these tests in patients who are doing well with antiepileptic therapy is debatable. A single assessment of serum levels may be useful when titration appears to be successful to document the appropriate level for the patient. This level may then be maintained. If seizure control decreases or side effects increase, serum levels of medication should be assessed. Remember the tried and true aphorism: "Treat the patient, not the laboratory." Patients occasionally do best (no seizures or side effects) at levels below or above the usual laboratory range.

14. What is status epilepticus?
Convulsive status epilepticus is a life-threatening emergency defined as generalized tonic-clonic seizure or a series of generalized tonic-clonic seizures without return of consciousness over a period of 30 minutes. Nonconvulsive status epilepticus involving partial or absence seizures is not associated with the poor outcomes common to generalized status epilepticus.

15. Do women with epilepsy have increased obstetric risks?
Because of the many misunderstandings about pregnancy in patients with epilepsy, it is important to educate all women of childbearing age who have seizure disorders. Whereas approximately 2% of all births in the United States involve fetal malformation, the incidence in infants born to epileptic mothers is 4–6%. This increased risk may be attributed to three causes: the underlying illness, if any, that created the mother's seizure disorder; the seizures themselves; and the medications taken by the mother to control the seizures.

As long as the mother does not experience trauma secondary to a seizure, nonconvulsive seizures have little, if any, significance to the fetus. Generalized tonic-clonic seizures in the mother have been shown to be associated with decelerations in fetal heart rate and thus place the fetus at significant risk. Therefore, patients with generalized tonic-clonic seizures should continue with antiepileptic medications from conception through delivery. The risks and benefits must be assessed on a case-by-case basis.

Folic acid supplementation is recommended for all pregnant women, but for women taking valproic acid or carbamazepine, a higher dose of 1 mg/day is generally recommended. Carbamazepine, phenytoin, and barbiturates may cause a transient and reversible deficiency of vitamin K clotting factors in neonates. Therefore, a 20-mg oral dose of vitamin K is recommended in the last few weeks of pregnancy along with 1 mg of intramuscular vitamin K for the neonate immediately after birth.

16. Should antiseizure medications be changed during pregnancy?

Although the teratogenicity of the various anticonvulsant medications differs, the current recommendation is to continue the regimen that has been most effective (best control with least toxicity) in the past. Because of changes in hepatic function, it is usually necessary to make gradual incremental changes in dosages of medications metabolized in the liver. Serum levels during the mother's monthly prenatal visit should guide drug dosage. At the time of delivery, the dosage should be restored to prepregnancy levels.

The use of divalproex sodium has been considered a contraindication in pregnancy because of a higher risk of neural tube defects. It turns out this an effect from folic antagonism, which can be counteracted with the appropriate use of folic acid. Unfortunately, information on the newer medications is not yet available. The general rules of good prenatal care, including prenatal vitamins, along with using the best agent with the least toxicity still guides therapy.

Epileptic mothers taking ethosuximide or barbiturates should be advised that these medications appear in breast milk in significant concentrations; thus, breast-feeding is inadvisable.

17. May patients with epilepsy drive a car?

The laws regarding driving (not including commercial or interstate driving) vary from state to state. Epileptics should not drive until it is clear that medication completely controls their seizures. The usual standard is a seizure-free period of 6–12 months.

18. What advice should be given to patients with epilepsy?

Routine "seizure precautions" include the advice to abstain from all activities, situations, or circumstances in which the patient may be injured (or injure others) in the event of a seizure. Although certain risky activities, such as using power tools, climbing ladders, or swimming, are likely to be self-evident, other less obvious activities, such as exposure to hot tap water, may pose significant risk to patients with an active seizure disorder.

19. Can surgery fix epilepsy?

Certain types of epilepsy can be helped by surgery. Most commonly, anterior temporal lobe resection can remove a particularly unresponsive epileptic focus. The tissue removed is usually not functioning properly because of the focal epileptic discharges; thus, there is commonly an improvement in functioning and IQ, not a decrease. Alternatively, tumors, hemorrhages, or vascular malformations sometimes trigger epilepsy. The removal of these does not necessarily mean the epilepsy will be either easier to control or cured, but sometimes that can happen.

Vagal nerve stimulation (VNS) has long been known to be effective in reducing seizures in the laboratory. Recently, an implantable device that stimulates the vagal nerve has been developed that reduces the number of seizures that a patient gets. Although this typically will not take refractory patients into a seizure-free state, the reduction in seizures often allows a great reduction in medications, allowing the patient to have a better life. Because some patient seem to get a feeling of well being from VNS, clinical trials are starting to test this agent in refractory depression.

20. Do epileptics need to quit their jobs?

No. Most patients with epilepsy are able to continue working. Similar to patients with other chronic health problems, they are well advised to understand the Americans with Disabilities Act. Because of old fears and ignorance, employers, teachers, and family members may also benefit from education.

21. Where can patients with epilepsy get more information?

The Epilepsy Foundation of America, which can be reached at (800) EFA-1000, may be of importance to patients, families, caregivers, and clinicians who provide medical care for patients with seizure disorders.

Disclaimer: All treatment guidelines are made with the understanding that the ultimate responsibility for all evaluation and treatment decisions rests exclusively with the treating physician. The authors take no responsibility for outcome or appropriateness of treatment guidelines.

BIBLIOGRAPHY

1. Delgado-Escueta AV, Janz D: Consensus guidelines: Preconception counseling, management, and care of the pregnant woman with epilepsy. Neurology 42(suppl 5):149–160, 1992.
2. Dodson WE: Level off [editorial]. Neurology 39:1009–1010, 1989.
3. Hauser WA, Hesdorffer DC: Epilepsy: Frequency, Causes and Consequences. New York, Demos Publications, 1990.
4. Hauser WA, Kurland LT: The epidemiology of epilepsy in Rochester, Minnesota, 1935 through 1967. Epilepsia 16:1–66, 1975.
5. Mattson RH, Cramer JA, Collins JF, et al: Comparison of carbamazepine, phenobarbital, phenytoin, and primidone in partial and secondarily generalized tonic-clonic seizures. N Engl J Med 313:145–151, 1985.
6. Salazar AM: Jabbari B, Vance SC, et al: Epilepsy after penetrating head injury. I: Clinical correlates: A report of the Vietnam Head Injury Study. Neurology 35:1406–1414, 1985.
7. Sato S, White BG, Penry JK, et al: Valproic acid versus ethosuximide in the treatment of absence seizures. Neurology 32:157–163, 1982.
8. Spitz MC, Towbin JA, Shantz D: Risk factors for burns as a consequence of seizures in patients with epilepsy. Epilepsia 35:764–767, 1994.
9. Temkin NR, Dikmen SS, Wilensky AJ, et al: A randomized, double-blind study of phenytoin for the prevention of post-traumatic seizures. N Engl J Med 323:497–502, 1990.
10. Treiman DM, Meyers PD, Walton NY, et al: A comparison of four treatments for generalized convulsive status epilepticus. Veterans Affairs Status Epilepticus Cooperative Study Group. N Engl J Med 339:792–798, 1998.
11. Turnball DM, Rawlins MD, Weightman D, Chadwick DW: A comparison of phenytoin and valproate in previously untreated adult epileptic patients. J Neurol Neurosurg Psychiatry 45:55–59, 1982.
12. Weiss GH, Salazar AM, Vance SC, et al: Predicting posttraumatic epilepsy in penetrating head injury. Arch Neurol 43:771–773, 1986.
13. Yerby MS: Pregnancy, teratogenesis, and epilepsy. Neurol Clin 12:749–764, 1994.
14. Young B, Rapp RP, Norton JLA, et al: Failure of prophylactically administered phenytoin to prevent late posttraumatic seizure. J Neurosurg 58:236–241, 1983.

XII. Common Disorders of the Chest

82. DYSPNEA

Jeanette Mladenovic, M.D., Benjamin T. Suratt, M.D.,
and Elizabeth L. Aronsen, M.D.

1. Define dyspnea.

Simply defined, dyspnea is the uncomfortable sensation of breathing. Normally breathing is an automatic function that involves no conscious effort. Patients may describe the symptom variously as "difficulty getting air in," "chest tightness," a feeling of "breathlessness," or perhaps a lack of "good air" or "air hunger." Some characteristic descriptions by patients may prove helpful in attempting to focus on an underlying cause. For example, patients with heart failure may complain of a feeling of suffocation or air hunger; patients with chronic obstructive pulmonary disease (COPD) may feel as if they cannot get a deep breath; patients with asthma may feel as if their chest is tight; and patients who experience dyspnea with exercise caused by deconditioning may complain of heavy breathing. Patients with acidosis may not have dyspnea at all or only when the acidosis is very severe.

2. What are the pathophysiologic mechanisms of normal breathing?

1. **Cortical brain.** The sensory cortex receives and processes afferent signals.

2. **Brain stem.** Chemoreceptors in the medulla respond to changes in hydrogen ion, carbon dioxide, and oxygen concentrations.

3. **Carotid body.** This peripheral chemoreceptor signals changes in hydrogen ion, carbon dioxide, and oxygen concentrations.

4. **Respiratory muscles.** Muscle spindles in intercostal muscles release afferent signals to spinal reflexes. Central respiratory drive is influenced by tendon organs in the diaphragm.

5. **Mechanoreceptors.** The airways and lung parenchyma have at least three types of mechanoreceptors that influence respiration:

- Stretch receptors respond to changes in lung volume.
- Irritant receptors along the bronchial walls respond to inhaled substances.
- C-fibers in the interstitium respond to changes in interstitial fluid.

3. What is the differential diagnosis of acute dyspnea?

The entire list of causes of dyspnea is extensive. However, acute dyspnea arising over minutes to hours is fairly limited in diagnostic possibilities and frequently is associated with complaints that help clarify the diagnosis. These can be considered in the following broad categories:

1. **Cardiac:** left ventricular failure caused by ischemia, tamponade

2. **Pulmonary:** acute bronchospasm, embolus, upper airway obstruction, pneumothorax, alveolar filling (pneumonia, bleeding, edema)

4. What are the causes of chronic dyspnea?

The list of potential causes is extensive and, in addition to diseases of the lung and heart, includes anemia, thyroid disease, deconditioning, and occasionally acidosis. However, the mostly likely diagnoses in patients with chronic dyspnea are:

Myocardial dysfunction
Asthma
COPD
Interstitial lung disease

5. How is dyspnea affected by position?

Postural effects on dyspnea are frequent and likely caused by changes in respiratory mechanics or gas exchange (ventilation-perfusion mismatching) related to body position. Positional dyspnea is described as (1) **orthopnea** (dyspnea in a supine position), (2) **trepopnea** (dyspnea in the right or left lateral decubitus position), (3) **platypnea** (dyspnea that worsens in the upright position and improves in the supine position).

6. Describe a reasonable and cost-effective work-up of the patient with dyspnea.

Work-up of any chief complaint begins with a complete history and physical examination, which leads to a correct diagnosis approximately two thirds of the time. Diagnostic tests may then be used to narrow the differential diagnosis or to confirm the diagnosis.

History. The characteristics and circumstances of the dyspnea may provide clues to the principal diagnosis and the mechanism of the dyspnea. Associated symptoms, current and recent medications (including over-the-counter, illegal, or herbal compounds), potential toxic exposures, and medical history are also important.

Physical examination. Although it should always be complete, the physician may want to focus especially on the head and neck, neurologic, cardiopulmonary, and skin exams.

Chest radiograph (CXR). Many patients may have an entirely normal physical exam but an abnormal CXR that accounts for the dyspnea. If one has not been performed previously while the patient has been dyspneic, a CXR should be done at the initial evaluation.

Electrocardiogram (ECG). Because cardiac abnormalities account for a great number of causes of dyspnea, a resting ECG should be performed early in the assessment.

Resting and exercise saturation by pulse oximetry (R/E SpO_2). Although some offices are not equipped to perform R/E SpO_2, it is helpful to perform this test early in the evaluation of dyspnea. Most cardiopulmonary causes of dyspnea result in exercise desaturation, whereas many noncardiopulmonary causes do not.

Laboratory tests. Laboratory tests may include a hemogram to exclude anemia or leukemia, chemistries to evaluate renal, liver, or metabolic causes of dyspnea, and assessment of thyroid-stimulating hormone.

7. What is hyperventilation syndrome (HVS)?

Hyperventilation syndrome (HVS) is a poorly understood entity that predominantly affects young women without underlying cardiopulmonary disease or other causes of dyspnea. It is characterized by fluctuating, recurrent episodes of dyspnea (often described as "breathlessness") without relation to exertion, often associated with atypical chest pain and other vague complaints. Stress at home or at work can precipitate an episode. Secondary complaints, often related to respiratory alkalosis caused by hyperventilation, include dizziness, faintness, or tingling and numbness of the fingers and toes. The only laboratory abnormality typically is respiratory alkalosis with a normal alveolar-arterial (A-a) gradient on arterial blood gas. HVS is a diagnosis of exclusion.

8. What is the differential diagnosis of dyspnea in patients with cancer?

Fifteen percent of patients with cancer present with dyspnea as the initial complaint. Dyspnea occurs in as many as 65% during the course of the illness. For these reasons it is important to have in mind an understanding of cancer-specific dyspnea. Causes include the tumor itself, treatment of the malignancy, and anxiety relating to the diagnosis.

1. **Cancer-related causes**
   - Upper airway obstruction
   - Superior vena cava syndrome

- Lung effacement by tumor
- Pleural effusion
- Pericardial effusion
- Lymphangitic spread of tumor
- Ascites or hepatomegaly obstructing normal diaphragmatic excursion

2. **Treatment-related causes**
   - Radiation pneumonitis
   - Lung injury from chemotherapies
   - Pulmonary insufficiency following lobectomy or pneumonectomy

9. What more specialized testing is used to evaluate dyspnea?

Causes of dyspnea not diagnosed by routine testing generally require consultation with a subspecialist. However, further tests often include:

1. **Pulmonary function tests (PFTs).** Full PFTs include spirometry or lung mechanics, lung volumes, diffusing capacity, flow-volume loop, and, if requested, arterial blood gases (ABGs).

2. **High-resolution computed tomography of the chest (HRCT).** HRCT provides a detailed examination of lung interstitium without the morbidity of tissue biopsy and is often performed in patients with suspected interstitial lung disease even with a normal CXR.

3. **Cardiopulmonary exercise testing (CPET).** CPET may be used to distinguish occult cardiac and pulmonary diseases from simple deconditioning.

10. When should the patient with chronic dyspnea be referred for cardiopulmonary exercise testing?

1. When the exact cause of dyspnea remains unclear despite complete pulmonary function testing.

2. When the patient has both pulmonary and cardiac disease and the contribution of either needs to be determined.

3. When the patient's symptoms are out of proportion to the severity of physiologic impairment.

4. When obesity, deconditioning, or anxiety is suspected as a cause of chronic dyspnea.

11. What serum test may help in the diagnosis of congestive heart failure (CHF)?

The diagnosis of CHF may prove difficult using only the history, physical examination, and CXR. However, with chronic increases in left filling pressure, an increase in both atrial and brain natriuretic peptide (BNP) occurs. A measurement of the BNP has recently been used to help distinguish CHF from other causes of dyspnea in patients seen in the emergency department. Very high levels (> 400 pg/mL, BNP) were seen in patients with CHF, whereas levels < 100 pg/mL were seen in patients with other causes of dyspnea.

12. What therapeutic modalities may be used to help alleviate dyspnea associated with COPD?

Based primarily on our current understanding of the pathophysiology of dyspnea in COPD, three general approaches may be pursued:

1. **Improve ventilatory capacity** by standard therapeutic methods, which include bronchodilation, anti-inflammatories, and respiratory muscle training. Bronchodilation is achieved with beta agonists, anticholinergics, and theophylline. Anti-inflammatory agents include cromolyn, nedocromil, and inhaled or systemic steroid. Respiratory muscle training is usually most effective in patients with demonstrable muscle weakness.

2. **Reduce ventilatory demand** by supplemental oxygen therapy, with exercise training to enhance mechanical efficiency and, in certain circumstances, with anxiolytic and dyspneolytic agents such as benzodiazepines or opiates.

3. **Mechanically unload inspiratory muscles** with negative pressure ventilation or low-level continuous positive-pressure ventilation.

13. Are narcotics or anxiolytics useful in the treatment of profoundly dyspneic patients?

Treatment of the underlying disease is obviously the first choice in the therapy of dyspnea. Relief of breathlessness is often incomplete, however, leading to consideration of pharmacologic agents to improve symptoms of profound dyspnea. Narcotics and anxiolytics may alter the perception of breathlessness, although they do not treat the underlying cause. Concern about their use centers on their potential to depress respiratory function and to worsen gas exchange. Most of the knowledge about such agents results from treatment of patients with COPD (dyspnea refractory to standard medical therapy) or patients with terminal cancer and intractable dyspnea.

Narcotics. Opiates have been used with variable efficacy to relieve dyspnea. Their major mechanism of action is respiratory depression through direct effects on the respiratory center of the brainstem. They not only alter the perception of breathlessness but also may reduce ventilatory drive. Exercise tolerance may increase without increased sensation of breathlessness. However, because of their frequent side effects (e.g., nausea, vomiting, constipation, drowsiness) and potential for addiction, they should be used only for the most severe cases of dyspnea in preterminal patients.

Anxiolytics. Anxiety and panic are often confounding factors in severely dyspneic patients. Because benzodiazepines act as anxiolytics and reduce respiratory drive, they are potentially beneficial in the treatment of refractory dyspnea. Early reports showed a subjective improvement in both dyspnea and exercise tolerance. However, the majority of the literature has not demonstrated consistent benefit in improving symptoms of breathlessness, exercise tolerance, or arterial blood gas values. In general, benzodiazepines are not indicated in treatment of dyspnea and should be used with extreme caution in patients with profound breathlessness and anxiety.

CONTROVERSY

14. Is the disproportionate dyspnea seen in some patients with breathlessness psychological in origin?

It has been suggested that depression, anxiety, and hysterical reactions may cause disproportionate symptoms. In patients with COPD and comparable degrees of respiratory impairment, the severity of breathlessness may vary considerably. Such variations in the level of dyspnea probably occur because dyspnea is a subjective sensation dependent on numerous factors, including past behavioral influences, the situation in which breathlessness occurs, and the patient's ability to describe breathlessness.

For: Comparisons between patients with and without disproportionate dyspnea found that significant numbers of patients with disproportionate breathlessness have depression (52%), anxiety (22%), and hysterical reactions (26%), whereas the other group suffers from no formal psychiatric disorder. Furthermore, successful treatment of the psychiatric disorder 2–3 years later revealed complete or partial resolution of dyspnea in patients with disproportionate symptoms. Finally, some data suggest that the threshold for detection of resistive ventilatory loads is greater in anxious patients.

Against: Differences among patients in perception of changes in respiratory effort, thoracic displacement, or respiratory muscle force offer a physiologic explanation for differences in the sensation of dyspnea. In addition, successful treatment of psychiatric symptoms with no improvement in disproportionate dyspnea has been reported. This suggests that the psychiatric disorders are a consequence and not a cause of dyspnea.

BIBLIOGRAPHY

1. American Thoracic Society: Dyspnea: Mechanism, assessment, and management: A consensus statement. Am J Respir Crit Care Med 159:321–340, 1999.
2. Bredin M, Corner J, Krishnaswamy M, et al: Multicentre, randomized, controlled trial of nursing intervention for breathlessness in patients with lung cancer. BMJ 318:901–904, 1999.
3. Cherniak NS, Altose MD: Mechanisms of dyspnea. Clin Chest Med 8:207–214, 1987.
4. Dudgeon DJ, Rosenthal S: Management of dyspnea and cough in patients with cancer. Hematol Oncol Clin North Am 10:157–171, 1996.

5. Harver A, Mahler DA: The symptom of dyspnea. In Mahler DA (ed): Dyspnea. Mount Kisco, NY, Futura, 1990, pp 1–53.
6. Mahler DA: Diagnosis of dyspnea. In Mahler DA (ed): Dyspnea. New York, Marcel Dekker, 1988, pp 221–253.
7. Mahler DA, Harver A, Lentine T, et al: Descriptors of breathlessness in cardiorespiratory diseases. Am J Respir Crit Care Med 154:1357–1363, 1996.
8. Maisel A: B type natriuretic peptide levels: Diagnostic and prognostic in congestive heart failure: What's next? Circulation 105:2328–2331, 2002.
9. Maisel AS, Krishnaswamy P, Nowak RM, et al: Rapid measurement of B type natriuretic peptide in the emergency diagnosis of heart failure. N Engl J Med 347:161–167, 2002.
10. Manning HL, Schwartzstein RM: Pathophysiology of dyspnea. N Engl J Med 333:1547–1553, 1995.
11. O'Donnell DE: Breathlessness in patients with chronic airflow limitation: Mechanisms and management. Chest 106:904–912, 1994.
12. Smith K, Cook D, Guyatt GH, et al: Respiratory muscle training in chronic airflow limitation: A meta-analysis. Am Rev Respir Dis 145:533–539, 1992.
13. Smoller JW, Pollack MH, Otto MW, et al: Panic anxiety, dyspnea, and respiratory disease. Theoretical and clinical considerations. Am J Respir Crit Care Med 154:6–17, 1996.

83. HEMOPTYSIS

Jennifer A. LaRosa, M.D.

1. Define mild, moderate, and massive hemoptysis.
Hemoptysis is defined by the amount of blood expectorated from the lower respiratory tract within a 24-hour period. The classifications are based on the fact that mortality from hemoptysis can be correlated most closely with the rate of blood loss.

- **Mild:** < 20 mL blood/24 hours
- **Moderate:** 20–600 mL blood/24 hours
- **Massive:** > 600 mL blood/24 hours or any degree of hemoptysis that causes airway compromise (e.g., asphyxiation, airway obstruction), hypotension, or requirement for blood transfusion

The following conversions may help in approximating a patient's hemoptysis:

1 teaspoon = 5 mL
1 tablespoon = 15 mL
1 cup = 240 mL

2. Define pseudohemoptysis, identify some common causes, and explain how to differentiate true hemoptysis from pseudohemoptysis.
Pseudohemoptysis is the expectoration of blood that does not originate in the lower respiratory tract. The following are common causes of pseudohemoptysis and how to differentiate them from true hemoptysis:

- **Bleeding from the upper respiratory tract (epistaxis).** This bleeding is generally worse in the supine position and is often noted on awakening from sleep.
- **Upper gastrointestinal (GI) bleed.** Many patients cannot differentiate between heavy coughing and vomiting; in fact, coughing and vomiting often occur simultaneously. Blood from the GI tract often contains food particles and has a lower pH because of the presence of gastric acid.
- **Pulmonary infection with *Serratia marcescens*.** This organism produces an unusual red pigment that can be mistaken for blood.
- True hemoptysis generally has an **alkaline pH** and is often accompanied by **pus** or a **foamy appearance.**

3. List the five most common causes of hemoptysis in descending order.

Bronchitis > malignancy > bronchiectasis > pneumonia > pulmonary tuberculosis. In the early 20th century, pulmonary tuberculosis, lung abscess, and bronchiectasis comprised the most common causes of hemoptysis. A surge in the use of antimicrobials and the abuse of cigarettes caused a shift to more nonacute noninfectious etiologies (i.e., those listed above).

4. List additional causes of hemoptysis based on anatomic location.

AIRWAY	PARENCHYMAL	VASCULAR	SYSTEMIC	IATROGENIC
Bronchitis	Diffuse alveolar	Arteriovenous	Amyloidosis	Bronchoscopy:
Bronchiectasis	hemorrhage	malformation	Behçet's disease	endobronchial
Broncholithiasis	Drugs and toxins	Pulmonary	Coagulopathy	biopsy, transbronchial
Foreign body	(e.g., trimellitic	emboli	Cystic fibrosis	biopsy, brushings,
Malignancy	anhydride;	Pulmonary	Endometriosis	lavage
Ruptured	cocaine)	hypertension	Goodpasture's	Pulmonary artery
bronchus	Interstitial lung		disease	catheter-induced
	disease		Mitral stenosis	rupture of a
	Pulmonary		Osler-Weber-	pulmonary artery
	contusion		Rendu	
			hemorrhagic	
			telangiectasias	
			SLE	
			Wegener's	
			granulomatosis	

Note that this list in not exhaustive. SLE = systemic lupus erythematosus.

5. Define and differentiate between idiopathic (cryptogenic) hemoptysis and idiopathic pulmonary hemosiderosis.

Idiopathic hemoptysis is a diagnosis of exclusion that can be made only after an extensive search, including bronchoscopy. A small percentage of these patients are subsequently diagnosed with carcinoma, but in most the prognosis is excellent, and the 5-year survival exceeds 90%.

Idiopathic pulmonary hemosiderosis is also a diagnosis of exclusion, but it has a very different pathogenesis and prognosis. It occurs most commonly in infants and children, especially those who have a sensitivity to gluten or milk. In adults, it occurs three times more often in men, and it manifests clinically as fever, weight loss, hemoptysis, and iron deficiency anemia. Within 5 years of diagnosis, more than 30% of patients succumb to the condition.

6. When identifying a bleeding site in hemoptysis, knowing the two vascular systems that supply the lungs will help localize the bleeding to one of the two pulmonary circulations. Name the two vascular systems that supply the lungs and define the areas that each system supplies.

1. **Bronchial circulation** is subset of the systemic circulation that originates from the aorta or intercostal arteries. These vessels feed most of the lungs, including the airways, hilar lymph nodes, and visceral pleura; they are the causative vessels in most cases of hemoptysis. Bleeding from these vessels tends to be more significant because they are under systemic level pressures.

2. **Pulmonary circulation** is an isolated vascular system the main purpose of which is to oxygenate the blood as it traverses the lungs. This is a low-pressure system that feeds only the terminal bronchioles and more distal structures.

Absolute differentiation between these two systems is made by angiography.

7. Virtually all patients presenting with hemoptysis deserve at least a minimal work-up. What should be included in this work-up?

- A complete history including questions about environmental or occupational exposures, tobacco use, preexisting lung disease, and inherited or medication-induced coagulation defects
- A complete physical examination

- Blood work: complete blood count, metabolic panel (including renal and liver function studies), coagulation studies, and arterial blood gas
- Urinalysis
- Chest x-ray

For moderate or massive hemoptysis, patients require a more extensive work-up as well as admission to a monitored setting (usually the intensive care unit). If airway control is compromised, these patients should be intubated early. The lung affected with hemoptysis should be in a dependent position. For example, if the bleeding is localized to the left lung, the patient should lie on his or her left side to minimize aspiration of blood into the right lung. In severe cases, a double lumen endotracheal tube and two distinct ventilation systems may be necessary.

8. In order to define the exact site and cause of bleeding, patients often have a computed tomography (CT) scan of the chest, bronchoscopy, or both. What are the advantages of each?

CT scan of the chest has become an increasingly important modality in the diagnosis of pulmonary disorders, especially since the advent of high resolution CT, spiral CT, and contract enhanced CT. CT scanning is superior to bronchoscopy in identifying malignancies (especially if peripheral), airway abnormalities, bronchiectasis, and interstitial lung disease. It also aids the bronchoscopist in identifying specific regions of the lung to examine more closely during bronchoscopy.

Bronchoscopy is ideal for visualizing endobronchial lesions and diffuse mucosal abnormalities. Bronchoscopy also has the unique advantage of allowing the physician to obtain microbiologic and pathologic samples and to control some bleeding sites directly. It is most effective in identifying a bleeding site when used within 48 hours of the onset of hemoptysis. The overall ability of bronchoscopy to diagnose the cause of bleeding is highly variable and ranges from 0% to 60%; this value is lower than the overall diagnostic yield of CT scanning.

9. Describe the bronchoscopic techniques that aid in the treatment of hemoptysis.

- In **balloon tamponade,** an inflatable balloon is passed through the bronchoscope and can directly tamponade a bleeding site for up to 48 hours.
- **Epinephrine injection** to a bleeding site (concentration 1:20,000) causes local vasoconstriction.
- **Iced saline lavage** is another means to promote local hemostasis and vasoconstriction.
- Through high-energy cautery of bleeding tissue, **laser therapy** allows direct control of the bleeding site.

10. Which nonbronchoscopic modalities aid in the diagnosis and treatment of hemoptysis?

Pharmacologic therapy for hemoptysis is limited. By suppressing cough, antitussives may limit ongoing tissue damage and disruption of new clots. In addition, any patient with suspected or proven infection should receive antimicrobial therapy because treating the underlying infection often results in prompt resolution of the hemoptysis. More invasive strategies are as follows.

Pulmonary or bronchial artery embolization. This modality is highly successful (up to 90% control of bleeding). The bleeding site is identified by angiography, and the bleeding vessel is embolized using gel foam, steel coils, or hyperosmolar contrast. Although this modality is very successful, care must be taken to avoid the rare but serious complication of bronchial artery embolization; the anterior spinal artery may originate from the bronchial arteries and, if embolized, will terminate spinal blood flow.

Surgical resection. Patients with localized bleeding, hemodynamic stability, medical failure, and adequate lung function are candidates for surgical resection. Mortality ranges from 10% to 50% and is highest among those with active bleeding at the time of surgery and in those who undergo emergent surgery. Even though the mortality rates are high, surgical resection may represent the only chance for survival for some patients with massive hemoptysis.

Radiation. This modality works by creating local edema and subsequent tamponade of the bleeding site. It has been used most successfully in cases of hemoptysis secondary to carcinoma and aspergilloma.

BIBLIOGRAPHY

1. Cahill BC, Ingbar DH: Massive hemoptysis. Clin Chest Med 15:147–168, 1994.
2. Ingbar DH: Causes and Management of Massive Hemoptysis. Wellesley, MA, UpToDate, 2002.
3. Lenner R, Schilero GJ, Lesser M: Hemoptysis: Diagnosis and management. Comprehens Ther 28:7–14, 2002.
4. McGuinness G, Beacher JR, Harkin TJ, et al: Hemoptysis: Prospective high-resolution CT/bronchoscopic correlation. Chest 105:1155–1162, 1994.
5. Naidich DP, Funt S, Ettenger NA, et al: Hemoptysis: CT-bronchoscopic correlations in 58 cases. Radiology 177:357–362, 1990.
6. Tasker AD, Flower CDR: Imaging the airways: Hemoptysis, bronchiectasis, and small airways disease. Clin Chest Med 20:761–773, 1999.
7. Thompson AB, Teschler H, Rennard SI: Pathogenesis, evaluation, and therapy for massive hemoptysis. Clin Chest Med 13:69–81, 1992.
8. Wedzicha JA, Pearson MC: Management of massive haemoptysis. Respir Med 84:9–12, 1990.

84. COUGH AND SPUTUM PRODUCTION

Carlos E. Girod, M.D., and Michael E. Hanley, M.D.

1. What are the components of the cough reflex?

The cough reflex protects the lungs from injury and infection by clearing large bronchial airways of foreign materials and accumulated secretions. The cough reflex requires interaction of three components: the sensory nerves, the cough center in the central nervous system, and the motor nerves. The sensory component of the cough reflex includes cough receptors located not only in the respiratory system but also in extrapulmonary sites, including the pleura, ear canal, nose, paranasal sinuses, stomach, pericardium, and diaphragm.

2. What pathophysiologic stimuli contribute to cough?

Activation of the cough reflex occurs through inflammatory, mechanical, chemical, and thermal stimuli. Inflammation of the pharynx, upper airway, trachea, and bronchi activates the cough reflex by exposing superficial sensory nerves that are abundant throughout the epithelium of the respiratory system. Mechanical stimuli, such as foreign objects, impacted mucopurulent material, postnasal drip, and airway manipulation, activate the cough reflex through stimulation of myelinated or nonmyelinated sensory nerves in the larynx or the rapidly adapting stretch receptors in the lung. Examples of chemical stimuli that may activate the cough reflex include gastric acid from gastroesophageal reflux, chlorine gas, and other irritant reducing and oxidizing agents. Thermal stimuli (cold or hot air exposure) promote cough in patients with underlying reactive airway disease. The involuntary cough reflex is primarily conducted through the vagus nerve.

3. What are the current definitions of cough?

Cough is classified by its duration as acute, subacute, or chronic.

Acute cough is defined as a cough lasting < 3 weeks. Acute cough is usually caused by an upper respiratory tract infection, common cold, chronic obstructive pulmonary disease exacerbation, or allergic rhinitis.

Subacute cough is defined as a cough lasting > 3 weeks but < 8 weeks. This recent classification was added to include the large number of patients with postviral or postinfectious cough.

After recovering from an acute respiratory infection, these patients develop a bothersome cough that can last up to 8 weeks. Postinfectious or postviral cough is believed to be mediated by postnasal drip, rhinitis, or tracheobronchitis. Reversible bronchial hyperresponsiveness has been demonstrated by methacholine inhalation challenge in a large number of patients with postinfectious or postviral cough. Other causes of subacute cough include *Bordetella pertussis* infection, bacterial sinusitis, and asthma.

Chronic cough has recently been redefined as cough lasting more than 8 weeks. This chapter primarily focuses on the diagnosis and treatment of chronic cough.

4. What are the most common causes of chronic cough?

Cough is one of the most common complaints encountered by office-based physicians and pulmonologists. The prevalence of chronic cough in nonsmoking adults ranges from 14% to 23%. More than 95% of patients with chronic cough have one or more of the following causes: postnasal drip syndrome, 41%; occult asthma, 24%; gastroesophageal reflux, 21%; chronic bronchitis, 5%; and bronchiectasis, eosinophilic bronchitis, or use of an angiotensin-converting enzyme (ACE) inhibitor in the remainder. A large percentage of patients have a nonpulmonary disorder as the main cause of cough. Therefore, the diagnosis of chronic cough usually can be made without referral to a pulmonologist.

5. What are the less common causes of chronic cough?

Less common causes of chronic cough include bronchogenic carcinoma, metastatic carcinoma, left ventricular failure, sarcoidosis, esophageal diverticula, tuberculosis, and chronic aspiration. Most of these conditions can be diagnosed by careful history, physical examination, and chest radiograph. Nevertheless, some authors report that even after extensive work-up for chronic cough, 12% of patients remain undiagnosed.

Other rare causes of chronic cough, such as vocal cord dysfunction, laryngeal polyps, foreign body aspiration, bronchostenosis, and broncholithiasis, may require invasive, specialized procedures for diagnosis (e.g., direct laryngoscopy or bronchoscopy). On the other hand, chronic cough may be caused by a trivial diagnosis such as loose hair in the external ear canal that impinges on the tympanic membrane and stimulates cough receptors located in the auditory canal mucosa.

6. What drugs may be associated with chronic cough?

The awareness that certain drugs may promote cough has increased. Beta-blockers were once the most common medications associated with chronic cough, especially in patients with underlying or previously asymptomatic bronchial hyperreactivity. The mechanism is bronchoconstriction through direct blockade of beta-2 receptors in the airways.

More recently, ACE inhibitors, a class of widely used drugs with vasodilator and antihypertensive effects, have been associated with a high incidence (5–25%) of chronic cough. ACE inhibitor–induced cough may occur as early as 3 weeks or as late as 1 year after start of therapy. The pathophysiologic mechanism is believed to be the accumulation of prostaglandins, kinins, or substance P, which directly or indirectly excites cough receptors that initiate the cough reflex. The diagnosis can be eliminated or confirmed with a short 4-day trial of withdrawal of the medication and careful observation for resolution or improvement of cough. Therapy consists of removal of the offending medication. Attempts to treat ACE inhibitor cough with the addition of nonsteroidal inflammatory agents or change to another ACE inhibitor are not recommended. Substitution of the ACE inhibitor with an angiotensin II receptor antagonist is the best option because these newer agents are not associated with chronic cough.

7. What are the roles of sinus radiographs, pulmonary function tests, and other laboratory evaluations in the diagnosis of chronic cough?

The most helpful part of the evaluation of patients with chronic cough are the history and physical examination. In a study of 102 patients, Irwin et al. delineated the clinical usefulness of the following tools in the diagnosis of chronic cough:

1. History	70%	5. Upper GI series	21%
2. Physical exam	49%	6. Esophageal pH monitoring	16%
3. Pulmonary function tests	26%	7. Sinus radiographs	15%
4. Methacholine inhalation	23%	8. Chest radiograph	7%
challenge		9. Bronchoscopy	4%

Sinus radiographs, pulmonary function tests, methacholine inhalational challenge, upper GI series, and ambulatory pH monitoring are helpful only if the initial history and physical examination suggest sinus disease, occult asthma, or gastroesophageal reflux, respectively.

8. What is the most studied and reliable diagnostic protocol for the evaluation of chronic cough?

The Anatomic Diagnostic Protocol was devised by Irwin and colleagues to serve as a systematic approach to the evaluation of chronic cough. It is based on the careful evaluation of the history and physical examination with further testing focused on the suspected anatomic location of the irritated cough receptor. This diagnostic protocol has been validated by various prospective studies with a diagnostic accuracy of 88–100% in obtaining the cause of chronic cough.

1. All patients must receive a careful history and physical examination focused on the anatomic location of cough receptors. Chest radiograph is recommended for all patients.

2. In smokers, patients with occupational or environmental exposures, and those taking an ACE inhibitor, initial steps should include smoking cessation, elimination of the irritant, or discontinuation followed by observation. No further diagnostic studies are indicated for at least 4 weeks.

3. Other imaging studies and pulmonary physiologic evaluation depend on the suspected cause after initial evaluation by history, physical examination, and chest radiograph. For example, if postnasal drip and chronic sinus disease are suspected, a sinus radiograph and allergy evaluation should be ordered first. If occult asthma is suspected, pulmonary function tests and methacholine inhalation challenge are recommended. If no cause is suggested by the history and physical examination, the next appropriate step is pulmonary function testing before and after administration of a bronchodilator or methacholine challenge.

4. If the above strategy suggests no cause, tests for the evaluation of gastroesophageal reflux are recommended, including an esophagogram and, if available, ambulatory pH monitoring, even in the absence of symptoms. If the study results are negative, other tests that may be obtained include sputum cytology for malignancy, sputum sample for eosinophilia (eosinophilic bronchitis), bronchoscopy, computed tomography (CT) of the chest, and noninvasive cardiac studies.

5. Determine the cause of the chronic cough by instituting a specific therapy and observing for resolution of cough. If one or more possible causes of chronic cough are discovered, specific therapy should be sequentially added to pinpoint the exact cause (or causes) of the cough.

9. How does a history of excessive sputum production help in the evaluation of chronic cough?

Previously, it was believed that chronic cough accompanied by excessive sputum production indicated a primary pulmonary condition such as chronic bronchitis, bronchiectasis, and cystic fibrosis. However, a prospective study reported by Smyrnios et al. (1995) clearly demonstrated that this is not the case. The most common cause of chronic cough with excessive sputum production continued to be postnasal drip syndrome (PNDS) in 40% of patients. Other common causes paralleled those seen in patients with no sputum production and chronic cough: asthma, 24%; gastroesophageal reflux disease, 15%; bronchitis, 11%; bronchiectasis, 4%; left ventricular failure, 3%; and miscellaneous causes, 3%. Therefore, the diagnostic work-up should proceed as for all patients with cough. However, the evaluation may be more extensive and require longer to reach a specific diagnosis in patients with excessive sputum production.

10. When does a cough that follows an upper respiratory tract illness warrant evaluation?

Postinfectious cough is the most common cause of subacute cough (3–8 weeks' duration). Viral or bacterial infections of the upper respiratory tract may promote or activate the cough reflex by injuring the airway epithelium and exposing sensory nerves that represent the afferent loop of the cough reflex. Approximately 77% of patients affected by an upper respiratory tract infection have a cough that lasts up to 3 weeks. In such patients, bronchial hyperactivity, as demonstrated with inhalational challenge, persists for up to 7 weeks after viral infection. In a significant number of patients, cough may last up to 8 weeks from the onset of the upper respiratory tract infection. Therefore, full diagnostic evaluation for cough that follows an upper respiratory tract infection is not recommended unless the cough lasts longer than 8 weeks or is significantly troublesome to the patient. Persistent cough after upper respiratory tract illness is best treated by a short course of corticosteroid or inhaled ipratropium bromide or both.

11. When does a cough in a cigarette smoker require evaluation?

The evaluation of chronic cough in smokers may lead to multiple unnecessary and expensive diagnostic procedures. Useful guidelines for full evaluation of chronic cough in a smoker include (1) change in or development of sputum production; (2) increase in frequency of cough; (3) hemoptysis; or (4) constitutional symptoms, such as weight loss and fatigue. Evaluation should focus on exclusion of lung cancer, emphysema, and chronic bronchitis. Physicians must also use this opportunity to reinforce the need for smoking cessation.

Evaluation should follow the diagnostic protocol described in question 8, focusing on history, physical exam, and chest radiograph. If the results are negative, no other diagnostic tests are recommended before complete cessation of smoking. If cough persists after 4 weeks of smoking cessation, bronchoscopy should be considered.

12. Can chronic cough be the sole presenting symptom of gastroesophageal reflux disease (GERD)?

Yes. Approximately 43–75% of patients with cough caused by GERD fail to report other classic reflux symptoms, such as heartburn, acid reflux into the mouth, and indigestion. GERD has been reported as the cause of chronic cough in 8–40% of patients. Reflux can activate the cough reflex by direct irritation of the upper respiratory tract without aspiration or by irritation of the lower respiratory tract by aspiration. Most importantly, cough caused by GERD is most commonly directed through a third pathway called the *esophageal bronchial cough reflex*. Reflux into the distal esophagus activates an esophageal cough receptor with afferent and efferent transmission of the reflex through the vagus nerve to the cough center. In fact, a direct communication between the esophagus and the trachea via sensory nerves has recently been reported.

A diagnosis of GERD-mediated cough is most reliably made with the use of 24-hour esophageal pH monitoring. This technique has a reported negative predictive value (NPV) of 100% and a positive predictive value (PPV) of 89%. Based on its limited availability and difficult interpretation, most experts recommend an empiric trial of GERD therapy with proton pump inhibitors (PPIs) for a duration of 2 weeks. If this treatment fails to relieve the cough, further investigation for GERD is still recommended before excluding this diagnosis as the cause.

13. What is eosinophilic bronchitis? What is its association with chronic cough?

Eosinophilic bronchitis was first reported by Gibson and colleagues in 1989. Recently, it has been reported as the cause of chronic cough in up to 13% of referred patients. Despite its association with tracheal eosinophilia and steroid responsiveness, it is not considered to be part of the asthma syndromes. Patients with eosinophilic bronchitis suffer from chronic cough but have normal spirometry and negative methacholine inhalational challenge. Diagnosis is made by cytologic analysis of expectorated sputum for eosinophilia. Patients usually respond to inhaled steroids but may require a course of oral prednisolone at a recommended dose of 30 mg per day for 2–3 weeks.

14. What complications are associated with cough?

1. Musculoskeletal: torn chest muscle, rib fractures
2. Pulmonary: pneumothorax, pneumomediastinum

3. Psychological: self-consciousness, fear of public appearances
4. Cardiovascular: syncope or near syncope
5. Neurologic: cough headache
6. Genitourinary: urinary incontinence
7. Constitutional: fatigue, poor appetite, weight loss
8. Miscellaneous: wound dehiscence, hoarseness

15. When and how should chronic cough be treated empirically?

The anatomic diagnostic protocol delineated by Irwin et al. (see question 8) leads to a specific diagnosis and treatment for chronic cough in more than 90% of patients. Failure of specific therapy is likely due to incorrect diagnosis or undertreatment. Therefore, empirical therapy for chronic cough is seldom necessary.

When complications are serious or diagnostic tests are not available, chronic cough should be treated in the absence of a diagnosis. However, the cough reflex should not be suppressed if it benefits the patient by clearing the airway of purulent secretions. When empirical therapy is indicated, the most studied and efficacious nonspecific antitussives should be used: narcotics (codeine or codeine-derived cough suspensions), nonnarcotics (most commonly dextromethorphan), and inhaled ipratropium bromide.

Certain clinical scenarios of chronic cough also merit empirical therapy. In some patients, diagnosis of gastroesophageal reflux may require 24-hour ambulatory pH monitoring, which is not readily available in most medical centers. Therefore, in patients suspected of having gastroesophageal reflux, empirical therapy with histamine-2 receptor blockers or, preferably, proton pump inhibitors should be instituted with careful observation of changes in the cough pattern.

Because of the high incidence of chronic cough due to occult asthma, many authors recommend a short course of oral corticosteroids for chronic cough with no obvious cause. Empiric steroids also may be helpful in treating postviral or postinfectious cough by relieving the associated airway inflammation and reactivity.

16. What is the role of mucolytic therapy in the management of chronic cough and sputum production?

Conditions associated with chronic cough and accompanied by sputum production include emphysema, chronic bronchitis, bronchiectasis, cystic fibrosis, and diseases of the large airways. Although its benefits have not been well documented, mucolytic therapy frequently is used in such clinical settings. Most common mucolytic agents work by thinning hyperviscous mucus. Examples include nebulized water and hypertonic electrolyte solutions, iodides and organic iodine compounds, guaifenesin, ipecacuanha, bromhexine, N-acetylcysteine (Mucomyst), and proteolytic enzymes. Clinical studies have shown that many of these agents have no benefit in the treatment of chronic sputum-producing conditions, and most must be given at high, nauseating doses to achieve mucolytic action. Nevertheless, mucolytic agents may be helpful in short-course treatment of acute viral respiratory infections and in acute exacerbations of chronic sputum disorders.

CONTROVERSIES

17. Is bronchoscopy of value in the evaluation of chronic cough?

In the early 1970s, chronic, severe, unexplained cough was an indication for bronchoscopy. Most of the controversy surrounding bronchoscopy for chronic cough is due to this uncorroborated indication, which was based on anecdotal reports of high yields of endobronchial abnormalities or carcinoma. In the 1980s and 1990s, many careful studies of patients with chronic cough demonstrated that bronchoscopy in a patient with a normal chest radiograph results in a low diagnostic yield (approximately 4%). Irwin et al. performed bronchoscopy in 51 of 109 patients with chronic cough and made a diagnosis of occult bronchogenic carcinoma in only one. Bronchoscopy is recommended if the chest radiograph is abnormal, but it should not be included routinely in the evaluation of chronic cough.

On the other hand, Sen and Walsh performed bronchoscopy in 25 patients with undiagnosed chronic cough despite careful examination, chest radiograph, and trial of empirical therapy. Fifty percent of the patients were older (age > 50 years) smokers with extensive prior work-up for cough. In approximately 25%, bronchoscopy yielded a diagnosis of broncholithiasis, tracheo-bronchopathia, tuberculous bronchostenosis, laryngeal dyskinesis, or laryngeal polyps. The authors recommend bronchoscopy in selected older patients with undiagnosed cough that lasts more than 2 months and is refractory to empirical therapy.

18. Can the history obtained from patients delineating the character, timing, quality, and complications of chronic cough determine its cause?

For: The medical literature has many examples of features of the history that suggest the cause of chronic cough: paroxysms of cough suggest asthma; cough in supine position or sleep, gastroesophageal reflux; sputum production, chronic bronchitis or bronchiectasis; and a loud "brassy" cough, large airway diseases.

Against: A prospective study conducted by Mello et al. (1996) demonstrated only two statistically significant correlates: (1) "wet" or productive cough was associated with bronchiectasis, and (2) "barking" or paroxysmal cough negatively correlated with asthma. Other historical features did not correlate with a specific etiology for chronic cough.

BIBLIOGRAPHY

1. Brightling CE, Ward R, Goh KL, et al: Eosinophilic bronchitis is an important cause of chronic cough. Am J Respir Crit Care Med 160:406–416, 1999.
2. Fuller RW, Jackson DM: Physiology and treatment of cough. Thorax 45:425–430, 1990.
3. Irwin RS, Curley FJ: The treatment of chronic cough: A comprehensive review. Chest 99:1477–1484, 1991.
4. Irwin RS, Curley FJ, Pratter MR: The effects of drugs on cough. Eur J Respir Dis 71(suppl 153):173–181, 1987.
5. Irwin RS, Curley FJ, French CL: Chronic cough: The spectrum and frequency of causes, key components of the diagnostic evaluation, and outcome of specific therapy. Am Rev Respir Dis 141:640–647, 1990.
6. Irwin RS, Madison JM: Anatomical diagnostic protocol in evaluating chronic cough with specific reference to gastroesophageal reflux disease. Am J Med 108:126S–130S, 2000.
7. Irwin RS, Madison JM: The diagnosis and treatment of chronic cough. N Engl J Med 343:1715–1721, 2000.
8. Irwin RS, Madison JM: Symptom research on chronic cough: A historical perspective. Ann Intern Med 134:809–814, 2001.
9. Irwin RS, Richter JE: Gastroesophageal reflux and chronic cough. Am J Gastroenterol 95(suppl 8):S9–S14, 2000.
10. Irwin RS, Zawacki JK, Curley FJ, et al: Chronic cough as the sole presenting manifestation of gastroesophageal reflux. Am Rev Respir Dis 140:1294–1300, 1989.
11. Israili ZH, Hall WD: Cough and angioneurotic edema associated with angiotensin-converting enzyme inhibitor therapy: A review of the literature and pathophysiology. Ann Intern Med 178:234–242, 1992.
12. Mello CJ, Irwin RS, Curley FJ: Predictive values of the character, timing, and complications of chronic cough in diagnosing its cause. Arch Intern Med 156:997–1003, 1996.
13. O'Connell EJ, Rojas AR, Sachs MI: Cough-type asthma: A review. Ann Allergy 66:278–282, 1991.
14. Ours TM, Kavaru MS, Schilz RJ, Richter JE: A prospective evaluation of esophageal testing and a double-blind, randomized study of omeprazole in a diagnostic and therapeutic algorithm for chronic cough. Am J Gastroenterol 94:3131–3138, 1999.
15. Patrick H, Patrick F: Chronic cough. Med Clin North Am 79:361–372, 1995.
16. Poe RH, Harder RV, Israel RH, Kallay MC: Chronic persistent cough: Experience in diagnosis and outcome using an anatomic diagnostic protocol. Chest 95:728–732, 1989.
17. Poe RH, Israel RH, Utell MJ, Hall WJ: Chronic cough: Bronchoscopy or pulmonary function testing? Am Rev Respir Dis 126:160–162, 1982.
18. Sen RP, Walsh TE: Fiberoptic bronchoscopy for refractory cough. Chest 99:33–35, 1991.
19. Smyrnios NA, Irwin RS, Curley FJ: Chronic cough with a history of excessive sputum production. Chest 108:991–997, 1995.
20. Widdicombe JG: Mechanisms of cough and its regulation. Eur J Respir Dis 153(suppl):173–181, 1987.
21. Zanjanian MH: Expectorants and antitussive agents: Are they helpful? Ann Allergy 44:290–295, 1980.

85. THE COMMON COLD AND ACUTE SINUSITIS

Larry I. Lutwick, M.D.

I contemplate a joy exquisite
In not paying you for your visit.
I did not call you to be told
My malady is a common cold.
　　　　　　from "Common Cold" by Ogden Nash (1902–1971)

A desire to take medicine is, perhaps, the great feature which
distinguishes man from animals.
　　　　　　Dr. William Osler, 1891

1. How common is the common cold, and what does the illness actually have to do with cold temperatures?

Although poked fun at in verse by Ogden Nash, the common cold is a major burden on society. This infection represents about 50% of all human illness and 75% of those in young children. In the United States, as many as 1 billion colds occur annually, with 50–60 million cases requiring restricted activity or medical attention. Tens of millions of lost school and work days result, causing huge monetary losses.

There is no clinically demonstrable relationship between the acquisition of a cold virus or the development of symptoms and a preceding chill from, for instance, not wearing adequate clothing in winter. The increased frequency of the common cold during the winter is, therefore, not explained by this old wives' tale.

2. What agent or agents cause the common cold?

Rhinoviruses, with more than 110 non–cross-protecting serotypes, are the most frequent cause of the common cold, accounting for 60–70% of the illnesses in which a viral cause is determined. Coronaviruses are also common. The three or four human serotypes of coronaviruses are difficult to study because they are difficult to cultivate *in vitro*. Most studies of the common cold, therefore, are done with rhinoviruses. A list of viruses associated with the common cold is shown in the table.

The Common Cold Viruses*

MAJOR CAUSES	OTHER CAUSES†
Rhinoviruses	Parainfluenza viruses
Coronaviruses	Respiratory syncytial virus (RSV)
	Adenoviruses
	Influenza viruses
	Miscellaneous (e.g., enteroviruses, ECHO viruses)

*As many as 30% of exposures are thought to be due to as yet unidentified groups or strains of viruses.
†In small children, infections with the group A beta-hemolytic streptococcus may be difficult to distinguish from the common cold.

3. Describe the epidemiology of the common cold.

The cold season in the United States spans from September through May, roughly corresponding to the school year. The major reservoirs of this disease are small children who spread

436

the agents to siblings, school classmates, and children in child care settings. The viruses are then passed to other family members, particularly the parents, at home.

On average, during peak season in the U.S., the common cold infection rate is 5–8 colds per 1000 persons per day, which decreases to 2–3 in the summer. The summer cold, therefore, occurs not uncommonly. Overall, in the U.S., adults have 2–4 colds/year and children 6–8, but 10–15% of children have at least 12 colds per year. The frequency of common colds decreases with increasing age, reaching adult levels by adolescence. This diminution relates to a combination of cumulative immunity to an increasing number of cold virus strains and less exposure to young children.

As a whole, boys have a somewhat higher incidence of illness compared with girls until adolescence, when the reverse occurs. This change is likely to be caused by the higher exposure of women to small children. Adults living with small children at home or with occupations associated with exposures to the reservoir have more colds than those without such exposure.

The risk of the common cold is not decreased by tonsillectomy or increased by exercise, diet, quality of sleep, alcohol use, or cigarette smoking. Smokers do, importantly, have a somewhat more severe illness. Psychological stress, however, does increase the incidence of both virus infections and clinical colds in a dose-response manner.

4. How does the rhinovirus produce disease?

No consistent direct histopathologic effects of rhinovirus replication in the nasal epithelium are found. The host response to rhinovirus infection, therefore, has been thought to have a significant role in the production of cold symptoms, including increased amounts of inflammatory mediators such as bradykinin and interleukins such as IL-6 and IL-8. Therapeutically relevant is that no detectable increase in histamine occurs in the nasal fluids during rhinovirus infection.

5. In what ways are the cold viruses acquired?

Cold viruses, as demonstrated particularly with the rhinovirus, are produced primarily in the nasal secretions, with peak viral amounts and infectivity occurring between the second and fourth days of illness.

Experimental studies with rhinoviruses have found that direct contact between people is the most efficient mode of transmission but that large-particle aerosols and fomites may also transmit the virus. Indeed, one study found that the use of a virucidal substance on the hands significantly decreased rhinovirus transmission, stressing the importance of handwashing as a method to decrease hand-to-hand transmission. Infection is best spread via the nasal and conjunctival mucosae rather than orally.

Although rhinovirus-associated common colds are quite frequent, the virus appears not to be terribly efficient in transmission. In one study, a transmission rate of only 44% from infected donors to susceptible contacts could be found after 150 contact-hours. About 25% of rhinovirus infections are asymptomatic.

6. Describe the natural course of the common cold and how it is different from a seasonal allergy.

After an incubation period of 1–2 days (slightly longer with coronaviruses), the common cold often begins with a scratchy throat that resolves over 1–2 days. The nasal symptoms of sneezing, rhinorrhea and nasal obstruction become prominent on day 2, peaking in intensity over 2–3 days. A cough may occur, especially as the nasal symptomatology is diminishing. Fever is generally minimal but can be more prominent in young children. Although the illness caused by rhinovirus, coronavirus, parainfluenza virus, and RSV are often quite similar in both adults and children, parainfluenza and RSV may well cause more lower respiratory infections such as bronchiolitis, croup, and viral pneumonia in young children. Influenza viral infection, which may produce an illness indistinguishable from a rhinovirus cold, more classically is associated with a febrile, more systemically ill, patient. The common cold usually resolves over 7 days but may persist in some for another week.

Allergic rhinitis is associated with prominent, red, itchy eyes and not usually with sore throat. Allergies are often seasonal, especially in the summer, but the common cold does occur, albeit less frequently, during this season. An illness with rhinitis lasting more than 2 weeks is much more likely to be allergic in origin unless the person has been sequentially infected with several cold viruses.

7. Do persons with an inadequate immune system have a more serious form of the common cold?

Frequent colds do not generally indicate the presence of any underlying immunologic defect. Instead, the frequency reflects the amount of exposure to the large number of viruses that can cause the illness.

There is minimal information regarding the role of the more frequent of the cold viruses, rhinoviruses, and coronaviruses regarding this issue. Overall, however, it is believed that in most cases with rhinovirus infection in the immunocompromised host, the virus remains limited to the upper respiratory tract. The length of symptoms, however, can be more prolonged, and bacterial pneumonias more common in these individuals.

Some of the less common viruses associated with the common cold, however, such as RSV, adenovirus, and parainfluenza virus as well as influenza, can have more severe illnesses with higher mortality rates associated with dissemination and viral pneumonia as well as bacterial and fungal superinfection.

8. What medications can be used in the treatment of the symptoms of the common cold?

- **Nasal congestion**—This is best managed with topical (oxymetazoline or xylometazoline) or oral (pseudoephedrine) adrenergics.
- **Rhinorrhea**—This may be treated with ipratropium nasal spray, which has decreased this symptom by about 30% over placebo in natural colds. First-generation antihistamines (FGAHs) have a modest effect on rhinorrhea caused by the common cold, but the newer nonsedating drugs do not. Because histamine release is not a feature of the common cold, any effect of FGAHs may be related to an anticholinergic effect.
- **Cough**—Cough suppressants based on guaifenesin are not effective. Indeed, this derivative of creosote has never been shown to be an antitussive in any situation. Neither codeine nor dextromethorphan has been studied in this setting. Persistent cough after a cold may be treated with bronchodilation therapy.
- **Sneezing**—FGAHs are effective in blocking the sneeze reflex, but the newer nonsedating drugs are not. This difference may be attributable to the ability of the former groups of drugs to pass through the blood–brain barrier and have an effect on both histaminic and muscarinic receptors.
- **Sore throat**—This usually can be managed with mild analgesia.

There is no evidence that either part of the old adage "feed a cold and starve a fever" has any validity. The use of "steaming" vapors in the form of beverages such as hot tea or chicken soup and a heated air humidifier may, however, have some value, at least in noncontrolled, nonrandomized studies.

9. Are there more specific antiviral medications potentially on the horizon for the common cold?

Specific antiviral therapy in the future may include intranasal interferon, which has been useful when combined with ipratropium and nonsteroidal antiinflammatory drugs (NSAIDs). Additionally, because many serotypes of rhinoviruses bind to intercellular adhesion molecule 1 (ICAM 1), the virus–receptor interaction may be able to be blocked by using antibody to ICAM 1 or soluble receptor to bind to the viral component.

10. Complementary and alternative medicines have become quite popular. Are any effective in the treatment of the common cold?

Zinc lozenges and echinacea have been suggested to be useful in the treatment or prevention of the common cold. It can be difficult to compare studies of these products because of differences in form, purity, and preparation. Overall, although there may be some effect, the benefits are not without side effects, and most trial data unconvincing. Vitamin C has been studied for the longest time period for prevention or treatment of the common cold. At best, ascorbic acid has a modest effect in treatment but no use in prevention.

11. What is the relationship between the common cold and acute sinusitis?

In fact, sinus involvement is a part of the common cold, better referred to as an acute viral rhinosinusitis. Computed tomography (CT) scans in patients affected by the common cold show evidence of sinus involvement in about 90% of individuals. This process is self-limited over several weeks. Bacterial sinusitis, however, can develop subsequently as a consequence of impaired mucociliary clearance and obstruction of the sinus ostia. About 0.5–2.0% of common colds are estimated to result in acute bacterial sinusitis.

Most, but not all, cases of bacterial sinusitis are a result of a viral infection. Infection may spread to a paranasal sinus from an adjacent focus such as an infected maxillary molar or be introduced directly into the sinus via injury or during oropharyngeal or dental surgery that inadvertently penetrates the sinus wall.

12. How does one recognize acute bacterial sinusitis (ABS)?

Clinical criteria to diagnose ABS can be quite unreliable because clinically suspected disease is confirmed, when based on direct sinus aspiration, in only 30–40% of cases. The most predictive symptomatology is a purulent nasal discharge associated with unilateral maxillary tooth or facial pain that increases after a period of improvement. Fever is present only 10–15% of the time. Although complete sinus opacification or an air–fluid level can be useful radiographic findings, the high prevalence of radiographic abnormalities in viral rhinosinusitis makes sinus x-rays of limited diagnostic value. ABS involving the deeper paranasal sinuses, particularly the sphenoid, may have no real localizing signs other than a poorly localized headache with or without fever.

13. Which microorganisms are common causes of ABS?

The most common bacteria to be associated with ABS are all organisms that can be found in the human upper airway. *Streptococcus pneumoniae* (the pneumococcus), *Haemophilus influenzae*, and *Moraxella* (formerly *Branhamella*) *catarrhalis* are the most common, in descending order. These organisms can manifest resistance to penicillin and ampicillin, the latter two by beta-lactamase production. Other streptococci, oral cavity anaerobes, and *Staphylococcus aureus* can also be significant.

14. In what ways should acute sinusitis be treated?

Over and above the desire Dr. Osler described (see epigraph), which can be expressed by physicians and patients alike, treating clinically suspected ABS with an antimicrobial agent is fraught with uncertainty because many of the cases do not have a bacterial cause. Additionally, in analyzing randomized, double-blind trials, only a small benefit of antimicrobial drug use can be found, and most individuals receiving placebo improve without antimicrobial therapy. Because of these observations, patients with suspected ABS with mild symptoms should be treated with nasal adrenergics and analgesia. Antimicrobial interventions together with symptomatic therapy are reasonable for those with systemic toxicity, substantial fever, immunodeficiency, or any features suggesting extrasinus spread. In these studies, no serious complications occurred in the placebo groups. Despite potential resistance, amoxicillin, doxycycline, or trimethoprim–sulfamethoxazole is suggested as an initial choice for therapy.

15. How do complications of ABS occur?

The relatively benign nature of ABS is reflected in the difficulties in decisions regarding the need for antimicrobial use. Uncommonly, however, ABS is complicated by the spread of infection outside of the sinus cavity proper. This can be a devastating event such as cavernous sinus thrombosis related to sphenoid ABS, epidural empyema from frontal sinusitis, or orbital cellulitis from the spread of maxillary or ethmoid disease. Additionally, brain abscess or meningitis may occur as a complication of ABS. Pott's puffy tumor, a frontal bone subperiosteal abscess related to osteomyelitis, can also occur.

BIBLIOGRAPHY

1. Cohen S, Tyrrell DAJ, Smith AD: Psychological stress and susceptibility to the common cold. N Engl J Med 325:606–612, 1991.
2. Douglas RM, Chalker EB, Treacy B: Vitamin C for preventing and treating the common cold. Cochrane Database Syst Rev 2:CD000980, 2000.
3. Ernst E: The risk-benefit profile of commonly used herbal therapies: Ginkgo, St. John's wort, ginseng, echinacea, saw palmetto, and kava. Ann Intern Med 136:42–53, 2002.
4. Gwaltney JM: The common cold. In Mandell GL, Bennett JE, Dloin R (eds): Mandell, Douglas, and Bennett's Principles and Practice of Infectious Diseases, 5th ed. Philadelphia, Churchill Livingstone, 2000, pp 1940–1948.
5. Hendley JO, Gwaltney JM: Mechanisms of transmission of rhinovirus infections. Epidemiol Rev 10:243–258, 1988.
6. Hirschmann JV: Antibiotics for common respiratory tract infections in adults. Arch Intern Med 162: 256–264, 2002.
7. Meschievitz CK, Schultz SB, Dick EC: A model for obtaining predictable natural transmission of rhinoviruses in human volunteers. J Infect Dis 150:189–194, 1984.
8. Muether PS, Gwaltney JM: Variant effect of first- and second-generation antihistamines as clues to their mechanism of action on the sneeze reflex in the common cold. Clin Infect Dis 33:1483–1488, 2001.
9. Singh M: Heated humidified air for the common cold. Cochrane Database Syst Rev 4:CD001728, 2001.
10. Sinus and Allergy Health Partnership: Antimicrobial treatment guidelines for acute bacterial rhinosinusitis. Otolaryngol Head Neck Surg 123:S1-S32, 2000.
11. Snow V, Mottur-Pilson C, Hickner JM: Principles of appropriate antibiotic use for acute sinusitis in adults. Ann Intern Med 134:495–497, 2001.
12. Turner RB: Epidemiology, pathogenesis, and treatment of the common cold. Ann Allergy Asthma Immunol 78:531–540, 1997.
13. Whimbey E, Englund JA, Couch RB: Community respiratory virus infections in immunocompromised patients with cancer. Am J Med 102(3A):10–18, 1997.

86. ASTHMA AND CHRONIC OBSTRUCTIVE PULMONARY DISEASE

Michael E. Hanley, M.D., and Jerry A. Nick, M.D.

1. What are the important historical considerations in asthma?

Asthma is usually easy to diagnose by its periodicity and characteristic symptoms. Chest tightness, breathlessness, and wheezing are reported most commonly. In some patients, especially children and adolescents, cough may be the only symptom. After the diagnosis is made, emphasis should turn to identification of triggers that may be avoidable or treatable. A personal or family history of atopy, with symptoms triggered by inhalation of readily identifiable allergens, is common. Exercise, cold air, and inhaled irritants or fumes are other common triggers. Esophageal reflux and chronic sinusitis may worsen asthma; a history of such disorders should be pursued aggressively. Some patients may have poor control because of concomitant use of beta-blockers or nonsteroidal drugs. Others may experience symptoms after exposure to metabisulfite in wines and salad bars. If the patient works in a high-risk occupation or reports improvement in symptoms during holidays and weekends, occupational asthma should be suspected.

2. Is there a difference in the pathophysiology of intrinsic and extrinsic asthma?

No. Asthma is an inflammatory disease of the airways characterized by reversible airflow limitation. The pattern of inflammation is similar in allergic (extrinsic) and nonallergic (intrinsic) asthma. The airways are infiltrated with eosinophils and lymphocytes. Release of inflammatory mediators results in airway edema, smooth muscle hypertrophy, and mucus secretion. Mast cell activation and histamine release are probably important in the early bronchoconstrictor response to allergens and other stimuli but not critical in the more chronic late-phase inflammatory reaction, which causes bronchial hyperresponsiveness.

3. When is bronchoprovocation testing useful in the diagnosis of asthma?

The pathophysiology of asthma includes both reversible airflow obstruction and airway hyperreactivity. Demonstration of reversible airflow obstruction by spirometry is highly supportive of the diagnosis of asthma. However, many patients have normal spirometry between exacerbations even though they remain mildly symptomatic. In this setting, demonstration of hyperreactive airways by bronchoprovocation testing is highly suggestive of the diagnosis. Testing involves measuring spirometry before and after inhalation of escalating doses of nonspecific irritants (methacholine or histamine). Patients with airway hyperreactivity experience significant declines in spirometry at much lower doses than normal subjects.

4. Is airway hyperreactivity unique to patients with asthma?

No. Chronic obstructive pulmonary disease (COPD), respiratory dysfunction after inhalation of smoke or chemical irritants, chronic bronchiectasis, sarcoidosis, and chronic lung disease after an episode of acute respiratory distress syndrome are characterized by airway hyperreactivity. In general, however, asthma is associated with the most severe degrees of airway hyperreactivity.

5. Should patients with asthma undergo inhalation challenge to identify offending allergens?

No. Identification of potential allergens by inhalation challenge may provoke acute, life-threatening bronchospasm. It should be performed only in extreme circumstances in laboratories specially staffed and equipped to handle respiratory emergencies.

6. When may patients benefit from immunotherapy for asthma?

Immunotherapy may have a role in treating extrinsic asthma when a patient's history correlates well with skin-test results, when avoidance of allergens is not possible, or when symptoms are difficult to control with inhaled corticosteroids and bronchodilators. If desensitization therapy is selected, higher doses of antigen and longer duration of treatment probably produce the best results. However, evidence that some asthmatics improve with desensitization therapy is limited.

7. When should a diagnosis of occupational asthma be considered?

Occupational asthma is characterized by reversible airflow limitation that results from exposure to certain chemicals and antigens in the workplace. More than 200 substances are known to produce the syndrome. Symptoms usually develop within a few years of steady exposure. The typical patient experiences relief outside the workplace (e.g., over the weekend or during vacations) but relapses on return to work. Frequent peak flow monitoring throughout the workday and on weekends for 3–4 weeks may be necessary to make the diagnosis because patients with predominantly late-phase asthmatic reactions do not become symptomatic until hours after exposure, typically when they are at home. Patients with preexisting asthma who experience exacerbations caused by nonspecific irritants in the workplace do not qualify for the diagnosis of occupational asthma. Treatment hinges on avoidance of the antigen; continued exposure may translate into progressive disease. If changing jobs is not an option, the use of a respirator and standard asthma therapy must be strongly considered.

8. What are the goals of pharmacotherapy in asthma?

Treatment of asthma depends on its severity. Patients with mild intermittent asthma have infrequent symptoms and rare exacerbations. They can be managed adequately with short-acting inhaled bronchodilators as needed. Mild, moderate, and severe persistent asthma are characterized by escalating severity and frequency of symptoms and exacerbations. The principal goals of pharmacotherapy in such patients is to prevent acute exacerbations by improving airway hyperreactivity and to maintain near-normal daily lung function while avoiding the unwanted effects of polypharmacy. Patients with mild persistent asthma generally can be managed with a single, low-dose anti-inflammatory agent (either inhaled corticosteroid or, in children, cromolyn) administered daily; a short-acting inhaled bronchodilator is used on an as-needed basis for breakthrough symptoms. For moderate persistent asthma, the dose of daily inhaled corticosteroid is increased. In addition, a long-acting bronchodilator (preferably inhaled) is also prescribed on a daily, regularly scheduled basis. Patients with severe persistent asthma require daily high-dose inhaled corticosteroids and a long-acting inhaled bronchodilator administered on a regularly scheduled basis. Patients with severe persistent asthma whose symptoms are not well controlled on this regimen may also need daily oral corticosteroids. However, before beginning therapy with chronic oral corticosteroids, inhaled corticosteroid and long-acting bronchodilator therapy should be maximized, metered-dose inhaler (MDI) technique should be evaluated, and a careful search for reversible triggers should be made.

9. What long-acting bronchodilators are available for the treatment of asthma?

Sustained-release theophylline, oral sustained-release albuterol, and inhaled long-acting beta-agonists (LABA) are all long-term bronchodilators. Of these medications, inhaled LABAs are the agents of choice based on the strength of their bronchodilating effects and low toxicity. Their sustained effect makes them especially valuable in patients with moderate and severe persistent asthma and those with significant nocturnal symptoms. However, because the onset of action of these medications is slow, patients must still be prescribed and educated on using a short-acting inhaled bronchodilator for breakthrough symptoms. Salmeterol is the only inhaled LABA currently available in the United States, although formoterol may also be available soon.

10. What are leukotriene modifiers?

Leukotriene modifiers are new anti-inflammatory agents that interrupt the inflammatory cascade by blocking leukotriene receptors or inhibiting the production of leukotrienes. They also have modest bronchodilating effects. Most of the clinical trials evaluating their efficacy in asthma have been conducted in patients with mild to moderate persistent asthma. These studies indicate that leukotriene modifiers may be an alternative to low-dose inhaled corticosteroid therapy in mild asthma. Although it is becoming increasing popular to add these drugs as an additional anti-inflammatory agent in patients with severe persistent asthma, their efficacy in this setting has not been studied.

11. Is magnesium indicated in the management of status asthmaticus?

Intravenous magnesium sulfate 1–2 g administered over 20 minutes, has been advocated as rescue therapy in patients with status asthmaticus. However, multiple large, randomized, placebo-controlled trials have yielded conflicting results regarding its efficacy. A number of trials have not shown any improvement in hospitalization rates, duration of emergency department treatment, or changes in peak expiratory flow rate (PEFR) or forced expiratory volume in 1 second (FEV_1) in magnesium-treated and untreated patients. Recent studies have suggested, however, that the administration of magnesium may be associated with improvement in emergency department (ED) FEV_1 and subsequent hospitalization rates, especially in patients with severe status asthmaticus ($FEV_1 < 25\%$ predicted).

12. How should patients with asthma be educated?

Patient education is a critical component of management of asthma, especially for patients with moderate to severe persistent disease. Education involves helping patients to understand the disease and to practice the skills necessary to manage it. Information should include the patho-physiology of asthma, especially its signs and symptoms, and the need to identify and avoid triggers. In addition, the importance of close monitoring of airway function with peak flow meters and early intervention when attacks begin must be stressed. Finally, patients must be educated about therapeutic approaches, including the mechanism of action of medications, potential side effects of acute and chronic use (including misconceptions), proper use of inhalers, indications for emergency care, and written plans for managing acute exacerbations.

13. Is peak flow monitoring useful in asthma?

Studies have suggested a reduction in the severity of asthma and reduced airflow variability when peak flows are monitored for several months and therapy is adjusted accordingly. Peak flow meters simply measure the maximal rate of expiratory airflow after inspiration to total lung capacity. Because peak flows are highly dependent on personal effort, patients must be well motivated. If effort is good, serial peak flows provide an objective measurement of airway function and are useful in monitoring respiratory trends in patients with moderate and severe asthma. Such monitoring is important because many patients cannot subjectively detect changes in airflow. Optimal benefit from peak flow monitoring requires keeping a diary that records simultaneous symptoms. Patients should record peak flows each morning and evening (before and after use of a bronchodilator) and whenever chest symptoms occur. Normally, some diurnal variation is seen, with morning values lower than evening values. The degree of hyperresponsiveness in asthmatics has been shown to correlate with early morning peak flows, the gap between morning and evening values (normally $< 15\%$), and the amount of improvement in flow rates after bronchodilator use. If a trend toward increased hyperresponsiveness is seen, the dose of inhaled steroid may be augmented. The converse also may be true.

14. Does a reduced peak flow rate always indicate asthma?

No. Determinants of air flow include airway resistance, driving pressure, and the lung volume at which airflow was measured. Other obstructive lung diseases, such as COPD, poor efforts caused by neuromuscular disease or lack of motivation, and restrictive lung disease associated with diminished lung volumes, may all result in reduced PEFRs.

15. When should a patient with asthma be hospitalized?

The decision to hospitalize an asthmatic patient depends on several factors, including the nature and persistence of the inciting stimulus, the severity of prior attacks (e.g., history of hospitalizations, intubation, steroid dependence), severity of symptoms, severity of airflow obstruction, medication use at the time of the exacerbation, access to medical care, adequacy of support at home, and psychiatric stability. Indicators of severe obstruction include tachycardia (> 110 bpm), extensive use of accessory muscles of respiration, pulsus paradoxus ≥ 15 mmHg, and inability to complete a sentence. An $FEV_1 < 40\%$ of the predicted value is an ominous sign. Impending cardiac arrest is suggested by cyanosis, altered mental status, normal to high $PaCO_2$, low pH, exhaustion, bradycardia, or a silent chest. If signs and symptoms do not improve within 20–30 minutes of aggressive beta-adrenergic therapy, the patient should be admitted. If discharge from the ED is considered, improvement in symptoms and spirometry must be significant and sustained with an increase in FEV_1 to at least 40% of the predicted value after 60–90 minutes. With a history of brittle asthma, relapsing course over the previous weeks or months, or prior ED visits during the current exacerbation, the patient should be considered for ED admission, regardless of the acute response to bronchodilators and steroids.

16. What is the proper way to use an MDI?

After shaking the inhaler, the patient should exhale normally to functional residual capacity (FRC), place the device about 4 cm in front of the mouth, simultaneously depress the canister, and begin a slow inhalation. Inspiration continues to total lung capacity (TLC), at which point the breath is held for at least a few seconds. Inspiration faster than 4–5 seconds causes excessive deposition of particles in the oropharynx and large airways. Breath holding is also crucial to allow aerosolized particles to settle on the mucosal surface of the targeted small airways. When used properly, MDIs are at least as effective as nebulizers. Spacers decrease the amount of medication lost to the air or deposited in the oropharynx and should be used routinely during severe exacerbations when slow inspiration and prolonged breath holding are difficult to perform. They also are useful if proper MDI technique cannot be mastered.

17. What is COPD?

COPD has no precise definition. It is a nonspecific term that refers to conditions generally characterized by cough expectoration, dyspnea, and progressive reduction in expiratory air flow. The term refers to a spectrum of disease that includes asthmatic bronchitis, chronic bronchitis, and emphysema and recognizes that these diseases share a common pathophysiology with varying clinical presentations. Chronic bronchitis is a clinical diagnosis defined as the presence of a productive cough for 3 or more months in at least 2 consecutive years without a known underlying cause other than cigarette smoking. Histologically, inflammation of the airway mucosa and hypertrophy of submucosal glands occurs as a result of chronic exposure to inhaled irritants. Emphysema is a pathologic diagnosis defined as the irreversible enlargement of airspaces distal to terminal bronchioles with destruction of gas-exchanging surfaces. As alveolar septae are destroyed, radial traction on small airways is lost. This loss of elastic recoil results in hyperinflation, excessive collapse of airways during expiration, and chronic airflow limitation. Cigarette smoking is by far the most important risk factor in the development of COPD, but only 10–15% of smokers develop clinically significant disease.

18. Is it important to differentiate clinically or physiologically between "blue bloaters" and "pink puffers"?

Patients with chronic bronchitis, often referred to as "blue bloaters," present with cough and copious sputum production. They are typically overweight and tend to have more upper respiratory infections as well as worse matching of ventilation and perfusion than patients with emphysema. Hypoxemia and hypercapnia are worse, and complications such as cor pulmonale and polycythemia are more prevalent. Because patients with predominant bronchitis are not markedly hyperinflated and have a tendency toward superimposed hypoventilation, dyspnea (which is related to work of breathing) may not be a major complaint.

Patients with predominant emphysema, often referred to as "pink puffers," are typically thin. Their lung volumes are considerably elevated because of air trapping, and dyspnea is a major complaint. Pursed-lip breathing and use of accessory muscles of respiration are common, and breath sounds are markedly diminished. In contrast to patients with chronic bronchitis, diffusing capacity may be severely reduced, indicating a major disturbance at the alveolar–capillary interface. Ventilation and perfusion deficits are relatively balanced, however, resulting in only mild or moderate hypoxemia. Hypercapnia usually occurs only during acute exacerbations or in end-stage disease. Consequently, emphysematous patients experience fewer complications of chronic hypoxia and hypercapnia and generally live longer but have more disability related to breathlessness.

Although pure examples exist, chronic bronchitis and emphysema typically coexist in varying proportions within the same patients. In end-stage patients, it is particularly difficult to distinguish between the two.

19. What is the National Lung Health Education Program (NLHEP)?

NLHEP is an ambitious new national education program aimed at primary care providers. A major focus of NLHEP is to improve early identification and intervention in COPD and related disorders through reduction of risk factors. This program was motivated in large part by the Lung Health Study, which confirmed that smokers most at risk for developing COPD can be identified before the onset of clinical disease by office spirometry and that smoking cessation in this group successfully alters the natural course of the disease. A critical concept of this project is that pulmonary function in smokers most at risk for developing COPD is characterized by acceleration of the age-related decline in the FEV_1 to FVC ratio. The Lung Health Study proved that the excessive rate of decline in FEV_1 in this population can be stopped by smoking cessation. The NL-HEP encourages primary care providers to perform office spirometry on smoking patients and to redouble efforts at risk reduction (primarily but not exclusively smoking cessation) in patients with evidence of early airflow obstruction. Patients should "test your lungs, know your numbers."

20. What are the "GOLD Guidelines"?

The **G**lobal Initiative for Chronic **O**bstructive **L**ung **D**isease is a collaborative effort between the National Heart, Lung and Blood Institute and the World Health Organization. The objectives of the GOLD project are to (1) increase awareness about COPD among health care professionals and the general public; (2) improve diagnosis, management, and prevention of COPD; and (3) stimulate research regarding COPD. The GOLD Guidelines include evidence-based treatment strategies emphasizing escalating therapy related to the severity of disease. Specific recommendations may be found at the GOLD website: www.goldcopd.com.

21. What concerns arise in administering oxygen therapy in patients with COPD?

A common worry associated with administering oxygen in patients with COPD is that life-threatening hypercapnia will result from increased dead-space ventilation. When oxygen is administered, hypoxic bronchoconstriction is reduced throughout the lung, including areas that are poorly perfused because of destruction of septal capillaries. The result is increased dead-space ventilation, usually accompanied by a modest increase in carbon dioxide tension. In general, however, the increase in dead-space ventilation and $PaCO_2$ is minimal. Indeed, some patients show an increase in minute ventilation as a result of the increasing $PaCO_2$. When oxygen therapy is instituted, the flow rate should be titrated gradually upward to maintain a PaO_2 of 60 and oxygen saturation of 90% without overcorrection. Any adjustment should be accompanied by measurement of arterial blood gases. Oxygen must not be withheld from a hypoxic patient because of fear of an increasing $PaCO_2$.

22. Are bronchodilators indicated in patients with COPD if spirometry does not improve acutely after their administration?

Unfortunately, many patients with COPD are labeled as nonresponders in the pulmonary testing laboratory when, on one occasion, they fail to show improvement after beta-adrenergic treatment. Although patients with COPD rarely respond to bronchodilators as dramatically as patients with asthma, most have a component of airway hyperreactivity that improves with treatment. Benefit may be indicated over a few weeks of treatment by improvement in FEV_1, decreased hyperinflation (with or without improved flow rates), reduction in dyspnea, or improved exercise tolerance. Additionally, in patients with stable COPD, anticholinergic agents such as ipratropium bromide produce more bronchodilation than conventional doses of beta agonists and do not lose efficacy over time. Anticholinergics are especially useful in patients with chronic bronchitis because these agents reduce the volume of sputum without changing its viscosity. However, because maximal benefit is not achieved for 30 minutes or more after use, these agents are less convenient for testing and often are not used in the pulmonary function laboratory.

23. Are oral corticosteroids effective in patients with chronic, stable COPD?

Although corticosteroid therapy in some form is essential in managing all patients with moderate or severe asthma, it is often ineffective in patients with COPD. A meta-analysis of 43 studies indicated that only 10% of patients with chronic, stable COPD experienced an increase of ≥ 20% in FEV_1 after being prescribed oral corticosteroids. It is difficult to predict who will respond to corticosteroids. A clinical trial is therefore warranted in patients with moderate to severe disease after cessation of smoking and institution of maximal bronchodilator therapy. Pulmonary function testing should be performed before and after the trial to assess objectively the effect on airflow limitation. Prednisone, 40 mg/day (or the equivalent) for 4 weeks, is a reasonable trial. If the patient shows significant objective improvement, the dose should be tapered to the lowest effective maintenance level. If no improvement occurs with corticosteroid therapy, it should be discontinued.

24. What can be done to improve quality of life in patients with severe COPD?

Despite cessation of smoking and optimal medical therapy (including oxygen), patients with severe COPD often continue to complain of breathlessness. Patients begin to avoid physical activity because of anticipated dyspnea, and their level of conditioning worsens. Some patients reap great benefits from a program of education and rehabilitation that addresses these issues. After screening for heart disease and exercise-induced hypoxia, daily exercise training may be initiated (e.g., stationary bicycle, walking) to build endurance and to increase the patient's ability to perform activities of daily living. Instruction in diaphragmatic and pursed-lip breathing may be of further assistance. Occupational therapists often suggest energy-saving devices and help to plan daily schedules that include rest periods. Furthermore, mental health professionals may play a key role in managing the reactive depression that is common in patients with severe COPD.

25. What is lung volume reduction surgery (LVRS)?

LVRS is an experimental surgical therapy for COPD. It is based on the concept that lungs in patients with COPD anatomically consist of areas of well-preserved lung tissue interspersed with regions with enlarged airspaces (bullae). Bullae contribute to dyspnea through hyperinflation, represent wasted ventilation that does not contribute to gas exchange, and further worsen gas exchange by compressing adjacent areas of normal lung. Goals of LVRS include improvement of symptoms and gas exchange through surgical resection of bullae with decompression of neighboring lung units. Studies evaluating the efficacy of this surgical approach have been hampered by lack of appropriate randomized controls and a potentially significant placebo effect. Although preliminary studies suggest that surgery results in at least a transient improvement in clinical symptoms and spirometry, it is not known whether this effect persists over the long term or translates into improved survival.

CONTROVERSIES

26. Are inhaled corticosteroids beneficial in COPD?

For: Use of inhaled corticosteroids in moderate COPD ($FEV_1 < 50\%$ predicted) may be associated with reduced symptoms and fewer exacerbations. In addition, patients with a high degree of reversibility or recent use of steroids are frequently excluded from effectiveness trials. These may be the very patients who benefit most from inhaled corticosteroids.

Against: The early introduction of inhaled corticosteroids does not affect the rate of decline in FEV_1 in COPD. In addition, effectiveness of inhaled corticosteroids in severe COPD ($FEV_1 < 800$ mL) has not been studied. Although relatively safe, use of higher doses of more potent inhaled corticosteroids may be associated with increased bone turnover, suppression of the pituitary–adrenal axis, and cataract formation.

27. Is theophylline beneficial in the management of patients with asthma and COPD?

For:

- Patients with prominent nocturnal symptoms may be greatly helped by 24-hour theophylline preparations given once daily in the early evening.
- Theophylline may be used as a steroid-sparing measure in patients with chronic severe asthma.
- Theoretical benefits include reduced diaphragmatic fatigability, positive inotropy, and improved mucociliary clearance.
- Theophylline is a central respiratory stimulant and may benefit a subset of patients with COPD who hypoventilate even though their resistive loads are not extreme (i.e., blue bloaters).

- Some studies suggest improved performance and quality of life not necessarily related to improved spirometry.

Against:

- During acute exacerbations, no improvement in spirometry or symptoms results when theophylline is added to maximal beta-agonist therapy, but side effects usually increase.
- Theophylline has a narrow therapeutic window, and levels may be affected by many commonly prescribed drugs as well as by smoking.
- The theoretical benefits are modest at best and of uncertain clinical importance.

28. Are oral beta agonists indicated in patients with asthma?

For:

- Long-acting preparations are particularly useful for relief of nocturnal asthma.
- Many small children and some adults cannot be trained to use MDIs effectively.

Against:

- At doses resulting in equivalent bronchodilation, oral beta agonists have four times the incidence of side effects as inhaled agents.
- For patients who cannot use MDIs properly, spacer devices, nebulizers, and rotacaps are available as an alternative to oral beta agonists.
- Long-acting inhaled beta agonists, such as salmeterol, are available for the treatment of nocturnal symptoms.

BIBLIOGRAPHY

1. Alsaeedi A, Sin DD, McAlister FA: The effects of inhaled corticosteroids in chronic obstructive pulmonary disease: A systematic review of randomized placebo-controlled trials. Am J Med 113:59–65, 2002.
2. Anthonisen NR, Connett JE, Kiley JP, et al: Effects of smoking intervention and the use of an inhaled anticholinergic bronchodilator on the rate of decline of FEV_1: The Lung Health Study. JAMA 272:1497–1505, 1994.
3. Bousamra M, Haasler GB, Lipchik RJ, et al: Functional and oximetric assessment of patients after lung reduction surgery. J Thorac Cardiovasc Surg 113:675–681, 1997.
4. Clark NM, Evans D, Mellins RB: Patient use of peak flow monitoring. Am Rev Respir Dis 145:722, 1992.
5. Fein A, Fein AM: Management of acute exacerbations in chronic pulmonary disease. Curr Opin Pulm Med 6:122–126, 2000.
6. Gomez FP, Rodriguez-Roisin R: Global Initiative for Chronic Obstructive Lung Disease (GOLD) guidelines for chronic obstructive pulmonary disease. Curr Opin Pulm Med 8:81–86, 2002.
7. Gross NJ: Leukotriene modifiers: What place in asthma? J Respir Dis 19:245–261, 1998.
8. Guidelines for the Diagnosis and Management of Asthma. Expert Panel Report II. Bethesda, MD, National Institutes of Health, 1997, NIH publication 97–4051.
9. Kornmann O, Beeh KM, Beier, L et al: Newly diagnosed chronic pulmonary disease. Clinical features and distribution of the novel stages of the Global Initiative for Obstructive Lung Disease. Respiration 70:67–75, 2003.
10. McEvoy CE, Niewoehner DE: Corticosteroids in chronic obstructive pulmonary disease. Clinical risks and benefits. Clin Chest Med 21:739–752, 2000.
11. O'Riordan TG: Inhaled corticosteroids in chronic obstructive pulmonary disease: New trials and old practices. J Aerosol Med 16:1–8, 2003.
12. Petty TL: The National Lung Health Education Program. Chest 113:123S–161S, 1998.
13. Petty TL, Weinmann GG: Building a national strategy for the prevention, management, and research in chronic obstructive pulmonary disease. JAMA 277:246–253, 1997.
14. Ries AL, Kaplan RM, Limberg TM, Prewitt LM: Effects of pulmonary rehabilitation on physiologic and psychosocial outcomes in patients with chronic obstructive pulmonary disease. Ann Intern Med 122:823–832, 1995.
15. Silverman RA, Osborn H, Runge J, et al: IV magnesium sulfate in the treatment of acute severe asthma. A multicenter randomized controlled trial. Chest 122:489–497, 2002.

87. PULMONARY FUNCTION TESTS

Michael E. Hanley, M.D.

1. When are pulmonary function tests (PFTs) indicated?

The primary purposes of PFTs are diagnostic (to uncover clinically undetected disease and to determine the nature of physiologic dysfunction), quantitative (to determine the severity of dysfunction), and monitory (to follow response to therapy or progression of disease). Common indications for pulmonary function testing in the primary care setting include evaluation of patients with unexplained dyspnea, cough, hypoxemia, right-sided congestive heart failure, or abnormal chest radiograph suggestive of diffuse lung disease. PFTs are particularly useful for chronic monitoring of patients with conditions characterized by infiltrative processes or airflow limitation.

2. Describe the myriad of PFTs.

Simple spirometry, lung volumes, diffusion capacity of the lungs for carbon monoxide (DLCO), flow-volume loops, and arterial blood gases are available in most laboratories. More extensive tests, including pressure–volume curves, airway resistance and conductance, inhalational challenge, exercise testing, ventilatory drive studies, maximum inspiratory and expiratory pressures (PI_{max} and PE_{max}), and polysomnography, are available in specialty laboratories.

3. What constitutes simple spirometry?

Simple spirometry consists primarily of forced vital capacity (FVC), forced expiratory volume in one second (FEV_1), FEV_1/FVC ratio, forced expiratory flow between 25% and 75% of vital capacity ($FEF_{25-75\%}$), and peak expiratory flow rate (PEFR). Simple spirometry also includes measurement of these parameters after bronchodilator treatment. Additional flow rates, such as forced expiratory flow at 25%, 50%, and 75% of vital capacity ($FEF_{25\%}$, $FEF_{50\%}$, and $FEF_{75\%}$) are occasionally reported but do not add significantly to the sensitivity of the other tests.

4. How is simple spirometry interpreted?

The patient's ability to perform the tests must be evaluated first. Abnormal results are occasionally obtained because patients are either unable (because of poor comprehension of instructions, altered mental status, or abnormal oral anatomy that precludes a good spirometer interface) or unwilling to cooperate with testing. Clues to poor patient cooperation include inability to produce consistent results (spirometry is generally measured at least three to five times during a test session), the presence of artifacts on flow–volume loops or spirograms, and written comments of the technician performing the tests. Although all parameters measured in simple spirometry depend on patient effort, the FEV_1 and FVC are the most reproducible and therefore offer the most reliable information.

If patient cooperation is good, the next step is to determine if the results are normal. Absolute PFT values obtained in normal subjects are influenced by several factors, including age, height, and sex. Regression equations are used to calculate published predicted normal values for a given patient on the basis of these factors. Other factors, particularly race, also influence predicted normal values but are not routinely considered in published standards. In general, predicted values for patients of African or Asian heritage tend to be 8–13% lower than those for those of European ancestry, but the optimal correction factors are controversial and not well defined.

Finally, if the results of FEV_1 or FVC are not within the normal range, the pattern of dysfunction should be determined by consideration of the FEV_1/FVC ratio and other flow rates (see questions 5 and 6).

5. Define *obstructive* lung diseases. How are they diagnosed?

Obstructive lung diseases are characterized anatomically and physiologically by obstruction of airflow (airflow limitation). Airflow depends on the lung volume at which it is measured (lower rates occur at smaller lung volumes), resistance of the airways, and pressure that generates flow (driving force determined by elastic recoil of the lung-thoracic cage unit). Common obstructive lung diseases caused primarily by increased airway resistance include asthma, chronic bronchitis, and chronic bronchiectasis; airflow limitation in emphysema is largely secondary to decreased elastic recoil. Because the FEV_1 depends on the rate of airflow more than the FVC, the FEV_1 is generally decreased out of proportion to the FVC in obstructive lung processes. Thus, the FEV_1/FVC ratio is decreased, usually below 0.7.

6. What are restrictive lung diseases?

Restrictive lung diseases are characterized by a reduced total lung capacity (TLC). The differential diagnosis is complex but can be simplified by organizing restrictive disorders into four categories: (1) parenchymal infiltrative disease (interstitial or alveolar), (2) chest wall abnormalities, (3) pleural disease, and (4) neuromuscular weakness involving ventilatory muscles.

Restrictive diseases are characterized by decreased lung volumes and, with the exception of neuromuscular weakness, increased elastic recoil of the lung-thoracic cage unit. Thus, although absolute measures of airflow are decreased (because of lower lung volumes), airflow corrected for lung volume is normal or increased. The FEV_1/FVC ratio is, therefore, normal or increased in patients with restrictive lung disease.

7. Define lung volumes.

Lung volumes measure the absolute volumes of the lungs at various points in the respiratory cycle. Commonly reported volumes include TLC (volume of gas in the lungs after total inspiration), residual volume (RV; volume of gas in the lungs after total expiration), and function residual capacity (FRC; volume of gas remaining in the lungs at end expiration during tidal volume breathing). When FRC is measured by body plethysmography (body box), it is referred to as thoracic gas volume (TGV).

As with simple spirometry, normal values are influenced by age, height, sex, and race. Thus, results are reported as both absolute values and as a percentage of the predicted normal value.

8. What approach is used in interpreting lung volumes?

Measurement of lung volumes is especially sensitive to patient effort. Of the three commonly measured volumes, FRC (or TGV) is the least effort dependent and the most reliable; thus, it should be considered first. In severe obstructive lung diseases, all three volumes are usually increased, but in severe restrictive diseases, they are usually decreased. Demonstration of a decreased TLC and an increased RV (regardless of FRC) suggests poor patient effort (e.g., inability or unwillingness to perform the maneuver).

9. When are lung volumes indicated?

Simple spirometry differentiates obstruction from restriction in most patients. Similarly, spirometry alone is adequate to monitor most patients' clinical condition and response to therapy over time. Therefore, lung volumes, which add significant expense to PFTs, are seldom required. Lung volumes are indicated (1) to evaluate patients with pulmonary symptoms and normal spirometry; (2) to quantitate more accurately the severity of restriction or obstruction; (3) to evaluate patients with both obstruction and restriction; and (4) to evaluate patients with severe obstruction and a markedly reduced FVC. In patients in the fourth category, lung volumes can clarify whether the decrement in FVC is attributable to obstruction alone or a coexistent restrictive process.

10. What does DLCO measure?

DLCO measures the diffusion of carbon monoxide (CO) across the alveolar-capillary membrane and is thought to reflect the efficiency of gas exchange. Although the permeability (and therefore thickness) of the membrane affects the value of DLCO, other factors are also important, including the surface area of the membrane (and therefore the lung volume at which it is measured), the hemoglobin (Hb) concentration in blood (Hb binds CO), and matching of ventilation and perfusion. Absolute values for DLCO are usually corrected for some of these factors. Specifically, DLCO-Hb corrects DLCO for hemoglobin concentration, and DLCO/VA corrects for the lung volume at which it is measured.

11. What diseases are associated with an abnormal DLCO?

DLCO is decreased in lung diseases characterized by thickening of the alveolar-capillary membrane (pulmonary infiltrative disorders), destruction of the membrane (emphysema or pulmonary vasculopathies), and mismatching of ventilation and perfusion. Thus, an abnormal DLCO is nonspecific. Conditions characterized by increased DLCO include congestive heart failure (prolonged capillary blood transit time increases the time for absorption of CO) and significant alveolar or airway hemorrhage.

12. What is the value of screening spirometry in asymptomatic cigarette smokers?

Smokers most at risk of developing chronic obstructive pulmonary disease (COPD) experience a long, asymptomatic period characterized by an accelerated loss of pulmonary function. Such patients can be identified by measuring the FEV_1/FVC ratio with office spirometry. Several studies have demonstrated that PFTs in patients with the most rapid decline in pulmonary function are characterized by an FEV_1/FVC ratio $< 70\%$. The low FEV_1/FVC ratio exists before measurable declines in FEV_1 develop. Successful intervention during this time interval can return patients to the normal age-related rate of pulmonary function decline before the onset of symptomatic COPD.

13. What is the effect of smoking cessation on pulmonary function in smokers most at risk of developing COPD?

FEV_1 declines at a rate of 70–90 mL/year in asymptomatic smokers who have an FEV_1/FVC ratio $< 70\%$. The 5-year Lung Health Study demonstrated that the rate of change in FEV_1 returned to the normal age-related rate of 20–30 mL/year after smoking cessation. In addition, FEV_1 increased significantly during the first 2–3 years after smoking cessation.

14. Should PFTs be obtained in acutely ill patients?

The timing of PFTs depends on the clinical scenario. Physiologic evaluation during an acute exacerbation of a chronic illness may be valuable to diagnose the cause of previously unexplained dyspnea, hypoxemia, or cough or to monitor response to therapy in exacerbations of chronic obstructive disease. However, if the diagnosis is already known or readily apparent from other clinical data, PFTs in acutely ill patients add little useful information but considerable unnecessary expense. For comparative purposes, it is generally more valuable to determine the severity of illness when patients are at baseline function. Return to baseline may require up to 6 weeks of convalescence after an acute exacerbation of obstructive disease. In addition, response to therapy in acutely ill patients is more efficiently and economically accomplished by monitoring PEFR alone.

15. Is the diagnosis of asthma confirmed by demonstration of improved airflow after administration of bronchodilators?

One of the clinical hallmarks of asthma is reversibility of airflow obstruction. Reversibility is indicated by significant improvement in FEV_1, FVC, or both after administration of an inhaled bronchodilator, usually a beta-2 agonist. *Significant* is defined as an increase > 15–20% with an absolute increase of ≥ 200 mL in either parameter. However, patients with other obstructive lung diseases, such as chronic bronchitis and emphysema, occasionally demonstrate similar improvement. Furthermore, PFTs in patients with severe asthma may not demonstrate acute reversibility until parenteral corticosteroids have been administered for several months. Thus, the diagnosis of asthma requires thorough consideration of all available clinical, physiologic, radiographic, and pathologic data and not solely the response to bronchodilator therapy.

16. What other physiologic clues help differentiate asthma from emphysema?

The DLCO in asthma may be mildly increased, normal, or decreased, but it is usually severely reduced in advanced emphysema. The pressure–volume curve in both conditions is shifted up and to the left when compared with normal. However, the slope of the curve is usually steeper than normal in emphysema but normal in asthma. Both conditions are also characterized by airway hyperreactivity (documented by measuring spirometry after inhaling escalating doses of methacholine); however, the degree of hyperreactivity tends to be greater in asthma.

17. How do flow volume loops identify the site of large airway obstruction?

Abnormalities in the expiratory or inspiratory limb of the flow volume curve help identify the site of obstruction because extrathoracic and intrathoracic airways behave differently during inspiration and expiration. Extrathoracic airways narrow during inspiration and expand during expiration. In contrast, intrathoracic airways become larger during inspiration and narrow during expiration. Thus, a variable (e.g., the degree of obstruction changes during the respiratory cycle) extrathoracic airway obstruction is characterized by flow limitation during inspiration but not expiration; the inspiratory flow loop has a plateau, but the expiratory loop appears normal. Variable intrathoracic airway obstruction is characterized by flow limitation during expiration; the expiratory flow loop has a plateau shape, but the inspiration loop is normal. A fixed (the degree of obstruction remains constant throughout the respiratory cycle) large airway obstruction is characterized by plateaus in both the expiratory and inspiratory flow loops.

BIBLIOGRAPHY

1. Anthonisen NR, Connett JE, Kiley JP, et al: Effects of smoking intervention and the use of an inhaled anticholinergic bronchodilator on the rate of decline of FEV_1. The Lung Health Study. JAMA 272:1497–1505, 1994.
2. Burrows B, Knudson RJ, Camilli AE, et al: The "horse-racing effect" and predicting decline in forced expiratory volume in one second from screening spirometry. Am Rev Respir Dis 135:788–793, 1987.
3. Cotton DJ, Soparker GR, Grahan BL: Diffusing capacity in the clinical assessment of chronic airflow limitation. Med Clin North Am 80:549–564, 1996.
4. Crapo RO: Pulmonary-function testing. N Engl J Med 331:25–30, 1994.
5. Culver BH: Preoperative assessment of the thoracic surgery patient: Pulmonary function testing. Semin Thorac Cardiovasc Surg 13:92–104, 2001.
6. Official Statement of the American Thoracic Society: Lung function testing: Selection of reference values and interpretive strategies. Am Rev Respir Dis 144:1202–1218, 1991.
7. Petty TL: The predictive value of spirometry. Identifying patients at risk for lung cancer in the primary care setting. Postgrad Med 101:128–140, 1997.
8. Smetana GW: Preoperative pulmonary assessment of the older adult. Clin Geriatr Med 19:35–55, 2003.
9. Subramanian D, Guntupalli KK: Diagnosing obstructive lung disease. Why is differentiating COPD from asthma important? Postgrad Med 95:69–85, 1994.
10. Townsend MC: ACOEM position paper. Spirometry in the occupational setting. American College of Occupational and Environmental Medicine. J Occup Environ Med 42:228–245, 2000.
11. Wanger J, Irvin CG: Office spirometry: Equipment selection and training of staff in the private practice setting. J Asthma 34:93–104, 1997.

88. HYPOXEMIA AND OXYGEN THERAPY

Michael E. Hanley, M.D., and Jerry A. Nick, M.D.

1. List the five pathophysiologic causes of hypoxemia.

1. Reduction in inspired partial pressure of oxygen (P_iO_2)
2. Hypoventilation
3. Diffusion impairment
4. Ventilation-perfusion (V-Q) mismatch
5. Shunting

2. When does decreased inspired PO_2 contribute to hypoxemia?

1. In patients receiving an inadequate fraction of oxygen in inspired gas (FiO_2) on mechanical ventilation.

2. In persons who travel to or live at an altitude at which inspired PO_2 is decreased because of lower barometric pressure.

3. How does hypoventilation cause hypoxemia?

Arterial PO_2 is determined in part by the partial pressure of oxygen in the alveolus (P_AO_2). P_AO_2, in turn, is determined by the total pressure in the alveolus (essentially barometric pressure) and the fraction of alveolar gas that is oxygen. Hypoventilation results in increased alveolar carbon dioxide (CO_2). As alveolar CO_2 increases, the proportion of alveolar gas that is oxygen decreases. Therefore, P_AO_2 is lower, and hypoxemia develops.

4. Why is isolated diffusion impairment unlikely to cause hypoxemia?

In diseases such as pulmonary fibrosis, an abnormally thickened alveolar-capillary membrane may impair oxygen diffusion. However, blood in the pulmonary capillaries of normal people is in contact with the alveolus approximately 3 times longer than is necessary to reach oxygen equilibrium. Thus, abnormalities in the alveolar-capillary membrane must be quite severe before hypoxemia results from diffusion impairment alone. In addition, diffusion impairment does not occur alone. Parenchymal lung processes that cause diffusion impairment generally are also associated with either V-Q mismatch or shunt.

5. What is the most common cause of hypoxemia?

V-Q mismatch is the most common cause of clinically noted hypoxemia. Optimal gas exchange requires balanced ventilation and perfusion throughout the lung. Blood passing through poorly ventilated areas of the lung is inadequately oxygenated and contributes to hypoxemia. Because of the characteristics of the oxygen dissociation curve, hyperventilation of normal areas of the lung cannot correct the hypoxemia.

6. When does shunt occur?

Shunt occurs when blood crosses the venous to the arterial circulation without receiving ventilation. Anatomic defects such as atrial or ventricular septal defects, patent ductus arteriosus, or arteriovenous malformations result in shunting. More common causes of shunting include atelectasis and airspace-filling disorders, such as pneumonia or pulmonary edema.

7. When should acute hypoxemia be suspected?

Clinically, acute hypoxemia is manifest by abnormal function in some organs and compensatory changes in others. Disturbance of the central nervous system (CNS) is usually the first clinical sign of hypoxemia. Initially, malaise and impairments of short-term memory and judgment are detectable. As hypoxemia worsens, cognitive and motor function become more compromised until eventually the patient loses consciousness. Cardiovascular compensation for mild-to-moderate hypoxemia includes tachycardia and increased stroke volume, but as hypoxemia worsens, rhythm disturbances develop. Hypoxic stimulation of the carotid body results in increased minute ventilation. Severe hypoxemia results in declining renal function and urine output and development of metabolic acidosis caused by anaerobic metabolism. Many patients who are hypoxemic appear cyanotic. Cyanosis, a bluish discoloration of the skin and mucous membranes, is present when the concentration of reduced hemoglobin in capillary blood reaches 5 g/100 mL.

8. What are the pitfalls in the observation of cyanosis?

Because the detection of cyanosis is determined by the amount of reduced hemoglobin in capillaries, a severely anemic patient may not appear cyanotic despite significant hypoxemia because of insufficient hemoglobin. Conversely, a patient with polycythemia may have hemoglobin in excess of oxygen-carrying needs and appear cyanotic despite a normal blood oxygen content. Furthermore, cyanosis may be caused by disorders other than systemic hypoxemia, such as peripheral vasoconstriction (e.g., Raynaud's disease) and methemoglobinemia.

9. What physical signs and laboratory results suggest chronic hypoxemia?

Hypoxemia results in pulmonary vasoconstriction, which, when chronic, causes pulmonary hypertension. Pulmonary hypertension increases right ventricular workload and eventually leads to right heart failure. In addition, chronic hypoxemic states result in elaboration of erythropoietin, which causes polycythemia. A patient with chronic hypoxemia may manifest signs of pulmonary hypertension and right heart failure, depending on the extent and duration of hypoxemia. Such signs include a right ventricular heave, loud pulmonic component to the second heart sound, right ventricular S_3, murmur of tricuspid regurgitation, jugular venous distention, hepatojugular reflux, and lower extremity edema. Laboratory tests reveal polycythemia. The electrocardiogram shows signs of right ventricular hypertrophy.

10. What is critical hypoxemia?

The first issue that must be addressed in hypoxemic patients is whether the hypoxemia is acute or chronic. Acute and subacute hypoxemia frequently require immediate hospitalization to diagnose and treat the cause. A $PaO_2 < 50$ places the patient at risk for arrhythmias and further decompensation. Hospitalization also should be considered for patients with clinical signs or organ dysfunction, such as tachypnea, tachycardia, or CNS disturbance. Chronic hypoxemia, if severe enough, has long-term detrimental effects but usually does not require urgent intervention.

11. What factors may lead to false analysis of arterial blood gas (ABG) samples?

Air bubbles in the syringe, if $> 5\%$ of the sample size, may artifactually raise PaO_2 and lower $PaCO_2$ readings toward ambient air values. In addition, if ABGs are not processed promptly, gas may diffuse through plastic syringe walls, altering readings. Lastly, extreme leukocytosis may result in pseudohypoxemia because of oxygen consumption by the white blood cells (WBCs) in the syringe. This is sometimes referred to as "leukocyte larceny."

12. How is the alveoloarterial oxygen (A-a O_2) gradient calculated? When is it useful?

The A-a O_2 gradient is the difference between the alveolar PO_2 (P_AO_2) and the arterial PO_2 (PaO_2). The arterial PO_2 is measured on routine blood gas analysis, but the alveolar PO_2 must be calculated with the alveolar air equation:

$$P_AO_2 = FiO_2 (P_B - P_{H_2O}) - \frac{PaCO_2}{0.8}$$

where FiO_2 is the proportion of oxygen in inspired air, P_B is barometric pressure, P_{H_2O} is water vapor pressure (normally 47 mmHg at 37°C), and $PaCO_2$ is the CO_2 tension in arterial blood. A normal A-a O_2 gradient is 5–15 mmHg. The gradient helps to distinguish hypoxemia attributable to cardiopulmonary disorders from other causes and to identify patients with significant lung pathology but a "normal" arterial oxygen tension because of hyperventilation.

13. How does the A-a gradient help differentiate between the various pathophysiologic causes of hypoxemia?

An elevated A-a O_2 gradient reflects an abnormality in gas transfer between alveoli and pulmonary capillaries. The A-a O_2 gradient is normal if hypoventilation or decreased FiO_2 is present. Hypoventilation is distinguished from decreased inspired O_2 by the presence of elevated $PaCO_2$. Most patients with V-Q mismatch, diffusion impairment, or shunt are able to increase minute ventilation sufficiently to normalize $PaCO_2$ in acute or subacute settings. Therefore, as long as an increased minute ventilation is maintained, blood gases reveal hypoxemia with normal or low $PaCO_2$. V-Q mismatch and shunt can be distinguished by assessing the effect of supplemental O_2 on hypoxemia. Increasing the FiO_2 improves hypoxemia if V-Q mismatch is the cause but does not significantly alter hypoxemia caused by shunting.

14. What are the limitations of pulse oximetry?

Oxygen saturation is estimated in pulse oximetry by measuring optical differences between oxidized and reduced hemoglobin. Because it is rapid, noninvasive, and simple to perform, it is commonly used in emergency departments, intensive care units, and office practices as a method of assessing patients for hypoxemia. It is accurate within 3–5% in patients with saturations above 70%. The main limitation of pulse oximetry is that it provides no measure of $PaCO_2$, a value that is critical both diagnostically and therapeutically. For example, an oxygen saturation of 96% is considered normal unless it is associated with a reduced $PaCO_2$, indicating that the patient must hyperventilate to maintain normal saturation. In addition, carboxyhemoglobin, methemoglobin, abnormal acid–base status, poor perfusion, and bright external light may complicate the interpretation of pulse oximetry.

15. How severe must chronic obstructive pulmonary disease (COPD) be before hypoxemia results?

In general, there is a poor correlation between the severity of COPD, as determined by spirometry, and alterations in blood oxygen tension. Patients with severely reduced forced expiratory volume in 1 second FEV_1 may maintain normal oxygen tension, but others with less severe airflow limitation may be hypoxic. This poor correlation is caused by two factors:

1. Although the primary mechanism of hypoxemia in patients with COPD is V-Q mismatch, alterations in airflow as measured by spirometry do not necessarily parallel alterations in V-Q balance. Emphysema and chronic bronchitis, which contribute to airflow limitation to varying degrees, do not result in equivalent degrees of V-Q mismatching. Thus, a patient whose obstruction is primarily emphysematous may not have as severe a V-Q disturbance as a patient with equal obstruction caused primarily by chronic bronchitis.

2. Individual patients have varying abilities to compensate for hypoxemia related to pulmonary parenchymal abnormalities by recruiting minute ventilation or cardiac output.

16. When is oxygen therapy indicated?

Supplemental oxygen is used for treatment of tissue hypoxia. Clinical scenarios characterized by presumed tissue hypoxia include acute myocardial infarction, acute anemia, carboxyhemoglobinemia, methemoglobinemia, conditions in which oxygen transport is compromised, and hypoxemia with a $PaO_2 < 60$ mmHg or arterial O_2 saturation $< 90\%$. In chronic settings, long-term oxygen therapy should be initiated if a clinically stable patient on an optimal medical regimen demonstrates a $PaO_2 \leq 55$ mmHg or a $PaO_2 \leq 59$ mmHg in the presence of cor pulmonale or polycythemia. Many authorities also recommend supplemental oxygen therapy for patients who are not hypoxemic at rest but desaturate with exertion or during sleep.

17. What three questions must be answered in patients considered for long-term oxygen therapy?

1. Will the patient benefit from home oxygen therapy?
2. What delivery system is best for the patient?
3. What oxygen flow rate is required at rest, with sleep, and during exertion?

18. What are the advantages and disadvantages of different home oxygen supply and delivery systems?

Home oxygen supply systems include bulk supplies stored as either liquid oxygen or compressed gas and oxygen concentrators. Oxygen concentrators extract oxygen from ambient air. They require less frequent servicing (there is no tank that needs to be refilled) but are more expensive, not readily portable within the home, and require a dependable electrical source. Oxygen concentrators are most appropriate for patients requiring only nocturnal oxygen or sedentary patients on lower oxygen flow rates. Most home oxygen is supplied as liquid oxygen. Liquid oxygen reservoirs have three times the capacity as compressed gas tanks and require less frequent refilling. Liquid oxygen reservoirs are also more portable (the reservoirs have wheels that allow them to be moved easily around the home environment), easier to use to fill portable tanks, and less bulky. However, liquid oxygen is more expensive than compressed gas oxygen.

Oxygen is delivered by either face mask or nasal cannula. Face masks are used primarily in patients requiring a very specific fraction of inspired oxygen or extremely high fractions of inspired oxygen. Masks are uncomfortable and poorly tolerated, limiting their long-term application. Most patients receive home supplemental oxygen via a nasal cannula.

19. What are oxygen-conserving devices?

Most long-term home oxygen therapy is delivered as continuous-flow oxygen. This type of delivery is inefficient because oxygen continues to flow throughout the respiratory cycle. Oxygen that flows during expiration is wasted. Oxygen-conserving devices limit the flow of oxygen to inspiration. They consist of pulsed inspiratory flow monitoring devices and reservoir systems. Pulsed inspiratory metering systems sense each breath and limit flow only to inspiration. Reservoir systems pool oxygen in a reservoir near the nose that fills during expiration and empties during inspiration. The advantage of these systems is that adequate oxygen saturation can be achieved at lower flow rates, resulting in less frequent servicing of stationary equipment and increased longevity of portable systems.

20. Should all patients with COPD who are newly diagnosed with hypoxemia be placed on chronic supplemental oxygen?

As many as 50% of patients with COPD who are hypoxic but not on medical therapy are no longer hypoxic after proper therapy is established. Therefore, only patients who are clinically stable and receiving appropriate medical therapy should be considered for supplemental oxygen. Such patients should be placed on long-term supplemental oxygen if the criteria listed in question 16 are met. Chronic supplemental oxygen is associated with improved survival, hemodynamics, and neuropsychological function in chronically hypoxemic patients. Maximal benefit is achieved with continuous oxygen delivery (i.e., 19–24 h/day).

21. What is transtracheal oxygen therapy? List its benefits and risks.

Transtracheal oxygen therapy is an oxygen delivery system in which a catheter is placed transcutaneously into the trachea at the level of the second or third tracheal ring. The transtracheal delivery system has been shown to have several benefits: improved cosmesis and comfort, decreased oxygen flow rate requirement, improved exercise tolerance, improved patient compliance, and fewer hospitalizations. The most common complications include accidental catheter displacement, obstruction of the end of the catheter with a mucus plug, and mild local cellulitis.

22. What issues are involved with air travel in patients with pulmonary disorders?

Although commercial aircraft cruise between 22,000 and 44,000 feet, passenger cabins are maintained at pressures equivalent to altitudes of 5000–8000 feet. It is difficult to estimate the PaO_2 of a particular patient at these altitudes because of patients' varying abilities to compensate. However, in a stable normocapneic patient with COPD, a sea level $PaO_2 > 72$ mmHg usually results in a $PaO_2 > 50$ mmHg at 8000 feet. The patient's expected PaO_2 at a particular altitude can be determined more accurately with the hypoxia altitude simulation test (HAST), which uses normobaric hypoxic breathing to simulate altitude and may be performed in PFT laboratories.

23. What advice should be given to a patient with pulmonary disorder who wishes to travel to the mountains?

Atmospheric oxygen is fairly constant at 21% of total barometric pressure at any altitude. However, barometric pressure decreases as altitude increases, resulting in a lower partial pressure of inspired oxygen P_iO_2. The P_iO_2 is 149 mmHg at sea level but decreases by approximately 4 mmHg/1000 feet of elevation. Normal persons respond to the acute hypoxia of altitude by increasing minute ventilation to maximize alveolar PO_2. A healthy person can maintain a PaO_2 of 50–60 mmHg at 8000–10,000 feet. Mild tachycardia also develops, increasing cardiac output and maintaining oxygen delivery to tissues. Blood flow to the brain is maintained as hypoxic vasodi-latation overcomes the vasoconstrictor effect caused by respiratory alkalosis. Such issues should be kept in mind in counseling patients with pulmonary diseases about travel to high altitudes. Patients with borderline oxygenation at sea level may become hypoxic, depending on the altitude to which they travel. Such patients may require supplemental oxygen, especially if they have a history of comorbid conditions such as angina pectoris, congestive heart failure, or cerebrovascular disease. In addition, patients already receiving supplemental oxygen may need to increase their oxygen flow rate.

24. Is chronic supplemental oxygen therapy indicated for patients who desaturate only with exercise or during sleep?

Many patients with COPD have normal or near-normal oxygen tension at rest but desaturate with exercise and during sleep. No clinical trials have evaluated the benefits of oxygen therapy on survival in this subset of patients. Therefore, the role of supplemental oxygen in this setting is not well defined. Because patients with COPD generally spend only a small percentage of their day participating in exercise, it may be unlikely that exercise desaturation contributes significantly to morbidity or mortality. However, some patients report an increase in exercise tolerance with supplemental oxygen. To the extent that supplemental oxygen improves quality of life, it may be reasonable to prescribe oxygen for such patients. Small studies have demonstrated that nocturnal oxygen prevents sleep-associated transient increases in pulmonary artery pressure and reduces the frequency of dysrhythmias. Although it is not known whether this benefit translates into long-term clinical benefit, many authorities use this rationale to justify the use of nocturnal oxygen in patients who desaturate only during sleep.

BIBLIOGRAPHY

1. Crockett AJ, Cranston JM, Moss JR, Alpers JH: A review of long-term oxygen therapy for chronic obstructive pulmonary disease. Respir Med 95:437–443, 2001.
2. Danztker DR: Pulmonary gas exchange. In Bone RC, et al (eds): Pulmonary and Critical Care Medicine. St. Louis, Mosby, 1993.
3. DesRosiers A, Russo R: Long-term oxygen therapy. Respir Care Clin North Am 6:625–644, 2000.
4. Gong H: Air travel and oxygen therapy in cardiopulmonary patients. Chest 101:1104–1113, 1992.
5. Hagarty KM, Skorodin MS, Langbein E, et al: Comparison of three oxygen delivery systems during exercise in hypoxemic patients with chronic obstructive pulmonary disease. Am J Respir Crit Care Med 155:893–898, 1997.
6. Phillips Y, Kristo D, Kallish M: Writing the take-home oxygen prescription in COPD. J Crit Illness 13:112–120, 1998.
7. Ram FS, Wedzicha JA: Ambulatory oxygen for chronic obstructive pulmonary disease. Cochrane Database Syst Rev 2:CD000238, 2002.
8. Rochester CL, Ferranti R: Long-term oxygen therapy: What benefits for your patient? J Respir Dis 19:133–151, 1998.
9. Sinex JE: Pulse oximetry: Principles and limitations. Am J Emerg Med 17:59–67, 1999.
10. Williams AJ: ABC of oxygen: Assessing and interpreting arterial blood gases and acid-base balance. Br Med J 317:1213–1216, 1998.
11. Zielinski J: Effects of long-term oxygen therapy in patients with chronic obstructive pulmonary disease. Curr Opin Pulm Med 5:81–87, 1999.

89. SOLITARY PULMONARY NODULE

Michael E. Hanley, M.D.

1. Why is it important to distinguish between a pulmonary nodule and a pulmonary mass?
   A solitary pulmonary nodule (SPN) is a well-circumscribed, approximately round lesion on chest radiogram that is < 4–6 cm in diameter. By definition, it is completely surrounded by aerated lung, thus excluding pleural- or mediastinal-based lesions. It is distinguished from a pulmonary mass by size (mass > 4–6 cm in diameter). Although this distinction is arbitrary, it has clinical significance in that the probability of malignancy increases with the size of the lesion.

2. Does a coin lesion differ from an SPN?
   No. *SPN* and *coin lesion* are synonymous terms. Coin lesion, however, is a misnomer, because it implies a two-dimensional lesion, but SPNs are three dimensional.

3. What is the differential diagnosis of an SPN?
   The differential diagnosis of SPNs is quite extensive. The major diagnostic consideration is to distinguish benign from malignant processes.

Neoplastic lesions

Malignant
   1. Primary lung
      Bronchogenic carcinoma
      Alveolar cell carcinoma
      Adenoma
      Sarcoma
      Lymphoma
      Hodgkin's disease
   2. Solitary metastases

Benign
   1. Hamartoma
   2. Teratoma

Nonneoplastic lesions

Infection
   1. Tuberculosis
   2. Coccidioidomycosis
   3. Histoplasmosis
   4. Blastomycosis
   5. Nocardiosis
   6. Actinomycosis

Inflammatory process
   1. Wegener's granulomatosis
   2. Organizing pneumonia
   3. Rheumatoid necrobiotic nodule
   4. Pulmonary infarct

Vascular lesions
   1. Arteriovenous malformations
   2. Pulmonary vein varix

Miscellaneous
   1. Bronchial cyst
   2. Bronchopulmonary sequestration
   3. Pulmonary hematoma
   4. Lipoid pneumonia
   5. Other

4. What is the differential diagnosis of an SPN in HIV-seropositive patients?
   Although HIV-seropositive patients may have an increased incidence of primary bronchogenic carcinoma, SPNs in this population most commonly have an infectious cause. In a review limited by a small number of patients, 60% of the SPNs in HIV-seropositive patients were caused by infections (*Pneumocystis carinii* pneumonia, cryptococcosis, nocardiosis, cytomegalovirus, mucormycosis, hydatidosis). The incidence of non-Hodgkin's lymphoma presenting as an SPN was only 10%.

5. Which three constellations of factors favor a benign nodule?

Calcifications of the lesion, absence of a history of tobacco use, and age younger than 35 years are important factors that strongly correlate with benign nodules. Noncalcified lesions may be benign or malignant. Absence of smoking history does not entirely exclude a malignant process because of potential exposure to other carcinogens (e.g., radon gas, asbestos, chromium) and second-hand smoke (passive smoking). Indeed, 15% of primary lung cancers occur in nonsmokers. Patients younger than age 35 years are more likely to have a benign lesion; however, this association is not absolute. A diagnostic workup may be necessary in the presence of other malignant risk factors, such as enlarging lesions or heavy tobacco use beginning at an early age.

6. Why is regular follow-up of a calcified pulmonary nodule important?

Patterns of calcification are more easily observed on computed tomography (CT) scans than plain chest radiographs. Six common patterns of calcification of SPNs are recognized: diffuse, central, popcorn, laminar, stippled, and eccentric. The first four are almost always benign, whereas the latter two may be either benign or malignant. However, even benign calcification does not exclude the presence of coincidental malignancy in adjacent tissue or the subsequent degeneration of a previously benign process into a malignant lesion ("scar" carcinoma). For this reason, close observation with serial chest radiographs every 6 months for at least 2 years is prudent for nodules with benign patterns of calcification.

| A. Diffuse | B. Central | C. Popcorn | D. Laminar, Concentric | E. Stippled | F. Eccentric |

Six common patterns of calcification occur in SPNs. Patterns A–D are associated with benign conditions; patterns E and F occur in both benign and malignant conditions. (Adapted from Web WR: Radiologic evaluation of the solitary pulmonary nodule. AJR 154:701–708; with permission.)

7. What other radiographic clues help to differentiate between benign and malignant lesions?

Cavitating lesions, lesions with multilobulated or spiculated contours, and lesions with shaggy or extremely irregular borders tend to be malignant. However, none of these associations is strong enough to determine accurately the nature of a lesion.

8. What is the most valuable test in evaluating an SPN?

The most valuable diagnostic test is comparison with an old chest radiograph. Benign nodules tend to grow at either very slow or very rapid rates. In contrast, malignant processes grow at steady, predictable, exponential rates. The growth rate of a nodule is conventionally defined as the doubling time (i.e., the time required for its *volume* to double) and corresponds to an increase in diameter by a factor of 1.26. In general, doubling times > 16 months or < 1 month (20–25 days) are associated with benign processes. Intermediate doubling times require additional evaluation to determine the nature of the lesion. If a nodule has not increased in size over a 2-year period, the probability that it is benign is > 99%. Occasionally, neoplasms such as bronchoalveolar cell and atypical carcinoids appear stable over 2 years. Lesions that appear radiographically stable should, therefore, continue to be monitored by radiograph on an annual basis for several more years.

9. What other radiographic tools may help to differentiate between malignant and benign SPNs?

Both high-resolution computed tomography (HRCT) and positron emission tomography (PET) have been proposed as additional tools to aid in differentiating between malignant and benign pulmonary nodules. Enhancement of the lesion by infusion of iodinated contrast during HRCT correlates with a higher probability of a malignant cause. In preliminary studies, contrast enhancement had a sensitivity approaching 100%, a specificity of 70%, and a positive predictive value of 90%. The negative predictive value was 92%. Uptake of 18F-fluorodeoxyglucose (FDG) during PET imaging also correlated with a malignant etiology. The sensitivity of FDG-PET imaging for SPN > 2 cm in diameter was 81% with a specificity of 80–100%. FDG-PET imaging was significantly less reliable if the lesion was < 2 cm. PET scanning may also improve clinical staging by identifying occult extrapulmonary malignant disease. In one study, extrathoracic malignant lesions were identified in 14% of patients thought to have limited stage thoracic disease by whole-body PET scans.

10. Does sputum cytology aid in the diagnosis of an SPN?

Sputum cytology has a low yield (5–20%) and is of limited value.

11. What are the pros and cons of the invasive tests available for diagnosing an SPN?

Absolute determination of the true nature of an SPN necessitates obtaining tissue for histologic evaluation. Three options are available:

1. Resection of the nodule by either **open thoracotomy or video-assisted thoracoscopy** (VAT) unequivocally determines the nature of the lesion but is associated with significant perioperative morbidity and occasional mortality.

2. **Fiber-optic bronchoscopy with transbronchial biopsy** is relatively safe (incidence of pneumothorax and significant hemorrhage < 3%), but its sensitivity in diagnosing malignancy depend on the size of the lesion. Overall, the yield is approximately 10–40% for lesions 1–2 cm in diameter, 60% for lesions 2–3 cm, and 80% for lesions > 3 cm. These figures, however, depend heavily on the operator's skill. Addition of transbronchial brushing, washing, and needle aspiration improves the yield.

3. **Percutaneous transthoracic needle aspiration** has a higher sensitivity in diagnosing malignancy than transbronchial biopsy but is associated with more morbidity. The diagnostic yield exceeds 90% for malignancy. However, subsequent pneumothorax occurs in 25% of patients, 50% of whom require tube thoracostomy. In addition, the sensitivity for diagnosing benign lesions is even lower than that for transbronchial biopsy. Because the specific yield of both transbronchial biopsy and transthoracic needle aspiration for benign lesions is low, nonmalignant but nonspecific results do not exclude malignancy with certainty.

12. When should a patient with an SPN be referred for invasive tests?

Initial evaluation of an SPN by the primary care provider consists of a thorough history and physical examination, laboratory tests to screen for potential metastases, and comparison with previous chest radiograms. If the presence or pattern of calcification is not readily apparent on a plain chest radiogram, CT of the chest should be obtained. Patients with a high probability of malignancy should be referred for invasive tests. Patients with a low probability of malignancy (based on characteristics of the nodule and risk factors) should have a repeat chest radiograph in 1 month. If no change is seen, the patient should be followed closely with a serial chest radiogram (every 3–6 months) until radiographic stability of the nodule has been demonstrated for at least 2 years.

13. What factors determine whether a malignant SPN should be resected?

Issues that determine whether resection should be performed include the potential for cure and whether the patient can tolerate surgery. The potential for cure is influenced by the histologic nature of the lesion as well as the clinical stage. Ascertaining the ability of a patient to tolerate surgery requires an assessment of cardiovascular and pulmonary risk factors. This assessment includes, at minimum, performance of a detailed history and physical examination and analysis of the patient's electrocardiogram, chest radiograph, arterial blood gases, and pulmonary function tests. Any abnormalities in these parameters should prompt referral to a cardiologist or pulmonologist for additional evaluation.

CONTROVERSIES

14. What is the value of CT screening for lung cancer?

The value of CT screening for lung cancer in high-risk populations remains controversial. Preliminary studies suggest that low-dose CT scans can detect malignant lesions at an early stage. However, the effect of screening on mortality is unknown, and it is unclear what should be done when subcentimeter lesions are detected. Some authorities have recommended monitoring lesions smaller than 0.4 cm in diameter with serial CT scans but aggressively evaluating larger lesions with PET scans, CT-guided percutaneous biopsy, or surgical resection. The appropriate approach likely includes a combination of these modalities and is driven by radiographic and historical risk factors for malignancy as described above.

15. Should patients who have an SPN with a high risk of cancer and who also are good surgical candidates be managed by immediate resection of the nodule by either open thoracotomy or video-assisted thoracoscopy (VAT) rather than subjected to invasive, exclusively diagnostic procedures?

For: Diagnosis of malignancy by transbronchial biopsy results in subsequent referral for therapeutic thoracotomy, whereas nonmalignant results are usually nonspecific, do not exclude malignancy, and result in referral for a diagnostic thoracotomy. Results of several studies indicate that staging fiberoptic bronchoscopy rarely identifies airway lesions that preclude surgery and potentially curative resection.

Against: Prethoracotomy fiber-optic bronchoscopy allows staging of the major airways by screening for metachronous endobronchial malignancies that may preclude or alter the extent of subsequent surgery. In addition, 5% of malignant SPNs are small-cell carcinomas that are not treated with surgery. Finally, morbidity and mortality are much lower for transbronchial biopsy and percutaneous transthoracic needle aspiration than for thoracotomy; although the yield for benign lesions is low, the higher risk of thoracotomy justifies an attempt at diagnosis by less invasive approaches, especially for patients who are psychologically reluctant to undergo surgery or are at high risk from thoracotomy or VAT.

BIBLIOGRAPHY

1. Dewan NA, Shehan CJ, Reeb SD, et al: Likelihood of malignancy in solitary pulmonary nodules: Comparison of Bayesian analysis and results of FDG-PET scan. Chest 112:416–422, 1997.
2. Gasparini S, Ferretti M, Secchi EB, et al: Integration of transbronchial and percutaneous approach in the diagnosis of peripheral pulmonary nodules or masses. Experience with 1,027 consecutive cases. Chest 108:131–137, 1995.
3. Hartman TE: Radiologic evaluation of the solitary pulmonary nodule. Semin Thorac Cardiovasc Surg 14:261–267, 2002.
4. Henschke CI, Yankelevitz DF, Libby DM, et al: Early lung cancer action project: Annual screening using single-slice helical CT. Ann N Y Acad Sci 952:124–134, 2001.
5. Lillington GA: Solitary pulmonary nodules: new wine in old bottles. Curr Opin Pulm Med 7:242–246, 2001.
6. Miller DL: Management of the subcentimeter pulmonary nodule. Semin Thorac Cardiovasc Surg 14:281–285, 2002.
7. Murthy SC, Rice TW: The solitary pulmonary nodule: A primer on differential diagnosis. Semin Thorac Cardiovasc Surg 14:239–249, 2002.
8. Ost D, Fein A: Evaluation and management of the solitary pulmonary nodule. Am J Respir Crit Care Med 162:782–787, 2000.
9. Ost D, Fein AM, Feinsilver SH: Clinical practice. The solitary pulmonary nodule. N Engl J Med 348:2535–2542, 2003.
10. Stroobants S, Verschakelen J, Vansteenkiste J: Value of FDG-PET in the management of non-small cell lung cancer. Eur J Radiol 45:49–59, 2003.
11. Swensen SJ: What is the significance of finding calcifications in pulmonary masses on CT scans? Am J Roentgenol 164:505–506, 1995.
12. Tang AW, Moss HA, Robertson RJ: The solitary pulmonary nodule. Eur J Radiol 45:69–77, 2003.
13. Worsley DF, Celler A, Adam MJ, et al: Pulmonary nodules: Differential diagnosis using 18F-fluorodeoxyglucose single-photon emission computed tomography. Am J Roentgenol 168:771–774, 1997.

XIII. Common Disorders of the Skin

90. ECZEMATOUS DERMATITIS

Loren E. Golitz, M.D., and Meg A. Lemon, M.D.

1. Define eczema.
Eczema is the final common manifestation of dermatitis of several causes, including atopic dermatitis, allergic and irritant contact dermatitis, and various other clinical forms of dermatitis. Papules, macules, and vesicles often coalesce with weeping and crusting. Eventually, thickening and scaling, called lichenification, result.

2. What rules should be considered in using topical steroid therapy?
1. Topical steroid preparations of low, mid, and high potency must be carefully distinguished. Examples include desonide 0.05% (low), triamcinolone acetonide 0.1% (mid), fluocinonide 0.05% (high).
2. Ointments are more effective than creams on dry, thickened skin.
3. Potent topical steroids (especially fluorinated ones) should not be applied to intertriginous areas or to the face and neck.
4. Potent topical steroids should be avoided in young children because of the possibility of systemic absorption.
5. Potential side effects from the prolonged use of potent topical steroids include cutaneous atrophy, development of striae, and suppression of the hypothalamus-pituitary-adrenal (HPA) axis. The risk of systemic absorption and suppression of the HPA is increased by high-potency preparations, prolonged use, application to large areas, and occlusive dressings.

3. When are systemic corticosteroids indicated?
In general, systemic steroids are indicated in otherwise healthy patients with self-limited, steroid-responsive disorders who present acutely with severe symptoms. For example, prednisone may be started at a dose of 40 mg/day and tapered over 3 weeks in acute, severe cases of contact dermatitis (e.g., poison ivy). A rapid taper over 5 days will result in recurrence of rash. Systemic steroids should be avoided, if possible, in chronic illnesses such as psoriasis and atopic dermatitis.

4. What substances are the most common causes of allergic contact dermatitis?
Poison ivy, poison sumac, and poison oak are the three most common plants that cause contact dermatitis in the United States. Topical medications, including neomycin, ethylenediamine, topical anesthetics, and thimerosal, are commonly implicated. Nickel is a common culprit because of its ubiquitous use in jewelry. Chromium may be implicated in patients with industrial exposures to substances such as cement. Rubber, epoxy glue, cosmetics, perfumes, and formaldehyde also may cause allergic contact dermatitis. Paraphenylenediamine in permanent black hair dye may cause severe scalp dermatitis.

5. How is contact dermatitis diagnosed?
The clinical history, including exposures at work and at home, is the most important element in making the diagnosis. The acute episode often follows contact with the allergen by approxi-

mately 48 hours. Hobbies are an important source of contact allergens. Any chemical that gets on the hands is readily transferred to the eyelids and genitalia.

6. Describe the classic presentation of poison ivy.

Poison ivy presents with a mixture of vesicles, bullae, and crusting. The blisters often appear in a linear arrangement at points where the broken stem or leaf of the plant has touched the skin. The rash is associated with intense pruritus.

7. Which parts of the hands and feet are commonly affected by contact dermatitis?

Contact dermatitis of the hands and feet usually involves the dorsal aspects because the palms and soles are relatively protected by thick layers of keratin.

8. What treatments are effective for contact dermatitis?

Treatment of allergic contact dermatitis includes cool compresses with a Burow's solution (a 1:20 solution is made by diluting 1 package of powder in 1 pint of cold water). The area should be soaked for 10–15 minutes and then patted with a towel. A topical steroid in the form of a cream or ointment may be applied to the skin 2–4 times/day. After a patient is allergic to a specific chemical, the allergy is maintained throughout life; thus, avoidance of contact with the agent is important.

9. In what instances are patch tests useful?

Patch testing may establish the specific cause of an allergic contact dermatitis. Screening trays allow testing of multiple potential allergens. Tests normally are read 48 or 72 hours after application. Patch tests may be used to support the diagnosis of contact dermatitis, to identify the specific allergen, or to exclude the diagnosis. Difficulties include false-positive and false-negative results as well as positive results with unclear clinical significance. Test results must be correlated with the patient's exposures. A common cause of false-negative testing is a delayed reaction after the usual 48-hour reading. A second reading 4–7 days after the application is recommended. Patch tests should not be used during episodes of severe extensive dermatitis.

10. Does atopic dermatitis affect adults?

Usually atopic dermatitis is a disease of infancy and childhood, beginning before age 6 months and diminishing in adulthood. However, up to 60% of patients with childhood atopic dermatitis have some form, albeit more limited, in adulthood. Pruritus, the major symptom, is accompanied by dry, lichenified patches on the flexor surfaces of the elbows, knees, wrists, ankles, and the periorbital region. The condition is usually idiopathic; exacerbating factors include extreme temperature, dry climates, cutaneous infections, and chemical irritants (e.g., soap).

11. What is the relationship of atopic dermatitis to other atopic states?

Up to 70% of patients have a personal or family history of asthma, hay fever, or dermatitis. Severe atopic dermatitis is seen in the hyper–immunoglobulin E (IgE) syndrome. Thus, diagnosis is usually made by the clinical and family history; examination of the lesions; and, in severe cases, assessment of the IgE level.

12. What is the mainstay of treatment of atopic dermatitis?

The mainstays of treatment are skin hydration and topical steroids. Patients should apply emollients to damp skin after bathing and repeatedly during the day. Topical steroids should be applied 2–4 times each day; ointments of mid to high potency, such as triamcinolone acetonide 0.1%, may be required. Occlusive dressings may be used to treat stubborn lesions.

13. What is new in atopic dermatitis therapy?

The latest breakthrough in treating atopic dermatitis is a new class of drugs know as topical immune modulators. Tacrolimus and pimecrolimus have received approval by the Food and Drug

Administration (FDA) as topical therapy for atopic dermatitis. These drugs directly inhibit the T cells that cause atopic dermatitis. These agents are not steroids and do not cause epidermal atrophy. They are useful when topical steroids have failed or when using topical steroids chronically is contraindicated.

14. What possibilities should be considered when atopic dermatitis fails to respond to therapy?

1. The patient is not meticulous about the frequency of therapy or is noncompliant with routine hydration and lubrication of the skin.

2. The patient is allergic (sensitized) to the topical agent. This possibility is especially likely when the treated area coincides with worsening disease.

3. Superinfection with *Staphylococcus aureus* is present. True infection is difficult to determine in the absence of cellulitis. However, vesicles, pustules, and large exudative lesions may warrant therapy with systemic antistaphylococcal agents.

4. The diagnosis is allergic contact dermatitis rather than atopic dermatitis, and the patient continues to be exposed to the allergen. Patch testing may be diagnostic.

15. What causes pruritic, dry, and scaly dermatitis in elderly patients?

Pruritic, dry, and scaly dermatitis in elderly patients, usually called asteatotic eczema or "winter itch," is related to decreased skin lipids. Drying climate, frequent bathing, and diuresis exacerbate the areas of dryness. Skin fissuring and erythema, most commonly on the anterior legs, dorsum of the hands, and interscapular region, are accompanied by pruritus. Emollients to hydrate the skin, low-potency topical steroids, and decreased soap use usually provide relief.

Rarely, new-onset ichthyotic dermatitis (scaling, dry skin) is associated with internal malignancy such as lymphoma. Itching can also be caused by cholestasis, thyroid dysfunction, renal insufficiency, and liver disease. Appropriate history, physical examination, and laboratory evaluation can rule out these causes.

16. Who is at risk for irritant hand dermatitis?

Irritant hand dermatitis, as opposed to allergic contact dermatitis, appears on the palmar aspect of the hand. Persons at risk include (1) patients with a history of atopic dermatitis or other skin diseases and (2) housekeepers, health care professionals, and others who chronically expose their hands to water and detergents.

17. Describe the therapy for irritant hand dermatitis.

Hand dermatitis may prove particularly difficult to clear, but the following steps are usually helpful:

1. Use of vinyl gloves, avoidance of chemicals, and addition of lubricants and barrier creams
2. Use of cool compresses and midpotency steroids
3. Aggressive treatment of secondary bacterial infection

In addition, dermatophyte infection should be ruled out with a potassium hydroxide (KOH) preparation and fungal culture.

18. How are antibiotics useful in flareups of dermatitis?

When the epidermal barrier is disrupted in disease states (e.g., atopic, irritant, and contact dermatitis; psoriasis), fissures in the skin allow bacteria to enter and cause local infection. Antigenic portions of these bacteria stimulate the immune response (specifically, T cells) and worsen the dermatitis. A 10–14-day course of oral antibiotics with good staphylococcal and streptococcal coverage (e.g., dicloxacillin, cephalexin, erythromycin) shortens the recovery period.

BIBLIOGRAPHY

1. Freedberg I, et al (eds): Fitzpatrick's Dermatology in General Medicine, 6th ed. New York, McGraw-Hill, 2003.

2. Halbert AR, Weston WL, Morelli JG: Atopic dermatitis: Is it an allergic disease? J Am Acad Dermatol 33:1008–1018, 1995.
3. Hanifin JM, Ling MR, Langley R, et al: Tacrolimus ointment for treatment of atopic dermatitis in adult patients: Part I: Efficacy. J Am Acad Derm 44:S28–S38, 2001.
4. Jung T: New treatments for atopic dermatitis. Clin Exp Allergy 32:347–354, 2002.
5. Leung DY: Atopic dermatitis: Immunobiology and treatment with immune modulators. Clin Exp Immunol 107(suppl 1):25–30, 1997.
6. Rothe MJ, Grant-Kels JM: Atopic dermatitis: An update. J Am Acad Dermatol 353:1–13, 1996.
7. Sulzberger MB: The patch test: Who should and should not use it and why. Contact Dermatitis 1:117–119, 1975.

91. MACULOPAPULAR ERUPTIONS

Tatiana Khrom, M.D.

1. What are macules and papules?

A macule is a flat, circumscribed skin discoloration (< 0.5 cm in diameter) that lacks surface elevation or depression. A papule is an elevated, solid lesion < 0.5 cm in diameter.

2. What is a morbilliform eruption?

A morbilliform rash comprises macules and papules in a symmetric distribution. They may become confluent and may involve the palms, soles, trunk, and mucous membranes. Morbilliform eruptions may be the most common manifestation of a drug-induced reaction. On the other hand, many viral exanthems (skin eruptions caused by viruses) are also morbilliform in nature. Therefore, a viral exanthem or a drug eruption should always be included in the differential diagnosis of a morbilliform rash.

3. What are the most common presentations of cutaneous drug eruptions?

As described above, the most common drug eruption is a morbilliform rash on the trunk, extremities, palms, and soles. The rash may become confluent and is usually quite pruritic. Mild fever may accompany the eruption. The reaction usually begins within 1 week of starting the drug and may last up to 2 weeks. Drug eruptions also may manifest as urticarial or photosensitive eruptions. Most drugs are suspect, but common etiologic agents include penicillin, barbiturates, allopurinol, and trimethoprim-sulfamethoxazole (TMP-SMX; a common cause of drug rashes in patients infected with the human immunodeficiency virus [HIV]).

4. How are drug rashes treated?

Treatment involves discontinuation of the drug and avoidance of further exposure. Desensitization is effective in some cases and may be considered when alternative regimens are ineffective (e.g., TMP-SMX desensitization in patients with AIDS who need *Pneumocystis carinii* prophylaxis). Pruritus is treated with antihistamines such as hydroxyzine hydrochloride, 25–50 mg four times/day. Severe, generalized drug eruptions may be treated with a short course of oral prednisone.

5. What is toxic epidermal necrolysis (TEN), and how is it managed?

TEN is a rare exfoliative disease of the skin and mucous membranes. It starts with diffuse tender erythema of the skin followed by sloughing of the epidermis (outermost layer of the skin). This disease is life threatening because it can affect 20–100% of the skin surface, thereby making patients highly susceptible to infection. On examination, patients have necrolysis (full-thickness skin detachment resulting in a red, glistening, and denuded skin surface), blisters, and erosions of the mucous membranes. The skin may denude when lateral pressure is applied (positive Nikolsky's sign)

About 80% of the time, the disease is caused by a drug. The culprits typically involved are the anticonvulsants (barbiturates, carbamazepine, phenytoin), allopurinol, antibiotics (amoxicillin, ampicillin, cephalosporins, sulfonamides), and nonsteroidal antiinflammatory drugs (NSAIDs). Patients with TEN should be managed in the burn unit with supportive treatment (intravenous [IV] fluids and nutritional support; monitoring for infection and pain control). The use of corticosteroids is controversial. A new modality recently reported to be beneficial in arresting the progression of the syndrome is treatment with IV immune globulin (IVIG).

6. What is a drug hypersensitivity reaction?

This complex drug reaction is seen most commonly with anticonvulsants; allopurinol; long-acting sulfonamides; and minocycline, a drug commonly used for treatment of acne. Patients with drug hypersensitivity may present with fever; a morbilliform rash; diffuse lymphadenopathy; eosinophilia; hepatitis; nephritis; and, rarely, involvement of the brain, lungs, or heart. The reaction may be delayed, occurring even after the causative agent has been discontinued. This kind of reaction is thought to be caused by an accumulation of a toxic metabolite that cannot be degraded by the affected patient. *Note:* Several anticonvulsants (phenobarbital, phenytoin, carbamazepine) lead to production of the same toxic intermediate and, therefore, cannot be substituted for one another.

7. How do viruses cause exanthems?

It is thought that the virus disseminates through the blood to the skin surface and the lesions of the exanthem arise from the local cutaneous response of the host to the virus.

8. Which three classic childhood exanthems result in a predominant morbilliform rash?

1. **Measles.** A rash beginning on the forehead and hairline follows a prodrome of coryza, cough, and development of small white lesions with blue centers on the oral mucous membranes (Koplik's spots).

2. **Rubella.** Pale maculopapular lesions start on the face and spread downward; lymphadenopathy (occipital and postauricular) is a consistent finding.

3. **Fifth disease (erythema infectiosum).** This parvovirus infection presents with a slapped-cheek appearance and often is accompanied by a mild fever, followed by a diffuse, reticular rash that spreads to the extremities.

9. What other viral entities cause morbilliform exanthem?

Epstein-Barr virus, coxsackievirus, echovirus, and adenovirus.

10. What diagnosis is suggested when a morbilliform rash develops in a patient treated with ampicillin for pharyngitis?

The probable diagnosis is infectious mononucleosis, which is caused by Epstein-Barr virus. In this instance, a drug–virus interaction results in the eruption. This interaction occurs with much greater frequency ($\leq 95\%$ of patients treated) than a reaction to ampicillin alone.

11. What diagnosis should be considered when a maculopapular eruption of the palms, soles, ankles, and wrists follows a febrile syndrome?

The initial eruption of **Rocky Mountain spotted fever** follows this distribution. Although lesions eventually become classically purpuric, early recognition of this tick-borne infection is important to appropriate management. **Atypical measles** also may present in this manner, especially in immunized adults.

12. Why is it important to consider the diagnosis of Kawasaki's disease in a child with a morbilliform or scarlatiniform rash?

Kawasaki's disease is a multisystem disorder of young children that results in coronary artery aneurysms in as many as 25% of patients. Early recognition of the disease may permit appropriate therapy (high-dose IV gammaglobulin and aspirin) to reduce the incidence of coronary arteritis. Hallmarks of the disease include rash (often leading to desquamation), conjunctival injection, nonsuppurative cervical lymphadenopathy, oral erythema with strawberry tongue, and fever.

13. What is scabies, and how is it treated?

Scabies is a contagious infection caused by the mite *Sarcoptes scabie*. The female mite burrows into the upper epidermis, lay her eggs, and dies after about 1 month. The infestation is transmitted from person to person by direct contact and by fomites. Patients complain of severe itching. On physical examination, one sees red, papulovesicular lesions, predominantly in the axillae, periumbilical area, groin, inner thighs, and interdigital webs of the fingers. One can also see characteristic linear burrows in the same areas, and the diagnosis is made by scraping the burrow with mineral oil and the identification of the mite or fecal matter under a microscope. If the host immune response is inadequate (AIDS or transplant patients as well as institutionalized patients), a variant called Norwegian scabies can develop. This variant is a massive infestation with innumerable mites characterized by asymptomatic crusting and eczematous dermatitis. The treatment for scabies is Elimite (5% permethrin cream) applied from the neck down, left on overnight and washed off in the morning. The treatment has to be repeated in 1 week. All linens and clothes have to be washed with warm water and dried. In pregnant or lactating women, 10% sulfur ointment in petrolatum should be used once a day for 3 days. If the infestation is severe, oral ivermectin, 200 µg/kg, should be taken once.

14. Do other mites affect humans?

Occasionally, cat and dog mites (*Chylietella* spp.) may bite humans but do not cause invasive disease as scabies does. The diagnosis is made when the patient's veterinarian finds mites on the family pet.

15. What is miliaria rubra?

Miliaria is a common finding in neonates, especially in warm climates. In miliaria rubra, there is a blockage of seat ducts that often occurs after periods of excessive warming (occlusive dressings or overdressing in warm weather). The blockage produces an inflammatory response that gives rise to erythematous papules and sometimes pustules. One should not confuse this common eruption with viral or drug eruptions. Miliaria rubra resolves spontaneously with cooling of the skin.

BIBLIOGRAPHY

1. Dover JS, Arndt KA, Jackson, BA, et al: Cutaneous Medicine and Surgery. Philadelphia, W.B. Saunders, 1996.
2. Fitzpatrick JE, Aeling JL: Dermatology Secrets in Color, 2nd ed. Philadelphia, Hanley & Belfus, 2001.
3. Freedberg I, Eisen AZ, Wolff K, et al (eds): Fitzpatrick's Dermatology in General Medicine, 6th ed. New York, McGraw-Hill, 2003.
4. Habif TP, Campbell JL, Quitadama MJ, Zug KA: Skin Disease Diagnosis and Treatment. St Louis, Mosby, 2001.

92. PAPULOSQUAMOUS SKIN LESIONS

Alison B. Gruen, M.D.

1. What characterizes papulosquamous skin lesions?

This major category of skin disorders is characterized by raised (papular) lesions with scales (squamous). They may or may not be pruritic.

2. Name the three most common diseases seen in primary care practice that present with a generalized papulosquamous rash.

Psoriasis, pityriasis rosea, and lichen planus. These diseases are often mistaken for tinea. A potassium hydroxide (KOH) preparation of dead skin cells helps to clarify the diagnosis.

3. Describe the presentation of psoriasis.

Psoriasis is a chronic inflammatory disease of the skin with onset in the third decade of life. It is characterized by sharply demarcated erythematous plaques covered with silvery scales that are symmetrically distributed over extensor surfaces of elbows, knees, gluteal cleft, and scalp. When the scales are removed, a few drops of blood may appear, a specific finding known as the Auspitz sign.

4. When is the Koebner phenomenon seen?

The Koebner phenomenon is commonly seen in patients with psoriasis and lichen planus. It refers to the development of plaques in an area of previous trauma. For example, lesions may line up over an excoriation or a scar or around a tattoo.

5. What other findings are associated with psoriasis?

Nail pitting is found in over 50% of patients, along with onycholysis and thickened nails. "Oil spots" or yellow-brown discoloration of the distal nail plate, may also occur. Joint manifestations are typically rheumatoid factor negative, asymmetric, and often limited to the distal interphalangeal joints. Arthritis mutilans, a rare form of arthritis, causes severe destruction of the phalanges with resultant telescoping of the digits.

6. What should be the initial therapy for psoriasis?

Skin hydration and midpotency steroids are standard therapy for limited skin plaques. A kerolytic agent (salicylic acid), topical retinoid (tazarotene), or tar gel may enhance steroid effectiveness. When the disease becomes less responsive or widespread (especially if erythroderma is present), more aggressive treatment with ultraviolet light, systemic methotrexate, or oral retinoids may be required. Such patients should be seen by a dermatologist to consider the most appropriate mode of therapy.

7. Describe the herald patch and the "Christmas tree" pattern in pityriasis rosea.

1. The herald patch is the initial lesion of pityriasis rosea that heralds the onset of the eruption by a few days. It is an annular salmon-pink patch with a rim or collarette of fine scale. It measures 2–6 cm in size and is larger than the lesions that follow it.

2. "Christmas tree" pattern describes the distribution of the oval papulosquamous lesions whose long axis follows the lines of skin cleavage. On the back, this arrangement resembles the shape of a Christmas tree.

8. What causes pityriasis rosea?

The cause of this self-limited, seasonal disease (seen in spring and fall) is unknown. A viral cause has been postulated but never proven. Treatment for pruritus is symptomatic; topic steroids may be used, if needed. Resolution is expected by 6–8 weeks.

9. What disease may pityriasis rosea mimic?

The lesions of pityriasis are similar to those of secondary syphilis, which is another papulosquamous disease. However, pityriasis rosea does not involve the palms and soles, both of which are commonly involved in secondary syphilis. If there is acral involvement or high clinical suspicion, serologic testing should be performed to exclude syphilis.

10. Where do lesions of lichen planus occur?

The pruritic, violaceous, papulosquamous lesions of lichen planus favor the wrists, shins, lower back, and genital area. Such lesions also commonly involve the oral mucosa, presenting as a white reticulated patch in the buccal area. Scalp involvement may lead to hair loss.

11. What causes lichen planus?

The cause of lichen planus is unknown. Outside the United States, it has been associated with hepatitis B and C virus. Similar lichenoid eruptions may result from a reaction to several drugs, including diuretics, antimalarials, and phenothiazines. Most cases, however, are idiopathic and spontaneously remit within 2 years. Topical steroids are often helpful.

12. What disease is characterized by dandruff and greasy yellow scale over the central area of the face?

Seborrheic dermatitis. It characteristically involves the glabella and the nasolabial folds and may also affect the external ears, eyebrows, and central chest.

13. What types of people are particularly susceptible to seborrheic dermatitis?

1. Infants ("cradle cap")
2. Patients with Parkinson's disease
3. Patients who previously suffered a cerebrovascular accident
4. Patients infected with the human immunodeficiency virus (HIV)

14. How should seborrheic dermatitis be treated?

1. Nonfluorinated topical steroids of low potency (e.g., hydrocortisone 1%) are most effective on glabrous skin. Nizoral 2% cream is particularly effective in patients with HIV because of the overgrowth of *P. orbiculare* in these individuals.

2. Shampoos with ketoconazole, selenium sulfide, tar, or zinc pyrithione used 2–3 times per week

15. What is the role of infection in seborrheic dermatitis?

Many investigators believe that *Pityrosporum orbiculare* is a causative organism in patients with seborrheic dermatitis. *P. orbiculare* (or *Malassezia furfur*) is a yeastlike fungus that lives in the stratum corneum. The addition of topical antifungal creams to the treatment regimen frequently helps to clear the eruption.

16. Why should a chronic scaly patch or plaque in the swimming-trunk distribution be considered for biopsy?

Such nonspecific lesions, which often appear psoriatic or eczematous, may be a prodromal or heralding lesion of mycosis fungoides (a chronic cutaneous T-cell lymphoma). Although the trunk distribution is common, lesions also may appear on the extremities.

17. How is mycosis fungoides diagnosed?

The history and physical examination point to the diagnosis. Patients have usually been treated for "eczema" for a prolonged period (up to 10–20 years). The diagnosis is made histologically. Biopsy initially may be nonspecific, and multiple biopsies may be necessary before a definitive diagnosis is made. The presence of a mononuclear infiltrate extending into the epidermis is a typical histologic feature of the disease. Collections of these abnormal lymphocytes in the epidermis are termed *Pautrier's microabscesses*. Gene rearrangement studies to determine clonality may aid in diagnosis.

BIBLIOGRAPHY

1. Freedberg I, Eisen AZ, Wolff K, et al (eds): Fitzpatrick's Dermatology in General Medicine, 6th ed. New York, McGraw-Hill, 2003.
2. Hay RJ, Graham-Brown RA: Dandruff and seborrheic dermatitis: Causes and management. Clin Exp Derm 22:3–6, 1997.
3. Lebwohl M, Ali S: Treatment of psoriasis. Part 1. Topical therapy and phototherapy. J Am Acad Dermatol 45:487–501, 2001.
4. Millikan LE, Shrum JP: An update on common skin diseases. Postgrad Med 1:96–98, 101–104, 107–110, 1992.

5. Phillips TJ, Dover JS: Recent advances in dermatology. N Engl J Med 326:167–178, 1992.
6. Siegel RS, Pandolfino T, Guitart J, et al: Primary cutaneous T-cell lymphoma: Review and current concepts. J Clin Oncol 18:2908–2925, 2000.
7. Sinni-McKeehen B: Scaling skin disorders. Prim Care Pract 1:1–13, 1997.
8. Skinner RB Jr, Noah PW, Taylor RM, et al: Double-blind treatment of seborrheic dermatitis with 2% ketoconazole cream. J Am Acad Dermatol 12:852–856, 1985.

93. VESICULAR AND BULLOUS SKIN ERUPTIONS

Gina A. Taylor, M.D.

1. What is the difference between a vesicle and a bulla?

Both are blisters of the skin filled with serous fluid, but vesicles are < 0.5 cm and bullae are > 0.5 cm in diameter. Some diseases are predominantly vesicular or bullous, but others involve a spectrum of lesions.

2. What is the differential diagnosis of a disseminated vesicular rash in children?

A vesicular rash is varicella (chickenpox) until proven otherwise. The diagnosis is suggested by history of exposure (90% attack rate in seronegative people) and crops of maculopapular lesions that progress to individual vesicles, each on an erythematous base. Within hours, they begin on the trunk and face and accompanied by pruritus. The rash is described as having the appearance of "dew drops on a rose petal."

Other less likely possibilities, often distinguished by the appropriate history and setting, include (1) infections with coxsackievirus or echovirus, (2) rickettsial pox (which may be distinguished by a herald spot [an eschar] at the site of the mite bite), and (3) disseminated herpes simplex infection (which may be seen in patients with atopic dermatitis, when it becomes known as eczema herpeticum).

3. How is the varicella virus transmitted?

The virus is transmitted by airborne droplets and by direct contact. Patients are contagious 2–3 days before appearance of exanthem and until all vesicles become crusted.

4. What is the incubation period of primary varicella infection?

The mean incubation period is 14 days. (The range is 10–23 days.)

5. What advice should providers give to patients with chickenpox infections?

1. Lukewarm soaks and compresses relieve pruritus and prevent secondary infection.
2. Oral antihistamines may be used for further symptomatic relief.
3. Close clipping of fingernails prevents excoriations.
4. The intake of aspirin by children should be prevented because of the risk of Reye's syndrome.
5. Oral acyclovir should be given to adolescents and adults with chickenpox of < 24 hours' duration.
6. New-onset respiratory symptoms require medical assessment.

6. Who should receive the varicella vaccine (Varivax)?

Those at high risk for primary infection with varicella virus should be vaccinated. The high risk populations include normal varicella-zoster virus seronegative adults, children with leukemia, and patients with HIV or who are otherwise immunocompromised.

7. What is shingles?

Shingles (or herpes zoster disease) results from varicella-zoster virus that has been latent in the dorsal root or cranial nerve ganglia. It presents as isolated pain followed by a unilateral vesicular eruption in a dermatomal distribution. Shingles occurs sporadically in the elderly population but rarely recurs. Cranial nerves may be involved, leading to mucosal, ear, and eye lesions.

8. What can be done to decrease the incidence of postherpetic neuralgia?

Up to 50% of older patients have dermatomal pain months after resolution of the vesicular lesions of zoster infection. This pain may be prevented by treatment with 7–10 days of acyclovir; the efficacy of steroids is less clearly established. Symptomatic relief with analgesics and amitriptyline may be attempted.

9. Which patients are at high risk of dissemination from varicella-zoster virus infections?

Immunocompromised patients, including those with HIV/AIDS or Hodgkin's lymphoma, patients who receive bone marrow transplants, and newborns are at risk of dissemination from varicella virus. Immune prophylaxis should be given to exposed patients; intravenous acyclovir is indicated for evidence of disease.

10. What is a Tzanck preparation?

A Tzanck prep or smear involves scraping the fluid from the base of a vesicle or pustule and examining the cytology of the fluid under light microscopy. It is said to be a positive result if the presence of multinucleated giant cells is noted. Tzanck smears are positive in all herpesvirus infections and do not distinguish between herpes simplex 1, herpes simplex 2, and varicella-zoster viruses.

11. Which diseases should be considered in the differential diagnosis of a bullous eruption?

The most common bullous diseases are pemphigus vulgaris, bullous pemphigoid, and erythema multiforme, which often can be diagnosed by clinical appearance. Diagnosis is confirmed by routine biopsy or by immunofluorescence microscopy of frozen tissue. Because treatment is somewhat different for each disease, correct diagnosis is crucial.

12. What is the typical appearance of erythema multiforme?

Erythema multiforme, the most common of the classic bullous diseases, affects predominantly children and young adults. Cutaneous lesions vary from fixed erythematous papules to annular and bullous lesions. The classic lesion is the target (also termed *iris lesion*), which most often occurs on the distal extremities and is characterized by a dusky gray center and an erythematous rim. Involvement of mucous membranes, especially the oral mucosa, is common. The ocular and genital mucosa are less often affected.

13. What are the most common causes of erythema multiforme?

The most common cause of erythema multiforme minor is recurrent herpes simplex infection (about 90% of patients). The rash of erythema multiforme occurs 7–10 days after a lesion of herpes simplex. Because herpes simplex is frequently recurrent, erythema multiforme also may recur. The second most common cause of erythema multiforme minor is drugs, especially sulfa drugs, barbiturates, and antibiotics such as tetracycline.

14. What is Stevens-Johnson syndrome (SJS)?

SJS is a more severe form of erythema multiforme and is also known as erythema multiforme major. The diagnosis is made when erythema multiforme–like lesions are accompanied by the involvement of two or more mucous membrane sites in the clinical setting of severe systemic symptoms. Mucous membranes often show severe involvement. If the ocular mucous membranes are involved, an ophthalmologist should be consulted to prevent permanent eye damage. The majority of cases are caused by drugs, particularly sulfa drugs. Patients with SJS are often very ill and may require hospitalization.

15. What is the difference between SJS and toxic epidermal necrolysis (TEN)?

TEN is considered by most to be a maximal variant of SJS. Both may begin with targetlike lesions, but about 50% of TEN cases do not. SJS is defined as having $< 10\%$ body surface area (BSA) involved with epidermal detachment; TEN has $> 30\%$ epidermal detachment. Any patient with 10–30% epidermal detachment can be considered to be in the SJS/TEN overlap.

16. Describe the lesions of pemphigus vulgaris.

Pemphigus vulgaris is an autoimmune skin disease in which the patient forms antibodies to the cellular bridges between epidermal keratinocytes. The antibodies cause the epidermis to fall apart in response to shear forces. Almost all patients have oral erosions at some point in the disease. Cutaneous lesions show denuded skin, similar to a burn. The epidermis pulls away from the dermis with minimal friction. Flaccid bullae are occasionally seen, but they readily rupture, leaving the characteristic erosions. Sites of predilection include the scalp; face; chest; and the intertriginous areas of the axillae, groin, and umbilicus. There is extensive involvement of the back in bedridden patients.

17. How is pemphigus vulgaris treated?

Before the development of systemic corticosteroids, pemphigus vulgaris was considered to be a uniformly fatal disease. Therefore, treatment needs to be relatively aggressive to control the disease as quickly as possible. After the correct diagnosis is established, patients should be treated with prednisone, 60–80 mg in a single daily dose. In most cases, a steroid-sparing drug, such as azathioprine, should be started at the initiation of prednisone therapy. The full steroid-sparing effect of azathioprine requires approximately 6 weeks. After the cutaneous lesions of pemphigus vulgaris show complete healing, the dosage of prednisone is slowly reduced. The goal should be to keep the patient on the lowest dose of alternate-day prednisone that controls the disease. It may require several months before the prednisone and azathioprine can be completely discontinued.

18. What is the presentation and treatment of bullous pemphigoid?

Bullous pemphigoid is typically a disease of middle-aged and elderly patients. At one time, it was referred to as bullous disease of the aged. It is characterized by large, tense blisters with a predilection for the intertriginous areas such as the inner thigh and axillae. The blisters show much less tendency to rupture than those of pemphigus vulgaris. Blisters may occur in the mouth but, unlike pemphigus vulgaris, mucosal lesions usually follow the onset of skin disease. The tense blisters of bullous pemphigoid are often situated on red urticarial plaques. Bullous pemphigoid is less likely to be a life-threatening disease than pemphigus vulgaris. Therefore, the dose of oral prednisone and steroid-sparing agents, such as azathioprine, may be more conservative. An initial prednisone dose of 40–60 mg/day is usually adequate. The disease responds to treatment more rapidly than pemphigus vulgaris.

BIBLIOGRAPHY

1. Freedberg I, Eisen AZ, Wolff K, et al (eds): Fitzpatrick's Dermatology in General Medicine, 6th ed. New York, McGraw-Hill, 2003.
2. Moschella SL, Hurley HJ (eds): Dermatology, 3rd ed. Philadelphia, W.B. Saunders, 1992.
3. Phillips TJ, Dover JS: Recent advances in dermatology. N Engl J Med 326:167–178, 1992.
4. Rajan P, Rivers JK: Varicella zoster virus. Recent advances in management. Can Fam Physician 47:2299–2304, 2001.
5. Stella M, Cassano P, Bollero D, et al: Toxic epidermal necrolysis treated with intravenous high-dose immunoglobulins: Our experience. Dermatology 203:45–49, 2001.
6. Tatnall FM, Schofield JK, Leigh IM: A double-blind, placebo-controlled trial of continuous acyclovir therapy in recurrent erythema multiforme. Br J Dermatol 132:267–270, 1995.

94. URTICARIA

Tatiana Khrom, M.D.

1. What is the primary lesion of urticaria?

Urticaria is characterized by **hives,** which are pale to red, well-demarcated, evanescent, pruritic swellings of the skin, mouth, and genitalia. Superficial swellings of the dermis are called **wheals.** Individual lesions typically last less than 24 hours, which sets them apart from other cutaneous disorders presenting with a similar morphology.

2. What is angioedema?

Angioedema describes deeper swelling of the skin and subcutaneous tissue. Most often, it involves the eyelids, lips, tongue, and genitalia. It can also involve the mucosal lining of the gastrointestinal (GI) and genitourinary (GU) systems. Angioedema can occur with or without urticaria and can be acute or chronic.

3. How common is urticaria?

An estimated 15–25% of the population experience an urticarial illness in their lives. Of this group, up to 40% experience urticaria alone, 10% angioedema alone, and 50% will have both urticaria and angioedema.

4. What is the pathogenesis of urticaria and angioedema?

Degranulation of mast cells with histamine release is central to the development of wheals and angioedema. Histamine release causes an increase in capillary permeability, which allows proteins and fluids to extravasate. This results in the urticarial wheal.

5. What is acute urticaria?

Acute urticaria is characterized by evanescent wheals that individually last less than 24 hours and completely resolve within 6 weeks of onset.

6. Name the most common causes of acute urticaria.

Urticaria with or without angioedema may be immunologic, nonimmunologic, or idiopathic. The binding of antigen to immunoglobulin E (IgE) antibodies on mast cells (immunologic type) is probably the most common mechanism responsible for acute urticaria. The typical antigens in this kind of urticaria are foods, drugs, and infectious agents. Some nonimmunologic factors that typically induce urticaria are radiocontrast dye, opiates, polymyxin, and aspirin and other nonsteroidal anti-inflammatory drugs (NSAIDs). These agents typically cause a direct or indirect degranulation of mast cells. However, in the majority of patients, a definite cause is not identified.

7. What is the mainstay of treatment for acute urticaria?

Treatment involves elimination of the cause, if known. The mainstays of medical therapy are histamine-1 (H_1) receptor blockers, including classic H_1 antihistamines (e.g., diphenhydramine and hydroxyzine) and nonsedating H_1 antihistamines (terfenadine, astemizole, and loratadine). Such agents should be initiated at standard doses and titrated as tolerated. Doxepin hydrochloride, a tricyclic antidepressant with powerful H_1 antagonist activity, also may be useful. H_2 antihistamines administered in combination with H_1 blockers may be more effective than H_1 antihistamines alone in some patients. Disodium cromoglycate, terbutaline, and calcium channel blockers also may have a role in the treatment of some patients. In rare patients, a 1- to 2-week course of systemic corticosteroids may be needed. For progressive or highly morbid disease, one can consider treatment with azathioprine, cyclosporine, and interferon gamma.

8. What is the relationship between urticaria and anaphylaxis?

Anaphylaxis is a life-threatening response of a sensitized individual to a specific antigen. Symptoms may vary widely from mild pruritus and urticaria with or without angioedema to shock and death secondary to respiratory distress (caused by bronchospasm and laryngeal edema) as well as vascular collapse (caused by massive histamine release). Airway protection, epinephrine, fluids, and systemic corticosteroids may be required in severe cases.

9. Is epinephrine ever indicated in the treatment of acute urticaria?

Yes. In severe cases of urticaria or when anaphylaxis is suspected, subcutaneous epinephrine (0.3 mL of a 1:1000 solution) should be administered and may be repeated at 30-minute intervals for severe reactions. Intravenous or intramuscular administration of epinephrine is required in patients with airway involvement, anaphylaxis, or cardiovascular collapse.

10. What are the most common causes of anaphylaxis?

Drugs (penicillins and NSAIDs) and radiographic contrast agents are the most common causes of anaphylaxis. Hymenoptera stings are the next most frequent cause, followed by ingestion of shellfish and other food allergens.

11. What should be done for patients who manifest urticaria to beestings?

It is important to determine the patient's potential risk of anaphylaxis. If no history is easily obtainable to assess risk, a skin test should be considered. Potential for anaphylaxis correlates with a positive skin test result. After assessing the risk for anaphylaxis, the following steps should be provided:

1. **Instruction in prevention.** The patient's lifestyle should be modified to avoid exposure to bees (wearing of shoes; avoidance of eating or wearing perfume in high-risk areas; limitation of unnecessary yard work, especially hauling trash).

2. **Instruction in emergency measures.** Unexpired epinephrine kits should be readily available at home and in the car, and informational bracelets and tags should be used.

3. **Desensitization.** In patients with a history or serious risk of anaphylaxis, venom immunotherapy may be undertaken until the skin test is negative. Desensitization is not required for children who experience a systemic reaction limited to the skin because progression to anaphylaxis is unlikely.

12. What is chronic urticaria?

Any pattern of recurrent urticaria occurring at least twice a week for 6 weeks is called chronic urticaria.

13. What is the differential diagnosis of chronic urticaria?

- Systemic or subacute lupus erythematosus
- Erythema multiforme
- Erythema anulare centrifugum
- Bullous pemphigoid
- Drug eruptions
- Urticarial vasculitis, a form of leukocytoclastic vasculitis associated with hypocomplementemia

14. What are the most common causes of chronic urticaria?

Although in the past, the majority of cases of chronic urticaria were thought to be idiopathic, it is now recognized that many of these cases can be ascribed to autoimmunity via the production of histamine-releasing autoantibodies. Physical stimuli may produce urticarial reactions and represent approximately 15% of chronic urticarias. A small percentage of cases are caused by medications, chronic infections (e.g., sinusitis), and food and food additives. Approximately 50% of cases currently remain unexplained.

15. What are the types of physical urticarias?

The most frequent type of physical urticaria is dermatographism, followed by cholinergic urticaria and acquired cold urticaria. Less frequent types are delayed pressure, solar, aquagenic, exercise-induced, and vibratory urticarias.

16. What is dermatographism?

Dermatographism is the most common cause of physical urticaria. Linear wheals develop rapidly after blunt, firm stroking of the skin and resolve within 1 hour. About 5% of the population has asymptomatic simple dermatographism; symptomatic dermatographism is much less common. Patients with atopic dermatitis have an increased incidence of dermatographism. For symptomatic patients, the pruritic wheals may last for several hours. Treatment consists of oral antihistamines and avoidance of trauma to the skin. Delayed dermatographism presents with linear, red nodules that develop 3–6 hours after stimulation and persist for 24–48 hours.

17. Describe the initial evaluation of patients with chronic urticaria.

A thorough history and physical examination are the most important parts of the workup. Key historical features include the pattern of occurrence and relationship to medications, diet, and activity. Medication usage, including nonprescription drugs and home or "natural" remedies, should be reviewed. Physical should include a complete blood count, liver and renal function tests, erythrocyte sedimentation rate, and urinalysis. Further testing is usually not necessary, unless suggested by positive findings from the history or physical examination (e.g., antinuclear antibodies, stool for ova and parasites, hepatitis-B serology, thyroid function studies, thyroid antibodies).

18. What is the natural history of chronic urticaria?

Fifty percent of patients who experience chronic urticaria will be free of their disease after 1 year. Twenty percent of patients continue to experience lesions for more than 20 years.

19. What is the mainstay of treatments of chronic urticarias?

Apart from antihistamines, some specific agents have been found to be effective in treating chronic urticaria. Cyproheptadine has been reported to be effective in controlling acquired cold urticaria. Stanazolol therapy has been effective in treating some patients with cold urticaria. NSAIDs and corticosteroids prevent delayed pressure urticaria lesions. Propranolol is effective in treating adrenergic urticaria. A course of antibiotics has cleared patients whose urticaria was caused by chronic sinusitis or *Helicobacter pylori* infections.

20. When is a skin biopsy indicated?

If individual lesions of urticaria are purpuric or persist for days, a skin biopsy should be considered to rule out urticarial vasculitis or any other disease mistaken for urticaria.

21. What is urticarial vasculitis?

The lesions of urticarial vasculitis may be clinically indistinguishable from wheals. However, the presence of small blood vessel damage on histopathology differentiates this entity from plain urticaria. The lesions of urticarial vasculitis usually last several days, may bruise, and tend to burn rather than itch.

BIBLIOGRAPHY

1. Dover JS, Arndt KA, Jackson, BA et al: Cutaneous Medicine and Surgery. Philadelphia, W.B. Saunders, 1996.
2. Grattan CE, Sabroe, RA, Greaves MW: Chronic urticaria, CME. J Am Acad Dermatol 46:645–660, 2002.
3. Fitzpatrick JE, Aeling JL: Dermatology Secrets in Color, 2nd ed. Philadelphia, Hanley & Belfus, 2001.
4. Freedberg IM, Eisen AZ, Wolff K, et al (eds): Fitzpatrick's Dermatology in General Medicine, 6th ed. New York, McGraw-Hill, 2003.
5. Habif TP, Campbell, JL, Quitadama MJ, Zug KA: Skin Disease Diagnosis and Treatment. St Louis, Mosby, 2001.

95. SKIN INFECTIONS

Colleen M. Crandell, M.D.

1. What is sycosis barbae, and how is it treated?

Sycosis barbae, also known as sycosis vulgaris or barber's itch, is a chronic, perifollicular staphylococcal infection of the beard region. It is manifested by recurrent inflammatory papules and pustules. Often, the disease begins near the upper lip, with follicular pustules that heal with erythema. Shaving exacerbates the condition, and allows for its spread throughout the beard area. In severe cases of sycosis, eye involvement in the form of blepharitis or conjunctivitis is seen. Sycosis vulgaris must be differentiated from pseudofolliculitis barbae. Pseudofolliculitis barbae is due to ingrown beard hairs, and does not represent a primary infectious process.

2. Describe the presentation and treatment of impetigo contagiosa.

Impetigo contagiosa is an infectious disorder of the skin that begins as small red macules, which may quickly develop into vesicles or bullae. Erosions then appear, covered by thick, honey-colored crusts. Sites of involvement include exposed body parts: the face, hands, neck, and extremities. Streptococci, once the most common cause of impetigo, has been replaced by *Staphylococcus aureus*. Occasionally, both organisms play an etiologic role. Bullous impetigo, secondary to *S. aureus,* is a highly contagious variant most often seen in newborns. Impetigo is usually seen in young children and often complicates atopic dermatitis, pediculosis capitis, insect bites, and other pruritic skin diseases. Treatment includes warm soaks to remove crusts, followed by application of bacitracin or mupirocin ointment. In addition, systemic antibiotics are necessary; oral erythromycin, a first-generation cephalosporin, and dicloxacillin are most commonly used. For recurrent cases of impetigo, a bacterial culture of the anterior nares is indicated because staphylococci are often harbored in this region. If so, topical mupirocin applied to the anterior nares or a 5-day course of rifampin is required. Finally, cases of impetigo caused by certain strains of beta-hemolytic streptococci may be followed by acute glomerulonephritis. Unfortunately, early treatment of impetigo does not reduce the risk of acute glomerulonephritis.

3. What is ecthyma?

Ecthyma is similar to impetigo but is a deeper skin infection, producing a shallow ulcer covered by crust. *Streptococcus pyogenes* is thought to be the primary causative organism, with subsequent contamination by staphylococci. The lower legs (shins, dorsal feet) are most commonly affected, and the condition is more prevalent in warm, humid climates. Poor hygiene and minor trauma are predisposing factors. Localized lymphadenopathy and a low-grade fever may be present. Lesions tend to heal with scars. Treatment includes warm compresses, topical bacitracin or mupirocin, and oral erythromycin, a first-generation cephalosporin, or dicloxacillin.

4. What is ecthyma gangrenosum?

Ecthyma gangrenosum is a cutaneous manifestation of *Pseudomonas aeruginosa* septicemia. This most commonly occurs in debilitated and immunocompromised patients and is manifested by vesicles or pustules that quickly become hemorrhagic. Upon rupture, ulcers with necrotic black centers form. Lesions most often appear on the extremities or buttocks. Treatment is urgent, with intravenous antibiotics including an aminoglycoside and an antipseudomonal penicillin (piperacillin).

5. Describe the typical appearance and treatment of a dermatophyte infection of the scalp.

Tinea capitis ("ringworm") is a fungal infection of the scalp most commonly seen in school-aged children. Rarely, adults are infected. *Trichophyton* and *Microsporum* species are the causative agents. *T. tonsurans* is the most common causative organism in the United States; *M. canis* is the second most common. Infection is either within the hair shaft (endothrix) or around the hair shaft (ectothrix). Variants of tinea capitis include gray-patch tinea capitis, black-dot tinea capitis, inflammatory tinea capitis, and favus. Gray-patch tinea capitis presents as scaly patches around a hair shaft. It is usually caused by *Microsporum audouinii*. Black-dot tinea capitis presents as patches of alopecia containing multiple infected broken-off hairs. *T. tonsurans* is usually implicated. Inflammatory tinea capitis is most commonly caused by *Microsporum canis* and begins with red, scaly papules leading to broken-off hairs. The inflammatory reaction can be severe in this type on tinea capitis, and at times an edematous, pus-filled, boggy lesion can develop (kerion). A kerion is believed to represent a delayed-type hypersensitivity to the fungi and can culminate in scarring of the scalp. Favus, very rare in North America, consists of thick yellowish crusts on the scalp surrounding loose hairs. The crusts are referred to as *scutula* (singular is *scutulum*), are malodorous, and heal with atrophy and scarring. *Trichophyton schoenleinii* is the causative agent.

6. What simple tests help to make the diagnosis of tinea capitis?

During the physical examination, regional lymphadenopathy should be assessed. Patients with tinea capitis often have cervical, posterior auricular, or occipital lymphadenopathy. Diagnostic testing should include a Wood's lamp examination of suspected lesions. In a dark room, lesions caused by *Microsporum* species and those caused by *T. schoenleinii* will reveal bright green fluorescence of infected hairs. Tinea capitis caused by *T. tonsurans* will not fluoresce. In addition, hair shafts and scale should be obtained for microscopic examination and culture on Sabouraud's agar. Infected areas may be scraped with a scalpel, or hairs may be plucked. The specimen is examined microscopically after the addition of 20–25% potassium hydroxide (KOH) solution. Hyphae and spores are seen on or within the hair shaft.

7. How is a KOH preparation performed?

Unlike vaginal and mucosal KOH preparations, the keratinized epidermis requires special methods to see the hyphae within the cells. The simplest procedure is to use two glass slides, one to scrape dead skin cells and the other to "catch" the cells. The cells are then covered with a cover slip, a few drops of 20% KOH are added, and capillary action is allowed to pull the KOH under the cover slip. The specimen must then be heated gently (with a match lighter or alcohol lamp). Do not allow the KOH to boil because it will crystallize and destroy the specimen. The heat breaks down the keratinized cell wall and allows hyphae to be seen microscopically. Hyphae should cross cell walls. Focusing up and down with the microscope condenser helps to differentiate between cell walls and hyphal elements.

8. What is the differential diagnosis of tinea capitis?

Seborrheic dermatitis	Trichotillomania
Atopic dermatitis	Lichen planus
Psoriasis	Lichen simplex chronicus
Alopecia areata	Secondary syphilis

9. How should tinea capitis be treated?

Systemic antifungals are required for the treatment of tinea capitis. For children, ultramicronized griseofulvin is recommended at a dose of 10 mg/kg/day. For children requiring oral suspension, griseofulvin microsize is given at a dose of 20 mg/kg/day. It should be noted that treatment failures of tinea capitis are often caused by inadequate dosing. Treatment is continued for 2–4 months or until negative cultures are obtained. Griseofulvin should be taken with fatty food to enhance its absorption. Adults with tinea capitis should be treated with griseofulvin microsize at a dose of 1 g/day for a similar time frame. Several recent clinical trials demonstrate the efficacy of alternative oral antifungals, including fluconazole (6 mg/kg/day), itraconazole (5 mg/kg/day), and terbinafine (62.5, 125, 250 mg/day, if weight is 10–20 kg, 20–40 kg, or > 40 kg, respectively). In addition, family members should be treated with ketoconazole or selenium sulfide shampoo. Inflammatory tinea capitis (kerion) should be treated with the same dose of griseofulvin plus systemic steroids to reduce the inflammation that can result in scarring and permanent hair loss.

10. What is a dermatophytid?

A dermatophytid is a skin reaction (id reaction) to fungal antigen at some remote site. It may be localized or generalized and often complicates inflammatory tinea capitis and bullous tinea pedis. Most commonly, an id reaction manifests as extremely pruritic vesicles on the hands and sides of the fingers. More widespread id reactions with pruritic lichenoid papules on the trunk can occur. Lesions may become secondarily infected by bacteria. The id lesions themselves do not contain fungi. Therapy includes treatment of the primary fungal infection.

11. How do dermatophyte infections of the hands and feet present?

Tinea manuum and tinea pedis are fungal infections of the hands and feet, respectively. Tinea manuum refers to dermatophyte infection of the palms and interdigital spaces. Tinea pedis is a dermatophyte infection of the soles of the feet and the interdigital spaces. Infections are transmitted from one person to another. Many believe that tinea pedis is acquired from going barefoot in public facilities such as gyms, pools, and locker rooms. However, it remains unclear as to why certain individuals are more susceptible to acquiring tinea pedis than others.

Tinea manuum and tinea pedis share the same etiologic fungi—most commonly *Trichophyton rubrum* (which causes a dry, moccasin-type eruption), *Trichophyton mentagrophytes* (which causes an inflammatory tinea), and *Epidermophyton floccosum* (which is rare and usually infects toe webs). In addition, nondermatophyte infections of the hands and feet that appear clinically similar are caused by *Scytalidium* species. Often, tinea manuum affects only one hand and is seen in combination with a moccasin-type tinea pedis. This is referred to as "two feet-one hand syndrome." In addition, cases of tinea pedis with prominent interdigital maceration may become secondarily infected with bacteria. Diagnosis is based on the clinical appearance, positive culture, and a KOH preparation revealing branching, septate hyphae.

12. How are tinea pedis and tinea manuum treated?

- Excessive moisture should be reduced with talcum or antifungal powders.
- Topical antifungals such as clotrimazole, miconazole, ciclopirox, ketoconazole, econazole, oxiconazole, terbinafine, and naftifine are effective.
- Systemic antifungal agents may be effective, although recurrence is common.
- Keratolytic products containing salicylic, glycolic, and lactic acids or urea can aid in reducing the significant hyperkeratosis see in dermatophyte infections of the hands and feet.

13. Describe the appearance of tinea corporis.

Tinea corporis, commonly referred to as "ringworm," includes fungal infections of the glabrous skin, excluding the hands, feet, hair, nails, and groin. Generally, infection is limited to the stratum corneum. The most common etiologic agent is *Trichophyton rubrum,* followed by *T. mentagrophytes.* Tinea corporis may be acquired in one of three ways: human to human (anthropilic), animal to human (zoophilic), or soil spread to human (geophilic). Domestic animals, including cats and dogs, are often implicated in zoophilic cases of tinea corporis. Additional predisposing factors include personal history of tinea capitis or pedis, close contact with a person who has tinea capitis or pedis, recreational exposure in facilities such as gymnasiums, contact with contaminated clothing and furniture, and immunosuppression.

Prominent hair-bearing areas of the body may exhibit more pronounced infection, because dermatophyte infections often track down the hair follicles. Typical incubation ranges from 1 to 3 weeks. Lesions of tinea corporis most commonly present as annular plaques with erythematous scaly borders and some central clearing. Scale may be diminished if topical steroids have been wrongly applied for treatment, resulting in a condition known as *tinea incognito.* Majocchi's granuloma is a variant of tinea corporis usually seen on the legs of women who shave. It presents with perifollicular inflammation and pustules. The differential diagnosis of tinea corporis includes other ring-like eruptions, such as erythema annulare centrifugum, nummular eczema, and granuloma annulare.

14. Can dermatophyte infection involve the face?

Yes. Dermatophyte infection of the face is referred to as *tinea faciei*. This can mimic cutaneous lupus erythematosus, seborrheic dermatitis, and contact dermatitis. Microscopic examination of a KOH preparation should be performed from the active border of the lesion. Clinical diagnosis requires a high index of suspicion. Combining a fungal culture with KOH examination increase the likelihood of making the definitive diagnosis.

15. How are tinea corporis and tinea faciei treated?

Localized cases are treated with topical antifungals (see question 12), whereas widespread tinea corporis and inflammatory components (such as Majocchi's granuloma) often necessitate treatment with systemic antifungals. These include griseofulvin (10–20 mg/kg/day for 2–4 weeks), fluconazole (150–200 mg/week for 2–4 weeks), itraconazole (200 mg/day for 1 week), and terbinafine (250 mg/day for 1 week).

16. What is tinea cruris?

Tinea cruris is commonly referred to as "jock itch." It occurs intertriginously, in the groin fold and upper inner thighs. The three most common dermatophytes implicated in causing tinea cruris are *Epidermophyton floccosum, T. rubrum,* and *T. mentagrophytes.* Men more commonly develop tinea cruris, because the scrotum encourages a moist environment in which dermatophytes thrive. Tinea cruris is often seen concomitantly with tinea pedis; clothing brought over infected feet lies in direct apposition with the groin. Clinically, tinea cruris manifests as sharply demarcated erythematous plaques with raised borders. Infection may be unilateral or bilateral. Generally, the scrotal area is spared from involvement (which can aid in ruling out a candidal infection, which often involves the scrotum). With resolution, hyperpigmented patches may persist at prior sites of involvement for several months. Reduction of moisture with talcum or antifungal powders is beneficial, and topical antifungals (see question 12) are generally effective. In addition, wearing loose clothing and drying thoroughly after bathing are helpful preventive measures.

17. Describe the manifestations of cutaneous candidiasis.

Infections caused by *Candida* most commonly involve intertriginous areas, including the axillae, groin, inframammary, gluteal, perianal, and finger space areas. In addition, the scrotum and diaper area in infants are often infected. Candidiasis of the skin folds has a beefy erythematous color and often reveals satellite papules and pustules at the periphery of the lesion. Lesions may become erosive. Candidal infection of the finger webs is referred to *erosio interdigitalis blastomycetica*.

Mucocutaneous candidiasis includes oral thrush, perlèche (angular cheilitis), vulvovaginitis, and balanitis. Also, *Candida* can infect the nail and periungual regions.

Candida albicans is the most common offending agent, followed by *Candida tropicalis.* Immunocompromised patients often exhibit widespread and more severe involvement.

The diagnosis is based on clinical presentation and KOH preparation, which demonstrates round or oval budding yeast and pseudohyphae. The organism is easily cultures on Sabouraud's medium.

18. How is cutaneous candidiasis treated?

Treatment of cutaneous candidiasis includes correction of predisposing factors such as heat and moisture and application of topical antifungal creams such as miconazole, clotrimazole, ketoconazole, or econazole. Nystatin powder or cream is effective in treating cutaneous candidal infections; it is ineffective, however, against dermatophyte species. Occasionally, treatment of the gastrointestinal tract with oral nystatin, in combination with topical agents, is required to treat anogenital candidiasis. Oral nystatin is not absorbed and, therefore, is not by itself useful in treating cutaneous candidiasis. Systemic antifungals may be required for patients with chronic or extensive infections or in those with underlying immunosuppression. Oral itraconazole, ketoconazole, and fluconazole possess greater anticandidal efficacy than does systemic terbinafine. In addition, griseofulvin is not effective in the treatment of candidiasis.

BIBLIOGRAPHY

1. Abdel-Rahman SM, Nahata MC: Oral terbinafine. A new antifungal agent. Ann Pharm 31:445–456, 1997.
2. Aly R, Berger T: Common superficial fungal infections in patients with AIDS. Clin Infect Dis 22(suppl 2):S128-S132, 1996.
3. Bolognia JL, et al (eds): Dermatology. St. Louis, Mosby, 2003.
4. Freedberg IM, Eisen AZ, Wolff K (eds): Fitzpatrick's Dermatology in General Medicine, 6th ed. New York, McGraw-Hill, 2003.
5. Lesher JL Jr: Recent developments in antifungal therapy. Dermatol Clin 14:163–169, 1996.
6. Moschella SL, Hurley HJ (eds): Dermatology, 3rd ed. Philadelphia, W.B. Saunders, 1993.
7. Odom RB, et al (eds): Andrews' Disease of the Skin, 9th ed. Philadelphia, W.B. Saunders, 2000.
8. Wolverton SE: Comprehensive Dermatologic Drug Therapy. Philadelphia, W.B. Saunders, 2001.

96. ISOLATED SKIN LESIONS

Alison B. Gruen, M.D.

1. How do common warts present?

Common warts (verrucae vulgares) appear as sharply marginated keratotic papules with a rough surface. A classic feature is the presence of punctuate black dots representing thrombosed capillaries. The loss of dermatoglyphics (fingerprint lines) helps differentiate the lesion from a callus when it occurs on an acral surface. They may appear anywhere on the skin but are most common on the dorsal surfaces of the hand and fingers. Common warts are a neoplasm caused by the human papillomavirus.

2. Describe the two common treatments for warts.

1. Twice daily application of 17% salicylic acid solution (Compound W, Wart-Off) results in sloughing of keratin. Prolonged therapy is usually required. Salicylic acid plaster (Mediplast) can be trimmed to cover the wart and left in place for up to 1 week at a time. Gentle debridement of the dead tissue followed by retreatment with the plaster usually results in resolution of the wart within 6–8 weeks. Additionally, a thick tape such as duct tape can be used to cover the wart after the salicylic acid is applied. The tape is changed every 24 hours. This "adhesiotherapy" is often more effective than salicylic acid alone.

2. Cryotherapy with liquid nitrogen may be applied with a probe, pressurized spray, or cotton swab. Hyperkeratotic warts should be pared down before freezing. The wart and a narrow rim of normal skin should be frozen for 20–30 seconds, allowed to thaw, and frozen a second time. The treatment is associated with mild burning pain. The double freeze-thaw method should be repeated at 7–10-day intervals until the warts are eliminated. Patients should be told that formation of a blister is an expected effect. Combining in-office cryotherapy with nightly application of salicylic acid is more effective than either treatment alone.

3. What topical agents are useful in the treatment of genital warts?

Provider-applied therapies for genital warts (condyloma acuminata) include cryotherapy and podophyllin resin 10–25% in tincture of benzoin. Podophyllin must be washed off in 4–6 hours to avoid irritation. If a large area is to be treated, a 5% viscous lidocaine ointment may be given for relief of irritation after treatment. Podophyllin is less effective in relatively dry anogenital areas, including the penile shaft, scrotum, and labia majora. Cryotherapy may be of more benefit. Either treatment (or both) is repeated weekly until the condylomata are gone. Patient-applied therapies include podofilox and imiquimod. Podofilox 0.5% is applied twice daily for 3 days/week for 4–6 weeks. Imiquimod 5% cream stimulates the host's immune response and has shown high rates of clearance and low rates of recurrence. It is applied overnight, 3 nights on and 4 nights off.

4. How does basal cell carcinoma present?

Basal cell carcinoma, the most common cutaneous malignancy, is found predominantly in patients with a history of chronic sun exposure; 80–90% of lesions are found on the head and neck. Lesions typically are firm papules with a smooth pearly surface and telangiectatic vessels. Large lesions commonly have central ulceration and crusting and "rolled" borders. Basal cell carcinomas may be heavily pigmented and difficult to differentiate from malignant melanoma.

5. Describe the appearance of actinic keratosis.

An actinic keratosis is a red macule with a dry, rough, adherent scale. It is commonly seen on sun-exposed areas such as the forehead and dorsal forearms.

6. Why should actinic keratosis be distinguished from seborrheic keratosis?

Actinic keratosis is a premalignant lesion that may convert to squamous cell carcinoma at a rate of 0.25–1.0% per year. Seborrheic keratoses, which appear on both the face and trunk, are brown-gray papules with a "stuck-on," waxy appearance. They are of cosmetic concern only.

7. Describe the typical appearance of squamous cell carcinoma.

Squamous cell carcinomas also arise in sun-damaged skin such as the head, neck, or arms. Lesions appear as firm, skin-colored, or slightly erythematous patches or plaques with a distinct margin. The surface is rough or verrucous, and ulceration is common. Squamous cell carcinomas of the skin often develop from preexisting actinic keratoses.

8. How should patients with actinic keratoses and actinic sun damage be managed?

Sun protection is critical. This includes sun avoidance, daily use of broad-spectrum (ultraviolet A and ultraviolet B) sunscreen, and the wearing of hats and sunglasses. Treatment options for existing actinic keratoses include cryosurgery, curettage, or excision. For extensive actinic damage, topical fluorouracil or topical tretinoin cream may be applied every night or every other night before bedtime. Photodynamic therapy is a newer noninvasive treatment modality.

9. How are basal and squamous cell carcinomas diagnosed and treated?

The definitive diagnosis is based on histologic examination of a biopsy specimen. Metastases are rare in basal cell carcinomas and squamous cell carcinomas in chronically sun-damaged skin. However, both tumors may be locally aggressive. Treatments include surgical excision, curettage and electrosurgery, Moh's micrographic surgery, and radiotherapy. Referral to a dermatologist is appropriate.

10. What risks are associated with giant congenital nevi?

Giant congenital nevi (those that measure > 20 cm) are associated with an estimated 6% lifetime risk of developing melanomas. Most of these melanomas develop within the first 5 years of life. Nevi in an axial location are associated with a greater risk than those on the extremities. Leptomeningeal melanosis is another risk. In this case, ectopic melanocytes infiltrate the leptomeninges. This may result in increased intracranial pressure, spinal cord compression, seizures, hydrocephalus, and death, often before age 2 years. Diagnostic magnetic resonance imaging (MRI) and neurologic consultation are appropriate.

11. Who is at risk for the development of melanoma?

- People who are fair skinned, blue eyed, red-haired, and freckled
- People with dysplastic nevi (atypical moles)

- Patients with a family history of melanoma
- People with a large congenital melanocyte nevus
- Immunocompromised patients

12. What features of a pigmented skin lesion suggest the diagnosis of malignant melanoma?

The **ABCD rule** can be used to evaluate a pigmented lesion for the possibility of melanoma or melanoma precursor (dysplastic nevus):

Asymmetry
Border irregularity
Color variegation or dark color
Diameter > 0.6 cm

The ABCD features are more common in melanomas than in benign pigmented lesions. Ulceration, pruritus, pain, new lesions, or changes in existing pigmented lesions also should arouse suspicion.

13. How should pigmented skin lesions be evaluated?

Clinically, atypical lesions should be excised to the level of fat and submitted in their entirety for histologic evaluation. Sampling a portion of a pigmented lesion is not recommended because a sampling error may occur. Shave biopsies of potentially malignant lesions destroy the pathologist's ability to measure tumor depth and thus interfere with prognostication. Patients with many pigmented lesions or a personal or family history should be evaluated by a dermatologist with special interest in pigmented lesions.

14. How is the prognosis of melanoma established?

Definitive diagnosis of a suspicious lesion is made by excisional biopsy. Prognosis of localized melanoma (localized to the skin) is based largely on tumor thickness, which is measured histopathologically. Lesions < 0.76 mm in thickness are associated with a 96% 5-year survival rate. Sentinel node biopsy is used to identify nodal metastases in the immediate area of the primary tumor. This procedure is used in patients with primary cutaneous melanoma and clinically negative lymph nodes. It improves the accuracy of staging and has a significant impact on prognosis.

15. What treatment and follow-up are indicated for melanoma?

Stage I melanoma is treated with surgical excision. Recent studies have shown that wide surgical margins usually are not necessary. Lesions up to 1 mm thick can be treated with 1-cm margins, whereas 2-cm margins may be indicated for thicker lesions. Prospective, randomized studies of prophylactic regional lymph node dissection have shown no survival benefit. Patients should have regular follow-up for local recurrence, metastases, and second primary melanomas. Patients with melanoma are best followed by oncologists, dermatologists, or other specially trained physicians.

BIBLIOGRAPHY

1. DeDavid M, Orlow SJ, Provost N, et al: A study of large congenital melanocytic nevi and associated malignant melanomas. J Am Acad Dermatol 36:409–416, 1997.
2. Freedberg IM, Eisen AZ, Wolff K, et al (eds): Fitzpatrick's Dermatology in General Medicine, 6th ed. New York, McGraw-Hill, 2003.
3. Gallagher RP, McLean DI: The epidemiology of acquired melanocytic nevi: A brief review. Dermatol Clin 13:595–603, 1995.
4. Goldstein BG, Goldstein AO: Diagnosis and management of malignant melanoma. Am Fam Physician 63:1359–1368, 2001.
5. Nguyen TH, Ho DQ: Nonmelanoma skin cancer. Curr Treat Options Oncol 3:193–203, 2002.
6. Plasencia JM: Cutaneous warts: Diagnosis and treatment. Prim Care 27:423–434, 2000.
7. Russell-Jones R, Acland K: Sentinel nodes biopsy in the management of malignant melanoma. Clin Exp Dermatol 26:463–468, 2001.
8. Walsh P, Gibbs P, Gonzalez R: Newer strategies for effective evaluation of primary melanoma and treatment of stage III and IV disease. J Am Acad Dermatol 42:480–489, 2000.

97. ACNE

Alison B. Gruen, M.D.

1. Describe the pathogenesis of acne vulgaris.

The follicular orifices become plugged with sebum and desquamated follicular epithelial cells. This obstruction leads to the formation of a microcomedo, the precursor lesion of acne. The microcomedo may evolve into a comedone ("blackhead" or "whitehead") or an inflammatory papule, pustule, or nodule. Inflammation is caused by proliferation of the lipophilic bacteria *Propionibacterium acnes*. Hormonal influences contribute to the initiation of these lesions.

2. What external factors aggravate acne?

1. Trauma from overvigorous skin scrubbing or irritant contact (athletic gear, picking acne lesions)

2. Topical agents (cosmetics and industrial compounds that are comedone forming, such as lanolin, paraffin oil, and oleic acid)

3. What drugs may cause an acneiform eruption or exacerbate underlying acne?

Glucocorticoids (topical or systemic), phenytoin, phenobarbital, isoniazid, and lithium.

4. What topical agents are effective therapies for acne vulgaris?

Topical retinoids (e.g., tretinoin) should be considered first-line therapy for most forms of acne, both comedonal and inflammatory. Retinoids normalize desquamation of the follicular epithelium, thus preventing the development of the microcomedo. Tretinoin also increases the penetration of other topical agents, such as antimicrobials. Therefore, combination therapy enhances efficacy in most patients. Benzoyl peroxide, erythromycin, and clindamycin are all effective antibacterial and anti-inflammatory agents. The addition of benzoyl peroxide to either clindamycin or erythromycin helps diminish antibiotic resistance and resultant treatment failure.

5. What are the indications for oral antibiotics?

Oral antibiotics decrease the number of *Propionibacterium acnes* in the pilosebaceous units, thereby reducing inflammation. The use of systemic antibiotics depends both on the severity of inflammation and the extent of skin involvement. Acne that is moderate to severe and refractory to topical antibiotics or acne involving the chest, shoulders, or back may benefit from oral antibiotic therapy.

6. Describe a typical treatment regimen using oral antibiotics for acne.

Common choices for oral antibiotics include tetracycline, minocycline, and doxycycline. Average daily doses are 500–1000 mg for tetracycline and 50–200 mg for doxycycline or minocycline, often given in divided doses. The initial dose may be continued for 4–6 weeks. After new lesions are no longer developing, the dose may be tapered to once-daily dosing.

7. Which acne therapeutics are safe and which are contraindicated during pregnancy and nursing?

Topical erythromycin, clindamycin, azelaic acid, and salicylic acid are all pregnancy category B. Topical retinoids and benzoyl peroxide are pregnancy category C and have an associated risk. Tazarotene (a new topical retinoid) and oral isotretinoin are absolutely contraindicated in pregnancy.

8. Name and describe a life-threatening variant of acne.

Acne fulminans is a rare variant characterized by the sudden onset of large, tender ulcerating lesions on the chest and back of patients (especially young men) with preexisting inflammatory acne. Fever and leukocytosis occur and are often associated with polyarthralgia and osteolysis. A transient glomerulonephritis may ensue. The prompt initiation of systemic glucosteroids is imperative.

9. When should isotretinoin (Accutane) be used?

Isotretinoin is indicated for severe nodulocystic acne or inflammatory acne that is refractory to standard therapy. Newer practice also supports the initiation of Accutane in the presence of both physical and psychological scarring related to the disease. Because of potential severe side effects, patient reliability is important. Doses usually range from 0.5–1.0 mg/kg/day with doses up to 2.0 mg/kg/day for severe truncal involvement. Therapy should be continued for 15–20 weeks and discontinued after 70–80% improvement is achieved. The greatest chance for remission is with a cumulative dose of 120–150 mg/kg. Monthly visits with close monitoring of side effects, response, and blood work are usually necessary.

10. What are the most common side effects of isotretinoin therapy?

Cheilitis occurs in almost every case. Other side effects include dry mouth, xerosis, conjunctivitis, vertebral hyperostoses, elevated serum lipids, pseudotumor cerebri, and hepatic toxicity. The most important side effect is severe fetal malformation.

11. What precautions should be taken before prescribing isotretinoin to women of child-bearing age?

Women of childbearing age should receive isotretinoin only after reading the educational material provided by the manufacturer and giving informed consent because it has been associated with a 25-fold increase in the risk of severe fetal abnormalities. Women of childbearing age should use two reliable methods of birth control simultaneously and continuously, starting at least 1 month before initiation of therapy. Two negative serum pregnancy test results should be obtained before initiating therapy. Monthly contraception counseling and pregnancy testing are recommended. Conception is generally considered safe 1 month plus one menstrual cycle after completing isotretinoin therapy.

BIBLIOGRAPHY

1. Bershad SV: The modern age of acne therapy: A review of current treatment options. Mt Sinai J Med 68:279–286, 2001.
2. Berson DS, Shalita AR: The treatment of acne: The role of combination therapies. J Am Acad Dermatol 32:S31–S41, 1995.
3. Ellis CN, Drach KJ: Uses and complications of isotretinoin therapy. J Am Acad Dermatol 45:S150–S157, 2001.
4. Freedberg IM, Eisen AZ, Wolff K, et al (eds): Fitzpatrick's Dermatology in General Medicine, 6th ed. New York, McGraw-Hill, 2003.
5. Leyden JJ: Therapy for acne vulgaris. N Engl J Med 336:1156–1162, 1997.
6. Phillips TJ, Dover JS: Recent advances in dermatology. N Engl J Med 326:167–178, 1992.
7. Webster GF: Inflammatory acne. Int J Dermatol 29:313–317, 1990.
8. Webster GF: Topical tretinoin in acne therapy. J Am Acad Dermatol 39:S38–S44, 1998.

98. DISORDERS OF THE NAILS AND HAIR

Gina A. Taylor, M.D.

1. How does fungal infection of the nail present?

Fungal infection of the nail, also referred to as *onychomycosis,* can be caused by dermato-phyte organisms (the infection can then be called *tinea unguium*) or nondermatophytes. Most commonly, the causative organisms are the dermatophytes *Trichophyton rubrum, Trichophyton mentagrophytes,* and *Epidermophyton floccosum.* The three patterns of presentation are:

- Distal or lateral subungual onychomycosis (the most common presentation) with distal or lateral onycholysis, yellow discoloration, and subungual hyperkeratosis
- White superficial onychomycosis where the entire nail plate is whitened and brittle
- Proximal subungual onychomycosis (almost exclusive to immunocompromised hosts) with discoloration and separation of the nail plate at the proximal nail fold

Concomitant tinea pedis or tinea manuum is common. As a general rule, the feet and toenails should be examined when a patient presents with a rash of the hands or fingernails.

2. When is treatment of onychomycosis indicated?

Onychomycosis most commonly has cosmetic sequelae, but thickened nails can be painful and disabling. Treatment with griseofulvin and ketoconazole is common but results in high fail-ure and recurrence rates. New systemic antifungals (itraconazole, tertinadine) are more effective and safer to use. A positive fungal culture of nail keratin or a positive fungal stain of nail clip-pings is necessary before committing the patient to prolonged therapy because many other con-ditions may mimic onychomycoses. Topical therapy for fungal infection of nails or hair is inef-fective. Onychomycosis can have serious complications such as cellulitis, especially in patients with concomitant diabetes mellitus or in patients who are immunocompromised. Therefore, the treatment of onychomycosis in these situations is strongly indicated.

3. What diseases are associated with pitting of the nail bed?

Psoriasis causes large, deep, and irregularly scattered punctate depressions (or pits) on the surface of the nail plate due to involvement of nail matrix. Other nail plate abnormalities seen in psoriasis include discoloration, thickening, and distal onycholysis. Eczema of the posterior nail fold skin may also cause pitting or irregularity of the nail plate. Nail abnormalities are associated with alopecia areata, a form of patchy nonscarring hair loss, in which there may be regularly dis-tributed, geometric nail pitting and trachyonychia (twenty nail dystrophy).

4. What do Beau's lines signify?

Beau's lines are transverse grooves of the surface of the nail plate that result from a tempo-rary disruption in the mitotic activity of the nail matrix. Beau's lines are most commonly caused by mechanical injury or dermatologic diseases of the proximal nail fold. The presence of Beau's lines at the same level in all nails indicates acute systemic illness (e.g., systemic infection, thyro-toxicosis, or drug reaction). The distance of the Beau's lines from the proximal nail fold may date the patient's illness; nails grow at a rate of approximately 1 mm per month.

5. What does longitudinal melanonychia indicate?

Longitudinal melanonychia are longitudinal bands of melanin pigment in the nail plate. They vary in color from light-brown to black, and they vary in width from a few millimeters to the en-tire nail plate. They are commonly seen in individuals with darkly pigmented skin and are much less comon in white patients. Longitudinal melanonychia (or melanonychia striata) may be caused by activation of nail matrix melanocytes, melanocytic nevus of the nail matrix, or nail matrix melanoma. When evaluating melanonychia striata, an important sign to look for is Hutchinson's sign: brown-black periungual hyperpigmentation. In the setting of nail matrix melanoma, Hutchinson's sign represents horizontal growth of the tumor.

6. When a patient is diagnosed with alopecia, what key distinctions should be made about the type of alopecia?
  1. Whether the alopecia is scarring or nonscarring
  2. Whether the alopecia is patchy or diffuse

7. What are the common causes of scarring and nonscarring alopecia?
  In **nonscarring alopecia,** the skin appears and feels normal. Examination of the skin in patients with scarring alopecia reveals atrophy, lack of visible follicular openings, and often erythema and hyperpigmentation or hypopigmentation. Causes of nonscarring alopecia include alopecia areata, androgenic alopecia (male- and female-pattern baldness), and telogen effluvium (hair loss often seen in women 2–3 months after childbirth). Examples of **scarring alopecia** include discoid lupus erythematosus, lichen planopilaris (a form of follicular lichen planus), acne keloidalis nuchae, folliculitis decalvans, dissecting cellulitis of the scalp, and central centrifugal alopecia.

8. Name the common causes of patchy alopecia.
  1. **Alopecia areata,** which is postulated to be an organ-specific autoimmune disease, shows well-circumscribed, round or oval areas of nonscarring hair loss.
  2. **Trichotillomania,** which may be difficult to distinguish from alopecia areata, often occurs in children and adolescents and presents as patchy, usually nonscarring hair loss. However, careful examination of the patch of hair loss reveals broken hairs of variable length and, often, superficial excoriations and areas of scale. In addition to the scalp, eyebrows and eyelashes are commonly involved. Invariably, the patient denies pulling out the hair.
  3. **Discoid lupus erythematosus** of the scalp is a form of patchy, scarring hair loss. A round or disk-like area typically shows central hypopigmentation and atrophy with a violaceous or hyperpigmented active margin. The surface is scaly, and hair follicles often are plugged with keratin, resembling the open comedones seen in acne.
  4. **Secondary syphilis** may also cause a patchy alopecia, although it is less common. The classic presentation is a nonscarring alopecia with a "moth-eaten" appearance of the scalp hair. Other signs of secondary syphilis may or may not be present. A positive serologic test for syphilis confirms the diagnosis.

9. What causes alopecia at the periphery of the scalp?
  Occasionally, alopecia primarily involves the periphery of the scalp in the areas of the temples and above the ears. This form of alopecia usually occurs in women and is almost always secondary to traction, such as ponytails, braids, tight hair extensions, or tight hair curlers, and can eventually lead to scarring.

10. Which systemic illnesses may result in diffuse alopecia?
  Telogen effluvium (telogen defluvium) is the term given to the diffuse alopecia that results when many scalp follicles suddenly enter a resting phase, leading to fall-out of hair shafts from the roots. Typically, this change occurs 2–4 months after an acute severe illness, high fever, major surgery, childbirth, or other major life event. The skin appears normal and nonscarred. Patients can be assured that the process is self-limited and the hair will grow back, although regrowth may take several months. Hair grows at an average rate of 0.3 mm/day or 1 cm/month.

11. What nutritional deficiencies may contribute to hair loss?
  Biotin, iron, protein, and zinc.

12. Characterize androgenetic alopecia.
  Androgenic alopecia (male- and female-pattern baldness) is usually classified as diffuse, nonscarring alopecia, although hair loss is accentuated in the areas of the temples and crown. The

thickness of hair behind the ears usually appears normal. Most patients have a family history of first-degree relatives with significant androgenic alopecia. On rare occasions, alopecia areata may present as diffuse alopecia.

BIBLIOGRAPHY

1. Abdel-Rahman SM, Nahata MC: Oral terbinafine: A new antifungal agent. Ann Pharm 31:445–456, 1997.
2. Bolognia JL, Jorizzo JL, Rapini RP (eds): Dermatology. St. Louis, Mosby, 2003.
3. Freedberg IM, Eisen AZ, Wolff K, et al (eds): Fitzpatrick's Dermatology in General Medicine, 6th ed. New York, McGraw-Hill, 2003.
4. Hull PR: Onychomycosis—treatment, relapse, and re-infection. Dermatology 194(suppl I):7–9, 1997.

99. DERMATOLOGIC MANIFESTATIONS OF SYSTEMIC DISEASES

Jeanette Mladenovic, M.D., and Meg A. Lemon, M.D.

1. What conditions should be considered when a patient complains of pruritus yet no rash is present?

Chronic renal disease. Up to 80% of patients undergoing hemodialysis have pruritus. The cause is unclear, and pruritus has no clear relationship to renal function tests. Patients undergoing dialysis have an increased number of intradermal mast cells and increased pruritus in response to histamine injection. Treatment with antihistamines is usually ineffective. A recent study demonstrated a marked improvement of pruritus in patients treated with erythropoietin. In some patients with secondary hyperparathyroidism, the pruritus may resolve after parathyroidectomy. Therapy with oral psoralens and long-wave ultraviolet light (PUVA) has been effective in some patients with pruritus related to renal failure, possibly through an effect on cutaneous mast cells.

Cholestatic liver disease. Although itching is correlated with increased levels of unconjugated bilirubin, the amount of pruritus is not. Biliary drainage or treatment with bile salt binders (colestipol or cholestyramine) often improves the pruritus.

Endocrine diseases. Thyrotoxicosis may present with generalized itching. Pruritus in hypothyroidism is probably related to dryness of the skin. Diabetes mellitus is usually not a cause of itching, although it may be associated with candidiasis or folliculitis.

Malignancy. With the exception of Hodgkin's lymphoma and polycythemia vera (PV), malignancies rarely cause significant pruritus. One study of 360 patients with Hodgkin's lymphoma found that 5.8% presented with generalized pruritus. "Bath itch" is a diffuse prickling sensation that occurs 30–60 minutes after a bath or shower in 50% of patients with PV. The occurrence of pruritus may precede the development of PV by several years.

Senescence. Itching occurs in many older patients. Most cases are not associated with systemic disease and are believed to be related to dry skin. The mainstay of treatment is hydration of the skin with water and moisturizing creams and avoidance of drying soaps.

Psychogenic disorders. Generalized or localized pruritus (commonly anogenital) may be a manifestation of anxiety. The diagnosis is made after primary skin diseases and systemic disorders are excluded. Extensive excoriation may produce areas of neurodermatitis. Patients with severe psychiatric illnesses may present with parasitophobia manifested by the sensation of worms crawling on or under the skin.

2. Describe the evaluation of patients who have pruritus without rash.

The history should focus on medications, underlying diseases, and dry skin. The physical examination should evaluate for adenopathy and organomegaly. Screening laboratory tests may include complete blood count; chest radiograph; and liver, renal, and thyroid function tests. Patients who have pruritus without a rash should be followed for evaluation of symptoms. Therapy is based on treatment of the underlying disorder. In idiopathic cases, a trial of emollients and oral antihistamines, such as hydroxyzine hydrochloride, is indicated.

3. Why is it important to distinguish palpable purpura from purpuric lesions?

Palpable purpura is always a manifestation of systemic disease. Purpuric lesions may result from abnormalities in the clotting system or, less commonly, isolated dermatologic conditions (e.g., solar purpura, Schamberg's purpura).

4. What types of diseases should be considered in patients with palpable purpura?

Palpable purpura results from vasculitis or embolic disease. Lesions caused by vasculitis are seen in patients with polyarteritis nodosa and leukocytoclastic vasculitis. Embolic diseases include meningococcemia, disseminated gonococcemia, ecthyma gangrenosum (caused by *Pseudomonas* species or other gram-negative organisms), and Rocky Mountain spotted fever. Leukocytoclastic vasculitis is strongly associated with hepatitis C virus infection.

5. Describe livido reticularis. In what conditions is it seen?

As the name suggests, livido reticularis refers to a lacy, reddish-brown pattern that develops on the extremities, often in cold temperatures. It may be seen in patients with lupus erythematosus, the antiphospholipid syndrome, polyarteritis nodosa, or essential thrombocythemia. Livido reticularis of the lower extremities may be seen after manipulation of the large or renal vessels (i.e., angiography). Progression to ischemic ulceration caused by vascular occlusion may be seen.

6. Describe erythema nodosum.

Erythema nodosum presents as red subcutaneous nodules, most commonly on the shins. The nodules become bluish as they resolve. Erythema nodosum is often idiopathic; however, the most common systemic associations are streptococcal infection, sarcoidosis, inflammatory bowel disease, and (less commonly) fungal infections (e.g., coccidioidomycosis, tuberculosis, histoplasmosis) and drug toxicity.

7. What is the significance of acanthosis nigricans?

Acanthosis nigricans is an acquired velvety hyperpigmentation in the axilla and groin. It is most often associated with obesity, although it may be associated with other endocrinopathies as well as malignancy, usually of the gastrointestinal tract. Thus, in patients with idiopathic onset and no clearly ascribable cause, a search for malignancy (with attention to appropriate screening for age) should be considered.

8. What does vitiligo imply?

Patients with vitiligo have an increased incidence of autoimmune disorders, especially hypothyroidism, Graves' disease, and pernicious anemia. Less frequently, a variant of melanoma may present with truncal vitiligo.

9. What systemic diseases should be considered in patients with nonhealing ulcers?

In addition to evident vascular diseases (arterial insufficiency of any cause, microvascular disease of diabetes, venous insufficiency), nonhealing ulcers may be associated with (1) local malignancy, (2) hemoglobinopathies and blood dyscrasias (spherocytosis, cryoglobulin), (3) pyoderma gangrenosum (although the appearance of this entity is characteristic), and (4) vasculitis (rheumatoid vasculitis, Raynaud's phenomenon, Behçet's disease).

10. What diseases are characterized by photosensitivity reactions?

A number of skin diseases, lupus erythematosus, and dermatomyositis are aggravated by the sun. However, true acquired photosensitivity reactions evidenced by erythema, fragility, telangiectasias, recurrent blistering, bullae, and desquamation in sun-exposed areas is limited to a short differential diagnosis: drug sensitization (both topical and systemically administered), porphyria cutanea tarda, and, on rare occasions, acquired metabolic defects. Photoallergy differs in that an eczematous picture develops, again most commonly in response to drug sensitization.

11. What disorder is associated with yellow plaques surrounded by erythematous halos on extensor surfaces of the extremities?

Such lesions may represent xanthomata, which are associated with lipid disorders such as hypertriglyceridemia. Common xanthelasma of the eyelids is usually *not* associated with defects in lipid metabolism or cardiovascular disease.

12. A young woman presents with a recurrent papulovesicular rash over the extensor surfaces of her extremities and occasionally notices similar lesions on her abdomen. What disease is she likely to have in association with this rash?

This is a classic description of dermatitis herpetiformis. It is now known that a very high percentage (up to 85%) of individuals with dermatitis herpetiformis have underlying, often asymptomatic, celiac disease. The diagnosis is supported by the presence of tissue transglutimase antibodies (anti-tTg antibodies) in the serum or by finding granular IgA deposits along the subepidermal basement membrane upon skin biopsy. These lesions frequently respond to a gluten-free diet.

13. What skin diseases should trigger a screen for hepatitis C virus (HCV)?

- Porphyria cutanea tarda
- Lichen planus
- Leukocytoclastic vasculitis (seen as palpable purpura, likely caused by the essential mixed cryoglobulinemia of hepatitis C)

Although these entities are uncommon, when found, they have a high association with the presence of anti-HCV antibodies.

BIBLIOGRAPHY

1. Cacoub P, Renou C, Rosenthal E, et al: Extrahepatic manifestations associate with hepatitis C virus infection: A prospective multicenter study of 321 patients. The GERMKIVIC. Medicine 79:47–56, 2000.
2. Freedberg I, Eisen A, Wolff K, et al (eds): Fitzpatrick's Dermatology in General Medicine, 6th ed. New York, McGraw-Hill, 2003.
3. Sontheimer R, Provost T (eds): Cutaneous Manifestations of Rheumatic Diseases. Philadelphia, Lippincott, Williams & Wilkins, 1996.

XIV. Care of Special Patients

---

100. THE ADOLESCENT PATIENT

Roberta K. Beach, M.D., M.P.H.

---

1. What is special about adolescence?

Adolescence is a time of dramatic physical and developmental changes that challenge the coping skills of adolescents, families, health professionals, and communities to a greater degree than any other age. For convenience, the age range of 13–19 years is often specified as adolescence, but this transitional phase between childhood and adulthood lasts for more than a decade, beginning around age 10 years and extending through age 21 years or later. Dynamic changes in three areas are of special interest:

1. **Physical changes.** The growth spurt, development of adult body physique, hormonal changes, sexual development, and the ability to reproduce come with puberty, although there is marked variation in the timing and progression of physical growth.

2. **Psychosocial (developmental) changes.** Essential tasks of adolescence include emancipation from family, development of peer relationships and sexual intimacy, determination of educational and vocational goals, and establishment of identity and self-responsibility. Major social milestones are achieved. The legal rights to drive, vote, and drink and cultural rites of passage such as leaving school, leaving home, first sexual relationship, and first job have immense social significance to adolescents.

3. **Cognitive changes.** Adolescents progress from concrete operational thinking ("here and now") to abstract operational thinking with a maturing ability to engage in deductive reasoning, understand risks and benefits, and appreciate future consequences of current choices.

2. Characterize the adolescent personality.

Although adolescents are frequently portrayed as hostile, rebellious, and alienated, they actually have many positive attributes. Adolescents are intensely idealistic and often have a passion for fairness and social justice. They are energetic and enjoy peak physical health. They tend to be optimistic about the future and excited about dreams, plans, and goals. They have a tremendous resilience and capacity for growth, and even serious problems can be converted into learning experiences and opportunities for change. The majority (about 80%) of adolescents progress through this stage of life with only modest difficulty and without serious social problems.

3. How do I get an adolescent patient to talk to me?

Although caregivers often consider them difficult to interview, adolescents are actually eager to find someone "safe" to talk to about their concerns. Because they often believe that "no one understands me," they are highly sensitive to disapproval or being judged negatively. Several techniques help to establish a sense of trust that promotes the therapeutic alliance:

- **Privacy.** Interview the adolescent alone and with full attention in a setting free of interruptions.
- **Confidentiality.** Clarify the policy on confidentiality and assure patients that nothing will be shared without permission unless it is life-threatening (e.g., a suicide attempt) or legally mandated (e.g., child abuse).

- **Listening skills.** Listen much more than you talk; interrupt rarely; do not lecture; and pay attention to body language, both yours and the patient's.
- **Nonjudgmental approach.** Avoid assumptions, respect differences, and show genuine interest.
- **Open-ended questions.** Use open-ended, nonthreatening questions early in the interview ("Tell me what a typical day in your life is like.").
- **Third-person examples.** Lead into sensitive questions by using third-person examples ("Have any of your friends experimented with drugs?").
- **Direct questions.** After rapport is established, ask direct questions for specific information ("Have you had sex in the past 3 months? Do you think you could be pregnant?").
- **Hidden agenda.** Although the chief complaint is the entrée to care, an underlying concern frequently motivates the visit. Hidden agendas often relate to sexual concerns.
- **Reflective listening.** If the adolescent is unwilling to talk, reflective listening techniques are the most helpful approach ("You seem very sad," "You said you hate being here. . . . Hate?"). Wait patiently for answers.
- **Positive reinforcement.** Adolescents are hungry for honest praise and support ("It took a lot of courage for you to talk about this. Thank you.").

4. What are the three developmental stages of adolescence?

Psychosocial development is a dynamic process that continues throughout the lifespan. Adolescence is commonly divided into three developmental stages: **early** (11–14 years), **middle** (15–17 years), and **late** (18–21 years). Age ranges are approximate, and girls tend to progress through the stages earlier than boys. At each stage, characteristic changes take place in cognitive thinking, behaviors, typical health concerns, and the most effective caregiver approach to the patient. Behavioral issues are usually subdivided into the four task areas: family, peers, school and vocation, and self-perception and identity. The following table briefly summarizes the characteristics of each stage.

Adolescent Developmental Stages

	EARLY ADOLESCENCE (11–14 YEARS)	MIDDLE ADOLESCENCE (15–17 YEARS)	LATE ADOLESCENCE (18–24 YEARS)
Cognitive thinking	Concrete thinking: here and now Appreciate immediate reactions to behavior but no sense of later consequences	Early abstract thinking: inductive/deductive reasoning; ability to connect separate events; understand later consequences	Abstract thinking: adult ability to think abstractly; philosophical; intense idealism about love, religion, social problems
Psychosocial task areas			
1. Family—independence	Transition from obedient to rebellious Ambivalence about wishes (dependence vs. independence) Hero worship of adults	Insistence on independence, privacy May have overt rebellion or sulky withdrawal Much testing of limits	Emancipation (leave home) Reestablishment of family ties Become legally responsible for care
2. Peers—social and sexual	Same-sex "best friend" "Am I normal?" concerns Sexual intercourse not normal at this age; indicates family dysfunction	Dating Sexual experimentation Risk-taking actions Need to please significant peers (of either sex)	Partner selection (serial monogamy) Mature friendships True intimacy possible only after own identity is established
3. School—vocation	Middle school Need structured setting Goals unrealistic and changing	High school Need choices, electives, more flexibility	Full-time work or college Identify realistic career goals

Table continued on following page.

Adolescent Developmental Stages *(Continued)*

	EARLY ADOLESCENCE (11–14 YEARS)	MIDDLE ADOLESCENCE (15–17 YEARS)	LATE ADOLESCENCE (18–24 YEARS)
	Want to copy favorite role model	Beginning to identify skills, interests Start part-time jobs	Watch for apathy (no future plans) or alienation; correlated with negative outcomes, such as unplanned pregnancy or juvenile crime
4. Self-perception— identity	Poor self-image Losing child's role but do not have adult role; hence, low self-esteem Tend to use denial ("it can't happen to me")	Confusion about self-image Seek group identity Very narcissistic Impulsive, impatient	Realistic, positive self-image Able to consider others' needs, less narcissistic Able to reject group pressure if not in self-interest
5. Values	Stage II values (back scratching): good behavior in exchange for rewards	Stage III values (conformity): behavior that peer group values	Stage IV values (social responsibility): behavior consistent with laws and duty
Chief health issues (other than acute illness)	Psychosomatic symptoms Fatigue and "growing pains" Concerns about normalcy Screening for growth and development problems	Outcomes of sexual experimentation (prevention and pregnancy, STDs, AIDS) Health-risk behaviors (smoking, drugs, alcohol, driving) Crisis counseling (e.g., runaways, acting out, family problems)	Health promotion/ healthy lifestyle Contraception and STD/AIDs prevention Self-responsibility for health and health care Transition to adult care settings
Professional approach	Firm, direct support Convey limits— simple concrete choices Do *not* align with parents but be an objective, caring *adult* Encourage parental presence in clinic but interview adolescent alone	Be an objective sounding board (but let them solve own problems) Negotiate choices Ensure confidentiality Adapt system to walk-ins, impulsiveness, testing of limits	Allow mature participation in decisions Act as a resource Idealistic stage, convey professional image Can expect patient to examine underlying wishes and motives regarding behavior

5. What are the stages of physical growth?

Compared with the complexities of psychosocial development, physical development during adolescence tends to be orderly and straightforward. Growth is divided into five stages from pre-pubertal to adult. Originally called Tanner stages after John Tanner's classic descriptions, they are now referred to as sexual maturing ratings (SMR) 1 through 5. The onset of puberty is highly variable, but in girls, it normally begins between ages 8 and 14 years and in boys, between ages 9 and 16 years. Physical growth continues for 5–6 years until adult stature is achieved.

In girls, the progression usually begins with breast budding at **thelarche** (SMR 2), followed by pubic hair at **pubarche** (SMR 3), first menses at **menarche** (SMR 4), and completion of pubic hair and breast growth (SMR 5). The average age of menarche in American girls is 12.3 years. The peak female growth spurt occurs immediately before menarche (SMR 2–3). Bone epiphyses close approximately 2 years after menarche, and growth is completed.

In boys, the progressions begins with early enlargement of the testes (SMR 2), followed by growth of pubic hair (SMR 3), penile growth (SMR 3–4), peak growth spurt (SMR 3–4), and facial hair and completion of genital and pubic hair growth (SMR 5). The average age of first nocturnal emission (wet dream) in boys is 13–14 years. In both boys and girls, pubic hair extends onto the thighs during SMR 5 and heralds the completion of physical growth.

6. When is puberty considered precocious?

Sexual precocity is the appearance of sexual maturation before age 8 years in girls and age 9 years in boys. Pubertal development that is out of phase with peers is a cause of great concern to early adolescents. Whereas early pubertal development (too soon) is usually a concern of girls, delayed pubertal development (too late) is typically a concern of boys.

Breast budding in girls is normal from age 8 years. It may be unilateral at first, causing concern about a "breast tumor." However, a breast bud should *never* be biopsied (removal destroys future breast growth). Breast growth prior to age 6 is considered precocious and between ages 6 and 8 requires consideration of early puberty. Menarche may occur as early as age 9 or 10 years, especially in overnourished girls. Complete puberty in girls before the age of 8 years is termed **precocious puberty** and is caused by the presence of gonadotropins and sex hormones (estrogens and androgens). The differential diagnosis includes hormone-secreting tumors (brain, liver, adrenal gland, ovary); exogenous administration of estrogen, anabolic steroids, or androgens; and hypothyroidism, neurofibromatosis, congenital adrenal hyperplasia, and other rare disorders. Virilization of a young girl indicates an endocrine disorder.

7. When should delayed puberty be evaluated?

If there are no signs of puberty by age 16 years, delayed puberty should be evaluated. The most common causes of delayed puberty include familial short stature, constitutional growth delay, and chronic illness. A rare cause is gonadal failure (Kallmann syndrome) in which hypogonadotrophic hypogonadism results in permanent absence of pubertal development. Boys with genetic short stature tend to grow at a rate below but parallel to the third percentile throughout childhood and adolescence. They often begin puberty at the same time as their peers. They will always be short. In constitutional growth delay, the onset of puberty is delayed, but the patient eventually catches up in growth. Growth hormone deficiency should be considered if height is 3–4 standard deviations below the mean. In delayed puberty, the most important aspects of evaluation are the family history, past growth pattern, SMR stage, medical history, bone age radiographs, and measurement of 8 A.M. serum testosterone in boys or serum follicle-stimulating hormone in girls. Growth hormone deficiency is treatable.

8. Which chronic illnesses are responsible for delayed puberty?

Chronic illnesses that may delay puberty include severe asthma and other pulmonary disorders, renal disease, cardiac disorders, and inflammatory bowel disease.

9. What are the primary health issues of adolescents?

Major morbidity and mortality during adolescence relate to risk-taking behaviors and experimentation. Health concerns result from complex behavioral decisions and include pregnancy, substance abuse, sexually transmitted diseases (STDs), infection with human immunodeficiency virus (HIV), depression, suicide, violence, and motor vehicle injuries.

10. What are some ways to screen for adolescent substance abuse?

Primary caregivers should routinely screen adolescents for alcohol and other drug use. Studies show that 90% of high-school students have tried alcohol and 50% of students have used illicit drugs. Adolescent substance use occurs along a continuum, ranging from **experimental use** (a normal developmental variation) to **regular use** (often in a social context), **problematic use** (resulting in negative consequences), **substance abuse** (loss of control and continued use despite harm), and **addiction** (physiologic and psychological dependency). Interventions are most effective if adolescents who are risk of developing a substance abuse disorder can be identified during the first three stages. Four questions have good ability to predict which adolescents may be at risk are:

1. Do you smoke cigarettes?

2. Have you ever been suspended from school?

3. Has anyone (parent, teacher, friend) ever thought you had a problem with alcohol or drugs?

4. Have you ridden in a car driven by someone (including yourself) who had been using alcohol or drugs?

Adolescents at high risk also include those whose closest friends drink or use drugs or who have a close family member who has a problem with alcohol or drugs.

One of the most useful tools to screen for serious drug and alcohol problems is the **CAGE** series of questions validated in adults and modified for adolescents:

C = Have you ever felt the need to **cut down** on your use of alcohol or drugs?

A = Have you ever gotten **annoyed** by someone's criticism of your alcohol or drug use?

G = Do you ever feel **guilty** or bad about your alcohol or drug use?

E = Do you ever need an **eye-opener,** a drink or drinks in the morning before you go to school?

Two or more "yes" answers have a high degree of sensitivity and specificity in diagnosing substance abuse or dependency.

11. Which adolescents are at risk of suicide?

Suicide is the third leading cause of death among adolescents, exceeded only by motor vehicle accidents and homicide. Adolescent suicide rates have doubled in the past 25 years, and national studies indicate that 6% of boys and 19% of girls have attempted suicide. Suicide attempts have been found to be associated with depression, substance use, overall number of life stressors, gender, and impulsive behaviors. Clinicians should recognize that adolescents at risk of suicide often have a cluster of other health risk behaviors, including lack of seat belt use, physical fighting and gun carrying, tobacco use, and illicit substance use. A history of suicide in a close family member is another high-risk factor. The single biggest risk factor in the medical history is a previous suicide attempt.

Over one half of adolescents who attempt suicide make contact with a physician in the month preceding their attempt. Although no brief screening questionnaires have been validated to be highly predictive for suicide risk, two questions are widely recommended for office use:

1. Have you felt sad or depressed for more than 3 days in a row (or much of the time)?

2. Have you thought of killing yourself in the past 3 months?

More subtle warning signs include a history of declining school performance, increasing family conflict, and persistent psychosomatic complaints. Recognizing a suicidal adolescent is difficult, but if risk factors and warning signs are present, prompt intervention is essential.

12. How do health supervision visits for adolescents differ from traditional health maintenance visits for adults?

Primary care providers should respond to the health consequences of risk-taking behavior by making preventive services a major component of the clinical approach to adolescents. The American Medical Association, in cooperation with the Centers for Disease Control and Prevention, published *Guidelines for Adolescent Preventive Services* (GAPS), a comprehensive set of recommendations that provide a framework for the organization and content of preventive health services. Similar guidelines have been developed by other national organizations. Health supervision visits for adolescents differ from traditional health maintenance visits in six ways:

1. The provider actively complements health guidance that adolescents receive from school, family, and community.

2. Preventive interventions target "new morbidities," such as alcohol, drugs, and sexual risk taking, rather than emphasize biomedical problems.

3. The provider screens for "comorbidities," which are clusters of risk-taking behaviors, rather than treats categorical health conditions.

4. Annual health supervision visits are recommended to provide anticipatory guidance and early intervention rather than episodic visits such as those for immunizations or sports examinations.

5. Comprehensive physical examinations are recommended at each of the three stages of de-

velopment: early, middle, and late adolescence. Sexually active adolescents need annual screening for STDs, including an annual Papanicolaou test in sexually active young women.

6. Parents of adolescents should receive specific counseling about parental concerns and adolescent needs at least twice during their child's adolescence.

13. What are the most important positive health behaviors to stress?

Primary caregivers have a critical role in ensuring that all adolescents are competent and motivated to make wise choices as they form lifelong habits. The Centers for Disease Control Division of Adolescent and School Health selected six priority health behaviors for youth based on risk factors that are a major source of morbidity and mortality, and are highly prevalent, modifiable, and measurable. Other areas of great concern for mortality, such as suicide and homicide, are difficult to reduce to a single achievable behavioral goal and therefore are not addressed in the six priority behaviors.

Priority Health Behaviors for Adolescents*

1. Use seat belts.	4. Do not smoke.
2. Do not drink (or use drugs) and drive.	5. Eat a low-fat diet.
3. If you have sex, use condoms.	6. Get regular aerobic exercise.

*These six golden rules are the most effective and achievable lifetime behaviors that will reduce years of potential life lost to the major killers: motor vehicle accidents, AIDS, cardiovascular disease, and cancer.

14. How can anticipatory guidance (office counseling) be given without lecturing?

Office counseling is most effective if it actively engages the adolescent in problem solving. Four steps are involved:

1. **Define the problem.** Ask the adolescent to describe the situation and any feelings or fears about it ("What if your pregnancy test were positive today?").

2. **Explore the options.** Ask the adolescent to describe some ways to solve the problem. The provider simply listens ("Tell me at least three choices you would have if you were pregnant."). Suggest other options if appropriate.

3. **Analyze the consequences.** Ask the adolescent to review the most likely positive and negative consequences of the best solutions considered ("What will be the best thing and the worst thing for you if you placed your baby for adoption?"). Then mention any major consequences or responsibilities overlooked by the adolescent.

4. **Develop an action plan.** Ask the adolescent to identify the specific steps to take after leaving your office. Include a plan for follow-up.

Remember that adolescents are not motivated by the long-term consequences; they are more concerned about immediate rewards and consequences and are particularly motivated by what gives them status and prestige in the eyes of their peers.

15. List the most common medical diagnoses for adolescent office visits.

Common causes of adolescent medical visits include acne, asthma, headache, abdominal pain, fatigue, and musculoskeletal pain.

16. List four common principles applicable to the care of adolescents with symptomatic complaints.

1. Adolescents may have excessive concerns about "Am I normal?" Therefore, they need large amounts of reassurance.

2. Adolescents often have underlying anxiety that they are to blame for the condition because of some behavior about which they feel guilty, such as experimenting with sex or drugs.

3. Adolescents may be very concerned about confidentiality and often want to obtain care independently without parental involvement.

4. Adolescents may need extra support to achieve compliance with treatment plans. They frequently test limits, act impulsively, and discontinue treatment in an effort to "be like everyone else."

In general, adolescents require extra time, more education, and closer follow-up than people of other age groups.

17. Where do adolescents go for health care?

Of adolescents who have seen a physician in the past 2 years, approximately one third see pediatricians, one third see family practice or internal medicine providers, and one third utilize local emergency departments. Adolescents have long been recognized as an underserved population who are particularly difficult to reach with health services. Issues of emancipation, independence, and a desire for confidential care create significant barriers for adolescents in the traditional health care system. In general, adolescents visit a health care provider less than once every 2 years, and those visits tend to be for episodic illness or emergency care. With 5 million uninsured adolescents in America, many have no regular source for health care. Even insured adolescents underutilize care. In one large study, upper middle-class adolescents who could identify a private physician stated that they would be unwilling to visit that physician for many sensitive concerns, such as sexuality or drug problems, for fear that their parents would find out.

18. Should adolescents receive health care without parental involvement?

Although parental involvement is generally beneficial and should be encouraged, the ability to provide confidential care to adolescents, with the minor's own consent, is essential to ensure access to health care. Consent and confidentiality are separate legal issues. *Consent* is a basic legal requirement for the provision of health care to patients of all ages. In general, minors under age 18 years require parental consent for medical treatment. However, because of the compelling interest of the state in encouraging adolescents to seek early health care for pregnancy, STDs, and substance abuse, courts and legislatures have created exceptions to parental consent that enable adolescents to obtain care independently for these health concerns. Numerous studies have shown that adolescents 14 years and older are as competent as adults to make informed choices about health care.

Confidentiality refers to maintaining privacy of medical information. Many adolescents are reluctant or completely unwilling to seek care without the assurance of confidentiality. Some require privacy as part of the normal process of developing autonomy; others may face hostile or abusive reactions from alienated or dysfunctional families if sensitive information is disclosed. Medical record information is usually not released without the patient's permission in accordance with the adolescent's legal right to privacy. The Health Insurance Portability and Accountability Act (HIPAA) of 1996 does not address adolescent confidentiality. Every state has specific statutes related to a minor's access to health care. Careful analysis of state legislation requiring parental notification shows no beneficial effect on family communication. Adolescents unwilling to share private information with parents tend to delay care, avoid care, seek clandestine care, or use judicial bypass mechanisms to access medical care under their own consent. The major documented effects of such legislation are delay in timely diagnosis and treatment and increased medical risk. Other studies demonstrate that many adolescents willingly involve their families (even if there is no legal requirement) if they believe that their families will be supportive and nonjudgmental. The most effective means for parents to ensure involvement in their adolescents' health care decisions is to establish open, trusting communication from early childhood on.

19. How can adolescent access to health care be improved?

1. **School-based and school-linked clinics.** At local, state, and national levels, implementation of school-based and school-linked health services is seen as one means to overcome barriers to care. Services range from professional telephone consultations with school-based personnel to comprehensive onsite health clinics that provide primary care, mental health services, social services, and other support. Advantages of school-based clinics include accessibility and affordability as well as greater access to preventive care and intervention.

2. **Increased caregiver training in adolescent medicine.** Training programs in pediatrics, family practice, internal medicine, and obstetrics and gynecology have recognized the need to provide specific training in adolescent medicine. Nurse practitioner and physician assistant train-

ing programs have likewise added adolescent medicine to curriculum components. Specialty board certification in adolescent medicine became available in 1994. Such efforts should increase the adolescent medicine skills of the next generation of health care providers.

3. **Expanded health care insurance through new health care delivery systems.** A cornerstone for improving the health of adolescents will be mechanisms to reimburse a wide range of providers and service settings for the time-consuming care that adolescents require. Inclusion in capitated health insurance programs and health maintenance organizations may improve access. "Safety-net" features for homeless, emancipated, out-of-school, unemployed, and other disenfranchised youth are essential.

20. When do adolescents become sexually active?

Middle-to-late adolescence has always been the average age for initiation of sexual intercourse. The age of sexual debut has become increasingly younger since the late 1960s, but in the past decade the proportion of youth reporting sex before age 13 has declined by 35% (from 10% in 1991 to 7% in 2001). The 2001 National Youth Risk Behavior Survey of students in grades 9–12 demonstrated a decrease in sexual activity, with 46% of students reporting they had ever had sex, compared to the 1995 report (53%). Rates increase steadily during high school, with 35% of 9th graders and 61% of 12th graders reporting sexual intercourse. The median age of first intercourse reported by students is now 17.2 years for females and 16.3 years for males. Intercourse is only one aspect of sexual activity. A recent study found that of adolescents who are virgins, one third reported that they had engaged in genital touching of a partner and one tenth had participated in oral-genital sex.

21. Why is there so much concern about adolescent sexuality?

The medical consequences of adolescent sexual activity are a national health concern. Although U.S. teenage pregnancy, birth, and abortion rates have declined steadily since 1991 due to improved contraceptive use and reduced sexual activity, approximately 750,000 teenage women still become pregnant annually, although only 300,000 of them are school-aged minors (age 17 years and younger). More than 3,000,000 cases of STDs occur in adolescents annually. It is estimated that the number of adolescents with HIV infection doubles every 14 months; AIDS is now the seventh leading cause of death in the 15- to 24-year-old age group.

22. Should primary care providers support contraceptive use?

Yes. Health promotion goals for adolescents include postponement of sexual activity until psychosocial maturity and consistent use of condoms and contraceptives by those who engage in sexual intercourse. Abstinence is highly effective in preventing pregnancies and STDs if used consistently and correctly; in actual practice, however, abstinence has a failure rate of 24% in teenaged couples attempting to use it for 1 year. The level of condom use by adolescents has tripled since 1979; over 60% report use of condoms with their last coitus. The actual pregnancy rate in sexually active adolescents has decreased 20% since 1991, reflecting an increased use of contraception. Long-acting contraceptive methods including Norplant and Depo-Provera helped account for the decreased pregnancy rate. Newer birth control preparations that are easier to use and may have fewer side effects are becoming available, including transdermal patches (Ortho Evra), a vaginal contraceptive ring (NuvaRing), new hormone formulations (Yasmin), and emergency contraception (EC) options. If the social environment is supportive, adolescents can be highly effective contraceptive users, as demonstrated in other Western countries. Caregivers should ensure that all adolescents receive anticipatory guidance about safer sex practices and have access to condoms and contraceptives when needed. Despite the perception of crisis, responsible sexual behavior by adolescents has increased.

23. Should "abstinence only" be the sexuality education message for adolescents?

Adolescent sexuality remains a highly controversial issue. During the past decade, the majority of professional health and educational organizations achieved consensus about the need for comprehensive sexuality education. Recently, there has been a surge in political advocacy by proponents of abstinence-only education, and since 1997, over $250 million dollars in federal and matching state funds have been awarded to educational programs teaching abstinence only. By definition, these programs must teach that abstinence from sexual activity outside marriage is the expected standard for all school-aged adolescents, that a mutually faithful monogamous relationship in the context of marriage is the expected standard for human sexual activity, and that sexual activity outside the context of marriage is likely to have harmful psychological and physical effects. The funded programs may not discuss contraception or condom use. Proponents of abstinence-only education argue that discussion of contraception and condoms sends an inappropriate mixed message to youths. They propose that if you firmly tell young people to abstain from sexual intercourse, they will. Proponents of abstinence-only programs often state that their own evaluations show that "just-say-no" programs are effective. At present, no published studies in the professional literature indicate that abstinence-only programs will result in a significant delay of intercourse.

Proponents of comprehensive sexuality education ("abstinence-plus") also support educational programs emphasizing that sexual abstinence is a desirable objective and the most effective method for preventing unintended pregnancy and STD and HIV infections. In addition, they advise young people who engage in intercourse to use contraception and condoms. Effective comprehensive sexual education programs also help to develop cognitive decision-making abilities and teach young people communication and conflict resolution skills to resist peer pressure. Multiple reviews conclude that programs most effective in changing young people's behavior are those that address abstinence plus contraception and STD prevention.

Young people need support for abstaining from premature sexual activity, but they also need affordable, sensitive, and confidential reproductive health services and life opportunities that offer them reasons not to become teenaged parents. Rather than being confused about mixed messages, health professionals, families, and communities may offer one very clear message: protect your health and your future—either by abstaining from sexual intercourse or by using effective contraception and condoms.

BIBLIOGRAPHY

1. American Medical Association: Guidelines for Adolescent Preventive Services (GAPS): Recommendations Monograph. Chicago, American Medical Association, 1997.
2. Borowsky IW, Ireland M, Resnick MD: Adolescent suicide attempts: Risks and protectors. Pediatrics 107:485–491, 2001.
3. Brener N, Lowry R, Kann L, et al: Trends in sexual risk behaviors among high school students—United States, 1991–2001. MMWR 51(38):856–859, 2002.
4. Darroch JE, Singh S, Frost JJ, et al: Differences in teenage pregnancy rates among five developed countries: The role of sexual activity and contraceptive use. Fam Planning Perspect 33:244–250, 2001.
5. Elster AB: Comparisons of recommendations for adolescent clinical preventive services developed by national organizations. Arch Pediatr Adolesc Med 152:195–199, 1998.
6. Ford CA, Millstein SG: Delivery of confidentiality assurances to adolescents by primary care physicians. Arch Pediatr Adolesc Med 151:505–509, 1997.
7. Friedman SB, Fisher M, Schonberg SK (eds): Comprehensive Adolescent Health Care, 2nd ed. St. Louis, Mosby, 1997.
8. Hofmann AD, Greydanus DE: Adolescent Medicine, 3rd ed. Norwalk, CT, Appleton & Lange, 1997.
9. Joffe AJ, Blythe MJ (eds): Handbook of Adolescent Medicine. Adolescent Medicine: State of the Art Reviews, vol. 14, no. 2. Philadelphia, Hanley & Belfus, 2003.
10. Kaplowitz PB, Oberfield SE: Reexamination of the age limit for defining when puberty is precocious in girls in the United States: Implications for evaluation and treatment. Pediatrics 104:936–941, 1999.
11. Klein JD, Wilson KM: Delivering quality care: Adolescents' discussions of health risks with their provider. J Adolesc Health 30:190–195, 2002.
12. Neinstein LS (ed): Adolescent Health Care: A Practical Guide, 4th ed. Philadelphia, Lippincott Williams & Wilkins, 2002.
13. Purcell JS, Hergenroeder AC, Kozinetz C, et al: Interviewing techniques with adolescents in primary care. J Adolesc Health 20:300–305, 1997.
14. Rimsza ME: Counseling the adolescent about contraception. Pediatr Rev 24:162–169, 2003.
15. Sarigiani PA, Ryan L, Petersen AC: Prevention of high-risk behaviors in adolescent women. J Adolesc Health Care 25:109–119, 1999.
16. Schainker E, Grant L: Medical home meets educational home: How you can make the most of school health services. Contemp Pediatr 20:55–81, 2003.

17. Schuster MA, Bell RM, Kanouse DE: The sexual practices of adolescent virgins: Genital sexual activities of high school students who have never had vaginal intercourse. Am J Public Health 86:1570–1576, 1996.
18. Styne DM: New aspects in the diagnosis and treatment of pubertal disorders. Pediatr Clin North Am 44:505–529, 1997.
19. Thrall JS, McCloskey L, Ettner SL, et al: Confidentiality and adolescents use of providers for health information and pelvic examinations. Arch Pediatr Adolesc Med 154:885–892, 2000

101. THE ELDERLY PATIENT

Edmund Bourke, M.D.

1. Explain what is meant by functional assessment.

A key distinguishing feature of the geriatric approach to patient evaluation is the emphasis on function in contradistinction to pathophysiology. Without intending to overstate the case, practitioners of eldercare focus more on how satisfactorily patients can manage their domestic, occupational, and social activities than on physiologic parameters that are emphasized more in younger age groups. The functional assessment addresses three areas: activities of daily living (ADLs), instrumental activities of daily living (IADLs), and mobility (gait and balance).

2. What are the ADLs and why are they important?

The five principal ADLs are (1) **bathing and grooming,** (2) **dressing,** (3) **transferring** (e.g., bed to chair), (4) **toileting,** and (5) **feeding.** These basic self-care tasks are considered essential to independent living. They tend to go in the order stated (younger patients recovering from coma tend to do so in the reverse order). A frequent first sign of deteriorating self-care is the body odor of deferred hygiene. An informant, preferably a caregiver, may be required to corroborate the level of function. Sensitivity on the part of the clinician helps establish trust in the face of defensiveness that may be induced by personal questions (e.g., who buttons the patient's shirt or deals with toileting issues).

Evaluating ADLs is important for three reasons. First, quality care including appropriate discharge planning requires the clinician's awareness of the patient's capacity for independent living. Second, it gets right down to what the caregiver is coping with and shows that the physician understands and cares. Third, familiarity with and concern for such practical matters facilitates team leadership in the interdisciplinary setting. The nurse is usually the team member best qualified to report on ADLs.

3. What are the IADLs, and why are they important?

The seven principal IADLs are (1) **paying the bills and writing the checks,** (2) **using the telephone,** (3) **shopping,** (4) **cooking,** (5) **housekeeping and laundry,** (6) **managing transportation,** and (7) **taking medications.** They are important for the same three reasons as the ADLs. With a little elaboration one can gain real insight into the patient's level of functioning. For example, if the patient does not pay the various bills, why not and for how long? Can the patient get to the shop, remember the various items he or she set out to buy, and arrive home with the correct change? Caregivers and other family members respond with enthusiasm to the physician who shows an awareness of the implications of shortcomings in these areas, and the whole discussion on future action plans for the patient becomes more open and focused. In the interdisciplinary team, the social worker frequently brings the most detailed insights to bear on the IADLs.

4. How is mobility evaluated in the elderly?

The timed Get Up and Go test. The patient is asked to stand from the seated position in a hard-backed chair keeping his or her arms folded; then, the patient should walk 10 feet, turn, return to the chair, turn again, and sit back down, all within 10 seconds. Increased time to completion indicates a deficit in mobility attributable to disorders of gait or balance. Gait and balance disturbances require attention to footwear and possible assistive devices such as a cane or walker.

5. Is protein calorie malnutrition common in the elderly? How is it recognized clinically?

Yes; 10–20% of elderly outpatients are malnourished. Concurrent medical illness; depression; inability to shop, cook, or feed oneself; and financial insufficiency are the major reasons. Aside from visual inspection, a body mass index below 20 kg/m^2 is a red alert.

6. What are the major causes of visual impairment in the elderly?

Refractive errors, cataracts, macular degeneration, glaucoma, and diabetic retinopathy. From age 65 years onward, visual impairment, defined as a visual acuity < 20/40, increases progressively. Blindness, defined as a visual acuity = 20/200, also increases with age, affecting 2% of those 75 years and older.

7. How common and how important are these causes of impaired vision?

Refractive errors affect the majority of geriatric patients, presbyopia being the characteristic defect.

Cataracts represent the world's most common cause of blindness, although it is not in the United States where access to surgery is generally available. Approximately 50% of Americans older than 75 years have a cataract. Extraction plus lens implantation is an ambulatory procedure. The main complication, delayed opacification of the posterior capsule, responds to YAG laser.

Macular degeneration is the most common cause of blindness in the developed world, with a prevalence of 20% by age 70. It is more common in fair-skinned people. The minority, who develop exudative lesions, risk loss of sight. Argon laser photocoagulation helps some.

Glaucoma is the second most common cause of blindness in the developed world and is the most common in African Americans. Primary open angle glaucoma is the most frequent variant. Increased intraocular pressure is no longer considered an essential criterion, although it remains a useful screening tool. Glaucoma is now defined by a characteristic optic nerve damage plus visual field defect. A variety of eye drops, including the prostaglandin analog latanoprost and the alpha$_2$-agonist brimonidine, are beneficial. Other pharmacologic and surgical approaches can be successful in more recalcitrant cases.

Diabetic retinopathy is the second most common cause of blindness in African Americans. Its severity can be significantly delayed by maintaining the hemoglobin A$_{1C}$ below 7% and the BP ≤ 140/80.

8. How prevalent and important is hearing impairment among the elderly?

It is under-reported either because patients take it for granted as a part of aging or because patients feel it is a social stigma. Ten percent of Americans between the ages of 65 and 75 years and 25% of Americans older than 75 years have hearing impairment. It is too often regarded as a relatively minor issue, but this is wrong. The prevalence of anger, depression, low self-esteem, social withdrawal, and otherwise a poor quality of life make it an important target for assessment.

9. What are the causes of hearing impairment, and how is it diagnosed?

If history taking leaves any doubt, a hand-held audioscope with a tone generator has a sensitivity and specificity of about 90%, respectively, in the primary care clinic. In the absence of excess wax, inability to hear 40 dB at 1000 and 2000 Hz indicates significant hearing impairment and the need for formal audiometry. Hearing loss is classified as conductive or sensorineural. **Conductive hearing loss** implies a defect in the external ear (e.g., cerumen) or middle ear (e.g., otosclerosis, perforated tympanic membrane, cholesteatoma). **Sensorineural hearing loss** is most often caused by cochlear disease including Meniere's disease. Less commonly, acoustic neuromas, ototoxic medications, and, rarely but importantly because it could be alleviated by surgery, Paget's disease all need to be considered. However, in the elderly, the majority of hearing loss is a sensorineural condition termed *presbycusis*, which is attributable to loss of cochlear hair cells and has a characteristic audiogram.

10. How does one evaluate a change in mental status in the elderly?

A change in mental status is one of the most important clinical scenarios that requires evaluation in the elderly. The three causes are, conveniently, the three D's: **d**ementia, **d**elirium, and **d**epression (or other psychiatric illness). The approach to a change in mental status is outlined in Chapter 74, Dementia. Also summarized in that chapter is Folstein's Mini-Mental Status Examination (MMSE), which has proved particularly useful in establishing a baseline from which to assess a change in cognitive function. The chapters on delirium and depression should also be consulted because, although all three D's are particularly germane to the assessment of the elderly patient, they require a chapter unto themselves for adequate coverage.

11. Why do elderly people fall?

Usually a combination of circumstances causes falls, but it is worth dissecting them because falls increase linearly with the number of risk factors, and many of the risk factors are correctible or modifiable. A reasonable approach is outlined as follows:
- Exclude or confirm a role for syncope or presyncope, which has its own diagnostic approach (see Chapter 40, Dizziness and Syncope).
- Review other potential intrinsic causes including falls occurring during the course of acute illness (e.g., pneumonia, influenza); cognitive defects with impaired judgment; sensory deprivation including correctible visual defects or proprioceptive disorders; disturbance of power, gait, or balance that could be helped by assistive devices such as a cane or walker; and "drop attacks."
- Consider a podiatric cause, which may be partly intrinsic but ill-fitting or wrong shoes or orthotics may play a role.
- Identify and, when possible, discontinue an iatrogenic factor. The most notable factor polypharmacy when four or more drugs are used. Also, an array of medications, such as anxiolytics, hypnotics, antidepressants, and neuroleptics, is a consideration.
- Correct or avoid extrinsic factors such as throw rugs, slippery floors, poor lighting, the absence of a rubber mat in the bathtub or shower, and clutter.

12. What are the consequences of falls in the elderly?

1. **Injuries,** including hip fractures and head injuries
2. **Psychological** consequences—fear of another fall may lead to decreased mobility or social withdrawal
3. **Social** consequences—falls may be a factor in the decision to institutionalize the patient

13. When should elder abuse be suspected?

A first step to identifying elder abuse is to change the term to *elder mistreatment,* because it widens the concept and identifies cases that would otherwise be overlooked. For instance, serious neglect is more common than physical abuse. Signs that raise suspicion of elder mistreatment are classifiable under four headings:
- Suspect **abandonment** if the patient is brought to the health care facility by someone other than the caregiver or is left at the facility by caregiver.
- **Abuse** should be considered when bruises, especially those that are bilateral or on inner surfaces of limbs and in various stages of healing, are seen. Fractures are also signs of abuse.
- **Exploitation** is suggested when unexplained loss of social security or pension checks occurs. Evidence of belongings being taken in exchange for care or without consent should also raise suspicions.
- Indications of **neglect** include poor hygiene, pressure ulcers, malnutrition, apathy, inappropriate dress, and the patient not getting medication.

14. What are the risk factors predisposing to elder mistreatment?

Risk factors for mistreatment included cognitive impairment in patient or caregiver, dependency of the caregiver on the patient, family discord, family history of substance abuse or psychiatric illness, and financial or psychological stress in the home. If the suspicion is confirmed, intervention becomes the responsibility of the health care team. It can be a complex responsibility and usually includes reporting to Adult Protective Services or other agencies mandated by state law.

15. How important is physical activity in the elderly?

An impressive body of evidence has accrued demonstrating that the level of physical activity is a major determinant of chronic disease burden including cardiovascular disease, hypertension, diabetes, obesity, osteoporosis, colon cancer, and fall-related injury. Physical activity level is also an important determinant of functional limitations, dependency, and mortality, both cardiovascular and noncardiovascular. The benefits of physical activity in terms of morbidity, mortality, quality of life, and reduction of health care costs are substantial.

16. Define adequate physical activity in the elderly.

There are small differences in definitions of moderate physical activity. A reasonable definition would be walking for 30 minutes at 3–4 mph on 5–7 days per week. For those who have walking limitations, a substitute activity that would expend a similar 150–200 kcal/day within the same time frame would suffice. Alternatively, several shorter (e.g., 10 minute) bouts of exercise within the day may substitute for the 30 minutes in patients where symptoms such as arthritis pain are a limiting factor. If properly planned, older adults can also achieve significant activity in performing some household chores or gardening. Some older patients prefer exercise classes. Monitoring pulse rate can be useful. Although the optimal level of physical activity is not established in the elderly, it is reasonable to exceed the moderate recommendations in those individuals who are fit to do so. Running in nonhabitual runners, however, is generally not recommended in the elderly.

17. What screening and preventive indices are recommended in the elderly?

Evidence-based Preventive Services Recommended for the General Population Aged 65 and Older

PREVENTIVE ACTIVITY	FREQUENCY (YEAR)	CONDITION TO DETECT OR PREVENT
Screening		
Blood pressure	≤ 1	Hypertension
Mammography	2–3	Breast cancer
Fecal occult blood testing *and/or*	1	Colorectal cancer
flexible sigmoidoscopy *or*	3–5	Colorectal cancer
colonoscopy	Once	Colorectal cancer
Pap smear	≤ 3*	Cervical cancer
Height and weight	≤ 1	Obesity, malnutrition
Alcoholism questionnaire	**	Alcoholism
Serum lipids in persons with MI, angina	1	Recurrent CAD
Vision testing	1	Sensory deficits
Hearing ability	1	Hearing impairment
Counseling to encourage		
Low-fat, well-balanced diet	1	Obesity, CAD
Adequate calcium intake	1	Osteoporosis
Physical activity	1	Immobility, CAD, osteoporosis
Injury prevention	1	Injurious falls, motor vehicle crashes, burns, other injuries
Smoking cessation	†	COPD, many cancers, CAD
Regular dental visits	1	Malnutrition, oral cancers, edentulism
Immunization		
Influenza vaccination	1	Influenza
Pneumococcal vaccination	‡	Pneumococcal disease
Tetanus booster	10	Tetanus
Chemoprophylaxis		
Discussion, implementation of HRT	§	Osteoporosis
Aspirin therapy in persons with prior MI	Daily	Additional MI, TIA, or stroke

CAD = coronary artery disease; COPD = chronic obstructive pulmonary disease; HRT = hormone replacement therapy; MI = myocardial infarction; TIA = transient ischemic attack. For updates from the U.S. Preventive Services Task Force, see http:/www.ahrg.gov/clinic/prevenix.htm.

Table continued on following page.

Evidence-based Preventive Services Recommended for the
General Population Aged 65 and Older (Continued)

*May stop screening at age 65 if patient has regularly normal smears up to that age; if never tested prior to age 65, may stop after two normal annual smears.

**Should be performed at initial visit and whenever drinking is suspected.

†Should be discussed at every visit of patients who smoke.

‡Immunize once at age 65 for immunocompetent patients; revaccination after 7–10 years may be appropriate for high-risk immunocompromised patients.

§ Should be discussed at menopause and at least one more time after age 65.

Adapted from Cobbs EL, Duthie EH, Murphy JB (eds): Geriatric Review Syllabus: A Core Curriculum in Geriatric Medicine, 5th ed. Malden, MA, Blackwell Publishing for the American Geriatrics Society, 2002.

BIBLIOGRAPHY

1. Alexander NB: Gait disorders in older adults. J Am Geriatr Soc 44:434–451, 1996.
2. American College of Sports Medicine: Position stand: Exercise and physical activity for older adults. Med Sci Sports Exerc 30:992–1008, 1998.
3. American Geriatrics Society, British Geriatrics Society, and American Academy of Orthopedic Surgeons Panel on Falls Prevention: Guidelines for the prevention of falls in older persons. J Am Geriatr Soc 49:664–672, 2001.
4. Bird AC, Bressler NM, Bressler SB, et al: An international classification and grading system for age-related maculopathy and age-related macular degeneration. The International ARM Epidemiological Study Group. Survey Ophthalmol 39:367–374, 1995.
5. Boult C, Pacala JT: Care of older people at risk. In Calkins E, Boult C, Wagner EH, et al (eds): New Ways to Care for Older People: Building Systems Based on Evidence in Managed Care. New York, Springer Publishing, 1999, pp 65–84.
6. Calle EE, Thun MJ, Petrelli JM, et al: Body-mass index and mortality in a prospective cohort of U.S. adults. N Engl J Med 341:1097–1105, 1999.
7. Christmas C, Anderson RA: Exercise and older patients: Guidelines for the clinician. J Am Geriatr Soc 48:318–324, 2000.
8. Cohn ES: Hearing loss with aging. Clin Geriatr Med 15:145–161, 1999.
9. Edelberg HK, Wei JY: Primary care guidelines for community-living older persons. Clin Geriatr 7:42–55, 1999.
10. Ferris FL 3d, David MD, Aiello LM: Treatment of diabetic retinopathy. N Engl J Med 341:667–678, 1999.
11. Gillespie LD, Gillespie WJ, Cummings R, et al: Interventions for preventing falls in the elderly. Cochrane Database Syst Rev 2:CD000340, 2000.
12. Gill TM, Robison JT, Williams CS, et al: Mismatches between the home environment and physical capabilities among community-living older persons. J Am Geriatr Soc 47:88–92, 1999.
13. Kitler DP: Cachexia. Ann Intern Med 133:622–634, 2000.
14. Larson VD, Willam DW, Henderson WA: Efficacy of 3 commonly used hearing aid circuits: A crossover trial. JAMA 284:1806–1813, 2000.
15. Manson J, Hu FB, Rich-Edwards JW, et al: A prospective study of walking as compared with vigorous exercise in the prevention of coronary heart disease in women. N Engl J Med 341:650–658, 1999.
16. Mansour-Shousher R, Mansour WN: Neurosurgical management of hearing loss. Clin Geriatr Med 15:163–177, 1999.
17. National Center on Elder Abuse at the American Public Human Services Association (formerly the American Public Welfare Association) in Collaboration with Westat, Inc.: The National Elder Abuse Incidence Study: Final Report. Washington, DC, National Aging Information Center, 1998.
18. Posiadlo D, Richardson S: The timed "Up and Go": A test of basic functional mobility for frail elderly persons. J Am Geriatr Soc 39:142–148, 1991.
19. Rowe JW: Geriatrics, prevention and the remodeling of Medicare. N Engl J Med 340:720–721, 1999.
20. Stuck AE, Walthert JM, Nikolaus T, et al: Risk factors for functional status decline in community-living elderly people: A systematic literature review. Soc Sci Med 48:445–469, 1999.
21. Van Swerringen JN, Paschal KA, Bonino P, et al: Assessing recurrent fall risk of community-dwelling frail older veterans using specific tests of mobility and the physical performance test of function. J Gerontol A Biol Sci Med Sci 53:M457–M464, 1998.
22. Wolf SL, Catlin PA, Gage K, et al: Establishing the reliability and validity of measurement of walking time using the Emory Functional Ambulation Profile. Phys Ther 79:1122–1133, 1999.

102. THE OBESE PATIENT

Laura M. Lasater, M.D., and Daniel H. Bessesen, M.D.

1. What is obesity?

Obesity is a chronic disease characterized by degrees of overweight that are associated with increases in morbidity and mortality. The concept of "ideal body weight" originated with the Metropolitan Life Insurance studies, which demonstrated a J-shaped relationship between body weight and mortality. People who weighed less than or more than a certain amount experienced excessive rates of mortality. The association between lower weights and increased mortality is attenuated after controlling for smoking, eliminating subjects who die early, and after other attempts to control for occult disease. More recent studies suggest that the relationship between body weight and mortality is essentially linear when fat mass alone rather than the body mass index (BMI), which also reflects lean body mass, is the independent variable.

2. How is obesity diagnosed?

In 1997, the World Health Organization designated the BMI as the international standard for identifying overweight and obesity in adult populations. BMI is calculated by dividing weight in kilograms by height in meters squared. A BMI of less than 25 is normal. A BMI of 25–26.9 indicates overweight; 27–29.9, obesity; 30–34.9, moderate obesity; 35–39.9, severe obesity; and > 40, morbid obesity.

Body Weights in Pounds According to Height and Body Mass Index*

	BODY MASS INDEX (kg/m^2)													
	19	20	21	22	23	24	25	26	27	28	29	30	35	40
HEIGHT (IN)	◄─────────────────────── BODY WEIGHT, lb ───────────────────────►													
58	91	96	100	105	110	115	119	124	129	134	138	143	167	191
59	94	99	104	109	114	119	124	128	133	138	143	148	173	198
60	97	102	107	112	118	123	128	133	138	143	148	153	179	204
61	100	106	111	116	122	127	132	137	143	148	153	158	185	211
62	104	109	115	120	126	131	136	142	147	153	158	164	191	218
63	107	113	118	124	130	135	141	146	152	158	163	169	197	225
64	110	116	122	128	134	140	145	151	157	163	169	174	204	232
65	114	120	126	132	138	144	150	156	162	168	174	180	210	240
66	118	124	130	136	142	148	155	161	167	173	179	186	216	247
67	121	127	134	140	146	153	159	166	172	178	185	191	223	255
68	125	131	138	144	151	158	164	171	177	184	190	197	230	262
69	128	135	142	149	155	162	169	176	182	189	196	203	236	270
70	132	139	146	153	160	167	174	181	188	195	202	207	243	278
71	136	143	150	157	165	172	179	186	193	200	208	215	250	286
72	140	147	154	162	169	177	184	191	199	206	213	221	258	294
73	144	151	159	166	174	182	189	197	204	212	219	227	265	302
74	148	155	163	171	179	186	194	202	210	218	223	233	272	311
75	152	160	168	176	184	192	200	208	216	224	232	240	279	319
76	156	164	172	180	189	197	205	213	221	230	238	246	287	328

*Each entry gives body weight in pounds (lb) for a person of a given height and body mass index. Pounds have been rounded off. To use the table, find the appropriate height in the left hand column. Move across the row to a given weight. The number at the top of the column is the body mass index for the height and weight. (From NIH Technology Assessment Conference Panel: Methods for voluntary weight loss and control. Ann Intern Med 116:942–949, 1992.)

3. Is the distribution of body fat important in assessing health risk?

Yes. The health risks of obesity are related not only to the amount of fat but also to the distribution of fat. A growing number of studies have demonstrated that excessive adipose tissue that accumulates in a central or upper body distribution (android or male pattern) as opposed to lower body obesity (gynoid or female pattern) increases the risk for adverse health consequences independently of BMI. Central obesity can be diagnosed by calculating a ratio of the waist circumference (WC) divided by the maximal circumference of the hips. This so-called waist-to-hip ratio (WHR) defines central obesity if it is > 0.85 in women or ≥ 1.0 in men. Current studies, however, suggest that WC alone is a better indicator of abdominal fatness and cardiovascular disease than either BMI or WHR. The optimal value of WC ranges from 89 to 94 cm for men and 77 to 82 cm for women and is dependent on the prevalence of the cardiovascular risk factor being considered and the age of the individual. For convenience, 80 and 90 cm can be used as cutoff points for women and men, respectively, without significantly compromising the predictive power of the measure.

Classification of Weight Status and Risk of Disease*

| | | RISK OF DISEASE† | |
	BMI	WAIST CIRCUMFERENCE: ≤ 35 INCHES (WOMEN) ≤ 40 INCHES (MEN)	WAIST CIRCUMFERENCE: ≥ 35 INCHES (WOMEN) ≥ 40 INCHES (MEN)
Underweight	< 18.5		
Healthy weight	18.5–24.9		
Overweight	25.0–29.9	↑	↑↑
Obesity	30.0–34.9	↑↑	↑↑↑
Obesity	35.0–39.9	↑↑↑	↑↑↑
Extreme obesity	≥ 40.0	↑↑↑↑	↑↑↑↑

*If patient is ≥ 18 years old, use the BMI and waist circumference to estimate weight status and relative risk for diabetes, high blood pressure, or heart disease.
†Relative to having a healthy weight and waist size. An increased waist circumference may indicate increased disease risk even at a normal weight.
Adapted from Expert Panel: Clinical Guidelines on the Identification, Evaluation, and Treatment of Overweight and Obesity in Adults. Bethesda, MD, National Institute of Health, National Heart, Lung, and Blood Institute, U.S. Department of Health and Human Services, Public Health Service, 1998.

4. What are the health consequences of obesity?

Obesity is clearly associated with some of the most common illnesses, including diabetes; hypertension; hyperlipidemia; coronary artery disease; degenerative arthritis; gallbladder disease; and cancer of the endometrium, breast, prostate, and colon. The incidence of these conditions increases steadily as body weight increases. It is surprising how risks increase with even modest gains in weight. Increased BMI is also associated with decreased use of preventive health services (e.g., mammogram, clinical breast examinations, Pap smears, and number of physician visits). A BMI > 25 kg/m² before age 20 years is a strong predictor of obesity and ill health in adulthood. Health risks are magnified in people with a family history of obesity-associated diseases. Obesity is responsible for 300,000 deaths per year in the United States. After smoking, it is the leading cause of potentially preventable death.

Prevalence and Relative Risks of Common Comorbidities in Severely Obese Patients*

COMORBIDITY	PREVALENCE IN SEVERELY OBESE (%)
Osteoarthritis	50–65
Hypertension	25–60
Gastroesophageal reflux	30–50
Urinary stress incontinence	30–40

Table continues on following page.

Prevalence and Relative Risks of Common Comorbidities in Severely Obese Patients* (Continued)

COMORBIDITY	PREVALENCE IN SEVERELY OBESE (%)
Gallbladder disease	25–45
Depression	20–40
Dyslipidemia	20–35
Hypertriglyceridemia	25
Low HDL cholesterol	20
Diabetes	10–20
Hyperinsulinemia	10–20
Asthma	10–20
Sleep apnea	5–40
Congestive heart failure	7–12

COMORBIDITY	RELATIVE RISK† IN SEVERELY OBESE WOMEN	RELATIVE RISK† IN SEVERELY OBESE MEN
Atherosclerotic diseases		
Claudication	25.0–100.0	5.0
Chest pain	7.0–35.0	15.0
Myocardial infarction	0.7	5.0
Stroke	0.7	—
Hypertension		
>155/95 mmHg	1.5–5.3	1.8
>175/105 mmHg	1.2–4.2	2.3
Diabetes	8.0–20.0	5.0
Dyspnea	5.5	4.0
Back pain	1.5–2.0	2.0
Cholelithiasis	2.5	1.5

*BMI $\geq$ 35 kg/m^2; class III and above.
Relative risk expressed in relation to the general population. HDL = high-density lipoprotein.
Adapted from Kral J: Morbidity of severe obesity. Surg Clin North Am 81:1039–1061, 2001.

BMI and Body Weight Associated with 20% and 50% Increases in Mortality from All Causes and Mortality from Cardiovascular Disease (CVD)

	20% INCREASE				50% INCREASE			
	MORTALITY FROM ALL CAUSES		MORTALITY FROM CVD		MORTALITY FROM ALL CAUSES		MORTALITY FROM CVD	
	BMI*	WEIGHT (KG)†	BMI*	WEIGHT (KG)†	BMI*	WEIGHT (KG)†	BMI*	WEIGHT (KG)†
70-in. men								
30–44 yr	23.8	166	22.9	160	27.2	189	25.3	177
45–54 yr	24.2	169	23.2	162	28.1	196	26.0	181
55–64 yr	24.7	172	23.9	167	29.1	203	27.5	192
65–74 yr	28.2	197	26.5	185	37.0	258	33.2	232
75–84 yr	30.5	213	28.1	196	42.1	294	36.7	256
64-in. women								
30–44 yr	26.0	152	23.5	137	32.1	187	26.5	155
45–54 yr	24.8	145	23.2	135	29.4	171	25.8	151
55–64 yr	25.9	151	25.2	147	32.0	187	30.3	177
65–74 yr	29.9	174	29.0	169	40.8	238	38.7	226

*A body mass index of 21.0 was used as the reference value.
†For men, a height of 70 inches (178 cm) and weight of 146.5 lb (67 kg) were used as reference values. For women, a height of 64 inches (163 cm) and weight of 122.5 lb (56 kg) were used as reference values.
From Rosenbaum M, Leibel RL, Hirsch J: Obesity. N Engl J Med 337:396–407, 1997, with permission.

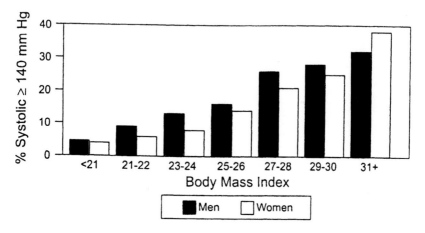

BMI and the risk of hypertension. (From Canadian Guidelines for Healthy Weights. Cat. No. H39-134 1989E: 1988:69.)

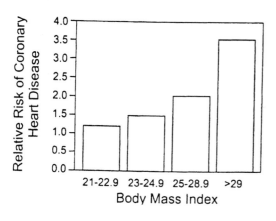

BMI and the risk of coronary artery disease. (From Colditz GA, Meir SJ, et al: A prospective study of obesity and risk of CHD in women. N Engl J Med 322: 882–890, 1990, with permission.)

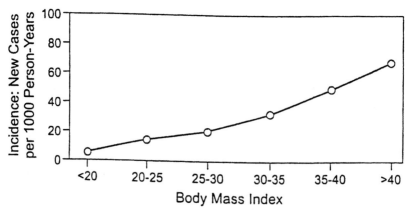

BMI and the risk of diabetes. (From Knowler WC, et al: Diabetes incidence in Pima Indians: Contributions of obesity and parental diabetes. Am J Epidemiol 113:144–156, 1981, with permission.)

5. What are the economic consequences of obesity?

In 1998, the National Heart, Lung, and Blood Institute estimated that 97 million adults in the United States were overweight or obese. The direct cost of obesity in 1995 was estimated to be $70 billion, or 7% of total health care costs. In addition, the loss in wages and productivity attributed to obesity approaches $50 billion per year. Finally, people attempting to lose weight spend $30–60 billion annually on weight-loss products, most of which have no proven benefit. A more recent study mandated by the American Obesity Association estimated the total cost of obesity to be $238 billion in 1999.

6. What are the psychological complications of obesity?

Situational depression and anxiety related to obesity are common. Obese people may suffer from discrimination that further contributes to difficulty with poor self-image and social isolation. In one study, obese adolescents were compared with adolescents who had other chronic health problems. Both groups were followed for 7 years. At the end of this period, obese women were 20% less likely to be married, made $6700/year less in income, and had 10% more poverty than control subjects. This effect was independent of baseline aptitude test scores and socioeconomic status. It may be difficult or impossible for care providers who have never experienced discrimination based on obesity to completely understand the experience of obese people. It is important for care providers to closely examine their own feelings about obesity and to consider how their feelings affect the care that they provide to obese patients.

7. How common is obesity?

Obesity has reached epidemic proportions in the United States. The most recent study of the prevalence of obesity (The National Health and Nutrition Examination Survey [NHANES III]) conducted by the federal government demonstrates that 60% of adult Americans are either overweight or obese. The NHANES studies have demonstrated that, despite a perception that consumption of low-calorie, low-fat foods and participation in regular exercise have increased, the prevalence of obesity has risen steadily over the past 30 years and dramatically in the last decade.

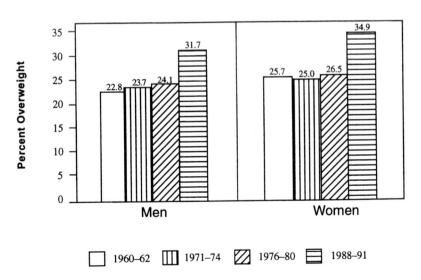

Percent of adult Americans who were overweight, 1960–1990. (From Kuczmarski RJ, et al: Increasing prevalence of overweight among U.S. adults. The National Health and Nutrition Examination Surveys, 1960–1991. JAMA 272:205–211, 1994, with permission.)

8. What causes obesity?

The regulation of body weight is complex. Maintaining energy balance is one of the most important jobs of any organism and involves assessing energy stores within the body and the nutrient content of the diet; determining whether the body is in negative energy or nutrient balance; and adjusting hormone levels, energy expenditure, nutrient movement, and consumatory behavior in response. These tremendously complex events involve thousands of gene products. Models of obesity in mice have provided new and fundamental insights into the mechanisms involved in body weight regulation.

Recent scientific developments have helped to foster a change in the way that people think about obesity. Professionals and lay people are increasingly viewing obesity as a chronic metabolic disorder much like diabetes or hypertension. This view requires a conceptual shift from the previous widely held belief that obesity is simply a cosmetic or behavioral problem. For obesity to develop, there must be a period of positive energy balance—that is, energy intake must exceed energy expenditure. The complex systems regulating body weight and composition must be altered, ultimately achieving a new steady state at a higher weight.

9. Do abnormal genes cause obesity?

The prevalence of obesity has dramatically increased in the past 60 years with minimal change in the human gene pool. The problem of human obesity is a classic gene–environment interaction. Genetic factors primarily determine the susceptibility to obesity, but environmental factors promote its phenotypic expression. The heritability estimate (fraction of the population variation in a trait that can be explained by genetic transmission) for obesity in large sample sizes is between 25% and 40% and as high as 70% in identical twins. A number of molecular-genetic approaches have been used to try to identify relevant genes. These efforts not only hold the promise of identifying physiologic mechanisms underlying the development of obesity but also may reveal novel targets for therapies.

10. What role does leptin play in obesity?

Leptin is a product of the *ob* gene locus. It is a circulating hormone produced by adipocytes that serves as the afferent component of a regulatory loop that adjusts energy balance through behavioral and metabolic effectors. Its absence triggers a series of neuroendocrine responses that conserve energy when food availability is limited. The main effect of leptin in inducing weight loss is mediated by its suppressive effect on food intake. Contrary to initial hypotheses, however, the majority of obese individuals have *high* circulating levels of leptin, whereas only a handful of severely obese individuals have been identified with either a congenital deficiency or a mutation in leptin or the leptin receptor. One study has demonstrated a dose–response relationship with weight and fat loss with subcutaneous recombinant leptin injections in both lean and obese subjects, even when baseline levels of leptin were high.

11. Does a decrease in energy expenditure play a role in the development of obesity?

For obesity to develop, there must be an imbalance between caloric intake and caloric expenditure. For fat mass to increase, there must be an imbalance between the amount of fat consumed compared with the amount of fat oxidized. One possibility is that people become obese because of a reduction in energy expenditure. There are three components to energy expenditure:

1. **Basal metabolic rate (BMR)** is the amount of energy needed to keep sodium and potassium where they belong, keep the body warm, pump blood, breathe, and perform other basic functions.

2. **Energy expended in activity (EA)** is the most variable and may account for as little as 10–20% of total energy expenditure in people who are bedridden or as much as 60–80% in training athletes.

3. **Thermic effect of food (TEF)** is a relatively small component of energy expenditure and represents the increase in energy expenditure that follows the consumption of meals.

Increasing evidence indicates that obesity is associated with a relative reduction in energy expended with activity. Evidence in favor of this hypothesis comes from the Pima Indians as well as obese caucasians and previously obese people placed on weight-reducing diets. The role that reductions in BMR play in weight gain is more controversial. Regardless of the absolute level of energy expenditure, obesity results when a person fails to accurately adjust energy intake to changes in energy expenditure.

12. What approaches are available for the treatment of obese patients?

Treatment options include diet, exercise, drugs, surgery, and combinations of these modalities.

13. What is an appropriate goal for a weight-reducing program?

This important question has no simple answer. Increasing evidence indicates that many obese people have unrealistic expectations about the amount of weight that they may lose through a weight-loss program. Most obese people would like to reach "ideal body weight" and to do so as quickly as possible. They are disappointed if they lose only 5–10% of their initial weight. These desires stand in stark contrast to the magnitude of weight loss that has been seen with all treatment modalities short of surgery. The most effective diet, exercise, or drug treatment programs give roughly a 10% weight loss in most people. This degree of weight reduction, although relatively small, has been associated with improvements in health-associated measures such as lower blood pressure (BP), reductions in low-density lipoprotein (LDL) cholesterol levels, improved functional capacity, and improved insulin sensitivity. It has been postulated that a feedback loop inhibits additional weight loss. As weight is lost by decreasing caloric intake, fat cells shrink, reducing expression of leptin. As leptin levels decrease, metabolic rate decreases, appetite increases, and further weight loss becomes more difficult. Most experts now believe that a sustained 5–10% weight loss (e.g., a 22-lb weight loss for someone who initially weighed 220 lb) is a realistic goal with probable medical benefits. It is important for providers to help patients set realistic goals before embarking on a diet and exercise program. These goals could include a gradual but sustained mild weight reduction. Alternatively, prevention of further weight gain may be an attainable goal, or the health care provider may encourage the patient to focus on eating and activity habits and not on a weight goal. In this manner, patients can succeed independently of weight loss, and if they go off the behavioral program, they have relapsed independently of what the scale says.

14. What is the role of diet in the treatment of obese patients?

The mainstays of dietary modification in weight loss therapy have been a diet low in fat and calories. Ultimately, however, it is caloric restriction, not diet composition, that determines weight loss. Whatever intervention is made must be lifelong to be beneficial. Therefore, it must be tolerable to the patient. The initial evaluation should include an assessment of whether the patient wants to change his or her diet; stages of change include precontemplative, contemplative, planning, action, and maintenance.

In addition, the primary care provider should assess the patient's current diet with a good nutritional history. This assessment can be done in a few minutes with a 24-hour dietary recall and a discussion of the composition of frequently eaten meals, including fast foods. Then slow, gradual dietary change should be encouraged. Simple dietary suggestions include (1) eating three meals per day, (2) eating only at meal times, (3) eating only one serving, and (4) making a conscious effort to eat slowly. These suggestions help patients to focus on what and how they are eating. Most people know what they should eat. The problem is that they either do not pay attention to what they eat, eat inappropriate portion sizes, eat too fast, or do not find a "good diet" palatable. A nutritionist can help to tailor a diet to the individual patient's needs. A nutritional consultation, however, does not take the place of ongoing discussion and encouragement from the primary care provider. Many settings do not allow sophisticated behavioral modification techniques to be taught.

The use of commercial programs such as Weight Watchers can provide reasonable nutritional counseling and social support. Many patients are surprised at the cost of these programs, which may be a deterrent to continued use. However, such programs involve no risk and may be cheaper in the long run than pharmacologic treatment. Unfortunately, many patients have already tried and failed at these approaches before they seek medical attention. The scientific literature supports the notion that, for many people, dietary approaches alone are not associated with a high level of success at achieving long-term weight loss.

15. What is the role of exercise in a weight loss program?

Exercise has a minor role in weight reduction but an important one in the maintenance of weight loss. The explanation is simple: the absolute caloric deficit produced by a moderate exercise program is simply insufficient to result in the degree of negative energy balance necessary for marked weight reduction. Another problem is that the patient may preserve or even increase lean body mass at a time when fat mass is decreasing; thus, the absolute amount of weight loss is reduced. However, over the long term, the success of a weight loss program is substantially greater if exercise is included. A recent study of people who had successfully lost weight and kept it off for more than 1 year found that the unifying feature was that all of them exercise regularly. Although most patients and physicians think of an exercise program as at least 30 minutes of high-intensity exercise at least three times per week, it is important to remember that the expenditure side of the energy balance equation is equal to the intensity of the activity multiplied by the time. Many Americans watch television for 3–4 hours/day (21–28 hours/week). The energy expended while watching television is roughly equal to a sleeping metabolic rate. If such people simply reduced the time spent watching television and worked more around the house, the net effect on total energy expenditure might be greater than a program of higher-intensity exercise for only brief periods one to three times a week. An important fact to emphasize to overweight or obese patients is that, independent of any effect on weight loss, exercise benefits them greatly by increasing cardiorespiratory fitness. Indeed, obese, fit men have a lower risk of cardiovascular mortality than do lean men with low levels of fitness.

16. What medications are available for the treatment of obesity?

Orlistat, a pancreatic lipase inhibitor, reduces the absorption of fat by roughly 30%. It is given as 120 mg three times a day after meals. Because it is not systemically absorbed, it is probably not associated with primary pulmonary hypertension (PPH). Its main side effects are gastrointestinal. Orlistat (Xenical) was approved by the Food and Drug Administration (FDA) in 1998. It is the only antiobesity agent that is noncontrolled and approved for prolonged use.

Sibutramine is a combination norepinephrine and serotonin reuptake blocker. Unlike fenfluramine and dexfenfluramine, it has no serotonin-releasing action and therefore is more similar to the serotonin-specific reuptake inhibitors currently used for treatment of depression. It is taken at doses of 10–40 mg/day and produces weight loss in the range of 8–10% at doses of 20 mg and higher, somewhat less than the weight losses generally seen with the combination of fenfluramine and phentermine. In humans, the drug works primarily by reducing appetite with minimal effects on energy expenditure. Sibutramine has been associated with an increase in BP in some people, particularly at higher doses. Sibutramine (Meridia) became available for use in 1998.

Others. New developments in the basic sciences suggest that a number of regulatory systems may be potential targets for pharmacologic therapies. Recombinant leptin is currently undergoing phase I trials. Similar to insulin, this peptide hormone must be administered parenterally. It may interact with cytokine receptors at the site of injection to induce a local inflammatory response, which may limit its usefulness. Other drug companies are looking at compounds that interact with the downstream portions of the leptin-signaling pathway, including drugs that interact with the neuropeptide Y receptor subtype responsible for feeding effects. Cholecytokinin (CCK) is a gut hormone that inhibits feeding. A number of long-acting CCK agonists have been synthesized and are in the early stages of clinical trials. Stimulation of the beta$_3$-adrenergic receptor subtype causes increases in thermogenesis and energy expenditure in rodents. With the recent identification of uncoupling protein 3 in human skeletal muscle, it is hoped that a beta$_3$ agonist will increase energy expenditure in humans and aid in weight reduction. A number of these compounds have been synthesized and are undergoing phase I clinical trials; however, bioavailability has been a major problem.

This partial list gives some sense of the broad range of targets currently being examined as well as the unforeseen difficulties that may limit the usefulness of such compounds. Medications may be considered in patients with a BMI > 27 if two or more comorbid conditions such as diabetes, hypertension, or degenerative arthritis are present or BMI > 30 in the absence of comorbid conditions.

17. Is liposuction an effective means for weight loss in obese individuals?
In the only controlled trial, weight lost by liposuction was regained. In some patients, the adipose tissue reaccumulated in the same site; in others, it reaccumulated elsewhere. Liposuction cannot be advocated as a weight loss strategy for patients with medically significant obesity.

18. What mechanical methods are available for the treatment of morbidly obese patients?
Surgical therapy offers the best long-term chance for reducing body weight in severely obese patients. A myriad of surgical procedures for the treatment of severe obesity exist. These can be classified as malabsorptive or restrictive. Malabsorptive procedures involve rearrangement of the small intestine to reduce the functional absorptive surface area for nutrients. Restrictive procedures involve decreasing the opening to or size of the stomach. American Society for Bariatric Surgery data for 1998 show that 82% of surgeons prefer a primary combination restrictive–malabsorptive procedure such as Roux-en-Y gastric bypass. The success rate for gastroplasty or gastric bypass is 60–70%, and the average weight loss is 30%. Criteria for surgical eligibility include BMI > 40 or BMI > 35 with obesity-related medical comorbidities, failure of aggressive medical therapy, stable psychiatric status, and understanding of the need for lifetime lifestyle modification. Many patients experience a marked improvement in preoperative morbidities, including resolution of diabetes, hypertension, and hyperlipidemia as well as improved rates of employment.

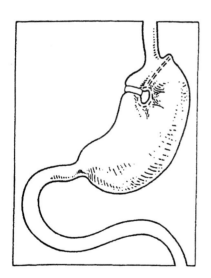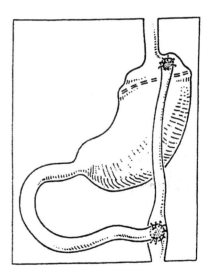

Gastroplasty *(left)* and gastric bypass *(right)* operations for the treatment of morbid obesity.

19. What is a very low-calorie diet (VLCD)? When should its use be considered?
AVLCD is a nutritionally complete diet of 800 kcal/day that produces weight loss. Experienced teams in supervised settings should administer such diets. When VLCDs are used in this manner, complications are rare. The long-term results with VLCDs are no better than with other dietary programs, which limits their usefulness. They may be helpful in patients who need a short-term weight loss to reduce the risk of a diagnostic or surgical procedure.

CONTROVERSIES

20. Can herbal medicines aid in weight loss?

The FDA became aware of the use of herbal medications purported to have the same mechanism of action as fen-phen without the side effects. These combinations usually include the herbal ingredient ephedra, commonly known as Ma Huang, and the herb *Hypericum perforatum*, also known as St. John's wort. The FDA does not approve of their use in obese patients, considers them "drugs" in a weight-loss program, and is taking regulatory action to remove them from the market because of the potential for serious side effects.

21. What are phen-fen and Redux?

Phen-fen is the combination of phentermine and fenfluramine. Redux is the trade name of dexfenfluramine. The two drugs were prescribed to more than 8 million people in an effort to help them lose weight. They were removed from the market because of serious side effects.

22. What side effects were observed with the use of phentermine-fenfluramine and dexfenfluramine?

Two serious, somewhat unexpected side effects were associated with the use of fenfluramine and dexfenfluramine: PPH and valvular heart disease. Although it is not clear how commonly PPH occurred, the best data suggest that, of 1 million people who took these medicines, between 28 and 50 will develop PPH, one half of whom will die from the condition even if the medications are stopped. The frequency of valvular heart disease as a complication is not clear. Echocardiography has demonstrated a prevalence of valvular disease ranging from 6% to 30%. Much of this variability between studies can be attributed to differences in the duration of drug exposure, because valvulopathy appears to be more common in people exposed to the drug for > 6 months. Use of a cohort design to exclude patients with preexisting FDA-defined aortic regurgitation (AR) or mitral regurgitation (MR) (at least mild AR or at least moderate MR) results in a much lower estimate of incidence at 2.6%. Aortic insufficiency is the most common lesion, and only 18% of affected people have an audible murmur by auscultation. Based on these findings, the drugs were voluntarily withdrawn from the market in 1997.

23. How should a patient who was treated with fenfluramine or dexfenfluramine be followed?

Definitive diagnostic and treatment guidelines are not yet available, but the U.S. Department of Health and Human Services has published interim recommendations. All patients with a history of use of fenfluramine or dexfenfluramine should undergo a careful history and cardiovascular physical examination. A transthoracic echocardiogram (two-dimensional and Doppler) should be done in patients with symptoms, cardiac murmurs, or other signs of cardiac involvement (e.g., widened pulse pressure or regurgitant c or v waves in the jugular venous pulse). Doppler echocardiography should be performed in patients for whom cardiac auscultation cannot be performed adequately because of body habitus. Asymptomatic patients without murmurs should undergo repeat physical examinations in 6–8 months. It has been advised that people with cardiac valvulopathy related to fenfluramine or dexfenfluramine should receive antibiotic prophylaxis if they undergo dental procedures. It is too early to know the natural history of this disease, although one small prospective study suggests the disease is not progressive after the drugs have been stopped and may actually improve over time.

24. How long do patients need to take a weight loss medicine?

In the past, the FDA would allow only short-term use of weight loss medicines. However, experts now believe that obesity is a chronic disease and that a medicine used to help lose weight will work only as long as it is taken. Patients who take a weight loss medicine, lose weight, and then stop the medicine are likely to regain the lost weight. The same effect is observed when someone goes on a diet for a certain period and then stops the diet. This so-called yo-yo effect is probably not good for health. Unfortunately, we do not have good data about the safety or effectiveness of weight loss medicines used for 10–20 years. In general, if a primary care provider and a patient decide to use a weight-loss medication, it should be used for a minimum of 3 months to determine whether the patient will lose at least 10% his or her of body weight. Then consideration should be given to some form of chronic use in view of the available information about the risks and potential benefits of the medications.

25. Does the weight loss provided by medications improve health?

We do not know the answer to this question. One reasonable approach is to wait until more research is done to answer this important question clearly. Other medicines developed for other conditions, such as ventricular arrhythmias, have turned out to hurt more than to help. We know that in some people, the weight loss accompanying the use of medicines is associated with decreases in BP, improved glucose control in patients with diabetes, reduced symptoms of degenerative arthritis, and reduced blood levels of cholesterol. Some people find that weight loss medicines reduce the occurrence of obsessive thoughts about eating, which may be their most important therapeutic effect. Although it makes intuitive sense that losing weight would improve health, it is not yet clear that losing weight *with medications* improves health. On the other hand, it is clear that increased weight is associated with health risks if nothing is done.

BIBLIOGRAPHY

1. Bonow RO, Carabello B, deLeon A, et al: Guidelines for the management of patients with valvular heart disease: Executive summary. A report of the American College of Cardiology/American Heart Association Task Force on Practice Guidelines. Circulation 98:1949–1984, 1998.
2. Bray GA: Obesity. Endocrinol Metab Clin North Am 25:781–1048, 1996.
3. Dobbelsteyn CJ, Joffres MR, MacLean DR, Flowerdew G, and The Canadian Heart Health Surveys: A comparative evaluation of waist circumference, waist-to-hip ratio and body mass index as indicators of cardiovascular risk factors. The Canadian Heart Health Surveys. Int J Obesity 25:652–661, 2001.
4. Expert Panel: Clinical Guidelines on the Identification, Evaluation, and Treatment of Overweight and Obesity in Adults. Bethesda, MD, National Institute of Health, National Heart, Lung, and Blood Institute, U.S. Department of Health and Human Services, Public Health Service, 1998.
5. Glazer G: Long-term pharmacotherapy of obesity 2000: A review of efficacy and safety. Arch Intern Med 161:1814–1824, 2001.
6. Kral JG: Morbidity of severe obesity. Surg Clin North Am 81:1039–1061, 2001.
7. Leermakers EA, Dunn AL, Blair SN: Exercise management of obesity. Med Clin North Am 84:419–438, 2000.
8. From NIH Technology Assessment Conference Panel: Methods for voluntary weight loss and control. Ann Intern Med 116:942–949, 1992.
9. Rish S, Rubin L, Walker A, et al: Anorexigens and pulmonary hypertension in the United States: Results from the Surveillance of North American Pulmonary Hypertension. Chest 117:870–874, 2000.
10. Rosenbaum M, Leibel RL, Hirsch J: Obesity. N Engl J Med 337:396–407, 1997.
11. Wei M, Kampert J, Barlow C, et al: Relationship between low cardiorespiratory fitness and mortality in normal-weight, overweight, and obese men. JAMA 282:1547–1553, 1999.
12. Wolf AM, Colditz GA: Social and economic effects of body weight in the United States. Am J Clin Nutr 63:466S–469S, 1996.

103. THE CIGARETTE SMOKER

Thomas D. *MacKenzie*, M.D., MSPH

1. What is the current prevalence of cigarette smoking among adults in the United States?

Cigarette smoking became the most popular form of tobacco consumption in the 1920s. Per capita cigarette consumption rose sharply during World War II and continued to rise until the

1950s. The first reports linking cigarette use with cancer emerged in the 1950s and were subsequently confirmed with other studies, leading to the famous *Surgeon General's Report on Smoking and Health* in 1964. Consumption eventually peaked in the late 1960s at more than 4000 cigarettes per capita per year and has declined annually since. The prevalence of cigarette smoking (percentage of the adult population who smoke regularly) peaked at 41% and declined annually until 1990, when prevalence reached 25%. Of great concern to public health officials is the fact that the rate of decline in cigarette smoking prevalence during the 1990s slowed considerably, resulting in a prevalence of 23.5% in 1999. Although the gender differential has narrowed over time, a higher percentage of men than women are current smokers (25.7% vs. 21.5%).

2. At what age do people start to smoke?
The average age of initiation of regular cigarette smoking has been declining since the 1920s. For persons born between 1910 and 1920, the average age of initiation was approximately 20 years. In 1992, 1 in 5 eighth graders reported smoking their first cigarette in fifth grade. Today the average age is 14.5 years.

3. How do you quantify a person's smoking history?
Multiply the average number of packs smoked per day by the number of years of smoking to get the number of pack-years of smoking. For example, a 55-year-old woman who began smoking at age 15 years and thinks that she smoked an average of 1.5 packs (30 cigarettes) per day has a 60 pack-year smoking history (1.5 packs $\times$ 40 years).

4. What is the prevalence of cigarette smoking among high school students?
It is important to recognize that "current smoking" is defined differently for teenagers and children than for adults. Research studies that report smoking prevalence among adults define current smokers as people who have smoked at least 100 cigarettes in their lives *and* who smoke every day or "some days." However, in surveys involving youth, most investigators define current smokers as anyone who has smoked a cigarette on any one of the preceding 30 days. "Frequent smokers" on youth surveys are kids who report smoking on at least 20 of the preceding 30 days.

With that in mind, the prevalence of current smoking among high school students increased from 27.5% in 1990 to 36.4% in 1997. Fortunately, data from the end of the decade suggest that prevalence has declined among high school students to 34.8%.

5. What are the five A's of smoking cessation counseling?
The Public Health Service (PHS)–sponsored clinical practice guidelines on treating tobacco use and dependence list five A's for office-based interventions:

1. **Ask** about tobacco use at every visit. Have a system in place to inquire and document tobacco use status on every patient. This raises the awareness of smokers, nonsmokers, and office staff members to the importance of cessation.

2. **Advise** all smokers to quit. Physician advice is a powerful and inexpensive tool for smoking cessation, especially when given in a "teachable moment" such as an office visit for bronchitis or a tobacco-related hospitalization. The message should be clear, strong, and personalized.

3. **Assess** willingness to make a quit attempt. This is the newest *A* of smoking cessation. Smokers who are willing to make a quit attempt should receive the fourth and fifth A's. Those who are not willing to make a quit attempt should receive a motivational intervention to improve their willingness to quit.

4. **Assist** patients in the quit attempt. Any health care provider can assist the patient in setting a quit date. The date should be set as soon after the initial counseling session as possible. With few exceptions (see question 7), pharmacologic treatment should be offered to all patients willing to make a quit attempt.

5. **Arrange** follow-up. A follow-up visit within in 1 week after the quit date can improve success rates. The vast majority of relapses occur within the first 2 weeks after cessation.

6. Why should cigarette smoking be considered a chronic disease?

It is tempting for clinicians to define tobacco dependence as a curable disorder. Many people think, "All the patient has to do is to stop smoking one day, and he will save himself a lifetime of morbidity from cigarettes." Unfortunately, tobacco dependence shows many features of a chronic disease. Few smokers are able to quit on their first attempt, and nearly half of all current smokers try to quit every year. Most smokers experience many cycles of relapse and remission in their attempts to be smoke free. If clinicians fail to recognize the chronicity of the illness, then unsuccessful quit attempts and relapse may be perceived as failure by the clinician or the patient. A much better approach is to recognize the chronicity of the dependence, anticipate relapse, and adopt a counseling style similar to that used for other chronic diseases such as diabetes, obesity, and hypertension.

7. Who should be offered pharmacologic treatment for smoking cessation?

All smokers *who are willing to make a quit attempt* should be offered some form of pharmacologic treatment with the following exceptions:
Patients with medical contraindications
Patients who smoke fewer than 10 cigarettes per day
Pregnant or breast-feeding women
Adolescents

8. What are the typical nicotine withdrawal symptoms?

Craving for nicotine, irritability, frustration, anger, anxiety, difficulty in concentrating, restlessness, increased appetite, and decreased heart rate.

9. What happens to pulmonary function tests with smoking cessation?

The forced expiratory volume in 1 second (FEV_1) has been used as the marker of pulmonary function in several studies. Among all men older than age 45 years, the FEV_1 typically declines at a rate of 20 mL/year as a natural consequence of aging. Smoking accelerates this age-related decline. For example, in the Honolulu Heart Program, men who continued to smoke showed a steeper rate of decline in FEV_1 of about 33 mL/year. Men who were able to quit in the first 2 years of the study rapidly reduced the rate of decline in FEV_1 to that of nonsmokers. Another study also showed that smoking intervention can significantly reduce the age-related decline in FEV_1 in middle-aged smokers with evidence of early chronic obstructive pulmonary disease (COPD).

10. What should I say to patients to help them quit smoking?

The message should be clear, strong, and personalized. If the patient presents with a smoking-related illness, tie the message to the current symptoms. Examples include:
- "I think it is important for you to quit smoking now, and I can help you."
- "Cutting down while you are ill is not enough."
- "As your clinician, I need you to know that quitting smoking is the most important thing you can do to protect your health now and in the future. The clinic staff and I will help you."
- "We know that smokers get bronchitis more often than nonsmokers; you might avoid this type of illness in the future if you quit smoking."

11. What are the major short-term health benefits of smoking cessation?

1. The excessive risk of premature coronary heart disease decreases by 50% within 1 year of abstinence.

2. Some of the toxic effects of cigarettes smoking that may lead to cardiac events, such as increased platelet activation, elevated carbon monoxide levels, and coronary artery spasm, are immediately reversible with cessation.

3. Pregnant women who stop during the first 3–4 months of pregnancy eliminate the risk of having a low–birth-weight baby.

12. Is inpatient smoking cessation treatment effective?

Four well-designed studies conducted with hospitalized smokers were reviewed for the PHS guideline. Inpatient counseling of varying intensity increased cessation rates by approximately 30%. The efficacy of the nicotine replacement therapy in hospitalized patients has not been well studied.

13. What are the major long-term benefits of smoking cessation?

1. Smoking cessation before age 35 years eliminates the excessive mortality associated with smoking and translates into 7 more years of life compared with continuing smokers.

2. People who stop smoking between the ages of 45 and 55 years can extend their lives by approximately 4 years and can cut the excessive risk of death in half over the next 15 years compared with continuing smokers.

3. Even for smokers who quit after age 65 years, there is significant improvement in overall survival compared with continuing smokers.

14. How much weight do people gain after they quit smoking?

In one large study of more than 2500 smokers, the mean weight gain attributable to smoking cessation was 2.8 kg (6.2 lbs) in men and 3.8 kg (8.4 lbs) in women. Major weight gain (> 13 kg or 28.6 lbs) occurred in 10% of men and 13% of women.

15. Which pharmacologic agents are approved by the Food and Drug Administration (FDA) for tobacco dependence?

Five therapies are approved for first-line use in the treatment of tobacco dependence:
1. Transdermal nicotine (the patch)
2. Nicotine gum
3. Nicotine nasal spray
4. Nicotine inhaler
5. Sustained release (SR) bupropion

Nortriptyline and clonidine can be used as second-line agents but are not approved by the FDA.

16. How effective is nicotine replacement therapy?

Two recent meta-analyses of randomized, placebo-controlled trials of nicotine replacement therapy demonstrate that both nicotine gum and transdermal nicotine are highly effective aids for smoking cessation. Both agents approximately double the smoking cessation rates at 1 year compared with placebo. Success rates are also influenced by the degree of nicotine dependence and the intensity of counseling (see question 24). Although fewer studies have been done on the nicotine inhaler and the nicotine nasal spray, they are both as effective as the gum and the patch.

17. How can a clinician assess the degree of tobacco dependency in an individual patient?

The Fagerström Test for Nicotine Dependence (FTND) is used to determine the degree of nicotine dependence for an individual patient. Studies have shown that highly dependent smokers benefit more from use of nicotine gum than less dependent smokers. However, the data for nicotine patches are mixed.

Fagerström Test for Nicotine Dependence

QUESTIONS	ANSWERS	POINTS
1. How soon after you wake up do you smoke your first cigarette?	Within 5 minutes	3
	6–30 minutes	2
	31–60 minutes	1
	After 60 minutes	0
2. Do you find it difficult to refrain from smoking in places where it is forbidden (e.g., in church, at the library, in the cinema)?	Yes	1
	No	0

Table continues on following page.

Fagerström Test for Nicotine Dependence (Continued)

QUESTIONS	ANSWERS	POINTS
3. Which cigarette would you hate most to give up?	The first one in the morning	1
	All others	0
4. How many cigarettes/day do you smoke?	≤ 10	0
	11–20	1
	21–30	2
	≥ 31	3
5. Do you smoke more frequently during the first hours after waking than during the rest of the day?	Yes	1
	No	0
6. Do you smoke if you are so ill that you are in bed most of the day?	Yes	1
	No	0

Adapted from Heatherton TF, Kozlowski LT, Frecker RC, Fagerström KO: The Fagerström test for nicotine dependence: A revision of the Fagerström tolerance questionnaire. Br J Addict 86:1119–1127, 1991.

18. Can pharmacotherapies for smoking cessation be combined?

Yes. Data suggest that combining nicotine patches with other forms of nicotine replacement can improve quit rates over a single agent alone. Also, limited data suggest that nicotine patches combined with bupropion is better than either agent alone.

19. What is the mechanism of action of nicotine gum?

The gum contains nicotine bound to an ion-exchange resin in a gum base, which allows the nicotine to be released slowly. A low pH impairs the release of the nicotine. After the nicotine is released, it is absorbed through the buccal mucosa. The systemic nicotine alleviates withdrawal symptoms normally associated with smoking cessation.

20. How is nicotine gum prescribed?

1. Use the FTND to determine the degree of dependence. Highly dependent (≥ 5) smokers are given 4-mg nicotine gum for 6 weeks and then 2-mg nicotine gum until completion of therapy. Smokers with moderate-to-low dependence are prescribed 2-mg nicotine gum. The mean nicotine content of a cigarette is 1.8 ± 0.4 mg.

2. Prescribe one piece of gum every hour while the patient is awake. The patient should be instructed to chew the gum until he or she senses that the nicotine has been released and then to park the gum to allow absorption through the buccal mucosa. An acid environment from drinking juice, soda, or coffee greatly impairs absorption of nicotine.

3. Remove the gum after 20 minutes.

4. Recommend tapering frequency of gum use after 3 months.

21. Discuss the length of treatment and dosing for nicotine patches.

Many randomized, controlled trials evaluating nicotine patches as an aid to smoking cessation suggest that the maximal benefit can be gained by using a 6- to 8-week course of daily patches. Although some patch manufacturers initially recommended nicotine patch use for up to 3 months, more recent studies have shown that end-of-treatment quit rates for 3 months of patch use are essentially the same as quit rates at the end of 4 weeks and worse than quit rates after 6 weeks of patch use. Studies suggest that 6–8 weeks is enough time for nicotine withdrawal symptoms to decrease and allows the patient to develop the new skills necessary to maintain abstinence. Many clinicians use high-dose patches uniformly in the initial 2–4 weeks and taper the dose at 2-week intervals thereafter. There is probably no significant difference in the efficacy of 24-hour versus 16-hour patches.

22. What is the correct dosing for bupropion SR?

Unlike the nicotine-replacement products, bupropion SR should be initiated approximately 1–2 weeks before the quit date. The dosage is 150 mg per day for 3 days and then 150 mg twice daily. Therapy should be continued for 7–12 weeks after the quit date. For patients who cannot afford twice-daily dosing, once-daily dosing is nearly as effective.

23. What are the contraindications and the common side effects of bupropion SR?
    Bupropion SR is contraindicated in individuals with a history of seizure disorder, a history of an eating disorder, who are using another form of bupropion (Welbutrin or Welbutrin SR), or who have used a monoamine oxidase (MAO) inhibitor in the past 14 days. The most common side effects reported by bupropion SR users are insomnia (35–40%) and dry mouth (10%).

24. What type of counseling is an effective adjunct to the use of nicotine patches?
    Although the patch appears to be effective for some patients without counseling, counseling along with the patch uniformly increases quit rates. A meta-analysis of 17 nicotine patch studies rated counseling intensity levels according to four criteria: (1) the goal of the meeting was smoking cessation; (2) one or more weekly meetings were held during the first 4 weeks of treatment; (3) the total number of meetings was greater than 7 in the first 12 weeks; and (4) counseling lasted more than 40 minutes. High-intensity counseling was shown to be more effective than low-intensity counseling. Furthermore, group counseling was more effective than individual counseling.

Abstinence Rates at 6 Months in a Meta-analysis of the Efficacy of Transdermal Nicotine by Format and Intensity of Counseling

	PLACEBO PATCH (%)	ACTIVE NICOTINE PATCH (%)
Counseling format		
Individual	7.7	20.0
Group	12.6	26.3
Counseling intensity		
Low	7.1	19.5
High	13.2	26.5

Adapted from Fiore MC, Smith SS, Jorenby DE, Baker TB: The effectiveness of the nicotine patch for smoking cessation: A meta-analysis. JAMA 271:1940–1947, 1994.

25. Can nicotine patches be used in patients with known coronary artery disease?
    It is generally believed that the patch can be used in patients with stable angina if the patient understands that the patch is a *substitute* for cigarettes and is motivated to abstain totally. In one study of 156 patients with stable coronary artery disease, 14-mg patches were compared with placebo for 5 weeks. Quit rates were 36% for active patch users versus 22% for placebo patch users. There was no increase in cardiac symptoms or complications in the active patch group. Patches are contraindicated in patients who have had a recent myocardial infarction or who have poorly controlled hypertension.

26. What strategies can be used to promote smoking cessation in a clinical setting?
    A meta-analysis of 39 controlled trials of smoking cessation strategies showed that smoking cessation programs using several modes of *repeated* counseling and intervention are most effective for initial and long-term cessation. Interventions included physician and nonphysician individualized counseling; setting a quit date; nurse telephone follow-up; group counseling and classes; and use of written materials, cassettes, and videos. Carbon monoxide monitors are often used to verify abstinence and may be useful in the initial counseling stages by demonstrating the "poison" that builds up in the blood of the smoker. The use of nicotine patches or nicotine gum should be considered in all patients.

27. What is the cost-effectiveness of smoking interventions?
    The cost-effectiveness of a therapy can be measured in dollars spent per quality-adjusted life year saved (QALY). Smoking cessation interventions are among the most cost-effective interventions in medicine. For comparison, hypertension screening costs $14,000–40,000 per QALY; annual mammography for women aged 50–69 years costs $46,000 per QALY. The table below shows that the cost per QALY for smoking cessation counseling is $1100–4000, depending on

the intensity of counseling. When you use the nicotine patch as adjunctive therapy, the cost effectiveness improves.

Costs and Cost-effectiveness Ratios for Smoking Cessation Counseling Interventions with and without Transdermal Nicotine*

| | COST/PARTICIPANT | | | |
INTERVENTION	SUCCESSFUL	FAILED	COST/QUITTER	COST/QALY[†]
Counseling alone				
Minimal	14.51	14.51	7922	4015
Full	75.55	75.55	2989	1515
Group intensive	53.14	53.14	2186	1108
Counseling with transdermal nicotine				
Minimal	246.25	141.40	4745	2405
Full	300.69	195.84	2715	1376
Group intensive	272.37	167.52	2310	1171

*Data from Cromwell J, Bartosch WJ, Fiore MC et al: Cost-effectiveness of the clinical practice recommendations in the AHCPR guideline for smoking cessation. JAMA 278:1759–1766, 1997.
†QALY = quality-adjusted life-year. Costs are discounted by 3% per year.

BIBLIOGRAPHY

1. Bartecchi CE, MacKenzie TD, Schrier RW: The global tobacco epidemic. Sci Am (May):26–33, 1995.
2. Bartecchi CE, MacKenzie TD, Schrier RW: The human costs of tobacco use. Part I. N Engl J Med 330:907–912, 1994.
3. Burchfiel CM, Marcus EB, Curb JD, et al: Effects of smoking and smoking cessation on longitudinal decline in pulmonary function. Am J Respir Crit Care Med 151:1778–1785, 1995.
4. Centers for Disease Control and Prevention: Cigarette smoking among adults—United States, 1999. MMWR Morb Mortal Wkly Rep 50:869–873, 2001.
5. Centers for Disease Control and Prevention: Cigarette smoking: Attributable mortality and years of potential life lost—United States, 1990. MMWR Morb Mortal Wkly Rep 42:230–233, 1993.
6. Centers for Disease Control and Prevention: Trends in cigarette smoking among high school students—United States, 1991–1999. MMWR Morb Mortal Wkly Rep 49:755–758, 2000.
7. Cromwell J, Bartosch WJ, Fiore MC, et al: Cost-effectiveness of the clinical practice recommendations in the AHCPR guideline for smoking cessation. Agency for Health Care Policy and Research. JAMA 278:1759–1766, 1997.
8. Doll R, Peto R, Wheatley K, et al: Mortality in relation to smoking: 40 years' observations in male British doctors. Br Med J 309:901–911, 1994.
9. Fiore MC, Bailey WC, Cohen SJ, et al: Treating Tobacco Use and Dependence. Clinical Practice Guideline. Rockville, MD, U.S. Department of Health and Human Services, Public Health Service, 2000.
10. Fiore MC, Kenford SL, Jorenby DE, et al: Two studies of the clinical effectiveness of the nicotine patch with different counseling treatments. Chest 105:524–533, 1994.
11. Fiore MC, Smith SS, Jorenby DE, Baker TB: The effectiveness of the nicotine patch for smoking cessation: A meta-analysis. JAMA 271:1940–1947, 1994.
12. Heatherton TV, Kozlowski LT, Frecker RC, Fagerström KO: The Fagerström test for nicotine dependence: A revision of the Fagerström tolerance questionnaire. Br J Addict 86:1119–1127, 1991.
13. MacKenzie TD, Bartecchi CE, Schrier RW: The human costs of tobacco use. Part II. N Engl J Med 330:975–980, 1994.
14. Surgeon General: The Health Benefits of Smoking Cessation. Washington, DC, Department of Health and Human Services, 1990, pp 473–515, DHHS Publication (CDC) 90–8416.
15. Surgeon General: Reducing the Health Consequences of Smoking: 25 Years of Progress: A Report of the Surgeon General: Executive Summary. Rockville, MD, Department of Health and Human Services, 1989, DHHS Publication (CDC) 89–8411.
16. Tang JL, Law M, Wald N: How effective is nicotine replacement therapy in helping people to stop smoking? Br Med J 308:21–26, 1994.
17. U.S. Preventive Services Task Force: Guide to Clinical Preventive Services, 2nd ed. Baltimore, Williams & Wilkins, 1996.
18. Williamson DF, Madans J, Anda RF, et al: Smoking cessation and severity of weight gain in a national cohort. N Engl J Med 324:739–745, 1991.

104. THE PATIENT WITH HUMAN IMMUNODEFICIENCY VIRUS

David W. Lehman, M.D., Ph.D.

1. When does a patient have acquired immunodeficiency syndrome (AIDS)?

AIDS is a clinical syndrome of acquired immunodeficiency resulting from infection with the human immunodeficiency virus (HIV). When a patient who is HIV positive develops an opportunistic infection, a specific neoplasm, or other specified condition, the patient has AIDS. The most common opportunistic infections are *Pneumocystis carinii* pneumonia (PCP), *Mycobacterium avium* complex (MAC), cytomegalovirus (CMV), *Mycobacterium tuberculosis* infection, candidal esophagitis, coccidioidomycosis, and other fungal infections. The most common neoplasms are Kaposi's sarcoma and non-Hodgkin's lymphomas, but invasive cervical carcinoma is also an AIDS-defining condition. Other AIDS-defining conditions include a CD4 < 200, pulmonary tuberculosis, recurrent pneumonia, HIV encephalopathy, and AIDS wasting syndrome.

Relative Risk of AIDS-defining Conditions as a Function of CD4 Count

May occur with higher CD4 counts (increased risk with lower counts)
Tuberculosis
Herpes simplex or zoster
Kaposi's sarcoma
Systemic fungal infection
Rare, unless CD4 count < 200 cells/μL
Pneumocystis carinii pneumonia
Non-Hodgkin's lymphoma
AIDS dementia complex
Progressive multifocal leukoencephalopathy
Wasting syndrome
Toxoplasmosis
Rare, unless CD4 < 50 cells/μL
Mycobacterium avium complex (MAC)
Cytomegalovirus disease

2. What risk factors for HIV disease should be assessed in primary care practice?

A complete history includes an assessment of HIV risk, which includes male homosexual behavior, intravenous drug use (specifically needle sharing), sex with IV drug users, prostitution, sex with prostitutes, history of blood transfusion between 1978 and 1985, history of sexually transmitted diseases (STDs), and history of multiple sexual partners. Potential risk may be clarified by determining the frequency of safe versus unsafe sex practices. The risk assessment process also may be used to educate patients about risk reduction, including safer sex and safer drug use.

3. When should a physician encourage a patient to be tested for HIV?

HIV testing should be recommended if a history of more than minimal risk is obtained. Because of the benefits of decreasing maternal–infant transmission with antiretroviral therapy, it is recommended that pregnant women be tested. Patients should be counseled about confidentiality issues and consent to testing. Some patients choose to be tested anonymously at an alternate test site.

4. How can a physician judge a patient's risk of transmission?

Parenteral blood products have the highest rate of transmission, estimated to be 95%. Higher viral loads (associated with primary infection, low CD4 count, or advanced disease) likely increase infectivity. Although condom failures have been reported, the consistent, correct use of condoms with nonoxynol-9 is nearly 100% effective in preventing HIV transmission. Among specific sexual behaviors, unprotected receptive anal intercourse with ejaculation is the highest risk, estimated at 3% (3 of 100) for each act of anal sex. The risk for insertive partners in rectal sex is somewhat lower. The risk of male-to-female transmission has been studied by evaluating the proportion of infected women among the steady partners of infected men. The estimated rate of infection in women for each act of unprotected vaginal sex varies widely but may be 1 in 500. Female-to-male transmission is probably lower, although the low prevalence in women has limited collection of suitable data. The risk of transmission of HIV by unprotected oral sex for performing and receiving partners is unquantified.

5. How accurate is HIV testing?

The joint false-positive rate of sequential enzyme-linked immunosorbent assay (ELISA) and Western blot testing is about 0.1%, depending on the experience of the laboratory. In a population with a low prevalence of HIV infection, this false-positive rate may correspond to positive predictive values of < 50%. False-negative tests in low prevalence populations are rare and result mainly from the window of time between infection and development of antibodies (usually < 3 months but rarely up to 6 months).

6. What are the natural history and prognosis of HIV infection?

On average, about 50% of untreated HIV-infected patients progress to AIDS in 10 years. Patients often gain a more positive outlook in learning that 50% of patients do *not* progress to AIDS after 10 years. Even in the asymptomatic stage, viral synthesis is very active, with as many as 10^{10} virions produced each day.

Mathematical models predict that > 95% of untreated HIV-infected patients will eventually progress to AIDS, but the data do not allow us to conclude that every HIV-positive person will inevitably develop AIDS. The HIV RNA viral load is the single best predictor of survival. CD4 cell count predicts outcome independently of viral load. The median survival after developing an AIDS-defining condition has increased to > 7 years with current therapy. The proportion of deaths caused by opportunistic infections has decreased markedly; liver disease (chronic hepatitis B or hepatitis C), kidney disease, and lymphoma have proportionately increased. A reasonable hope now exists that a significant number of patients can manage their HIV infection as a relatively stable, long-term chronic disease.

7. How should newly diagnosed HIV-positive patients be evaluated?

The complete history and physical examination for HIV-positive patients includes special emphasis on risk factors (timing of seroconversion, if possible); psychosocial issues; systemic issues (fever and weight loss); and targeted organs: skin, oropharynx, lungs, gastrointestinal (GI) tract, and lymph nodes. Routine laboratory evaluation includes chest radiograph; complete blood count with differential and platelet count; levels of aspartate aminotransferase (AST), alanine aminotransferase (ALT), lactate dehydrogenase (LDH), bilirubin, alkaline phosphatase (AP), albumin, total protein, and creatinine; serologic test for syphilis and toxoplasmosis; and assessment of HIV RNA viral load and T cells with subsets. Hepatitis status is evaluated with hepatitis A total antibodies, hepatitis C serology, and hepatitis B surface antigen (HBsAg), plus, if negative, hepatitis B total core antibodies. Vaccinations (including diphtheria–tetanus, Pneumovax, and influenza) are updated, and purified protein derivative (PPD) skin testing is done. Hepatitis B vaccine is recommended for HBsAg-negative and hepatitis B total core antibody–negative patients. Hepatitis A vaccine is recommended for hepatitis A total antibody–negative patients. Risk reduction behavior (e.g., tobacco cessation, alcohol moderation, IV drug cessation) should be encouraged. A nutritional evaluation and plan help patients to maintain a healthy weight.

8. How can a patient's clinical status, risk of disease progression, and response to therapy be determined?

The single best marker of clinical status is the viral load because it is the best predictor of progression to AIDS and death. The viral load is a measure of the number of copies of virus in a milliliter of blood. The combination of viral load and CD4 count gives a more accurate prediction of clinical status. For example, a patient with CD4 count > 750 and viral load < 500 has only a 3.6% risk of progressing to AIDS in 9 years; a patient with CD4 count of 201–350 and viral load of 10,000–30,000 has an 85% risk of progressing in 9 years and a 56% risk of progressing in only 3 years. Patients should be routinely monitored every 3–4 months. Because of intra-assay and biologic variability, the viral load should be repeated within 2–4 weeks after baseline measurement; after a change in therapy; or after a significant change in viral load, which would lead to an adjustment in therapy. A 0.5-log (threefold) decrease in viral load is the minimal change necessary for a positive response to therapy. Several drug regimens have been shown to decrease viral load by 1–2 logs (10- to 100-fold) or more. Treatment with antiretroviral drugs often leads to increases in CD4 count. A 1-log (tenfold) decrease in viral load on drug therapy (by week 8) is associated with a 65% decrease in risk of progression to AIDS. A 0.5-log increase or a return to within 0.5 log of baseline is an indication of treatment failure.

9. What are the goals of antiviral therapy?

Multiple goals have been proposed, ranging from eradication of infection (currently theoretical) to keeping the viral load undetectable or as low as possible (with CD4 count as high as possible) and the longer-term maintenance goal of keeping the patient healthy, functional, and free of side effects as long as possible. It is preferable to restore immune function rather than only to stop further deterioration, even if eradication becomes possible.

10. What antiretroviral drugs (ARV) are available?

Current ARV drugs represent four ways to prevent the synthesis of new HIV: nucleoside reverse transcriptase inhibitors (NRTIs), nonnucleoside reverse transcriptase inhibitors (NNRTIs), a nucleotide reverse transcriptase inhibitor (tenofovir), and protease inhibitors (PIs). The NRTIs are zidovudine, stavudine, lamivudine, didanosine, abacavir, and zalcitabine. The available NNRTIs are efavirenz, nevirapine, and delavirdine. The PIs are ritonavir, nelfinavir, indinavir, lopinavir, amprenavir, and saquinavir. Because of the high likelihood of the development of resistance to ARVs by HIV, monotherapy should not be used. Patients who choose to take drugs should take a combination of at least three drugs. A combination of two NRTIs and one PI reduced viral load below detectable levels in 90% of one small series of patients at 24 weeks. Prior patient experience with one or more ARVs may alter the likelihood that the patient already has drug-resistant virus and should be a factor in choosing an appropriate drug regimen. Cross-resistance between drugs is a major problem, increases with partial or suboptimal treatment, and may decrease the effectiveness of future drug regimens. Research is ongoing, and better drugs (more effective, improved dosing schedule, fewer side effects) will most likely be available in the next 1–5 years.

No single drug regimen is best for all patients. A combination of two NRTIs with one PI or one NNRTI is frequently used. Because of the ongoing rapid flow of new clinical outcomes data and subsequent changing recommendations for therapy, physicians should consult recent expert recommendations for assistance in choosing the best drug regimen for a particular patient.

11. When should ARV treatment be started?

The timing and choice of ARVs are areas with rapidly evolving data about which physicians disagree. Well-informed patients often state their own preferences, which should be a major factor in the therapeutic decision process. Several groups and individuals have proposed algorithms for starting ARV treatment. These recommendations are extrapolations from limited clinical data about treatment of certain HIV clinical status categories. Data are not available for all HIV clinical status categories. The data are limited because outcomes were usually evaluated at 1–2 years at most, yet patients need to be treated for much longer periods. Current Department of Health and Human Services guidelines are available on the Web (www.hivatis.org).

Because the drug regimens can be difficult to follow and because the likelihood of drug-resistant mutants is high and increases when suboptimal drug regimens are followed, the decision to start drugs should follow careful patient education about the risks and benefits of ARVs and the commitment of the patient to adhere to the drug regimen for at least 3 years and potentially for life. As patients live longer and anticipate taking ARVs for many years, the issue of side effects (most notably, changes in body fat distribution, hyperlipidemia, and glucose intolerance) has become more important. Present or past use of alcohol or other drugs should raise concerns about the patient's ability to make a long-term commitment to a complex drug regimen. Illicit drug use may counteract the benefits of ARVs and increase the likelihood of not completely following a drug regimen.

The current indications for treatment include viral load > 30,000 copies/mL, CD4 count < 350 cells/μL, symptoms suggesting progression, and symptoms of primary infection. A decreasing CD4 count (> 100 decrease in CD4/year) or an increasing viral load are also appropriate considerations in a decision to start treatment. Many patients and their physicians choose to start ARVs even though the viral load is low and the CD4 count is high. Because such patients have a good prognosis even without drugs, they need to take drugs for many years to realize a benefit and risk feeling worse in the interim because of drug side effects. Over such a long time, the likelihood of noncompliance and subsequent development of drug resistance increases.

12. Describe the common skin problems in HIV infection.

Up to 90% of HIV-positive patients have a skin disease. Kaposi's sarcoma is discussed in question 22 with other malignancies. The prevalence of skin infections is high. Among bacterial causes, *Staphylococcus aureus* is the most common, usually presenting as folliculitis or, less frequently, bullous impetigo, ecthyma, abscesses, or cellulitis. Among viral causes, herpes viruses (zoster and simplex) are the most common. The suggestion to assess HIV risk factors in all adults aged 18–50 years is especially applicable if such a patient (even up to 65 years) presents with zoster. **Molluscum contagiosum** is common and especially difficult to eradicate in HIV-positive patients.

By virtue of taking more drugs, HIV-positive patients and patients with AIDS are at increased risk of drug reactions. The most common is caused by trimethoprim–sulfamethoxazole (TMP-SMX) and presents as a diffuse maculopapular eruption. Other antibiotics, notably penicillins, are also common offenders. Among ARVs, nevirapine most often causes a rash.

13. What mouth problems are common in HIV infection?

Common oral lesions in HIV-positive patients have fungal, bacterial, viral, or neoplastic causes. The two most common types are hairy leukoplakia (white thickening of mucosal surfaces, often with vertical corrugations) and thrush (pseudomembranous candidiasis). Both have been shown to predict progression to AIDS independently of CD4 counts. Candidal infection also may present as angular cheilitis, candidal leukoplakia, or the erythematous form. Gingivitis and periodontitis are common bacterial complications of HIV disease. Kaposi's sarcoma may produce oral lesions.

14. What entities should be considered when an HIV-positive patient complains of dysphagia?

Candidal esophagitis is the most common cause of dysphagia; odynophagia and retrosternal chest pain are other frequent symptoms. Less common causes are CMV, herpes virus, and Kaposi's sarcoma. Response to empiric treatment for candidal infection with fluconazole sometimes provides a presumptive diagnosis. Endoscopy with biopsies is needed for a definitive diagnosis.

15. Describe the neuropsychiatric complications of HIV infection.

The common neurologic manifestations may be caused directly by HIV (e.g., AIDS dementia complex and peripheral neuropathy) or secondary to drugs or opportunistic disease, including fungal (*Cryptococcus* spp.), protozoan (toxoplasmosis), mycobacterial, and viral infections. Peripheral neuropathy presents as a painful sensation with limited sensory or motor deficits. *Cryptococcus neoformans* meningitis is the most common fungal infection of the central nervous system (CNS) in HIV-positive patients. Other fungal pathogens are histoplasmosis and coccid-ioidomycosis. *Toxoplasma gondii* causes encephalitis and focal intracerebral lesions, which are ring enhancing on computed tomographic (CT) scan. Progressive multifocal leukoencephalopa-thy (PML), caused by the human polyomavirus (JC), commonly presents insidiously over weeks with focal neurologic deficits. AIDS dementia complex is an organic mental disorder with cog-nitive deficits (confusion, memory loss, impaired concentration or mental slowing), behavioral manifestations (depressed affect or agitation), and motor symptoms (weakness, unsteady gait, or decreased coordination). The common psychiatric manifestations include adjustment, affective, and anxiety disorders. An increased prevalence of substance abuse is self-evident among IV drug users but also has been described empirically in the male homosexual population.

16. When should a primary care physician seek hematologic consultations for HIV disease?

Anemia, leukopenia, and thrombocytopenia may occur singly or in combination either as a direct manifestation of HIV disease or as a result of opportunistic infections or neoplasms, drug effects, or nutritional deficiencies. In many instances, the primary care physician may diagnose and manage the penias of HIV infection. Anemia is the most common abnormality, occurring in up to 85% of patients with AIDS. Isolated anemia is associated with *Mycobacterium avium* or parvovirus infection. Hemolytic anemia may occur in patients who are deficient in glucose 6-phosphate-dehydrogenase and treated with dapsone. Zidovudine may cause anemia that requires transfusions, neutropenia, and thrombocytopenia. Ganciclovir, pentamidine, trimethoprim, and cancer chemotherapeutic agents commonly cause neutropenia. Isolated immune thrombocytope-nia may occur as a manifestation of HIV infection or AIDS. Diagnosis and treatment of immune thrombocytopenia may require bone marrow biopsy and hematologic consultation. In some in-stances, treatment of appropriate patients (CD4 counts < 500) with AZT has led to marked im-provement of thrombocytopenia. In addition, the administration of growth factors (erythropoietin and granulocyte colony-stimulating factor [G-CSF]) may be helpful in some instances.

17. Contrast the clinical presentations and management of the various forms of pneumonia in HIV-positive patients.

Pneumocystis carinii pneumonia (PCP) is the most common AIDS-defining condition and usually occurs only in severely immunocompromised patients (CD4 < 200 cells/μL). Prophy-laxis against PCP has been shown to prolong life for HIV-infected patients. Several agents are available for PCP prophylaxis: TMP-SMX (first-line agent), dapsone, and aerosolized pentami-dine. Patients should be monitored for the occurrence of side effects that require a change to a dif-ferent agent. Clinical presentation includes fever, nonproductive cough, and progressive short-ness of breath; pleuritic chest pain is uncommon. Supportive evidence includes an elevated LDH, hypoxia or at least an increased alveoloarterial oxygen gradient, and a diffuse interstitial infiltrate on chest radiograph. Diagnosis is made by fluorescent antibody stain of induced sputum (64% sensitive) or, if necessary, bronchoalveolar lavage specimens (97% sensitive). Treatment options include TMP-SMX, pentamidine, TMP-dapsone, clindamycin–primaquine, and atovaquone with the addition of steroids for acute disease.

Bacterial pneumonia, which is an AIDS-defining condition if it is recurrent, occurs with in-creased frequency in HIV-positive patients. The most common pathogens include *Streptococcus pneumoniae, Haemophilus influenzae,* and *Moraxella catarrhalis.* The presenting symptoms—fever, productive cough, and dyspnea—are often acute and of short duration. The chest radio-graph more often shows lobar or segmental infiltrates. Blood cultures are positive for bacterial pneumonia in 40–80% of cases. The sputum Gram stain sometimes gives an immediate diagno-sis. Empiric treatment with TMP-SMX provides excellent coverage of the common bacterial agents as well as PCP, pending definitive diagnosis.

Mycobacterial infection, which occurs with pulmonary as well as systemic manifestations, is discussed in question 19. The herpes family causes pneumonia and infects other organs or occurs as a systemic disease (see question 20). Fungal agents include *Cryptococcus* spp., *Histoplasma* spp., and coccidioidomycosis.

18. Should HIV-positive patients be screened regularly for tuberculosis?

Yes. *Mycobacterium tuberculosis* has been found in 3.8% of patients with AIDS, with a disproportionate increase in extrapulmonary sites. IV drug users and ethnic minorities are at especially increased risk. The 1993 revised case definition added pulmonary tuberculosis as an AIDS-defining condition. Annual screening with PPD (a > 5-mm reaction is a positive result) is recommended for all HIV-positive patients who are not already known to be anergic. Because of frequent anergy, some physicians also recommend a screening chest radiograph, depending on local prevalence of tuberculosis. PPD-positive patients of any age should take prophylactic isoniazid. Initial empiric treatment for active tuberculosis includes isoniazid, rifampin, and pyrazinamide; further adjustment depends on the presence of extrapulmonary tuberculosis and the local prevalence of multidrug-resistant strains.

19. Which patients are susceptible to MAC?

Disseminated MAC is a frequent late complication of HIV infection ($\leq 53\%$ in one autopsy series). It occurs only in patients with < 100 CD4 cells (75% of patients in one series had < 19 CD4 cells). Antimicrobial prophylaxis against *M. avium* for patients with CD4 < 75 with prior opportunistic infections decreases the incidence of mycobacteremia and improves survival. Lifetime prophylaxis with clarithromycin, azithromycin, or rifabutin is recommended, although physicians must weigh the risks of drug toxicity, drug interactions, and detrimental effects on compliance of adding another drug to often complex medical regimens. The common clinical manifestations of MAC are fever, malaise, weight loss, anemia, neutropenia, chronic diarrhea, abdominal pain, and malabsorption. Diagnosis is by special blood culture techniques. Because of their low sensitivity and low positive predictive value, stool cultures are not recommended. MAC bacteremia is associated with increased risk of death. Various multidrug regimens have been recommended; the combination of clarithromycin, ethambutol, and rifabutin has been shown to improve clearance of *M. avium* bacteremia and to increase survival rates.

20. List the three most common viral infections in HIV-positive patients.

Herpes simplex infection has a high prevalence (95% seropositivity in homosexual men with AIDS) and sometimes has severe manifestations in HIV-positive patients, including esophagitis, pneumonia, and encephalitis. Some patients require chronic acyclovir suppression. **Herpes zoster** (recurrent varicella zoster infection) occurs frequently in HIV-infected patients, and the new diagnosis of zoster in any patient younger than 65 years should prompt a risk assessment and consideration of testing for HIV. Patients may experience multiple recurrences and systemic dissemination. **Active CMV** is a frequent late complication of AIDS (in one series, the median CD4 count was 19 cells/μL, and 75% of patients had < 46 CD4 cells). Clinical manifestations include retinitis, pneumonia, encephalitis, and severe diarrhea.

21. How should an HIV-positive patient with diarrhea be evaluated and treated?

First, a diagnosis should be sought to identify treatable causes of diarrhea. Stool should be cultured for bacteria and examined microscopically for parasites. *Mycobacterium avium intracellulare* (MAI) is best identified by blood cultures (see question 19). Common bacterial causes include *Salmonella, Shigella,* and *Campylobacter* species, *Giardia lamblia; Entamoeba histolytica,* and, less commonly, *Cryptosporidium* species and *Isospora belli* (parasitic agents). A toxin from *Clostridium difficile* should be considered when the patient has been taking antibiotics. In one series, CMV colitis was the most common cause of diarrhea; diagnosis requires identification of CMV and biopsy of mucosal ulcers. If no specific cause is identified, symptomatic treatment with nonspecific antidiarrheal drugs may provide significant benefit to patients.

22. Which malignancies are associated with HIV infection?

The AIDS-defining opportunistic malignancies are Kaposi's sarcoma (most common), non-Hodgkin's lymphoma, and invasive cervical carcinoma. Kaposi's sarcoma usually presents as violaceous, palpable nodules of the skin or oral mucosa; it also may involve the GI tract, lungs, and lymph nodes. About 70% of non-Hodgkin's lymphoma is B-cell lymphoma and usually presents as advanced extranodal disease. Seventy-five percent of patients with non-Hodgkin's lymphoma have CD4 counts < 80 cells/μL; the disease may present as a primary lymphoma of the CNS but usually not until patients are severely immunocompromised (CD4 < 50 cells/μL). Invasive cervical carcinoma was added as an AIDS-defining condition in the revised case definition of 1993.

23. Describe the special issues associated with HIV in women.

The rising prevalence, changing epidemiology, and severity of HIV infection in women present special issues. The fastest growing AIDS group is women. IV drug use is responsible for 59% of AIDS cases in women, either directly (39%) or indirectly (20%) through sex with an injection drug user. Minorities are disproportionately represented; 78% of women with AIDS are African American or Hispanic. AIDS is now the third most common cause of death among women of color ages 25–44 years in the United States and the fifth most common cause of death among all U.S. women in that age group. Among young people (ages 13–24 years), 47% of newly diagnosed HIV cases in 2000 were women. Women tend to present in more advanced stages of disease, in part because up to 50% of women with heterosexual sex as a risk factor were unaware of their risk. As in men, PCP is the most frequent AIDS-defining diagnosis. Some opportunistic infections, including PCP, *Streptococcus pneumoniae* infection, esophageal thrush, and CMV colitis, are more common in women than in men. Candidal vaginitis is the most frequent symptom of early immunodeficiency and may occur in the presence of CD4 counts > 500 cells/μL. HIV-infected women also appear to have vaginal warts and cervical dysplasia (associated with human papilloma virus) both more frequently and more severely than noninfected women. Treatment with AZT during pregnancy and delivery plus 6 weeks of AZT for the newborn reduces the risk of maternal–infant transmission from 23% to 8%. For treatment of pregnant women, guidelines should be consulted and cesarean section should be considered.

24. When and how should advance care directives be discussed with HIV-infected patients?

The 100% mortality rate associated with an AIDS diagnosis impels a discussion of advance care directives so that the extent and type of end-stage care complies with the patient's wishes. This discussion is best initiated by a caring primary care provider within a long-term provider–patient relationship. Postponing the discussion until emergent hospital admission and expecting the admitting house officer (unfamiliar to the patient and subject to frequent distractions) to help the patient understand the issues needed to make an appropriate decision is a disservice to the patient. Physicians must accept the responsibility to anticipate situations in which a clear advance directive will improve patient care and initiate discussion of this issue in a timely manner. There is increasing discussion of physician-assisted suicide. More than 80% of patients who request physician assistance to end their lives do not commit suicide. The request is often a call for help in dealing with a range of issues related to end-stage disease and needs to be evaluated for its broader implications.

BIBLIOGRAPHY

1. Bartlett JG, Gallant JE (eds): 2001–2002 Medical Management of HIV Infection. Timonium, MD, H & N Printing & Graphics, 2001.
2. Burman WJ, Reves RR, Cohn DL: The case for conservative management of early HIV disease. JAMA 280:93–95, 1998.
3. Cohen OJ: Antiretroviral therapy: Time to think strategically. Ann Intern Med 132:320–322, 2000.
4. Deeks SG, Smith M, Holodny M, Kahn JO: HIV-1 protease inhibitors. JAMA 277:145–153, 1997.
5. Department of Health and Human Services: Guidelines for the use of antiretroviral agents in HIV-infected adults and adolescents. Available at http://www.hivatis.org/guidelines.
6. Hirsch MS, Brun-Vezinet F, D'Aquila RT, et al: Antiretroviral drug resistance testing in adult HIV-1 infection: Recommendations of an International AIDS Society—USA panel. JAMA 283:2417–2426, 2000.
7. Hogg RS, Yip B, Chan KJ, et al: Rates of disease progression by baseline CD4 cell count and viral load after initiating triple-drug therapy. JAMA 286:2568–2577, 2001.

8. Kobayashi JS: The evolution of adjustment issues in HIV/AIDS. Bull Menninger Clin 61:146–188, 1997.
9. Kovacs JA, Masur H: Prophylaxis against opportunistic infections in patients with human immunodeficiency virus infection. N Engl J Med 342:1416–1429, 2000.
10. Lee LM, Karon JM, Selik R, et al: Survival after AIDS diagnosis in adolescents and adults during the treatment era, United States, 1984–1997. JAMA 285:1308–1315, 2001.
11. Levine AM: Evaluation and management of HIV-infected women. Ann Intern Med 136:228–242, 2002.
12. Martinez E, Mocroft A, Garcia-Viejo MA, et al: Risk of lipodystrophy in HIV-1-infected patients treated with protease inhibitors: A prospective cohort study. Lancet 357:592–598, 2001.
13. Mellors JW, Munoz A, Giorgi JV, et al: Plasma viral load and CD4+ lymphocytes as prognostic markers of HIV-1 infection. Ann Intern Med 126:946–954, 1997.
14. Moore RD, Chaisson RE: Natural history of opportunistic disease in an HIV-infected urban clinical cohort. Ann Intern Med 124:633–642, 1996.
15. Price RW: Neurological complications of HIV infection. Lancet 348:445–452, 1996.
16. Samet JH, Muz P, Cabral P, et al: Dermatologic manifestations in HIV-infected patients: A primary care perspective. Mayo Clin Proc 74:658–660, 1999.
17. Sande MA, Volberding PA (eds): The Medical Management of AIDS, 6th ed. Philadelphia, W.B. Saunders, 1999.
18. Yeni PG, Hammer SM, Carpenter CCJ, et al: Antiretroviral treatment for adult HIV infection in 2002: Updated recommendations of the International AIDS Society—USA Panel. JAMA 288:222–235, 2002.

105. THE PATIENT WITH ANOREXIA OR WEIGHT LOSS

Lawrence G. Smith, M.D.

1. What is medically important weight loss?

Any degree of weight loss can be significant, but most experts define loss of 5% of body weight over 6 months as medically important if the patient was not on a reduced calorie diet or undergoing diuretic therapy. Greater amounts of weight loss are more often associated with serious disease.

2. When does anorexia need to be evaluated?

Anorexia without weight loss is rarely the result of serious disease. Side effects of medication, changes in taste, gastrointestinal (GI) and liver disease, or psychiatric conditions need to be considered. However, the basic evaluation of serious anorexia parallels that of unintentional weight loss. Organic disease is predicted by age > 50 years, absence of psychiatric symptoms, presence of anemia, smoking, or localizing symptoms.

3. Is it important to verify weight loss?

Weight loss is a common complaint to primary care physicians. More than 50% of such patients have been found not to have sustained significant weight loss and need no evaluation. Verifying weight loss is essential; methods include comparison with earlier weights, demonstration of change in clothing size, clear confirmation from friends or relatives, or visible signs of cachexia.

4. What are the major causes of weight loss?

The data in the table below combine several studies. Of note is that studies of inpatients showed a higher percentage of serious organic disease, whereas studies of outpatients showed a higher percentage of psychiatric disease.

Causes of Weight Loss*

CAUSE	RELATIVE FREQUENCY (%)	CAUSE	RELATIVE FREQUENCY (%)
Psychiatric disease	4	Hyperthyroid disease	2
Malignancy	22	Other severe physical disease	10
Gastrointestinal disease	11	Medication effects	3
Food intake disorders	4	No cause found	24

*Estimates compiled from four studies with a total of 407 patients.

5. Do patients with serious illnesses often present only with weight loss?

Although most serious illnesses, such as cancer, end-stage heart disease, chronic obstructive pulmonary disease, arthritis, and renal failure, are associated with significant involuntary weight loss, this loss usually occurs long after the disease is diagnosed. It is rare for someone to have weight loss from a serious organic illness that is not obvious at the time of evaluation.

6. Does occult malignancy present as weight loss?

Most studies have shown that malignancy is an uncommon cause of isolated weight loss, and occult malignancy is very rare. In all series, most malignancies were obvious at initial visits, and all were diagnosed by 6 months after the first evaluation. Extensive evaluations searching for occult malignancy are not appropriate in patients with weight loss.

7. What causes weight loss and increased appetite?

Few conditions truly produce the combination of weight loss and increased appetite. Possibilities include hyperthyroidism, diabetes mellitus, pheochromocytoma, and perhaps malabsorption syndromes. Psychiatric disorders such as schizophrenia, mania, or a primary eating disorder also need to be considered.

8. Why do patients not maintain adequate food intake?

Anorexia is not the only reason for inadequate food intake. Pain associated with eating, as in esophageal and gastric diseases, may lead to aversion of food. Dental problems, taste disorders, neurologic difficulties, medication side effects, social conditions, financial problems, and many other factors may contribute to poor nutrition. In evaluating poor food intake, an open-minded approach is important.

9. How extensive should the initial evaluation be?

Serious organic disease is usually obvious at the time of presentation. All studies emphasize the high sensitivity of a good history and physical examination. The table below shows a typical initial screening panel of laboratory studies.

Initial Screen for Weight Loss

- Complete history
- Complete physical examination, including mental status and functional assessment
- Complete blood count
- Sequential multiple analysis—12 tests
- Urinalysis
- Chest radiograph
- Stool—occult blood
- Upper GI series if abdominal symptoms are present
- Thyroid tests if symptoms are suggestive or patient is elderly

10. When should physicians look extensively for occult disease?

The answer is probably never. Occult serious disease is rare and usually becomes evident quickly on follow-up. Specifically, computed tomography (CT) scans to discover unsuspected problems have not proved useful in the setting of weight loss. The exception may be patients with a high level of alkaline phosphatase and low level of serum albumin; in one study, the incidence of positive findings was high in such patients. Because of the high incidence of GI disease, any symptoms should trigger a full evaluation.

11. Approximately 25% of patients with weight loss have no specific diagnosis. How long does follow-up need to be continued?

If no illness is obvious at 6 months, it is highly unlikely that the weight loss is caused by un-diagnosed organic disease. Serious social or psychiatric problems, however, may have been missed.

12. What psychiatric disorders are associated with weight loss?

Most studies show depression as the most common psychiatric disorder in all patients with weight loss and the most common diagnosis overall in outpatients with weight loss. In addition, schizophrenia, conversion disorder, and the primary eating disorders of anorexia nervosa and bulimia are seen occasionally. Addiction to drugs and alcohol also may present with profound weight loss.

13. How are primary eating disorders recognized?

Patients with eating disorders are typically young adult white women of middle to upper so-cioeconomic class. Bulimic patients present at an older age than patients with anorexia nervosa. Symptoms are vague and usually result from weight loss (e.g., amenorrhea, fatigue, weakness) or vomiting (e.g., electrolyte abnormalities). Patients rarely seek help on their own and, despite being thin, perceive themselves as overweight. They are at risk for life-threatening problems from weight loss and vomiting. Bulimics frequently also abuse laxatives and diuretics. A team approach with psychiatric evaluation and nutritional support is essential.

14. What social conditions may present as weight loss?

Poverty, isolation, lack of transportation, and inability to cook or shop for food are some of the social problems associated with significant weight loss. If suspicion is high, a social service referral and a home visit may be valuable.

15. Are elderly patients of special concern?

Decreasing functional states, dementia, stroke, and decreasing taste for and interest in food are some of the geriatric problems that account for weight loss. A careful neurologic examina-tion, Mini-Mental Status evaluation, functional assessment, and screening for depression are par-ticularly useful in elderly individuals. Because hypothyroidism may present in its apathetic form in elderly patients, routine thyroid function studies are probably in order. Elderly people are also particularly susceptible to the anorectic side effects of medication. Nursing home residents are particularly prone to depression manifesting with significant weight loss.

16. Is weight loss a normal occurrence of aging?

It is true that most community-dwelling elderly patients show a gradual loss of weight at the extremes of age. However, studies have shown that the typical change in body weight is 0.5% per year. Weight loss > 5% almost always indicates a serious problem. Weight loss has been de-scribed as one of the earliest findings of dementia in community-dwelling adults along with other neurologic and psychological problems.

CONTROVERSIES

17. Does forced feeding benefit patients when weight loss is caused by serious organic illness?

Despite many clinical trials, especially among patients with terminal cancer, attempting to reverse cachexia with forced feeding, including total parenteral nutrition, has shown little evidence of overall benefit. Transient weight gain has been reported but without consistent benefit to functional status or survival.

18. Are medications effective in the weight loss associated with serious systemic illness?

Several interventions, including introgastric and parenteral nutrition as well as drug treatment with cyproheptadine and anabolic steroids, have failed to pass scientific scrutiny. However, several drugs have been evaluated in placebo-controlled trials and have shown to be effective in improving appetite, sense of well-being, and body mass in patients with cancer and AIDS. Examples include metoclopramide, megestrol acetate, corticosteroids (especially dexamethasone), and delta-9-tetrahydrocannabinol (THC).

BIBLIOGRAPHY

1. Barrett-Connor E, Edelstein S, Corey-Bloom J, et al: Weight loss precedes dementia in community-dwelling older adults. J Am Geriatr Soc 44:1147–1152, 1996.
2. Bilbao-Garay J, Barba R, Losa-Garcia JE, et al: Assessing clinical probability of organic disease in patients with involuntary weight loss: a simple score. Eur J Intern Med 13:240–245, 2002.
3. Bouras EP, Lange SM, Scolapio JS: Rational approach to patients with unintentional weight loss. Mayo Clin Proc 76:923–929, 2001.
4. Coodley G, Loveless M, Merrill T: The HIV wasting syndrome: A review. J Acquir Immune Defic Syndr 7:681–694, 1994.
5. Garfinkel P, Garner D, Kaplan A, et al: Differential diagnosis of emotional disorders that cause weight loss. Can Med Assoc J 129:939–945, 1983.
6. Huffman GB: Evaluating and treating unintentional weight loss in the elderly. Am Fam Physician 65:640–650, 2002.
7. Marton K, Sox H, Krupp J: Involuntary weight loss: Diagnostic and prognostic significance. Ann Intern Med 95:568–574, 1981.
8. McKinley M, Goodman-Black J, Lesser M, et al: Improved body weight status as a result of nutrition intervention in adult, HIV-positive outpatients. J Am Diet Assoc 94:1014–1017, 1994.
9. Nelson K, Walsh D, Sheehan F: The cancer anorexia-cachexia syndrome. J Clin Oncol 12:213–225, 1994.
10. Rabinovitz M, Pitlik S, Leifer M, et al: Unintentional weight loss. Arch Intern Med 146:186–187, 1986.
11. Reife C: Involuntary weight loss. Med Clin North Am 79:299–313, 1995.
12. Sullivan D, Martin W, Flaxman N, Hagen J: Oral health problems and involuntary weight loss in a population of frail elderly. J Am Geriatr Soc 41:725–731, 1983.
13. Thompson M, Morris L: Unexplained weight loss in the ambulatory elderly. J Am Geriatr Soc 39:498–500, 1991.
14. Von Roenn J: Management of HIV-related body weight loss. Drugs 47:774–783, 1994.
15. Wallace J, Schwartz R, LaCroix A, et al: Involuntary weight loss in older outpatients: Incidence and clinical significance. J Am Geriatr Soc 43:329–337, 1995.
16. Wise G, Craig D: Evaluation of involuntary weight loss. Where do you start? Postgrad Med 95:143–146, 149–150, 1994.

106. THE PATIENT WITH CANCER

Juan C. Iregui, M.D.

1. What pitfalls should be avoided in telling a patient that he or she has cancer?

Breaking the news to a patient newly diagnosed with cancer is one of the most challenging tasks encountered in clinical practice. The good news is that it is a learnable skill that requires awareness of a few simple principles that can be easily implemented in a busy practice. Remember that patients' dissatisfaction with their doctors' communication skills far outweighs any dissatisfaction with technical competence (e.g., the doctor who does not listen or appears not to listen, the doctor who uses jargon, the doctor who talks down to the patient).

The first principle is to provide the right physical setting for the interview. Privacy is essential. If possible, take the patient or relative to a separate room. If no room is available, close the doors of your office or, in an inpatient setting, pull the curtains closed. Find out who the patient wants to be present when the results become available; some patients want a relative or friend to be with them during the interview. The next step—and probably the most important rule for all important communications by health care professionals—is to sit down.

Once you and the family are comfortably settled, explore what the patient understands about what is wrong (e.g., "Before we go over the results, it would help me to know what you have been told about your medical situation so far" or "What is you understanding of the reasons we did the MRI?"). Knowledge of the gap between what the patient believes is happening and medical reality helps to tailor the discussion and anticipate the patient's emotional reaction.

Once you are ready to break the news, give the information in small chunks and gently bring the patient's perception of the situation as close to the medical facts as you know them. Use empathic responses to deal with the patient's emotions. For example, if a patient cries, move closer and offer a tissue. This strategy gives the patient overt permission to cry as well as a means to restore his or her face—and it gives you something to do if you feel embarrassed. Touch the patient only if both of you are comfortable with contact.

Make sure that you reinforce and clarify the information frequently. Repeat important points, and use diagrams and written or recorded materials. If you cannot answer a question, don't try. Instead, assist the patient in framing the questions and help him or her obtain information elsewhere.

One of the most difficult questions to answer is "How long do I have?" The basic rule of thumb is to find out what the patient means. Many patients want to know whether they will be around for specific events, such as weddings, graduations, or trips. Stay away from hard figures; you are very likely to be wrong. Many studies have shown that doctors are highly inaccurate in predicting survival. If the patient insists on a figure, use ranges rather than a single figure (e.g., "We may be looking at several weeks or a matter of months"). Also use the survival rates published in the literature, taking into account that the patient's performance status at the time of diagnosis is as important as staging of the tumor in predicting survival. Always acknowledge uncertainty, and verbalize that you are likely to be wrong to avoid future conflicts. Sometimes the best advice that you can give the patient is to hope for the best while preparing for the worst. This approach emphasizes the importance of dealing with personal matters early during the disease, particularly if loss of decision-making capacity is anticipated with progression of the disease.

Finally, at the end of the interview, summarize the important facts for the patient, and put together a plan that includes a combination of your agenda and the patient's concerns. This is an excellent opportunity to show the patient that you have been listening and that you have heard the main concerns and issues. Many patients fear abandonment by their physicians when they are diagnosed with cancer. If part of the treatment implies referrals to other physicians, reassure the patient that you will be available during the whole process and that you will continue caring for his or her other medical needs.

2. When a patient presents with a metastatic cancer of unknown primary site, what are the appropriate diagnostic tests to consider?

Although the initial impulse is to perform "head-to-toe" scans and endoscopic procedures in search of the primary origin, this approach has a low yield and does not improve outcomes. For the majority of patients who present with widespread carcinoma for which no obvious primary site is apparent, a complete history and physical examination (including pelvic and rectal exams) should be followed by a chest radiograph, a mammogram in women, and laboratory tests and radiographs designed to investigate symptoms or abnormal signs. Once a possible site is identified, every effort should be made to obtain a tissue diagnosis. The intervention to be planned will be based almost exclusively on the pathologic findings. Immunohistochemical stains performed on biopsy (e.g., common leukocyte antigen for leukemia and lymphoma, cytokeratin for carcinomas, vimentin for sarcoma, melanoma, and lymphoma), cytogenetic studies (e.g., estrogen/progesterone receptors and *Her-2/neu* overexpression for breast cancer, *K-ras* mutation for adenocarcinoma of the bone, B-cell/T-cell markers and *bcl-2* overexpression for lymphomas), and, occasionally, serum marker studies are used to determine the primary site.

Prostate-specific antigen is the only serum marker that is used in screening, staging, treatment evaluation, and follow-up of men with prostate cancer. Other markers, such as carcinoembryonic antigen, CA125, CA 27-29, Ca 19-9, alpha fetoprotein, and the beta-human chorionic gonadotropin (hCG) subunit should not be used in routine screening for malignancy of unknown origin because they have low sensitivity and specificity. However, in certain circumstances (e.g., medial chest lesions, beta-hCG), they are quite helpful.

Currently available treatments are limited, and the prognosis for this group of patients is usually dismal. Some might be candidates for ongoing clinical trials that have shown some success. Patients should be referred early after diagnosis, particularly if they have good performance status.

3. How should analgesics be initiated in patients with cancer?

The World Health Organization (WHO) recommends a simple and effective three-step process or ladder for titrating pharmacologic therapy; this approach provides effective pain relief for more than 90% of patients with cancer.

Step one is to use acetaminophen, aspirin, or other nonsteroidal anti-inflammatory drugs (NSAIDs) for relief of mild-to-moderate pain.

Step two is implemented when pain persists or increases and consists of adding a weak opioid such as codeine or hydrocodone to the NSAID for additive analgesia. Combination tablets are available and should be administered on an around-the-clock basis with additional as-needed booster doses to control breakthrough pain. When higher doses of codeine or hydrocodone are needed, separate dosage forms of the opioid and nonopioid are used to avoid the adverse side effects of high-dose acetaminophen and other NSAIDs.

Step three is to replace a weak opioid with a more potent opioid, such as morphine or hydromorphone, if pain persists or worsens.

Patients who at presentation to the physician are experiencing moderate-to-severe pain (intensity of 5 or 6 on the pain scale ranging from 0 to 10) are usually started at the second or third step of the ladder. Adjuvant drugs or coanalgesics (medications that have analgesic properties for specific types of pain even though they are usually not considered pain relievers, such as antidepressants, anticonvulsants, and steroids) may be used at any one of the steps to enhance analgesia or treat concurrent symptoms.

4. Summarize the general principles of pain management.

1. Use scheduled doses of analgesics. Provide a rescue dose of a short-acting opioid for control of breakthrough pain. This dose should be 10% of the total daily opioid dose and may be given every 1–2 hours as needed.

2. To assess and manage the patient's pain, use a pain scale. Adjust the dose frequently. The goal is to control the pain to a tolerable level within a few hours, if possible.

3. Follow patients closely, particularly when beginning or changing analgesics. Watch for the development of tolerance, and treat appropriately.

4. The oral route for analgesics is preferred.

5. Physicians are more likely to underestimate and undertreat pain in women, children, elderly patients, patients with a history of drug abuse, and Hispanic and black patients.

6. Follow the WHO three-step approach to pharmacologic pain management. Remember the different types of pain, and modify your therapeutic approach accordingly.

7. Prescribe a laxative whenever you use opioids. An antiemetic may be needed initially for opioid-naïve patients and when opioids are increased or rotated. Other less frequent but sometimes distressing narcotic side effects include urinary retention, pruritus, excessive sweating, and myoclonic jerking. Reassurance may be all that is necessary for the last three; urinary retention occasionally requires use of a urinary catheter.

8. Address common misconceptions about the use of opioids for treatment of pain. Many patients believe that opioids are dangerous and addictive, can shorten life, and are used only as a

last resort. Emphasize that opioids are safe, rarely if ever cause addiction in patients suffering from pain, and are the mainstay of pain treatment.

5. What is the maximal dose for opioids?

No evidence suggests the existence of a specific maximal dose. The maximal dose is whatever is required to achieve analgesia in an individual patient. Physiologic tolerance is an expected outcome of chronic opioid use and should be anticipated. Patients may require hundreds, even thousands, of milligrams per day, yet remain awake and even ambulatory. Respiratory depression and somnolence are rarely significant problems because of the rapid development of tolerance in the vast majority of patients. However, even if respiratory depression occurs, it may be viewed as a secondary effect and should not lead to hesitation on the part of the provider to use whatever dose is needed to control terminal pain or discomfort. Naloxone should be avoided in patients taking chronic narcotics because it precipitates immediate narcotic withdrawal symptoms and causes extreme pain and suffering.

6. Summarize the dosage equivalents for various narcotics.

ANALGESIC	ORAL DOSE (mg)	PARENTERAL DOSE (mg)
Morphine	30	10
Meperidine	300	75
Oxycodone (IR)*	20	NA
Oxycodone (SR)*	20	NA
Methadone	20	10
Hydromorphone	7.5	1.5
Levorphanol	2	1
Fentanyl patch[†]	NA	25 µg/hr

NA = not applicable, IR = immediate-release, SR = slow-release.
*Oxycodone is available primarily in combination with acetaminophen or aspirin. Recently IR and SR forms of oxycodone alone became available.
[†] Fentanyl patch dose is equivalent to 10–20 mg/day of parenteral morphine or 30–60 mg/day of oral morphine.

7. Summarize the properties of morphine sulfate, methadone, and fentanyl.

Morphine sulfate
Available routes of administration:
Oral, sublingual
Slow-release oral pill
Rectal
Intravenous, intramuscular, subcutaneous
Intrathecal
Intraventricular
Slow-release pills
8-, 12-, or 24-hour duration of analgesia
Ease of administration
Can be given rectally
Expensive

Methadone
Variable duration of analgesia
Duration of analgesia not equivalent to duration of sedating effects because of accumulation of metabolites
Cheap
Not cross-reactive in morphine-allergic patients

Fentanyl
Routes: topical (dermal absorptive) or intravenous
New product (Duralgesic): fentanyl transdermal patch
Excellent alternative to morphine infusion in patients unable to swallow
Expensive (but not as much as intravenous morphine)
Slow onset of action, depot effect in subcutaneous tissue, and variable rate of absorption

8. What pain syndromes occur in patients with cancer? How do they affect therapy?

Three types of pain can be recognized as separate syndromes requiring somewhat different management strategies:

Somatic or musculoskeletal pain arises from skin and subcutaneous tissues, bone, muscle, blood vessels, and connective tissue (e.g., arthritis, bone metastasis). It is constant, dull, and aching, increases with movement, and is localized to the area of the lesion. When somatic pain originates from bone metastases, the frequently associated inflammation may respond well to anti-inflammatory drugs. Combinations of opioids with anti-inflammatory drugs usually provide pain relief for the vast majority of patients.

Visceral pain arises from organs and the lining of body cavities (e.g., myocardial ischemia, liver metastasis); it is poorly localized, deep, cramping, twisting, or tearing. It may result from compression of autonomic nervous pathways, as in deep-seated tumors of the abdomen, or from obstruction of bowel or other visceral organs. This pain is often associated with other unpleasant sensations, such as nausea and vomiting. Opioids are the mainstay of treatment, usually at higher doses.

Neuropathic pain arises from peripheral nerves, the spinal cord, and the central nervous system; it is described as burning, sharp, shooting, tingling, electrical, or shock-like. Neuropathic pain is the most distressing and least responsive to opioids. Adjunctive medications such as tricyclic antidepressants or anticonvulsants are often needed. Corticosteroids as an adjunct to analgesics may be useful in both somatic and neuropathic pain syndromes. Opioids are less successful unless they are combined with tricyclics or anticonvulsants.

9. How are pharmacologic adjuncts to analgesics used to improve pain control in patients with malignancy?

1. Nonsteroidal anti-inflammatory agents may be used at standard doses as part of the treatment of bone pain due to malignancy.

2. Nortriptyline, desipramine, amitriptyline, imipramine, and doxepin at one-tenth to one-half the doses used for antidepressant effects may be prescribed for neuropathic pain, sleep, and depression associated with a diagnosis of cancer.

3. Lancinating pain and neuropathic pain may be treated with carbamazepine at 100–200 mg orally 2 or 3 times daily. Other anticonvulsants also have been used successfully.

4. Corticosteroids have been used at high doses (e.g., dexamethasone, 8–40 mg/day) for control of brain edema and resultant headaches and for nerve root or spinal cord compression symptoms. At low doses (e.g., dexamethasone, 0.75 mg/day, or prednisone, 10–20 mg/day) corticosteroids are sometimes helpful in treating pain from diffuse bone metastases or visceral pain from deep-seated intraabdominal tumors.

5. Antihistamines, cannabinoids, and amphetamines have been reported anecdotally to help alleviate pain.

6. Topical drugs, such as local anesthetics applied to ulcers or capsaicin cream applied to painful or dysesthetic intact skin, may be helpful.

7. Pamidronate, an intravenous biphosphonate that directly inhibits osteoclast activity, has been shown in randomized trials to improve bone pain significantly and to reduce skeletal fractures in patients with multiple myeloma and breast cancer metastatic to bone with lytic lesions.

10. Should any drugs be avoided in the management of cancer pain?

Mixed narcotic agonist–antagonist drugs, such as pentazocine (Talwin), should be avoided. Meperidine given orally has poor bioavailability. Parenteral meperidine is somewhat useful for acute pain, but the duration of action is too short for chronic pain; long-acting metabolites may cause confusion and precipitate seizures. Benzodiazepines as an adjunct to cancer pain may paradoxically sedate the patient enough to prevent the expression of pain but do little to abate the sensations.

11. How should the cancer patient with back pain be assessed?

Back pain in a patient with cancer is considered spinal cord compression until proven otherwise. Spinal cord compression is truly a medical emergency, and the overall outcome is influenced most directly by the patient's neurologic status at the time when treatment is initiated. With vertebral involvement, the metastatic tumor most often compresses the anterior (ventral) aspect of the dural sac. The most common symptom is pain, which usually increases in intensity with coughing, sneezing, or straining. After a few weeks of persistent pain (usually with no abnormal physical exam findings except perhaps for percussion tenderness over the affected vertebral body), weakness and sensory loss develop, followed rapidly first by urinary retention and constipation, then by paraplegia and loss of bowel and bladder continence. Once neurologic symptoms begin, progression to complete and permanent paraplegia may take only a few hours or days.

If the patient is treated while he or she is still ambulatory, the probability of remaining ambulatory is 89–94%. If the patient becomes paraparetic before therapy, the probability of regaining the ability to ambulate is only 39–51%. If the patient becomes paralyzed, the probability of regaining ambulation decreases to 10%.

12. Which malignancies most commonly metastasize to the spine?

The malignancies that most commonly metastasize to the spine are cancers of the lung, breast, and prostate; myeloma; lymphoma; and renal-cell carcinoma. Most often spinal cord compression occurs in a patient with a known cancer, but it is not uncommonly the presenting symptom of malignancy. The location of cord compression is most often the thoracic spine (70%), followed by the lumbar (20%) and cervical (10%) spines. More than one area of spine may be involved, and several locations may threaten the cord. Compression most often results from a mass that begins in the vertebral body or neural arch and extends into the spinal canal, compressing the epidural space. More rarely a tumor may form in the epidural or intradural spaces without bone involvement.

13. What should you do if a patient with cancer develops signs of cord compression?

Any patient with cancer and signs of cord compression requires immediate treatment, followed by imaging of the suspected area of involved spine and spinal cord. Intravenous dexamethasone should be given (10–20 mg) with a 4-mg dose repeated every 4–6 hours while immediate neurologic, neurosurgical, and oncologic consultations are arranged and before imaging studies are done. Some authors recommend high-dose dexamethasone for patients with impaired function of the spinal cord or cauda equina and patients with a high-grade radiologic lesion (100-mg intravenous bolus followed by 24 mg orally 4 times/day for 3 days, to be tapered over 10 days).

In patients with back pain and a plain film of the spine consistent with metastasis, the probability of invasion of the epidural space is approximately 70%. The presence of radiculopathy raises the probability to 90%. Emergency magnetic resonance imaging (MRI) is indicated in such patients, even when the neurologic exam is completely normal, especially in the presence of tenderness to spinal percussion. Some authors recommend MRI of the entire spine at presentation to rule out more than one epidural site affected by the tumor that needs to be included in the radiation field.

Once the diagnosis of spinal cord compression is confirmed, certain factors influence the choice of treatment. In general, radiation therapy is the treatment of choice for tumors known to be radiosensitive (e.g., lymphoma, cancer of the breast, prostate, and lung). Chemotherapy is indicated in chemotherapy-sensitive tumors and for relapse of cord compression after resection or radiation therapy. Finally, patients with pathologic vertebral fractures with instability, patients with tumors known to be radioresistant (e.g., renal cell, sarcoma, unknown primary), and patients with no response to or relapse after radiation therapy should be considered for vertebral resection (laminectomy alone has led to disappointing results).

14. What should be considered in a patient with cancer and change in mental status?

The patient with cancer who presents with a mental status change, either directly or by corroborative history from the caregiver, should undergo a careful neurologic examination. In the presence of focal abnormalities or complaints of headache, a structural cause should be assumed; however, many patients with structural central nervous system lesions have no focal findings on exam. Evaluation consists of metabolic screening laboratory tests, review of drug therapy, and an imaging study of the central nervous system (lumbar puncture, if indicated).

15. What is the most common metabolic paraneoplastic syndrome? How is it treated?

Hypercalcemia is the most frequent metabolic abnormality in patients with cancer. Symptoms of a high level of serum calcium include confusion, nausea, constipation, polydipsia, and polyuria. It is commonly associated with non–small-cell lung cancer, breast cancer, multiple myeloma, and bladder and prostate cancer. Malignancy-related hypercalcemia, even for patients with extensive bone metastases, is mediated locally by proteins produced by malignant cells that lead to bone destruction. Even in patients with known malignancy, adequate work-up for causes of hypercalcemia should be ordered, particularly during the first episode.

Once a diagnosis of cancer-related hypercalcemia is made, it is important to start therapy with vigorous hydration with normal saline at a rate of 200–400 mL/hr, as dictated by the patient's underlying cardiac status. Furosemide should be used cautiously. Pamidronate is the treatment of choice for most patients and may be safely given on an outpatient basis over 3–5 hours at a dose of 60–90 mg by vein. Its effects begin within 24–48 hours and last 3–6 weeks. Other less successful or more toxic options include gallium nitrate, plicamycin, calcitonin, and oral diphosphonates.

16. What are the common causes of dyspnea in a patient with cancer?

Patients with cancer are at risk for **pulmonary embolism**. A hypercoagulable state accompanies adenocarcinomas, particularly carcinoma of the prostate, pancreas, and breast. Patients with breast cancer who undergo chemotherapy are at especially high risk for thromboembolic events. Other patients at extremely high risk are adults with primary brain tumors.

The **superior vena cava (SVC) syndrome** usually presents with dyspnea as well as facial and arm swelling, conjunctival edema, venous engorgement on the chest wall or in the neck, and, on rare occasions, somnolence. The SVC may be blocked by extrinsic pressure, intravascular invasion, or thrombosis from an indwelling catheter, usually in association with lung carcinoma, mediastinal lymphomas, germ-cell cancer, and occasionally breast cancer. SVC syndrome is a diagnosis easily made by physical examination and chest radiograph; invasive studies are rarely necessary, and it is rarely a true emergency. If SVC syndrome is the first evidence of malignancy, empirical therapy with radiation or chemotherapy should not be initiated in the absence of a tissue diagnosis. Maintaining the patient in an upright posture is the most important initial step in management; occasionally gentle diuresis may help control the symptoms. Depending on the underlying tumor type, treatment may be radiation or chemotherapy; anticoagulation is recommended only when catheter-induced thrombosis leads to SVC syndrome.

Pleural and pericardial effusions caused by malignant studding of the serosal surface or by mediastinal lymphatic obstruction are also common causes of dyspnea. Lung, breast, and ovarian cancers are common causes of effusions, but lymphomas, leukemias, and many other tumors may involve the pleura or pericardium. A pleural effusion large enough to cause dyspnea is usually quite apparent on exam and chest radiograph. A pericardial effusion requires a higher index of suspicion. Patients with dyspnea and tachycardia with no other explanation should be carefully evaluated for both pericardial effusion and pulmonary embolus. Treatment includes drainage of the effusions while treatment of the underlying malignancy is started. If reaccumulation is anticipated, pleurodesis or pericardial window should be performed.

17. Describe the practical approach to the outpatient who is undergoing treatment for cancer and whose white blood cell counts are decreasing.

The majority of cancer therapy is safely given in an outpatient setting. One result is that many patients experience iatrogenic myelosuppression at home. Most chemotherapy regimens have a predictable peak time of cell death, which usually starts 7–10 days after drug administration and lasts for a few days. If a patient develops absolute granulocytopenia (< 500) but feels well and remains afebrile, no intervention is needed. The Infectious Diseases Society of America recommends against prophylactic antibiotics in patients with neutropenia without fever because of the lack of evidence that they improve end-points for morbidity and mortality. On the other hand, some data show an increase in the incidence of infections with resistant pathogens.

Patients should be instructed to check their temperature twice a day and to report fevers or symptoms of infection. The counts should be repeated daily or every other day until the absolute granulocyte count (AGC) increases above 1000. Patients with moderate fever and moderately low granulocyte counts (i.e., 500–1000) or patients who are "on the rise" probably can be safely placed on a broad-spectrum oral antibiotic but should be checked frequently.

18. When are empirical antibiotics used in patients with cancer? What is the rationale for their use?

Empirical antibiotics are now considered standard treatment for febrile granulocytopenic cancer patients. The risk is greatest for patients with a rapid decline in absolute neutrophil count, patients with neutrophil counts < 100 granulocytes/mL^3 of blood, and patients with protracted neutropenia (longer than 7–10 days).

Interventions such as chemotherapy not only decrease the number of neutrophils but also result in chemotactic and phagocytic defects. Breakdown of skin and mucosal barriers, which can result in bacteremia, often results from chemotherapy, radiation, peripheral and central intravenous lines, surgery, or tumor invasion. Mucositis develops throughout the alimentary system, and seeding of the bloodstream with endogenous flora in the gastrointestinal tract is believed to explain a majority of febrile neutropenic episodes. Obstruction of the lymphatics, biliary tract, and gastrointestinal or urinary systems by tumors or as a result of surgical procedures can also cause infections.

Granulocytopenia is defined as < 500 granulocytes/mL^3 of blood. The AGC is calculated by multiplying the total leukocyte count by the added percentage of neutrophils plus bands; it is also often referred to as the absolute neutrophil count (ANC). Granulocytopenic patients are at particular risk for spontaneous bacteremia. Historically, gram-negative bacilli, particularly *Pseudomonas aeruginosa,* were the most commonly identified pathogens. More recently there has been an increase in gram-positive infections. Of great concern is the increasing frequency of antibiotic-resistant organisms, including coagulase-negative staphylococci, methicillin-resistant *Staphylococcus aureus,* vancomycin-resistant enterococci, and penicillin-resistant *Streptococcus pneumoniae,* in addition to an increased prevalence of systemic fungal infections, particularly in patients with prolonged neutropenia and antibiotic use.

19. Which empirical antibiotics are appropriate?

Numerous antibiotic regimens have been studied as initial empirical therapy in febrile neutropenia, but none has been shown to be clearly superior. Most regimens fall into one of three categories: (1) monotherapy with ceftazidime, imipenem, meropenem, or cefepime, (2) double coverage with a beta-lactam and an aminoglycoside, or (3) double beta-lactams. No study has shown clear benefit with use of initial double coverage compared with monotherapy, and toxicity was increased in the combined therapy group, particularly when an aminoglycoside was used. Currently the initial approach is monotherapy with ceftazidime, imipenem, meropenem, or cefepime. Carbopenems are probably better than ceftazidime when the source of the fever is unknown, in patients who have received prophylactic antibiotics (particularly quinolones), in patients with severe neutropenia (ANC < 100 cells/mL), and in bone marrow transplant recipients. Antimicrobials with anaerobic coverage should also be considered, depending on the suspected source of infection. Ceftazidime as monotherapy can be used in stable patients who are at lower risk.

The addition of vancomycin should be considered in patients who are hemodynamically unstable on presentation, patients with severe mucositis, and patients with catheter site infection. The incidence of fungal infection (especially with *Candida* or *Aspergillus* species) increases with prolonged neutropenia; therefore, empirical antifungal therapy (e.g., amphotericin B) is recommended for patients with persistent fever despite 5 days of empirical antibiotics. Alternative amphotericin preparations or newer antifungals may be considered in patients at high risk for adverse reactions, especially nephrotoxicity, and in patients who are intolerant of or failed to respond to amphotericin B desoxycholate.

20. What is the role of nutritional support in the management of patients with cancer?

Several studies addressing the use of artificial nutrition in patients with cancer have shown no benefit except when the intervention is temporary and has specific goals. Such scenarios usually occur early in the course of illness when the patient is unable to eat or absorb food because of gastrointestinal disease due to cancer or its treatment (e.g., surgery, radiation- or chemotherapy-induced mucositis). In these scenarios the intervention is implemented because of anticipated reversibility of the underlying condition. The enteral route should be tried first, whenever possible, because parenteral nutrition has no advantages over enteral nutrition and is associated with more complications.

Food and water have great symbolic significance for patients and family members, who may ask for enteral or parenteral nutrition because they associate lack of intake with weakness or lethargy. In fact, for unclear reasons, patients in whom some nutritional parameters were improved by artificial nutrition showed no significant increase in strength or energy. For the patient with profound anorexia due to advanced cancer, being forced to eat is often burdensome and intrusive. This common end-of-life symptom may be an adaptive mechanism. Education of patients and family members as well as health care workers is crucial. Families must be helped to understand the lack of benefit and the potential harm of forced nutrition in a terminally ill patient. No effective appetite stimulant has yet been identified for cancer-associated anorexia.

21. Which patients with cancer are at risk for carrying a genetic defect?

Breast cancer occurs in approximately 12% of women who live to age 90. The most important risk factor for the development of breast cancer is a strong family history. A family history of breast cancer, however, is not synonymous with an inherited genetic mutation. Only 5–10% of all breast cancers are associated with inherited genetic mutations, such as mutations in *BRCA1* and *BRCA2,* which are autosomal dominant genes that act as tumor suppressors. Deleterious mutations to these genes interfere with their function and account for the majority of genetically related breast cancers. Pedigree studies have shown that families with multiple members who have breast or ovarian cancer, particularly at an early age, are at increased risk for carrying a genetic mutation.

Several different tools developed by the National Cancer Institute, the American Society of Clinical Oncology, and others are commercially available for risk stratification. Once a patient has been found to have a significant risk (10% is considered significant by the American Society of Clinical Oncology) of having a mutation in a breast cancer susceptibility gene, adequate counseling should be done before the test is ordered.

Hallmarks of a family with a possible cancer syndrome are early onset, three or more first-degree relatives with the same cancer, bilateral cancers in paired organs, and a pattern consistent with autosomal dominant inheritance. Families with a suspected familial cancer syndrome are best served by referral to a specialized center with oncologic and genetic expertise.

22. What are the major types of problems to expect in long-term survivors of successful cancer treatment?

1. **Social adjustments** are frequent in survivors of cancer. Many report problems with obtaining employment and with eligibility for health or life insurance. Many patients experience long-term anxiety about the possibility of relapse, especially at the time of visits to the doctor.

2. **Persistent physical problems** include sexual dysfunction manifesting as ejaculatory disturbances in men and vaginal dryness that leads to dyspareunia in women; infertility in both men and women; fibrosis or inflammation in irradiated areas or surgical scars; growth retardation and learning problems in children; cataracts in recipients of head or whole-body radiation; cardiomyopathy in persons treated with cardiotoxic drugs or chest radiation; accelerated atherosclerosis in radiation fields; and hypertension, Raynaud's phenomenon, and hypercholesterolemia in survivors of testicular cancer.

3. **Higher risk for the development of another cancer** or for second malignancies that are treatment-induced. Early after chemotherapy (< 5 years) for various cancers (best described af-

ter Hodgkin's disease), about 5% of patients develop chemotherapy-induced acute myelogenous leukemia or a myelodysplastic disorder. Patients treated with radiation, particularly in childhood or young adulthood, are at risk for second radiation-induced cancers in the treated areas. These second cancers may not begin to appear until the second or third decade after treatment.

23. Discuss the role of palliative care medicine in the management of cancer patients.

Palliative care is an interdisciplinary collaboration that focuses on patient-defined goals of care, relief of patient distress, and relief of family distress extending into the bereavement period after the patient's death. The concept of suffering in palliative care requires not only adequate knowledge of the physiopathology of the patient's disease but also an understanding of how the patient experiences his or her disease (e.g., how the disease affects body image, what the illness means to the patient and his or her family, how the disease affects spiritual beliefs). A study of bone marrow transplant recipients showed how psychological and social variables are significant predictors of the pain level after transplantation, emphasizing how the perception of discomfort is highly individualized and constructed by patients.

Among the several domain-based assessment tools that account for the variability of burden and preferences at the end of life, one of the simplest and most practical is the **PEACE Tool**, which assesses six domains:

- **P** = **P**hysical symptoms (e.g., pain, anorexia, incontinence, nausea and other gastrointestinal symptoms, dyspnea, cough, ulcerations, level of functioning, side effects of drugs)
- **E** = **E**motive (and cognitive) symptoms (e.g., sadness, anxiety, grief)
- **A** = **A**utonomy-related issues (e.g., Are we doing all of and only the things that you desire? Have you named a decision-maker? Do you know what to expect of your illness?)
- **C** = **C**ommunication, **C**ontribution to others, and **C**losure of life affairs (e.g., Is there anyone whom you have not seen in a long time and need to talk to? What would be left unfinished if you died today?)
- **E** = **E**conomic burden and other practical issues (e.g., Has your illness created a financial burden for you and your family? Do you have your financial affairs in order?)
- **T** = **T**ranscendental and existential issues (e.g., Is faith or spirituality important to you in this illness? What do you think will happen to you after death? Would you like a visit from the chaplain?)

Assessment of patients along several domains helps elucidate the nature of their suffering and facilitates the involvement of other members of the palliative care team.

24. How can we discuss palliative care while disease-remitting treatments are continued?

Early in the course of the disease, many patients choose to undergo surgery, chemotherapy, or other disease-oriented treatments; patients may trade short-term discomfort for the prospect of longer survival or a better quality of life. As the disease progresses, however, many patients decide not to make such trade-offs and choose palliation as the paramount goal of care.

Unfortunately, many doctors focus discussions with their patients solely on clinical decisions that need to be made while disease-remitting treatments are being implemented and typically talk about palliative care only after a decision to limit life-prolonging interventions has been made. This approach has resulted in the misconception that palliative care equals low-technology care at home.

Missed opportunities commonly encountered to introduce the topic of palliation include (1) when the patient is healthy and advanced directives are discussed during routine medical visits; (2) when the patient is facing the loss of a close relative, particularly when the patient has witnessed unnecessary suffering of loved ones; (3) when the patient has recently been in the hospital; (4) when therapies are ineffective or very burdensome; and (5) when the disease has progressed despite curative attempts.

Discussing palliative care with patients is useful throughout the course of serious, progressive chronic illness, because the patient's condition, needs, and concerns may change. At each visit, routinely ask open-ended questions to determine the patient's needs and suffering (e.g., Are you having discomfort or suffering that bothers you or limits what you do? How is treatment going for you and your family?). Physicians should take a *both/and* instead of an *either/or* approach to palliative and disease-oriented care. Relieving pain, promoting quality of life, and attending to the psychosocial aspects of illness are valid goals of care from the time of diagnosis until the bereavement period, during which the physician still has an opportunity to assist family members as they face loss. Discussion about palliative care can be put into the context of exploring patient and family concerns about the future and helping the patient retain control of his or her care.

Recent legal decisions about physician-assisted suicide have received widespread coverage in the lay and professional press. Patients with cancer may ask the physician's opinion about this issue or even request such a service. Ideally, this issue should never require implementation. A physician who is uncomfortable providing adequate symptom control to patients with terminal illness should consider referring the patient for evaluation, ideally by an interdisciplinary team (e.g., hospice). Physician-assisted suicide is not an appropriate surrogate for adequate pain and symptom control.

25. What is hospice?

For many patients and physicians, the term *hospice* means a place to go to die after the physician signs a form certifying a prognosis of less than 6 months of life. This misinterpretation persists, even though the majority of patients enrolled in hospice programs live in their own homes until they die. More than 80% of Americans polled in one survey indicated that they would like to die at home if they knew they had a life-threatening illness.

In reality, the word *hospice* is used in the United States to describe four different concepts:

1. A site of care for the dying, such as a freestanding facility or a dedicated unit in a hospital or nursing home.

2. An organization that provides care in a variety of settings, but usually in the patient's home.

3. A synonym for palliative care, referring to a multidisciplinary approach to the care of dying patients in all care sites and practices, including intensive care units if necessary.

4. A benefit available to Medicare beneficiaries and subject to regulations promulgated by the Health Care Financing Administration (HFCA).

In summary, the hospice philosophy is to ensure the best quality of care for patients with terminal illnesses. Patient and family always have access to a multidisciplinary team of nurses, social workers, nursing aides, chaplains, volunteers, and physicians (including the referring physician). Patients typically receive care at home, but 24-hour home nursing and hospitalization are available, if needed, for uncontrollable symptoms. The care is centered on the goals and values of patients and their families, and attention is paid to the physical, psychological, social, financial, spiritual, and existential causes of distress. Family also are assisted during the bereavement period.

For referral to hospice care, a patient must have a life expectancy of 6 months or less. Although the majority of patients carry the diagnosis of cancer, any patient with a terminal illness is eligible, regardless of the underlying diagnosis (e.g., congestive heart failure, chronic obstructive pulmonary disease, multiple sclerosis). It is usually not difficult to determine when patients with cancer are eligible for hospice care, but this determination can be difficult for patients with nonmalignant terminal illnesses. In 1996 the National Hospice Organization published guidelines to help physicians with this decision.

The sad reality is that most hospice referrals occur within days to weeks of death, giving little time for the patient and family to receive the full benefits of available services. Recent data have shown more favorable numbers.

BIBLIOGRAPHY

1. American Cancer Society: Important facts about cancer pain treatment. CA Cancer J Clin 51:365–366, 2001.
2. Anderson KO, Richman SP, Harley J, Palos G: Cancer pain management among underserved minority outpatients: Perceived needs and barriers to optimal control. Cancer 94:2295–2304, 2002.

3. Cherny N, Ripamonti C, Pereira J, et al: Strategies to manage the adverse effects of oral morphine: An evidence-based report. J Clin Oncol 19:2542–2554, 2001.
4. Emanuel LL, Alpert HR, Emanuel EE: Concise screening questions for clinical assessments of terminal care: The needs near the end of life care screening tool. J Palliat Med 4:465–474, 2001.
5. Feld R, DePauw B, Berman S, et al: Meropenem versus ceftazidime in the treatment of cancer patients with febrile neutropenia: A randomized double-blind trial. J Clin Oncol 18:3690–3698, 2000.
6. Greco FA, Burris HA, Erland JB, et al: Carcinoma of unknown primary site. Cancer 89:2655–2660, 2000.
7. Helweg-Larsen S, Sorensen PS, Kreiner S: Prognostic factors in metastatic spinal cord compression: A prospective study using multivariate analysis of variables influencing survival and gait function in 153 patients. Int J Radiat Oncol Biol Phys 46:1163–1169, 2000.
8. Hyers TM, Agnelli G, Hull RD, et al: Antithrombotic therapy for venous thromboembolic disease. Chest 119:176S–193S, 2001.
9. Joranson DE, Ryan KM, Gilson AM, Dahl JL: Trends in medical use and abuse of opioid analgesics. JAMA 283:1710–1714, 2000.
10. Kaplan R, Slywka J, Stagle S, Ries K: A titrated morphine analgesic regimen comparing substance users and non-users with AIDS related pain. J Pain Symptom Manage 19:265–273, 2000.
11. Lawlor PG: The panorama of opioid-related cognitive dysfunction in patients with cancer: A critical literature appraisal. Cancer 94:1836–1853, 2002.
12. Loblaw DA, Laperriere NJ: Emergency treatment of malignant extradural spinal cord compression: An evidence-based guideline. J Clin Oncol 16:1613–1624, 1998.
13. Marr KA: Empirical antifungal therapy: New options, new tradeoffs. N Engl J Med 346:278–280, 2002.
14. Mercadante S, Casuccio A, Fulfaro F, et al: Switching from morphine to methadone to improve analgesia and tolerability in cancer patients: A prospective study. J Clin Oncol 19:2898–2904, 2001.
15. Meuser T, Pietruck C, Radbruch L, et al: Symptoms during cancer pain treatment following WHO guidelines: A longitudinal follow-up study of symptoms prevalence, severity, and etiology. Pain 93:247–257, 2001.
16. Rockhill B, Spiegelman D, Bryne C, et al: Validation of the Dail et al. model of breast cancer risk prevention and implications for chemoprevention. J Natl Cancer Inst 93:358–366, 2001.
17. Rowell NP, Gleeson F: Steroids, radiotherapy, chemotherapy, and stents for superior vena cava obstruction in carcinoma of the bronchus (Cochrane review). Cochrane Database Syst Rev 4:CD001316, 2001.
18. Schumacher KL, Koresawa S, West C: Putting cancer pain management regimens into practice at home. J Pain Symptom Manage 23:369–382, 2002.
19. Silveira MJ, DiPiero A, Gerrity MS, Feudtner C: Patients' knowledge of options at the end of life: Ignorance in the face of death. JAMA 284:2483–2488, 2000.
20. Snyder L, Quill TE: Physicians Guide to End-of-Life Care. Philadelphia, American College of Physicians, 2001.
21. Strewler GJ: The physiology of parathyroid hormone-related protein. N Engl J Med 342:177–185, 2000.
22. Suarez-Almazor ME, Newman C, Hanson J, Bruera E: Attitudes of terminally ill cancer patients about euthanasia and assisted suicide. J Clin Oncol 20:2134–2141, 2002.

107. THE PREOPERATIVE PATIENT

Jeffrey Pickard, M.D.

1. What test(s) must be done before surgery?

The simple answer is that no test is considered essential for preoperative evaluation. In general, tests should be based on the type of surgery (e.g., urinalysis before urologic surgery) and the patient's current and medical history (e.g., chest radiograph for patients with chronic obstructive pulmonary disease [COPD]). Practically speaking, however, certain tests are ordered almost routinely because they can be obtained relatively easily and cheaply (e.g., complete blood count [CBC]; urinalysis; and, in the elderly, electrocardiogram [ECG] and chest radiograph).

2. How does age affect the outcome of surgery?

Recent studies have determined that age is a significant risk factor for adverse outcomes of surgery. Elderly patients ($\geq$ 70 years) are at increased risk for in-hospital mortality, perioperative cardiac events (including cardiogenic pulmonary edema, myocardial infarction [MI], ventricular arrhythmias), noncardiac events (bacterial pneumonia, respiratory failure), and prolonged hospital stay. Perioperative mortality, however, even in inpatients older than 80 years, is low.

3. What type of anesthesia is the safest?

There is a fairly common misconception that spinal anesthesia is safer and better tolerated than general anesthesia. However, both confer equal risks of postoperative fatal and nonfatal MI. Regional or local anesthesia may be less risky than general or spinal anesthesia. The type of anesthesia should be determined by the anesthesiologist.

4. Which types of surgery are inherently riskier than others?

Vascular surgery appears to carry the greatest risk, both because the procedures are physiologically stressful and because patients who require such procedures have a high incidence of coronary artery disease. Intrathoracic, intraperitoneal, and emergency procedures are also high risk.

5. What is meant by a patient's preoperative cardiac risk index?

The preoperative cardiac risk index refers to a quantitative assessment of a patient's risk of adverse cardiac outcome intra- or postoperatively; it is based on various preoperative clinical, historical, and laboratory variables. The first, and probably most widely used, of these indices was published by Goldman et al. in 1977 (see table). Although all of the published models of perioperative risk have a statistically significant ability to predict adverse outcomes, their ability to discriminate between those at risk and those who are not is poor.

Computation of the Cardiac Risk Index

CRITERIA	MULTIVARIATE DISCRIMINANT-FUNCTION COEFFICIENT	POINTS
1. History		
Age > 70 yr	0.191	5
MI in previous 6 mo	0.384	10
2. Physical examination		
S_3 gallop or JVD	0.451	11
Important VAS	0.119	3
3. Electrocardiogram		
Rhythm other than sinus or PACs on last preoperative ECG	0.283	7
> 5 PVCs/min documented at any time before operation	0.278	7
4. General status		
Po_2 < 60 or Pco_2 > 50 mmHg, K < 3.0 or HCO_3 < 20 mEq/L, BUN > 0.50 or Cr > 3.0 mg/dL, abnormal SGOT, signs of chronic liver disease or patient bedridden from noncardiac causes	0.132	3
5. Operation		
Intraperitoneal, intrathoracic, or aortic operation	0.123	3
Emergency operation	0.167	4
Total possible points		53

MI = myocardial infarction, JVD = jugular vein distention, VAS = valvular aortic stenosis, PACs = premature atrial contractions, PVCs = premature ventricular contractions, Po_2 = partial pressure of oxygen, Pco_2 = partial pressure of carbon dioxide, K = potassium, HCO_3 = bicarbonate, BUN = blood urea nitrogen, Cr = creatinine, SGOT = serum glutamic oxaloacetic transaminase.

Cardiac Risk Index

CLASS	POINT TOTAL	NO OR ONLY MINOR COMPLICATION (n = 943)	LIFE-THREATENING COMPLICATION* (n = 39)	CARDIAC DEATHS (n = 19)
I (n = 537)	0–5	542 (99%)	4 (0.7%)	1 (0.2%)
II (n = 316)	6–12	295 (93%)	16 (5%)	5 (2%)
III (n = 130)	13–25	112 (86%)	15 (11%)	3 (2%)
IV (n = 18)	> 26	4 (22%)	4 (22%)	10 (56%)

*Documented intraoperative or postoperative myocardial infarction, pulmonary edema, or ventricular tachycardia without progression to cardiac death.
Adapted from Goldman L, Caldera DL, Nussbaum SR, et al: Multifactorial index of cardiac risk in noncardiac surgical procedures. N Engl J Med 297:845–850, 1977.

6. How does a history of MI affect a patient's perioperative risk?

Traditionally, "recent" MI has been defined as an MI that has occurred within the previous 3 months and has been considered a high-risk period for surgery. Elective surgery has generally been delayed until at least 3–6 months after MI. More recent guidelines suggest that the high-risk periods are "acute" (1–7 days) and "recent" (1 week to 1 month) and that elective surgery should be delayed until after this period, assuming that an exercise treadmill test (ETT) does not indicate residual myocardium at risk.

7. Which patients should be evaluated for coronary artery disease (CAD) before surgery?

Patients who undergo high-risk procedures such as those listed above (especially vascular procedures that require cross-clamping of the aorta) may require additional evaluation for CAD, such as an ETT. Patients with unstable angina (new ECG changes [especially ischemic] or high cardiac risk indices), decompensated congestive heart failure, significant arrhythmias, or severe valvular heart disease should also should be considered for further cardiac evaluation. Patients who are unable to exercise (e.g., patients with peripheral vascular disease), have poor functional capacity, or have baseline ECG abnormalities may require a dipyridamole-thallium scan or dobutamine stress echocardiogram to detect ischemia. Patients with evidence of ischemic disease on noninvasive testing may require coronary angiography. Subsequent care should be determined based on the results of these evaluations. Further intervention should not be done specifically to "clear" a patient for surgery but only if it is indicated regardless of impending or potential surgery.

8. How should beta-blockers be used perioperatively?

Patients who have known CAD or who are at significant risk for CAD should receive beta-blockers perioperatively to reduce the risks of perioperative ischemia, MI, and total mortality. When possible, a cardioselective beta-blocker should be started days or weeks before elective surgery and the dose titrated to achieve a resting heart rate $\leq$ 65 bpm. Therapy with beta-blockers should continue postoperatively at least until discharge and possibly longer, if indicated.

9. How does the presence of hypertension affect perioperative risk?

Hypertension as an independent risk factor is notably absent from both Goldman's and Detsky's scoring systems. Mild to moderate hypertension appears to be generally well-tolerated during and after surgery. Although clear evidence is lacking, patients with diastolic blood pressure > 110 mmHg or systolic blood pressure > 170 mmHg are thought to be at increased risk of perioperative morbidity and should have their blood pressure controlled before going into surgery, if possible. The period of time required to adequately correct hypertension is not known, although it may take several weeks to correct some of the physiologic changes associated with severe hypertension. Patients with stage 1 or 2 hypertension who have no evidence of end-organ damage can generally proceed to surgery without further delay.

10. How should antihypertensive medications be adjusted in patients who are undergoing elective surgery?

Assuming adequate control of blood pressure, most antihypertensive medications should be continued until surgery and restarted postoperatively when the patient resumes oral intake. Guanethidine and monoamine oxidase (MAO) inhibitors are rarely used and probably should be avoided perioperatively. Earlier case reports suggested that abrupt withdrawal of both clonidine and beta-blockers was associated with rebound hypertension and ischemia and recommended that both agents should be tapered before surgery. According to current recommendations, however, these medications are continued during the perioperative period. If necessary, transdermal clonidine and intravenous (IV) beta-blockers may be used while oral intake is prohibited. Because of a concern for hypotension with general anesthesia, angiotensin-converting enzyme (ACE) inhibitors and angiotensin receptor blockers (ARBs) are generally not taken on the day of surgery.

11. Describe the perioperative management of patients taking medication for diabetes.

Ideally, patients should be euglycemic perioperatively, but this goal is often not practical because the risks of hypoglycemia may be substantial. Therefore, patients generally are allowed to be somewhat hyperglycemic. Patients taking insulin should be given approximately 50% of the usual morning dose of intermediate-acting insulin on the morning of surgery and should be maintained on a continuous infusion of dextrose until oral intake is resumed. Fingerstick glucoses should be obtained at regular intervals during prolonged procedures. Levels of blood sugar should be checked, either by fingerstick or phlebotomy, every 4–6 hours postoperatively until the patient is able to resume normal oral intake. Small doses of subcutaneous regular insulin may be used to maintain blood glucose levels between 150 and 200 mg/dL, if possible. Patients with type 1 diabetes and patients who are difficult to control may require insulin drips. Patients taking oral hypoglycemic agents usually do not require significant adjustment of medications. Some authors recommend discontinuing chlorpropamide 2–3 days before surgery because of its prolonged half-life and risk of hypoglycemia. However, this is an issue only in rare patients with type 2 diabetes who are euglycemic on oral medications.

12. What is the value of preoperative pulmonary function tests (PFTs)?

In patients with no history of pulmonary problems, PFTs are of little or no value and should not be routinely ordered. Although some authors believe that severely obese patients are at risk for postoperative pulmonary complications, few data support the use of PFTs as part of the preoperative evaluation. Patients with a history of lung disease (COPD, asthma, smokers with productive cough) or signs and symptoms of pulmonary dysfunction (wheezing, dyspnea) may be at risk for postoperative pulmonary complications. In such patients, PFTs may be helpful in identifying patients with severe disease (forced expiratory volume [FEV] = 0.5 L; hypercapnia) but otherwise are of little help in quantifying the risk of postoperative pulmonary complications.

13. How should patients with potential pulmonary problems be evaluated before surgery?

As stated previously, patients with pulmonary disease are at increased risk for postoperative pulmonary complications, and their respiratory status should be optimized before surgery. Chest radiographs are usually obtained for baseline values but rarely change management. Other risk factors may include length of surgery (> 3.5 hours), surgical factors (intrathoracic surgery and intra-abdominal procedures, especially those close to the diaphragm), age > 60 years, poor functional status, and smoking (> 20 years or > 1 pack/day actively). There is little difference in risk between general and spinal anesthesia, although procedures done under regional or local anesthesia may have lower risk.

14. How should you manage a patient with asthma perioperatively?

Assess the patient for signs and symptoms of airflow obstruction, such as awakening at night, increased use of bronchodilators, and recent steroid use (inhaled or systemic). Steroids should be considered for use both before (2–3 days) and after (taper over 1 week) surgery because perioperative asthma exacerbations increase the risk of pulmonary complications. Wound infections, pneumonia, and adrenal insufficiency are not increased in patients with asthma who are treated with steroids perioperatively.

15. How should cigarette smokers be counseled before surgery?

Although only a small percentage of smokers will quit when advised to do so by their physicians, all smokers should be advised to quit before elective surgery. Abstinence for at least 2 months and perhaps as long as 1 year may be necessary to decrease postoperative pulmonary complications significantly.

16. What are the important preoperative predictors of postoperative renal failure?

Patients with elevated serum creatinine (> 1.2 mg/dL) have a three- to fourfold increase in postoperative renal insufficiency compared with patients whose creatinine level is normal. A rising serum creatinine perioperatively and left ventricular dysfunction are also significant risk factors for postoperative renal failure.

17. How should patients on chronic anticoagulation be managed perioperatively?

There is no standard regimen to prepare patients on chronic warfarin therapy for surgery. Patients with an international normalized ratio (INR) < 2.9 rarely have significant postoperative bleeding problems. However, most patients on warfarin therapy should be taken off their medications 3–4 days before the procedure so that the INR is < 1.5 at the time of surgery and restarted postoperatively when oral intake is resumed. Patients at high risk for thromboembolic disease (e.g., patients who have had recurrent or recent thromboembolism) may be switched to heparin 3–4 days before surgery, but this is rarely necessary. In these patients, it may be prudent to use heparin in the immediate postoperative period until the INR is therapeutic on warfarin. Patients requiring dental surgery rarely bleed while on warfarin therapy; thus, discontinuance is unnecessary. Likewise, because routine cataract surgery is avascular, it does not necessitate reversal of anticoagulation. Accumulating data indicate that subcutaneous low-molecular-weight heparin may be superior to warfarin in preventing postoperative thromboembolism.

18. What are the perioperative risks associated with the use of herbal medications?

Herbal preparations are used by a significant number of people in the United States. Most patients who take herbals do not volunteer this information to their physicians and, therefore, should be specifically questioned about their use. The table below lists some of the more common herbal medications and their potential implications for patients undergoing surgery. In general, all herbal preparations should be stopped 1 week prior to surgery, if possible.

HERB	POTENTIAL EFFECTS
Ephedra	Tachycardia, hypertension, arrhythmias
Garlic	Bleeding
Gingko	Bleeding
Ginseng	Hypoglycemia, bleeding,
Kava	Increased sedation, possibly addicting
St John's wort	Induction of CYP450 liver enzymes

BIBLIOGRAPHY

1. Ang-Lee MK, Moss J, Yuan CS: Herbal medicines and perioperative care. JAMA 286:208–216, 2001.
2. Arozullah AM, Khuri SF, Henderson WG, Daley J: Development and validation of a multifactorial risk index for predicting postoperative pneumonia after major noncardiac surgery. Ann Intern Med 135:847–857, 2001.
3. Auerbach AD, Goldman L: β-Blockers and reduction of cardiac events in noncardiac surgery. JAMA 287:1435–1444, 2002.
4. Bach DS, Eagle KA: Prediction of perioperative risk: The glass may be three-quarters full. Ann Intern Med 133:384–386, 2000.

5. Eagle KA, Berger PB, Calkins H, et al: Guideline update for perioperative cardiovascular evaluation for noncardiac surgery—executive summary. A report of the American College of Cardiology/American Heart Association task force on practice guidelines. J Am Coll Cardiol 39:542–553, 2002.
6. Fleisher LA: Preoperative evaluation of the patient with hypertension. JAMA 287:2043–2046, 2002.
7. Goldman L, Caldera DL, Nussbaum SR, et al: Multifactorial index of cardiac risk in noncardiac surgical procedures. N Engl J Med 297:845–850, 1977.
8. Kearon C, Hirsh J: Current concepts: Management of anticoagulation before and after elective surgery. N Engl J Med 336:1506–1511, 1997.
9. Inzucchi SE: Glycemic management of diabetes in the perioperative setting. Int Anesthesiol Clin 40:77–93, 2002.
10. Jacober SJ, Sowers JR: An update on perioperative management of diabetes. Arch Intern Med 159:2405–2411, 1999.
11. Lawrence VA: Predicting postoperative pulmonary complications: The sleeping giant stirs. Ann Intern Med 135:919–921, 2001.
12. Polanczyk CA, Marcantonio E, Goldman L, et al: Impact of age on perioperative complications and length of stay in patients undergoing noncardiac surgery. Ann Intern Med 134:637–643, 2001.
13. Schein OD, Katz J, Bass EB, et al: The value of routine preoperative medical testing before cataract surgery. N Engl J Med 342:168–175, 2000.
14. Wahl MJ: Dental surgery in anticoagulated patients. Arch Intern Med 158:1610–1616, 1998.
15. Weitz HH: Postoperative medical complications. Med Clin North Am 85:1151–1169, 2001.

108. THE PREGNANT PATIENT

Jeffrey Pickard, M.D.

1. At 37 weeks' gestation, a 20-year-old primigravida who has received optimal prenatal care is noted to have proteinuria, edema of both upper and lower extremities, and a 5-pound weight gain over the preceding week. Her blood pressure (BP), which has been normal for pregnancy, now measures 136/92 mmHg. What is the diagnosis?

The triad of hypertension, edema, and proteinuria occurring late in pregnancy is a classic presentation of preeclampsia. Preeclampsia occurs six to eight times more commonly in primigravidas than in multigravidas and occurs in 5–10% of all pregnancies. It is almost never seen before 20 weeks' gestation (except with trophoblastic diseases) and usually occurs near term. Because it is seen so often in normal pregnancies, edema is no longer considered part of the clinical criteria for diagnosis.

2. How is preeclampsia managed?

The only definitive treatment of preeclampsia is delivery. Hypertension is only a sign of preeclampsia, and treatment of the BP does little to alter the course of the disease. Diuresis for edema likewise does not alter the underlying pathophysiology and may actually be counterproductive and adversely affect fetal outcome because intravascular volume is already depleted in women with preeclampsia.

The triad of proteinuria, edema, and hypertension is not specific for preeclampsia. Edema may be seen during normal pregnancy, as may low levels of proteinuria. Hypertension late in pregnancy may signify previously unrecognized chronic hypertension or gestational hypertension. If the fetus is not yet mature, it may be appropriate to monitor the pregnancy closely in hope of delaying delivery.

3. What laboratory evaluations should be done in a woman who presents with hypertension during the second half of pregnancy?

A complete blood count should be obtained. Hemoglobin and hematocrit levels may be elevated because hemoconcentration may occur in preeclampsia. Thrombocytopenia and evidence of hemolysis on the smear may suggest severe preeclampsia. Liver function tests (aspartate aminotransferase, alanine aminotransferase), uric acid, and creatinine also may be elevated in cases of severe preeclampsia.

4. Describe the evaluation of a woman who presents with hypertension before week 20 of gestation.

In addition to obtaining the laboratory data mentioned above, a careful history should be obtained with emphasis on duration of elevated BP, BP in previous pregnancies, previous diagnostic evaluation, and symptoms associated with secondary causes of hypertension. Pregnant women, especially young pregnant women, with chronic hypertension or hypertension during the first half of pregnancy are more likely than other patients to have secondary causes of hypertension. Pheochromocytoma, although rare, is associated with high maternal mortality, and appropriate screening should be done with even minimal suspicion.

5. What is the HELLP syndrome?

H = **H**emolysis
E = **E**levated
L = **L**iver enzymes
L = **L**ow
P = **P**latelets

This syndrome, associated with severe preeclampsia, is rapidly progressive and life threatening to both mother and baby. Regardless of the stage in pregnancy at which it occurs, the HELLP syndrome is an emergency and requires immediate termination of pregnancy.

6. How does the nonpharmacologic management of hypertension differ in pregnant and nonpregnant patients?

As in nonpregnant patients, mild to moderate hypertension should be treated with nonpharmacologic modalities first, especially when the diastolic BP is between 90 and 99 mmHg. However, nonpharmacologic strategies for BP control during pregnancy differ from those used in nonpregnancy.

Weight reduction is frequently recommended for BP control in nonpregnant patients but should not be recommended during pregnancy. Salt (sodium) restriction should not be recommended during pregnancy unless the patient has been on a sodium-restricted diet before becoming pregnant. Volume status may be important for maintaining uteroplacental perfusion in pregnant hypertensive patients, whose intravascular volume is usually lower than that in normotensive patients.

Because of its unknown effect on uteroplacental blood flow, exercise should be discouraged in pregnant women with hypertension. Whereas its effectiveness has not been well studied in chronic hypertension, bed rest during pregnancy enhances uteroplacental blood flow, reduces premature labor, lowers BP, and promotes diuresis in women with hypertension.

7. How should drugs be used to treat hypertension during pregnancy?

The goal of treating hypertension during pregnancy is to minimize short-term risks of elevated BP to the mother without compromising fetal well-being. Pharmacologic therapy may be necessary if nonpharmacologic maneuvers are unsuccessful in lowering BP or if diastolic BP exceeds 99 mmHg.

First-line therapy for hypertensive pregnant women not already taking medication is methyldopa, the only drug that is both efficacious for lowering maternal BP and is unquestionably safe for the fetus. Second-line therapy is usually hydralazine, because other than methyldopa, it is the drug with the most frequent use during pregnancy and generally is considered safe for the fetus. However, it is not highly effective as a single agent because of the reflex tachycardia and increased cardiac output that it causes. Other agents used to treat hypertension during pregnancy are beta-blockers, labetalol, and nifedipine. Nifedipine has not been associated with adverse fetal effects in humans, but studies in pregnant sheep have demonstrated fetal acidosis and hypoxia. Data in humans are limited to the second and third trimesters. Atenolol is rarely used in pregnancy because of one small study that suggested it caused fetal growth restriction.

Because of their theoretical effect on uteroplacental perfusion, thiazides are usually not begun during pregnancy but may be continued when already in use by a hypertensive woman who becomes pregnant. Angiotensin-converting enzyme (ACE) inhibitors are relatively contraindicated during pregnancy after the first trimester because of their association with high rates of fetal loss in animals and because of several case reports of anoxic renal failure, sometimes fatal, in neonates exposed *in utero.*

Antihypertensive Medications for Use in Pregnancy

MEDICATION	DAILY DOSE	COMMENTS
Methyldopa	500 mg–2 g	Drug of choice during pregnancy
Hydralazine	40–200 mg	Second-line therapy; associated with reflex tachycardia
Hydrochlorothiazide	25–50 mg	Potentially decreases uteroplacental perfusion; may be continued during pregnancy if patient already taking it
Beta-blockers (e.g., propranolol)	40–240 mg	Case reports of neonatal hypoglycemia, bradycardia, possible mild intrauterine growth restriction
Calcium channel blockers (e.g., nifedipine)	30–120 mg	Limited data in humans; fetal acidosis and hypoxia in sheep
Labetalol	200–1000 mg	Probably safe; limited data in humans
Angiotensin-converting enzyme inhibitors	—	Contraindicated; teratogenic in animals; anoxic renal failure in human neonates

8. What is the long-term prognosis of women who have hypertension during pregnancy?

Women with gestational hypertension during one pregnancy have recurrent hypertension in up to 10–15% of subsequent pregnancies as well as a higher likelihood of developing chronic hypertension in the future. In contrast, women who do not have hypertension during pregnancy, especially after age 25 years, have a low likelihood of developing chronic hypertension.

Women who develop preeclampsia-eclampsia during their first pregnancy have about a 10% chance of having preeclampsia in subsequent pregnancies. Their risk of developing chronic hypertension is no different from that of the general population. Women with chronic hypertension have an increased risk of developing preeclampsia when they become pregnant.

9. Describe normal maternal carbohydrate metabolism during pregnancy.

Early in pregnancy, usually at about 10 weeks' gestation, maternal fasting glucose levels decrease to as low as 50–60 mg/dL and usually remain at this level. This early decrease in maternal glucose levels occurs before the conceptus is large enough to have an effect and probably is due to an enhancement (increased sensitivity) of insulin-mediated glucose assimilation related primarily to the large increase in placental hormones (especially estrogen).

Basal insulin levels, which are normal during the first half of pregnancy, increase sharply (50–100%) during the second half of pregnancy. Throughout most of pregnancy, the stimulation of insulin in response to glucose load increases. Overall, insulin sensitivity in pregnancy is about 20% of that in the nonpregnant state. The mechanism for the decreased tissue responsiveness to insulin is not completely understood but probably relates to hormonal changes of pregnancy, such as elevated levels of prolactin, cortisol, and other counterregulatory hormones. The human placenta produces placental lactogen, an insulin antagonist, in increasingly larger amounts after 20 weeks' gestation. In addition to a decrease in insulin-receptor binding, postreceptor response to insulin at the tissue level also may be diminished.

10. How do the metabolic changes in a diabetic pregnancy affect the fetus?

Glucose crosses the placenta by facilitated diffusion so that fetal glucose levels are only slightly lower than the mother's. Maternal insulin does not cross the placenta. Maternal hyperglycemia, therefore, leads to fetal hyperglycemia. The fetal pancreas, which starts producing insulin between weeks 9 and 11, secretes large amounts of insulin to control glucose levels. Studies of fetal and infant pancreases exposed to diabetes *in utero* have documented beta-cell hypertrophy and hyperplasia. Amino acids are actively transported across the placenta and stimulate fetal secretion of insulin. These and other substrates are stored in adipose and other insulin-responsive tissues and lead to macrosomia as well as organomegaly of heart, lung, spleen, liver, and adrenal glands. Hyperinsulinemia at birth leads to neonatal hypoglycemia in as many as 75% of infants of diabetic mothers. Other consequences of poor metabolic control include neonatal hypercalcemia, polycythemia, hyperbilirubinemia, and respiratory distress syndrome (RDS).

11. What is the White classification?

This classification schema was devised by Priscilla White to categorize women with pregestational diabetes on the basis of duration of disease, age at onset, mode of therapy, and presence of vascular complications. Current modifications now include gestational diabetes, either as a separate category or as defined by treatment (diet vs. insulin). Classes A–D correlate with slight increases in fetal mortality, whereas classes F and higher are also associated with increased maternal risk.

White Classification

CLASS	AGE AT ONSET*/COMPLICATION	DURATION*	INSULIN
A_1	Any	Any	−
A_2	Any	Gestational[†]	+
B	≥ 20 years	< 10 years	+
C	10–19 years	10–19 years	+
D	< 10 years	≥ 20 years	+
R	Proliferative retinopathy or vitreous hemorrhage		+
F	Nephropathy		+
RF	Retinopathy and nephropathy		+
H	Heart disease, usually coronary artery disease		+
T	Renal transplant recipient		+

*Either age at onset or duration determines class.
[†]Gestational diabetes mellitus (GDM) is often classified separately. In the original White classification, class A was diabetes of any age or duration that did not require insulin.

12. Discuss the other possible adverse outcomes of pregnancy in women with diabetes.

The incidence of major congenital anomalies associated with type I diabetes is as high as 10% in some studies, an overall risk of two to four times that of control populations. Patients in poor metabolic control and patients with vascular disease are at higher risk. Most likely, metabolic disturbances (hyperglycemia, hypoglycemia) during the period of organogenesis (weeks 3–8) are responsible for the malformations (mostly sacral agenesis and complex cardiac defects). Women who are in good metabolic control at the time of conception and through the first trimester appear to be at much lower risk of having either infants with congenital anomalies or first-trimester spontaneous abortions. Women in class F, R, or RF of the White classification are more likely to have infants with intrauterine growth restriction as well as premature infants.

Maternal morbidity is increased in diabetic pregnant women with retinopathy or nephropathy. Nephropathy (defined by proteinuria) may worsen during pregnancy, but the worsening is rarely permanent. Retinopathy (especially proliferative changes) worsens in a substantial number of women during pregnancy and may not completely regress after delivery.

13. What is gestational diabetes mellitus (GDM)? How is it diagnosed?

GDM is diabetes that is first diagnosed during pregnancy (although it may have existed before pregnancy). Every woman should be screened for GDM, usually between 24 and 28 weeks of gestation, with a randomly administered 50-gram glucose load. Plasma glucose ≥ 140 mg/dL at 1 hour after ingestion indicates the need for further diagnostic testing, which consists of administering a 100-gm glucose load to a fasting woman and then measuring hourly glucose levels for 3 hours (see criteria below). If any two values are abnormal or if the fasting glucose level is elevated, the patient has GDM and is followed accordingly. The National Diabetes Data Group

(NDDG) criteria were first published in 1979. Revised criteria were recommended for adoption at the Fourth International Conference on Gestational Diabetes in 1998.

Three-hour Glucose Tolerance Test

	PLASMA GLUCOSE LEVEL (mg/dL)	
TIME	NDDG	Revised
Fasting	≥ 105	95
1 hour	≥ 190	180
2 hours	≥ 165	155
3 hours	≥ 145	140

14. What are the criteria for beginning medical therapy in women with GDM?

Some authors advise starting prophylactic insulin in all women diagnosed with GDM. Most clinicians, however, assess control of diabetes by regularly checking fasting and 2-hour postprandial levels of serum glucose. Adequate control is indicated by a fasting level < 105 mg/dL and a 2-hour postprandial level < 120 mg/dL. If either value is exceeded twice within 1 week, medical therapy is usually begun. Insulin has long been the standard therapy for treating GDM during pregnancy. However, in recent years, glyburide has been used as first-line therapy (usually after the first trimester).

15. Describe the changes in respiratory physiology during pregnancy.

Normal pregnancy is a state of mild, compensated respiratory alkalosis. During the first trimester, pregnant women hyperventilate by increasing tidal volume by ≤ 50%. Respiratory rate stays fairly constant. Arterial pH is normal (7.40–7.45) because of renal compensation so that levels of serum bicarbonate decrease. Such changes probably occur because of progesterone effects and remain constant throughout pregnancy. Both expiratory reserve volume (ERV) and residual volume (RV), which together make up the functional residual capacity (FRC), decrease by a total of 20%, mostly during the third trimester. Vital capacity (VC) is essentially unchanged.

16. How should asthma be managed during pregnancy?

Pregnancy changes the management of asthma very little. Medications used to treat asthma in nonpregnant patients also may be used during pregnancy. One exception is saturated solution of potassium iodide (SSKI), which occasionally has been used as a mucolytic. The iodine crosses the placenta easily and theoretically may cause fetal thyroid abnormalities. Because of the lack of data during pregnancy, the leukotriene inhibitors are also usually not used.

17. Describe the hemodynamic changes of pregnancy.

By early in the third trimester, cardiac output is increased by up to 50% over prepregnancy levels because of a marked increase in plasma volume (40–50%) and a lesser increase (20–30%) in red blood cell mass. This causes a physiologic anemia of pregnancy. Despite the marked increase in cardiac output, however, BP decreases early in pregnancy because of arteriolar vasodilation and a marked decrease in systemic vascular resistance. Pulmonary pressures are largely unchanged. Organs with the largest increase in perfusion are the kidneys, breasts, skin, and uterus.

18. How does pregnancy affect thyroid function?

Despite earlier reports to the contrary, the size of the normal thyroid gland usually does not change significantly during pregnancy when iodine intake is adequate. Because of the effects of estrogen, thyroid-binding globulin level increases two to three times above normal, and levels of total thyroxine (T_4) and total triiodothyronine (T_3) increase concomitantly. Levels of free T_4 and free T_3 stay within the normal to low-normal range. Levels of thyroid-stimulating hormone (TSH) may decrease slightly during early pregnancy because of the weak thyroid-stimulating activity of beta human chorionic gonadotropin (hCG) but return to normal during the second and third trimesters.

19. How does renal disease affect pregnancy?

Renal disease, especially moderate to severe renal disease (serum creatinine > 1.4 mg/dL) increases the risks of preterm delivery, cesarean section, fetal growth restriction, maternal hypertension, and preeclampsia. Fetal survival is moderately reduced ($\sim$93%). Maternal renal function may be markedly affected by pregnancy in women whose initial serum creatinine is > 1.4 mg/dL. Only 60% of these women have stable renal function 6 months after delivery. Thirty-five percent of women whose initial serum creatinine is ≥ 2.0 mg/dL are at risk for end-stage renal failure as a result of pregnancy.

20. How does pregnancy affect the diagnosis of thyrotoxicosis?

Diagnosis of thyrotoxicosis during pregnancy may be difficult because signs and symptoms such as palpitations, heat intolerance, emotional lability, and diaphoresis may be seen with normal pregnancy. Poor weight gain and persistent tachycardia along with a goiter suggest the diagnosis. Laboratory evaluation is made by demonstrating elevated values of free T_3 and free T_4 and suppressed TSH. Transient thyrotoxicosis also may be seen with hyperemesis gravidarum (persistent vomiting, tachycardia, and weight loss during pregnancy). Thyrotoxicosis in this setting is transient and rarely requires treatment.

21. How should women with epilepsy be treated during pregnancy?

Patients whose seizures are controlled by medication generally should continue medication during pregnancy. Although no antiepileptic agent is safe during pregnancy, uncontrolled seizures are harmful to both mother and fetus. If a woman has been seizure free for 2 years, she may attempt to discontinue medication before becoming pregnant. If withdrawal is successful, she may be followed expectantly during gestation.

If possible, women taking valproic acid should change to another medication before becoming pregnant. Although published data in humans are not completely clear, valproic acid has been implicated in a number of congenital anomalies. The major concern is neural tube defects, which occur within the first 4 weeks after conception. Carbamazepine is also associated with an increased risk of neural tube defects, so it is also usually avoided during the first trimester. Trimethadione, which is rarely used anymore, is clearly associated with a constellation of congenital anomalies and should be avoided during pregnancy.

22. How does infection with the human immunodeficiency virus (HIV) affect pregnancy?

The incidence of perinatal transmission is 20–30% without treatment. However, treatment of HIV-infected women with zidovudine during pregnancy and delivery has been shown to decrease the incidence of vertical transmission by about two thirds. Currently, pregnancy is not a contraindication for antiretroviral therapy. In general, pregnant women should receive combination antiretroviral therapy as if they were not pregnant, although not in the first trimester, if possible.

23. What is the significance of asymptomatic bacteriuria during pregnancy?

Asymptomatic bacteriuria may occur in up to 5–10% of pregnant women. Unlike their nonpregnant counterparts, up to 40% of these women may develop infections. Such infections may have a deleterious effect on pregnancy, especially if pyelonephritis ensues. Therefore, all pregnant women with asymptomatic bacteriuria should be treated with antibiotics. In women with recurrences, daily suppressive doses of antibiotics may be indicated until after delivery.

24. How should pregnant women with deep venous thrombosis be treated?

In general, warfarin should be avoided during pregnancy because it crosses the placenta and has been associated with fetal malformations as well as neurologic dysfunction. In pregnant women with a documented blood clot, acute therapy should be given with intravenous heparin followed by intermittent (2 or 3 times/day) subcutaneous heparin for several weeks in doses adequate to keep the midinterval partial thromboplastin time at 1.5–2.0 times control. Thereafter, the patient should be maintained on low-dose subcutaneous heparin (5000–10,000 U twice daily) until delivery. Warfarin is then generally substituted until 4–6 weeks after delivery, at which time anticoagulation may be discontinued. Woman taking warfarin may breastfeed.

Women who have had thrombosis in a prior pregnancy are generally considered to be at risk if they again become pregnant. They are treated with low-dose subcutaneous heparin throughout gestation. Although opinions differ as to the proper dose, heparin levels apparently decrease as pregnancy proceeds if the amount is not increased accordingly. Therefore, we recommend 5000 U subcutaneously twice daily in the first trimester; 7500 U twice daily in the second trimester; and 10,000 U twice daily in the third trimester. Because the risk of thromboembolic events may persist in the early postpartum period, warfarin is used as above.

Low–molecular-weight heparin (LMWH) may have some advantages during pregnancy because of its longer half-life, which may allow once-daily dosing with fewer bleeding complications. LMWH does not cross the placenta and has been used safely during pregnancy.

BIBLIOGRAPHY

1. Barbour LA, Pickard J: Management of thromboembolism in pregnancy. Prim Care Case Rev 3:96–104, 2000.
2. Davison J: Renal disorders in pregnancy. Curr Opin Obstet Gynecol 13:109–114, 2001.
3. Holmes LB, Harvey EA, Coull BA, et al: The teratogenicity of anticonvulsant drugs. N Engl J Med 344:1132–1138, 2001.
4. Lucas M: Medical complications of pregnancy. Obstet Gynecol Clin 28:513–536, 2001.
5. Langer O, Conway DL, Berkus MD, et al: A comparison of glyburide and insulin in women with gestational diabetes mellitus. N Engl J Med 343:1134–1138, 2000.
6. Luskin AT, Lipkowitz MA: Asthma and allergy during pregnancy: Immunol Allerg Clin North Am 20:745–761, 2000.
7. Mulder JE: Thyroid disease in women. Med Clin North Am 82:103–125,1998.
8. National Heart, Lung, and Blood Institute National High Blood Pressure Education Program: Report of the National High Blood Pressure Education Program Working Group on High Blood Pressure in Pregnancy. Am J Obstet Gynecol 183:S1–S22, 2000.
9. Pickard J, Barbour LA: Management of diabetes and hypertension in pregnancy. Prim Care Case Rev 3:87–95, 2000.
10. Pschirrer E, Monga M: Seizure disorders in pregnancy. Obstet Gynecol Clin North Am 28:601–611, 2001.
11. Walker J: Pre-eclampsia [seminar]. Lancet 356:1260–1265, 2000.
12. Watts DH: Management of human immunodeficiency virus infection in pregnancy. N Engl J Med 346:1879–1891, 2002.

XV. Patient Safety

109. HEALTH CARE AND PATIENT SAFETY

Jeanette Mladenovic, M.D.

1. Is patient safety synonymous with quality of patient care?

Not necessarily. All patient safety issues represent quality issues, but not all quality of care issues represent patient safety issues.

2. What is the definition of quality health care?

According to the IOM, quality of care is the degree to which health services for individuals and populations increase the likelihood of desired health outcomes and are consistent with professional knowledge. Thus, to fulfill these characteristics, health care should be accessible, effective, and safe.

3. What are some types of medical errors?

Errors usually occur because of multiple, confluent, often small, failures in a system of care. Some general categories of errors include the following:

- Diagnostic errors, which can lead to incorrect therapeutic choices, a failure to diagnosis, or a failure to act on abnormal results. Thus, these include errors of commission and omission.
- Equipment failures that can lead to delay in treatment or inappropriate treatment (e.g., a defibrillator with dead batteries or a faulty intravenous pump that allows too much medication)
- Infections, such as nosocomial and postsurgical wound infections
- Blood transfusion–related errors, such as giving a patient blood of the incorrect type
- Misinterpretation of medical orders or prescriptions

4. How frequent are medication errors?

An estimated 1 million medication errors are made per year. Twenty percent of these lead to adverse drug reactions, and an estimated 7000 patients die per year.

5. What are the most common reasons for medication errors?

- Illegibility
- Wrong dose caused by misplaced decimal points
- Failure to recognize drug interactions

The recognition of these types of errors has led to the belief that computerized order entry systems, which have decreased drug errors by 70–88% in two large institutions, would generally improve the safety of health care. Although expensive, the intuitive rationale for this system suggest that it is an appropriate way to decrease these avoidable systems errors.

6. Do all drug interactions result in an adverse drug reaction (ADR)?

No. A drug interaction does not necessarily result in an ADR, even with documentable changes in drug level or physiologic parameters. The specific definition of an ADR varies but usually addresses the following issues: severity of outcome; whether the drug met therapeutic indications; and whether the adverse reaction occurred after an overdose, on withdrawal, or as a failure of the expected pharmacologic action.

7. What is a reportable ADR?

A reportable ADR is defined as a reaction that is (1) suspected to be secondary to drug therapy; (2) uncommon or not described in the package insert; or (3) severe in nature, requiring treatment or prolonging hospitalization. All ADRs should be recorded in the progress notes of the patient's medical record, along with outcome and treatment. ADRs that fit these criteria should be reported to the institution through the mechanism approved by the local Pharmacy and Therapeutics Committee. If the institution does not have a mechanism for forwarding the information to the Food and Drug Administration (FDA), the physician may call the FDA directly at 1–800-FDA-1088. Such reports contribute to postmarketing surveillance of drugs.

8. How can I determine the likelihood that a drug caused an adverse event?

Perhaps the most important problem in assessing ADRs is determining whether there is a causal relationship between consumption of the drug and occurrence of an adverse event. Various algorithms are available to assist clinicians in determining the causal probability of a suspected ADR. The algorithms range from simple to complex; some have been automated and put into computer software format. Each clinician may find a different algorithm most useful in his or her practice setting. One time-tested, well-validated example of an ADR probability assessment scale is that of Naranjo et al., who suggested a list of 10 questions to assess ADR causality. The questions, answer choices, and score values are as follow:

QUESTIONS	YES	NO	DON'T KNOW
1. Are there previous *conclusive* reports of this reaction?	+1	0	0
2. Did the adverse event appear after the suspected drug was administered?	+2	−1	0
3. Did the adverse reaction improve when the drug was discontinued or a *specific* antagonist was administered?	+1	0	0
4. Did the adverse reaction reappear when the drug was readministered?	+2	−1	0
5. Are there alternative factors (other than the drug) that could have caused the reaction?	−1	+2	0
6. Did the reaction appear when a placebo was given?	−1	+1	0
7. Was the drug detected in the blood (or other fluids) in concentrations known to be toxic?	+1	0	0
8. Was the reaction more severe when the dose was increased or less severe when the dose was decreased?	+1	0	0
9. Did the patient have a similar reaction to the same or similar drugs in any previous exposure?	+1	0	0
10. Was the adverse event confirmed by any objective evidence?	+1	0	0

To calculate a causal probability for an ADR, sum the scores for the 10 questions and refer the total score to the following ranges:

Score	ADR Causal Probability
9–13	Definite
5–8	Probable
1–4	Possible
−4–0	Doubtful

The resulting causal probability category for the suspected ADR gives clinicians a crude but fairly reliable method for determining whether a drug has actually caused an adverse event. Several adverse event reporting systems in the United States use similar questions (if not the entire Naranjo algorithm) for determination and classification of ADRs.

9. What effect do closed intensive care units (ICUs) and staffing with intensivists have on patient safety and outcomes?

In more than seven studies, ICU staffing with ready availability of intensivists has decreased mortality. Additionally, providing this expertise in the care of patients in ICUs has decreased the length of stay and decreased numbers of inappropriate admissions to ICUs.

10. What are important characteristics to consider when referring a patient for a complex surgical procedure, such as a coronary bypass operation?

Although the skill of the surgeon is important, many studies have demonstrated the importance of surgical volume to patient outcome. Although many states publish mortality data for patients, others do not, and wide variation may exist. Some of the areas in which volume of procedures in the institution have been associated with improved patient outcome include: coronary artery bypass graft (CABG), endarterectomy, delivery of high-risk newborns, abdominal aneurysms, and outcomes of some cancer treatments. The health care environment, in addition to the skill set of the provider, is thought to improve patient outcomes.

11. What are the two most powerful predictors of hospital-acquired infections?

1. The patient's length of stay
2. The use of invasive devices

12. What is HIPAA?

The initials HIPAA stand for the Health Insurance Portability and Accountability Act, which was signed into law in August of 1996. Essentially, this law has directed the secretary of Health and Human Services to mandate the use of standards for common electronic administrative transactions and to establish a privacy standard for personal health information. Failure to comply with these standards, which were set to protect patients and to improve the efficiency of the administrative work of health care, carries stiff penalties for health care institutions and providers.

13. What does HEDIS measure?

HEDIS stands for health plan employer data and information set. These criteria are a set of performance standards for managed health care plans to measure themselves against. More importantly, these are one group of indicators used by the National Committee for Quality Assurance (NCQA), which compares the health care delivered among various managed care organizations.

14. What is evidence-based medicine (EBM)?

Sackett et al. define EBM as the "conscientious, explicit, and judicious use of current best evidence in making decisions about the care of individual patients." The application of EBM requires the knowledge of basic epidemiologic and statistical concepts that allows clinicians to interpret and apply studies to individual patients.

15. List four evidence-based clinical practices that decrease patient injury.

1. Venous thromboembolism prophylaxis
2. Perioperative use of beta-blockers in patients undergoing coronary artery bypass graft surgery
3. Antibiotics to prevent surgical postoperative site infections
4. Use of maximal sterile barriers during insertion of central venous catheters to prevent bacteremia

16. What benefits of computer-based clinical support systems have been demonstrated?

The use of these support systems has helped physicians improve the care that is provided to their patients in specific areas: drug dosing and preventive care. The effect on actual patient outcomes has not been well documented. However, because of the large amount of information overload, the use of technology is a logical extension of physicians' need to manage information, whether medical or patient.

BIBLIOGRAPHY

1. Agency for Healthcare Research and Quality: Making Health Care Safer: A Critical Analysis of Patient Safety Practices. Rockville, MD, AHRQ, 2001.

2. American Board of Internal Medicine Foundation: Physician Quality. Available at www.projectphysicianquality.org.

3. Burke JP: Patient safety: Infection control: A problem for patient safety. N Engl J Med 348:651–656, 2003.

4. Hunt DL, Haynes RB, Hanna SE, Smith K: Effects of computer-based clinical decision support systems on physician performance and patient outcomes. A systematic review. JAMA 280:1339–1346, 1998.

5. Ioannidis JP, Lau J: Evidence on interventions to reduce medical errors. An overview and recommendations for future research. J Gen Intern Med 16:325–334, 2001.

6. Kohn LT, Corrigan JM, Donaldson MS (eds): To Err Is Human: Building a Safer Health System. Washington, DC, Committee on Quality Health Care in America, Institute of Medicine, National Academy Press, 2000.

7. Leape L, Berwick D, Bates D: What practices will most improve safety: Evidence-based medicine meets patient safety. JAMA 288:501–507, 2002.

8. Naranjo CA, Busto U, Sellers EM, et al: A method for estimating the probability of adverse drug reactions. Clin Pharmacol Ther 30:239–245, 1981.

9. Sackett DL, Rosenberg WM, Gray JA, et al: Evidence based medicine: What it is and what it isn't. Br Med J 312:71–72, 1996.

10. Shojania KG, McDonald K, Wachter RM: Safe but sound: Patient safety meets evidence-based medicine. JAMA 288:508–513, 2002.

INDEX

Page numbers in **boldface type** indicate complete chapters.